P9-CFY-528

Evidence-Based Practice in Nursing & Healthcare

A Guide to Best Practice

Third Edition

Evidence-Based Practice in Nursing & Healthcare

A Guide to Best Practice

Third Edition

Bernadette Mazurek Melnyk,
PhD, RN, CPNP/PMHNP, FAANP, FNAP, FAAN

Associate Vice President for Health Promotion
University Chief Wellness Officer
Dean and Professor, College of Nursing
Professor of Pediatrics & Psychiatry, College of Medicine
The Ohio State University
Editor, Worldviews on Evidence-Based Nursing
Partner, ARCC llc; President, COPE for HOPE, Inc.; Founder, COPE2Thrive, llc

Ellen Fineout-Overholt,
PhD, RN, FNAP, FAAN

Mary Coulter Dowdy Distinguished Professor of Nursing
College of Nursing & Health Sciences
University of Texas at Tyler
Editorial Board, Worldviews on Evidence-Based Nursing
Partner, ARCC llc

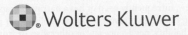 Wolters Kluwer

Philadelphia · Baltimore · New York · London
Buenos Aires · Hong Kong · Sydney · Tokyo

Acquisitions Editor: Chris Richardson
Product Development Editor: Meredith L. Brittain
Development Editor: Robin Bushing
Editorial Assistant: Zachary Shapiro
Production Project Manager: Marian Bellus
Design Coordinator: Holly McLaughlin
Illustration Coordinator: Jennifer Clements
Manufacturing Coordinator: Karin Duffield
Marketing Manager: Dean Karampelas
Prepress Vendor: Integra Software Services Pvt. Ltd.

3rd edition

9 8 7 6 5 4 3

Printed in China

Library of Congress Cataloging-in-Publication Data

Melnyk, Bernadette Mazurek, author.
  [Evidence-based practice in nursing & healthcare]
  Evidence-based practice in nursing and healthcare : a guide to best practice / Bernadette Mazurek Melnyk, Ellen Fineout-Overholt. — Third edition.
       p. ; cm.
  Preceded by: Evidence-based practice in nursing & healthcare / Bernadette Mazurek Melnyk, Ellen Fineout-Overholt. 2nd ed. c2011.
  Includes bibliographical references and index.
  ISBN 978-1-4511-9094-6
  I. Fineout-Overholt, Ellen, author. II. Title.
  [DNLM: 1. Evidence-Based Nursing—methods—Practice Guideline.   2. Nurse Clinicians—Practice Guideline.   WY 100.7]
  RT42
  610.73—dc23
                                   2014021179

LWW.com

I dedicate this book to my loving and understanding family, who has provided tremendous support to me in pursuing my dreams and passions: my husband, John; and my three daughters, Kaylin, Angela, and Megan; as well as to my father, who always taught me that anything can be accomplished with a spirit of enthusiasm and determination. It is also dedicated to all of the committed healthcare providers and clinicians who strive every day to deliver the highest quality of evidence-based care.

Bernadette Mazurek Melnyk

The third edition of this book is thoughtfully dedicated to all healthcare consumers. Particularly, I dedicate this edition to my precious family, Wayne, Rachael, and Ruth, and my Mom, Virginia Fineout, who are the primary consumers who inspire me to persist in partnering to transform health care and healthcare education to achieve best outcomes. Also, I dedicate this edition to the loving memory of my Dad, Art Fineout, my brothers Mark and Paul Fineout, and our baby, Wayne P. Overholt. The experiences with these losses continue to shape my commitment to best care.

Ellen Fineout-Overholt

Anne Wojner Alexandrov, PhD, RN, NVRN-BC, ANVP-BC, CCRN, FAAN
Professor and U.S. National Principal Investigator
International Stroke Nursing Research Collaboration
Australian Catholic University
Sydney, Australia
Professor
Nursing
University of Tennessee Health Science Center
Memphis, Tennessee
Program Director
NET SMART
Health Outcomes Institute
Fountain Hills, Arizona
Chapter 10, The Role of Outcomes and Quality Improvement in Enhancing and Evaluating Practice Changes

Karen Balakas, PhD, RN, CNE
Director
Research
St. Louis Children's Hospital
St Louis, Missouri
Chapter 16, Teaching Evidence-Based Practice in Clinical Settings

Marcia Belcher, MSN, BBA, RN, CCRN-CSC, CCNS
Clinical Nurse Specialist
The Ohio State University Wexner Medical Center
Evidence-based Practice Mentor
Clinical Instructor of Practice
The Ohio State University
College of Nursing
Columbus, OH
Making EBP Real, Unit 2

Michael J. Belyea, PhD
Research Professor
College of Nursing & Health Innovation
Arizona State University
Phoenix, Arizona
Making EBP Real, Unit 6

Cecily L. Betz, PhD, RN, FAAN
Clinical Associate Professor
University of Southern California
Los Angeles, California
Chapter 18, Disseminating Evidence Through Publications, Presentations, Health Policy Briefs, and the Media

Barbara B. Brewer, PhD, RN, MALS, MBA, FAAN
Associate Professor
The University of Arizona College of Nursing
Tucson, Arizona
Chapter 10, The Role of Outcomes and Quality Improvement in Enhancing and Evaluating Practice Changes

Terri L. Brown, MSN, RN, CPN
Assistant Director
Texas Children's Hospital
Houston, Texas
Chapter 9, Implementing Evidence in Clinical Settings

Jacalyn (Jackie) Buck, PhD, RN, NE-BC
Administrator, Health System Nursing Quality, Research, Education and EBP
The Ohio State University Wexner Medical Center
Clinical Assistant Professor
College of Nursing
The Ohio State University
Columbus, Ohio
Research Communications
Chapter 11, Leadership Strategies and Evidence-Based Practice Competencies to Sustain a Culture and Environment That Supports Best Practice

Donna Ciliska, PhD, RN,
Professor
Scientific Director of the National Collaborating
Centre for Methods and Tools
Co–Principal Investigator, McMaster Evidence
Review and Synthesis Centre
School of Nursing
McMaster University
Hamilton, Ontario, Canada
Chapter 13, Models to Guide Implementation
and Sustainability of Evidence-Based Practice

Robert E. Cole, PhD
Associate Professor of Clinical Nursing
University of Rochester
Rochester, New York
Chapter 19, Generating Evidence Through
Quantitative Research

John F. Cox III, MD
Assistant Professor
Clinical Medicine
University of Rochester School of Medicine
Rochester, New York
Chapter 15, Teaching Evidence-Based Practice in
Academic Settings

Laura Cullen, DNP, RN, FAAN
Evidence-Based Practice Scientist
University of Iowa Hospitals and Clinics
Iowa City, Iowa
Chapter 13, Models to Guide Implementa-
tion and Sustainability of Evidence-Based
Practice

Maria Cvach, DNP, RN, CCRN
Assistant Director
Nursing, Clinical Standards
The Johns Hopkins Hospital
Baltimore, Maryland
Chapter 13, Models to Guide Implementa-
tion and Sustainability of Evidence-Based
Practice

Deborah Dang, PhD, RN, NEA, BC
Director
Nursing
Johns Hopkins University School of Nursing
Baltimore, Maryland
Chapter 13, Models to Guide Implementa-
tion and Sustainability of Evidence-Based
Practice

Alba DiCenso, PhD, RN
CHSRF/CIHR Chair in Advanced Practice
Nursing
Professor, School of Nursing
Professor, Department of Clinical Epidemiology
& Biostatistics
McMaster University
Director of the Ontario Training Centre for
Health Services and Policy Research (OTC)
Hamilton, Ontario, Canada
Chapter 13, Models to Guide Implementation
and Sustainability of Evidence-Based Practice

**Lynn Gallagher-Ford, PhD, RN, DPFNAP,
NE-BC**
Director
Center for Transdisciplinary Evidence-Based
Practice
The Ohio State University
Columbus, Ohio
Chapter 7, Integration of Patient Preferences and
Values and Clinician Expertise Into Evidence-
Based Decision Making
Chapter 11, Leadership Strategies and Evidence-
Based Practice Competencies to Sustain a
Culture and Environment That Supports Best
Practice

**Doris Grinspun, RN, MSN, PhD, LLD (Hon),
OONT**
Chief Executive Officer
Registered Nurses' Association of Ontario
Toronto, Ontario, Canada
Chapter 8, Advancing Optimal Care With Rigor-
ously Developed Clinical Practice Guidelines
and Evidence-Based Recommendations

Tami A. Hartzell, MLS
Clinical and Translational Science Librarian &
Expert EBP Mentor
Rochester General Hospital
Rochester, NY
Chapter 3, Finding Relevant Evidence to Answer
Clinical Questions

**Marilyn J. Hockenberry PhD, RN, PNP-BC,
FAAN**
Bessie Baker Professor of Nursing
School of Nursing
Duke University
Durham, North Carolina
Chapter 9, Implementing Evidence in Clinical
Settings

Sheila Hofstetter, MLS, AHIP
Health Sciences Librarian
Arizona State University
Tempe, Arizona
Chapter 3, Finding Relevant Evidence to Answer
Clinical Questions

Diana Jacobson, PhD, RN, PNP-BC, PMHS
Assistant Professor
College of Nursing & Health Innovation
Arizona State University
Phoenix, Arizona
Making EBP Real, Unit 6

Stephanie Kelly PhD, RN, FNP-BC
Assistant Research Professor
College of Nursing & Health Innovation
Arizona State University
Phoenix, Arizona
Making EBP Real, Unit 6

Robin Kretschman, MSA, RN, NEA-BC
Vice president of Patient Care Services
Ministry Saint Joseph's Hospital
Marshfield, WI

June H. Larrabee, PhD, RN
Professor and Clinical Investigator
West Virginia University and West Virginia
University Hospitals
Charleston, West Virginia
Chapter 13, Models to Guide Implementation
and Sustainability of Evidence-Based Practice

Lisa English Long, PhD(c), RN, CNS
Expert Evidence-based Practice Mentor
Clinical Instructor
Center for Transdisciplinary Evidence-based
Practice
College of Nursing
The Ohio State University
Chapter 7, Integration of Patient Preferences and
Values and Clinician Expertise Into
Evidence-Based Decision Making

Pamela Lusk, DNP, RN, PMHNP-BC
Clinical Associate Professor
Psychiatric/Mental Health Nurse Practitioner-
Community Health Center
The Ohio State University College of Nursing
Yavapai County, Arizona
Making EBP Real, Unit 3

Tina L. Magers, MSN, RN-BC
Nursing Professional Development and Research
Coordinator
Mississippi Baptist Health Systems
Jackson, Mississippi
Making EBP Real, Unit 1

Kathy Malloch, PhD, MBA, RN, FAAN
President, KMLS, llc
Clinical Professor
The Ohio State University College of Nursing
Columbus, Ohio
Professor of Practice
Arizona State University College of Nursing and
Health Innovation
Phoenix, AZ
Chapter 12, Innovation and Evidence: A
Partnership in Advancing Best Practice and
High Quality Care

Flavio F. Marsiglia, Ph.D.
Southwest Interdisciplinary Research
Center
(SIRC) Director
Distinguished Foundation Professor of Cultural
Diversity and Health
Arizona State University
Phoenix, Arizona
Making EBP Real, Unit 6

**Dianne Morrison-Beedy, PhD, RN,
WHNP-BC, FNAP, FAANP, FAAN**
Professor
Senior Associate Vice President, USF
Health
Dean, College of Nursing
University of South Florida
Tampa, Florida
Chapter 19, Generating Evidence Through
Quantitative Research

Dónal P. O'Mathúna, DPO
Senior Lecturer in Ethics, Decision-Making and
Evidence
School of Nursing
Dublin City University
Glasnevin, Dublin, Ireland
Chapter 5, Critically Appraising Quantitative
Evidence for Clinical Decision Making
Chapter 22, Ethical Considerations for Evidence
Implementation and Evidence Generation

Elizabeth Ponder
Manager of Instruction and Information
Services
Mamye Jarrett Library
East Texas Baptist University
Marshall, Texas
Chapter 3, Finding Relevant Evidence to Answer
Clinical Questions

**Tim Porter-O'Grady, DM, EdD, ScD(h),
APRN, FAAN, FACCWS**
Senior Partner
TPOG Associates, Inc.
Atlanta, Georgia
Clinical Professor
The Ohio State University
Columbus, Ohio
Professor of Practice
Arizona State University
Phoenix, Arizona
Chapter 12, Innovation and Evidence: A
Partnership in Advancing Best Practice and
High Quality Care

Bethel Ann Powers, RN, PhD, FSAA, FGSA
Professor & Director, PhD Programs &
Evaluation Office
University of Rochester School of Nursing
Rochester, New York
Chapter 6, Critically Appraising Qualitative
Evidence for Clinical Decision Making
Chapter 20, Generating Evidence Through
Qualitative Research and Appendix D, Walking
the Walk and Talking the Talk

Brett W. Robbins, MD
Associate Professor
University of Rochester Medical Center
Rochester, New York
Chapter 15, Teaching Evidence-Based Practice in
Academic Settings

Cheryl Rodgers, PhD
Assistant Professor
Duke University School of Nursing
Durham, North Carolina
Chapter 9, Implementing Evidence in Clinical
Settings

Jo Rycroft-Malone, PhD, MSc, BSc (Hons), RN
Professor of Health Services and Implementation
Research
University Director of Research
School of Healthcare Sciences
Bangor University
Bangor, Gwynedd, United Kingdom
Chapter 13, Models to Guide Implementation
and Sustainability of Evidence-Based Practice

Alyce A. Schultz, RN, PhD, FAAN
Fulbright Senior Specialist
Consultant & Owner
EBP Concepts, LLC
Great Falls, Montana
Bozeman, Montana
Chapter 13, Models to Guide Implementation
and Sustainability of Evidence-Based Practice

Gabriel Q. Shaibi, PhD
Associate Professor and Southwest Borderlands
Scholar
College of Nursing and Health Innovation
Arizona State University
Phoenix, Arizona
Making EBP Real, Unit 6

Michelle Simon, BSN, RN, CCRN
Staff Nurse
The Ohio State University Wexner Medical
Center
Richard M. Ross Heart Hospital
Columbus, Ohio
Making EBP Real, Unit 2

**Leigh Small, PhD, RN, CPNP-PC, FNAP,
FAANP**
Department Chair and Associate Professor,
Family and Community Health Nursing
Virginia Commonwealth University
Richmond, Virginia
Making EBP Real, Unit 6

Kathryn A. Smith, RN, DrPH
Associate Director for Administration
USC University Center for Excellence in
Developmental Disabilities
Children's Hospital
Los Angeles, California
Associate Professor of Clinical Pediatrics
Keck School of Medicine
University of Southern California
Los Angeles, California
Chapter 18, Disseminating Evidence Through
Publications, Presentations, Health Policy Briefs,
and the Media

Cheryl B. Stetler, PhD, RN, FAAN
Consultant, EBP and Evaluation
Amherst, Massachusetts
Chapter 13, Models to Guide Implementation
and Sustainability of Evidence-Based Practice

Kathleen R. Stevens, RN, EdD, ANEF, FAAN
Professor and Director
University of Texas Health Science Center
San Antonio, Texas
Chapter 4, Critically Appraising Knowledge for
Clinical Decision Making
Chapter 13, Models to Guide Implementa-
tion and Sustainability of Evidence-Based
Practice

Susan B. Stillwell, DNP, RN, CNE, ANEF, FAAN
Associate Dean
Graduate Programs
University of Portland
Portland, Oregon
Chapter 2, Asking Compelling, Clinical
Questions
Chapter 15, Teaching Evidence-Based Practice in
Academic Settings

R. Terry Olbrysh, MA, APR
Independent Consultant in Marketing &
Communications
Phoenix, Arizona
Chapter 18, Disseminating Evidence Through
Publications, Presentations, Health Policy Briefs,
and the Media

Kathleen M. Williamson, PhD, RN
Chair & Associate Professor, Wilson School of
Nursing
Midwestern State University
Robert D. & Carol Gunn College of Health
Sciences & Human Services
Wichita Falls, Texas
Chapter 15, Teaching Evidence-Based Practice in
Academic Settings

For a list of the contributors to the Student and Instructor Resources
accompanying this book, please visit
http://thepoint.lww.com/Melnyk3e.

Anne Wojner Alexandrov, PhD, APRN,
CCRN, FAAN
Professor
University of Alabama at Birmingham
Birmingham, Alabama
Chapter 10

Karen Balakas, PhD, RN, CNE
Professor and Director of Clinical Research/EBP
Partnerships
Goldfarb School of Nursing
Barnes-Jewish College
St. Louis, Missouri
Chapter 14

Patricia E. Benner, PhD, RN, FRCN, FAAN
Professor Emerita (former Thelma Shobe
Endowed Chair in Ethical and Spirituality)
Department of Social and Behavioral Sciences
University of California San Francisco
San Francisco, California
Chapter 7

Donna R. Berryman, MLS
Assistant Director of Education and Information
Services
School of Medicine and Dentistry
University of Rochester
Rochester, New York
Chapter 3

Cecily L. Betz, PhD, RN, FAAN
Associate Professor of Clinical Pediatrics
Department of Pediatrics
Keck School of Medicine
Director of Nursing Training
Director of Research
USC Center for Excellence in Developmental
Disabilities
Children's Hospital
Los Angeles, California
Editor-in-Chief
*Journal of Pediatric Nursing: Nursing Care of
Children and Families*
Chapter 16

Barbara B. Brewer, PhD, RN, MALS, MBA
Director of Professional Practice
John C. Lincoln North Mountain Hospital
Phoenix, Arizona
Chapter 10

Terri L. Brown, MSN, RN, CPN
Research Specialist
Texas Children's Hospital
Houston, Texas
Chapter 9

Donna Ciliska, PhD, RN
Scientific Co-Director of the National
Collaborating Centre for Methods and Tools and
Professor
School of Nursing
McMaster University
Hamilton, Ontario, Canada
Chapter 11

Robert Cole, PhD
Associate Professor of Clinical Nursing
University of Rochester
Rochester, New York
Chapter 17

John F. Cox III, MD
Assistant Professor of Clinical Medicine
School of Medicine and Dentistry
University of Rochester
Rochester, New York
Chapter 13

Laura Cullen, MA, RN, FAAN
Evidence-Based Practice Coordinator
University of Iowa Hospitals and Clinics
Iowa City, Iowa
Chapter 11

Deborah Dang, PhD, RN, NEA-BC
Director of Nursing
Practice, Education, Research
Johns Hopkins Hospital
Baltimore, Maryland
Chapter 11

Alba DiCenso, PhD, RN
Professor
School of Nursing
McMaster University
Hamilton, Ontario, Canada
Chapter 11

Doris Grinspun, PhD, RN
Executive Director
Registered Nurses' Association of Ontario
Toronto, Ontario, Canada
Chapter 8

Marilyn J. Hockenberry, PhD, RN, PNP-BC, FAAN
Professor of Pediatrics, Hematology/Oncology
Baylor College of Medicine
Houston, Texas
Chapter 9

Sheila Hofstetter, MLS, AHIP
Health Sciences Librarian
Noble Science and Engineering Library
Arizona State University
Tempe, Arizona
Chapter 3

Linda Johnston, PhD, RN
Professor and Chair of Neonatal Nursing Research
The Royal Children's Hospital
Parkville
Deputy Head of School and Associate Head (Research)
School of Nursing
The University of Melbourne
Murdoch Children's Research Institute
Melbourne, Australia
Chapter 5

June H. Larrabee, PhD, RN
Professor and Clinical Investigator
West Virginia University and West Virginia University Hospitals
Charleston, West Virginia
Chapter 11

Victoria Wynn Leonard, RN, FNP, PhD
Assistant Professor
University of San Francisco School of Nursing
San Francisco, California
Chapter 7

Robin P. Newhouse, PhD, RN, CNAA, BC
Assistant Dean
Doctor of Nursing Practice Studies
Associate Professor
School of Nursing
University of Maryland
Annapolis, Maryland
Chapter 11

Dónal P. O'Mathúna, PhD
Senior Lecturer in Ethics, Decision-Making and Evidence
School of Nursing
Dublin City University
Glasnevin, Dublin, Ireland
Chapters 5 and 20

Bethel Ann Powers, RN, PhD
Professor and Director
Evaluation Office
University of Rochester School of Nursing
Rochester, New York
Chapters 6, 18, and Appendix C

Tom Rickey, BA
Manager of National Media Relations and Senior Science Editor
University of Rochester Medical Center
Rochester, New York
Chapter 16

Brett W. Robbins, MD
Associate Professor of Medicine and Pediatrics
University of Rochester
Rochester, New York
Chapter 13

**Jo Rycroft-Malone, PhD, MSc,
BSc (Hon), RN**
Professor of Health Services and Implementation
Research
School of Healthcare Sciences
Bangor University
Frowheulog, Bangor, United Kingdom
Chapter 11

Alyce A. Schultz, PhD, RN, FAAN
Consultant
EBP Concepts, Alyce A. Schultz & Associates,
LLC
Chandler, Arizona
Chapter 11

Kathryn A. Smith, RN, MN
Associate Director for Administration
USC University Center for Excellence in
Developmental Disabilities
Children's Hospital
Associate Professor of Clinical Pediatrics
Keck School of Medicine
University of Southern California
Los Angeles, California
Chapter 16

Julia Sollenberger, MLS
Director
Health Science Libraries and Technologies
University of Rochester Medical Center
Rochester, New York
Chapter 3

Cheryl B. Stetler, PhD, RN, FAAN
Consultant
EBP and Evaluation
Amherst, Massachusetts
Chapter 11

Kathleen R. Stevens, RN, EdD, FAAN
Professor and Director
Academic Center for Evidence-Based Nursing
The University of Texas Health Science Center at
San Antonio
San Antonio, Texas
Chapter 4

Susan B. Stillwell, DNP, RN, CNE
Clinical Associate Professor and Expert EBP
Mentor
College of Nursing and Health Innovation
Arizona State University
Phoenix, Arizona
Chapters 2 and 13

Nancy Watson, PhD, RN
Associate Professor and Director
John A. Hartford Foundation Community
Initiative & Center for Clinical Research on
Aging
University of Rochester School of Nursing
Rochester, New York
Appendix I

Kathleen M. Williamson, PhD, RN
Clinical Associate Professor and Associate
Director
Center for the Advancement of Evidence-Based
Practice
College of Nursing and Health Innovation
Arizona State University
Phoenix, Arizona
Chapter 13

Reviewers

Maureen Anthony, PhD
Associate Professor
University of Detroit Mercy
Detroit, Michigan

Dot Baker, RN, MS(N), PHCNS-BC, EdD
Professor
Wilmington University
Georgetown, Delaware

Jennifer Bellot, PhD, RN, MHSA, CNE
Associate Professor
Thomas Jefferson University
Philadelphia, Pennsylvania

Janie Best, DNP, RN, CNL, ACNS-BC
Assistant Professor/Nurse Scientist
Queens University of Charlotte
Charlotte, North Carolina

Billie Blake, EdD, MSN, BSN, RN, CNE
Associate Dean and Professor
Nursing
St. Johns River State College
Orange Park, Florida

Wendy Blakely, PhD, RN
Associate Professor
Capital University
Columbus, Ohio

Della Campbell, PhD, RN
Associate Professor
Felician College
Lodi, New Jersey

Robin Chard, PhD, RN, CNOR
Associate Professor
Nova Southeastern University
Fort Lauderdale, Florida

Kristina Childers, MSN, ARNP, FNP-BC
Senior Lecturer
West Virginia University
Charleston, West Virginia

Sara Clutter, PhD, RN
Associate Professor
Nursing
Waynesburg University
Waynesburg, Pennsylvania

Beth Crouch, MSN, RN, BS
Assistant Professor
Nursing
Milligan College
Milligan College, Tennessee

Connie Cupples, PhD, RN
Associate Professor
Nursing
Union University
Jackson, Tennessee

Marianne Curia, PhD, MSN, RN
Assistant Professor
University of St. Francis
Joliet, Illinois

Brenda W. Dyal, DNP, FNP-BC
Assistant Dean and Assistant Professor
Nursing
Valdosta State University
Valdosta, Georgia

Patricia Eckhardt, PhD, RN
Assistant Professor
Stony Brook University
Stony Brook, New York

Judith Floyd, PhD, RN, FAAN
Professor
Wayne State University
Detroit, Michigan

Patricia Gagliano, PhD, RN
Professor
Indian River State College
Fort Pierce, Florida

Jane Gannon, DNP, CNM, CNL
Clinical Assistant Professor
University of Florida
Gainesville, Florida

Mary Garnica, DNP, APRN, FNP-BC
Assistant Professor
Nursing
University of Central Arkansas
Conway, Arkansas

Valera Hascup, PhD, MSN, RN, CTN, CCES
Assistant Professor
Kean University
Union, New Jersey

Annette Hines, PhD, CNE
Assistant Professor
Queens University of Charlotte
Charlotte, North Carolina

Karyn Holt, CNM, PhD
Director
Online Quality
Drexel University
Philadelphia, Pennsylvania

Brenda Hosley, PhD, RN, CNE
Clinical Associate Professor
Arizona State University
Phoenix, Arizona

Marguerite Huster, MSN, RN
Assistant Professor and Simulation Center Coordinator
William Jewell College
Liberty, Missouri

Renee Ingel, PhD, MSN, BSN, RN
Assistant Professor
Carlow University
Pittsburgh, Pennsylvania

Selma Kerr-Wilson, RN, MS
Faculty
BSN Program
British Columbia Institute of Technology
Burnaby, British Columbia

Stefanie LaManna, PhD, ARNP, FNP-C
Assistant Professor
Nova Southeastern University
Palm Beach Gardens, Florida

Debra Pecka Malina, DNSc, MBA, CRNA, ARNP
Assistant Program Director Clinical Education
Anesthesiology Programs
Barry University
Hollywood, Florida

Cheryl Martin, BSN, MSN, PhD
BSN Programs Director
University of Indianapolis
Indianapolis, Indiana

Gretchen Mettler, PhD
Assistant Professor
Director
Nurse Midwife Education Program
Case Western Reserve University
Cleveland, Ohio

Diane Monsivais, PhD, CNE
Director
MSN in Nursing Education
The University of Texas
El Paso, Texas

Audrey Nelson, PhD, RN
Associate Professor
University of Nebraska Medical Center
Omaha, Nebraska

Marie O'Toole, RN, EdD, FAAN
Associate Dean and Professor
Rutgers School of Nursing
Stratford, New Jersey

Brenda Pavill, CRNP, PhD
Associate Professor
Misericordia University
Dallas, Pennsylvania

Michael Perlow, DNS
Professor of Nursing
Murray State University
Murray, Kentucky

Ruth Remington, PhD, AGPCNP-BC
Associate Professor
Framingham State University
Framingham, Massachusetts

Susan Rugari, PhD, RN, CNS
Associate Professor & Interim Department
Head
Tarleton State University
Stephenville, Texas

Lois Seefeldt, RN, PhD
Coordinator Executive
DNP Leadership Track
Concordia University
Mequon, Wisconsin

**Debra Shelton, EdD, MSN, BSN,
APRN-CNS, CNE, ANEF**
Director
Assessment and Evaluation
Northwestern State University
Shreveport, Louisiana

Ida Slusher, RN, PhD, CNE
Professor & Nursing Education Coordinator
Eastern Kentucky University
Richmond, Kentucky

Susan Van Cleve, DNP, CPNP-PC, PMHS
Associate Professor
Robert Morris University
Pittsburgh, Pennsylvania

Julee Waldrop, DNP, FNP, PNP, PMHS, CNE
Clinical Associate Professor
University of Central Florida
Orlando, Florida

Carole White, PhD, RN
Associate Professor
University of Texas Health Sciences Center
San Antonio, Texas

Cathy Williams, DNP, RN
Associate Professor
Albany State University
Albany, Georgia

Kathleen Wisser, PhD, RN, CPHQ, CNE
Assistant Professor
Nursing
Alvernia University
Reading, Pennsylvania

Threasia Witt, EdD
Professor
Nursing
Davis & Elkins College
Elkins, West Virginia

**Supakit Wongwiwathananukit, PharmD,
MS, PhD**
Associate Professor
Pharmacy Practice
University of Hawai'i
Hilo, Hawai'i

Julie Zadinsky, PhD
Assistant Dean for Research
Georgia Regents University
Augusta, Georgia

For a list of the reviewers of the Test Generator accompanying this
book, please visit http://thepoint.lww.com/Melnyk3e.

Like many of you, I have appreciated health care through a range of experiences and perspectives. As someone who has delivered health care as a combat medic, paramedic, nurse, and trauma surgeon, the value of evidence-based practice is clear to me. Knowing what questions to ask, how to carefully evaluate the responses, maximize the knowledge and use of empirical evidence, and provide the most effective clinical assessments and interventions are important assets for every healthcare professional. The quality of U.S. and global health care depends on clinicians being able to deliver on these and other best practices.

The Institute of Medicine calls for all healthcare professionals to be educated to deliver patient-centered care as members of an interdisciplinary team, emphasizing evidence-based practice, quality improvement approaches, and informatics. Although many practitioners support the use of evidence-based practice, and there are indications that our patients are better served when we apply evidence-based practice, there are challenges to successful implementation. One barrier is knowledge. Do we share a standard understanding of evidence-based practice and how such evidence can best be used? We need more textbooks and other references that clearly define and provide a standard approach to evidence-based practice.

Another significant challenge is the time between the publication of research findings and the translation of such information into practice. This challenge exists throughout public health. Determining the means of more rapidly moving from the brilliance that is our national medical research to applications that blend new science and compassionate care in our clinical systems is of interest to us all.

As healthcare professionals who currently use evidence-based practice, you recognize these challenges and others. Our patients benefit because we adopt, investigate, teach, and evaluate evidence-based practice. I encourage you to continue the excellent work to bring about greater understanding and a more generalizable approach to evidence-based practice.

Richard H. Carmona, MD, MPH, FACS
17th Surgeon General of the United States

The evidence is irrefutable: evidence-based practice (EBP) improves the quality of care and patient outcomes as well as reduces the costs of care across healthcare settings and the life span. Furthermore, although there are many published interventions/treatments that have resulted in positive outcomes for patients and healthcare systems, they are not being implemented in clinical practice. In addition, qualitative evidence is not readily incorporated into care.

The purpose of this third edition of *Evidence-Based Practice in Nursing and Healthcare* is to continue our efforts to help all clinicians, no matter their healthcare role, to accelerate the translation of research findings into practice and the use of practice data to ultimately improve care and outcomes. Although there has been some progress in the adoption of EBP as the standard of care in recent years, there is still much work to be done for this paradigm to be used daily in practice by point of care providers. The daunting statistic that it takes an average of 17 years or longer to move research findings into practice is still a reality in many healthcare institutions across the globe. Therefore, increased efforts are required to provide the tools that point of care clinicians need in order to use the best evidence from research and their practices to improve their healthcare system, practitioner, and patient outcomes.

We will always believe that anything is possible when you have a big dream and believe in your ability to accomplish that dream. It was the vision of transforming health care with EBP, in any setting, with one client–clinician encounter at a time and the belief that this can be the daily experience of both patients and practitioners, along with our sheer persistence through many "character-building experiences" during the writing and editing of the book, that culminated in this user-friendly guide that assists all healthcare professionals in the delivery of the highest quality, evidence-based care in order to produce the best outcomes for their patients.

The third edition of this text has been revised to assist healthcare providers with implementing and sustaining EBP in their daily practices and to foster a deeper understanding of the principles of the EBP paradigm and process. In working with healthcare systems and clinicians throughout the nation and globe and conducting research on EBP, we have learned more about successful strategies to advance and sustain evidence-based care. Therefore, you will find new material throughout the book, including new chapters, competencies, and tools to advance EBP.

As with the first and second editions, the third edition provides the knowledge for a solid understanding of the EBP paradigm or worldview, which is the foundation for all clinical decisions. This worldview frames the understanding of the steps of the EBP process, the clarification of misperceptions about the implementation of EBP, and the practical action strategies for the implementation of evidence-based care that can enhance widespread acceleration of EBP at the point of care. It is our dream that this knowledge and understanding will continue across the country and globe until the lived experience of practicing from the EBP paradigm becomes a reality across healthcare providers, settings, and educational institutions.

The book contains vital, usable, and relatable content for all levels of practitioners and learners, with key exemplars that bring to life the concepts within the chapters. At the end of each chapter, we now provide EBP Fast Facts, which are golden nuggets of information to reinforce important concepts and offer the opportunity for readers to double-check themselves or quickly identify key chapter content. Another new feature at the end of each unit, "Making EBP Real," provides real-life examples that help readers to see the principles of EBP applied. Furthermore, clinicians who desire to stimulate or lead change to a culture of EBP in their practice sites can discover functional models and practical strategies to introduce a change to EBP, overcome barriers in implementing change, and evaluate outcomes of change.

For clinical and academic educators, we have included specific chapters on teaching EBP in educational and health care settings (Chapters 15 and 16, respectively). Educators can be most successful as they make the EBP paradigm and process understandable for their learners. Often, educators teach by following chapters in a textbook through their exact sequence; however, we recommend using chapters of this third edition that are appropriate for the level of the learner (e.g., associate degree, baccalaureate, master's, or doctoral). For example, we would recommend that associate degree students benefit from Units 1, 3, and 4. Curriculum for baccalaureate learners can integrate all units; however, we recommend primarily using Units 1–4, with Unit 5 as a resource for understanding more about research generation and methods. Master's and doctoral programs can incorporate all units into their curricula. Advanced practice clinicians will be able to lead in implementing evidence in practice and thoughtfully evaluate outcomes of practice, while those learning to become researchers will understand how to best build on existing evidence to fill gaps in knowledge with valid reliable research. Another important resource for educators to use in tandem with the EBP book is the ***American Journal of Nursing*** EBP Step-by-Step series, which provides a real-world example of the EBP process from step 0 through step 6. A team of healthcare providers encounters a challenging issue and uses the EBP process to find a sustainable solution that improves healthcare outcomes. Educators can assign the articles before or in tandem with readings from this book. For example, the first three chapters of the book could be assigned along with the first four articles, which could offer an opportunity for great discussion within the classroom (see suggested curriculum strategy at this book's companion website, http://thepoint.lww.com/Melnyk3e). With these approaches in mind, we believe that this book will continue to facilitate changes in how research concepts and critical appraisal are being taught in clinical and academic professional programs throughout the country. Finally, researchers, clinicians in advanced roles, and educators may benefit from the chapters on generating quantitative and qualitative evidence (Chapters 19 and 20) as well as how to write a successful grant proposal (Chapter 21).

FEATURES

As proponents of cognitive-behavioral theory, which contends that how people think directly influences how they feel and behave, we firmly believe that how an individual thinks is the first step toward or away from success. Therefore, **inspirational quotes** are intertwined throughout our book to encourage readers to build their beliefs and abilities as they actively engage in EBP and accomplish their desired goals.

With the rapid delivery of information available to us, **web alerts** direct readers to helpful Internet resources and sites that can be used to further develop EBP knowledge and skills.

Content new to this edition includes:

- **EBP Fast Facts:** Important points highlighed at the end of each chapter.
- **Making EBP Real:** A successful real-world case story emphasizing applied content from each unit.
- **Updated** information on **evidence hierarchies for different clinical questions** because one hierarchy does not fit all questions.
- **Successful strategies for finding evidence,** including updates on sources of evidence.
- **Updated rapid critical appraisal checklists, evaluation tables, and synthesis tables** that provide efficient critical appraisal methods for both quantitative and qualitative evidence for use in clinical decisions.
- A **new chapter (7) on the role of a clinician's expertise and patient preferences/values in making decisions about patient care**.
- **EBP models updated by their original creators** (Chapter 13) to assist learners as they build a sustainable culture of EBP.
- **Updated approaches to evaluating outcomes** throughout the book, along with a **chapter (10)** on the role of evaluating practice outcomes.
- A **new chapter (11) on leadership strategies** for creating and sustaining EBP organizations.
- A **new chapter (12) on sparking innovation in EBP.**

- **Updated information on the role of the EBP mentor,** a key factor in the sustainability of an EBP culture, including evaluation of the role and its impact on care delivery.
- **Samples of established measures** of EBP beliefs, EBP implementation and organizational culture, and readiness for EBP within the service and educational setting.
- Updated chapter (14) that details how to **create a vision to motivate a change** to best practice.
- **A new framework for teaching EBP** to improve learner assimilation of the EBP paradigm as the basis for clinical decisions-the **ARCC-E model (Chapter 15).**
- Updated chapters (19 and 20) that provide step-by-step principles for **generating quantitative and qualitative evidence** when little evidence exists to guide clinical practice.
- Updated chapter (21) on how to **write a successful grant proposal** to fund an EBP implementation project or research study.
- Updated information on how to **disseminate evidence** to other professionals, the media, and policy makers.
- Updated chapter (22) that addresses the **ethics of evidence use and generation**.
- Many updated **usable tools that will help healthcare providers implement EBP,** in the appendix and online at this book's companion website, http://thepoint.lww.com/Melnyk3e.

ADDITIONAL RESOURCES

Evidence-Based Practice in Nursing and Healthcare, third edition, includes additional resources for both instructors and students that are available on the book's companion website at http://thepoint.lww.com/Melnyk3e.

Instructors

Approved adopting instructors will be given access to the following additional resources:

- An **E-Book** allows access to the book's full text and images online.
- **Brownstone test generator.**
- Additional **test and reflective questions, application case studies, and examples** for select chapters.
- **PowerPoint presentations**, including multiple choice questions for use with interactive clicker technology.
- **Guided lecture notes** present brief talking points for instructors, provide suggestions on how to structure lectures, and give ideas on organizing material.
- We can include the PhD and DNP in this list as well.
- **Sample syllabi** for all levels: RN to BSN, Traditional BSN, MSN, PhD, and DNP.
- The *American Journal of Nursing* EBP Step-by-Step Series, which provides a real-world example of the EBP process, plus a suggested curriculum strategy. (The series is an ancillary accessible to students; the curriculum strategy is an instructor asset.) See also information earlier in this preface about how this resource might be used.
- An **image bank,** containing figures and tables from the text in formats suitable for printing, projecting, and incorporating into websites.
- **Strategies for Effective Teaching** offer creative approaches.
- **Learning management system cartridges.**
- Access to all student resources.

Students

Students who have purchased *Evidence-Based Practice in Nursing and Healthcare*, third edition, have access to the following additional online resources:

- **Learning Objectives** for each chapter
- **Checklists and templates** including checklists for conducting an evidence review and a journal club, and a template for PICOT questions.

◆ **Journal articles** corresponding to book chapters to offer access to current research available in Wolters Kluwer journals
◆ The *American Journal of Nursing* **EBP Step-by-Step Series,** which provides a real-world example of the EBP process
◆ An example of a poster (to accompany Chapter 18)
◆ A **Spanish–English audio glossary** and **Nursing Professional Roles and Responsibilities**

See the inside front cover of this text for more details, including the passcode you will need to gain access to the website.

A FINAL WORD FROM THE AUTHORS

As we have the privilege of meeting and working with clinicians, educators, and researchers across the globe to advance and sustain EBP, we realize how important our unified effort is to world health. We want to thank each reader for your investment of time and energy to learn and use the information contained within this book to foster your best practice. Furthermore, we so appreciate the information that you have shared with us regarding the benefits and challenges you have had in learning about and applying knowledge of EBP. That feedback has been instrumental to improving the third edition of our book. We value constructive feedback and welcome any ideas that you have about content, tools, and resources that would help us to improve a future edition. The spirit of inquiry and life-long learning are foundational principles of the EBP paradigm and underpin the EBP process so that this problem-solving approach to practice can cultivate an excitement for implementing the highest quality of care. As you engage your EBP journey, remember that it takes time and that it becomes easier when the principles of this book are placed into action with enthusiasm on a consistent daily basis.

As you make a positive impact at the point of care, whether you are first learning about the EBP paradigm, the steps of the EBP process, leading a successful EBP change effort, or generating evidence to fill a knowledge gap or implement translational methods, we want to encourage you to keep the dream alive and, in the words of Les Brown, "Shoot for the moon. Even if you miss, you land among the stars." We hope you are inspired by and enjoy the following EBP RAP.

> *Evidence-based practice is a wonderful thing,*
> *Done with consistency, it makes you sing.*
> *PICOT questions and learning search skills;*
> *Appraising evidence can give you thrills.*
> *Medline, CINAHL, PsycInfo are fine,*
> *But for Level I evidence, Cochrane's divine!*
> *Though you may want to practice the same old way*
> *"Oh no, that's not how I will do it," you say.*
> *When you launch EBP in your practice site,*
> *Remember to eat the chocolate elephant, bite by bite.*
> *So dream big and persist in order to achieve and*
> *Know that EBP can be done when you believe!*

© 2004 Bernadette Melnyk
Bernadette Mazurek Melnyk and Ellen Fineout-Overholt

Note: You may contact the authors at
bernmelnyk@gmail.com
ellen.fineout.overholt@gmail.com

Acknowledgments

This book could not have been accomplished without the support, understanding, and assistance of many wonderful colleagues, staff, family, and friends. I would first like to acknowledge the outstanding work of my co-editor and cherished friend, Ellen—thank you for all of your efforts, our wonderful friendship, attention to detail, and ongoing support throughout this process—I could not have accomplished this revised edition without you. Since the first edition of this book, I have grown personally and professionally through the many opportunities that I have had to teach and mentor others in evidence-based practice across the globe—the lessons I have learned from all of you have been incorporated into this book. I thank all of my mentees for their valuable feedback and all of the authors who contributed their time and valuable expertise to this book. Along with my wonderful husband John and my three daughters, Kaylin, Angela, and Megan, I am appreciative for the ongoing love and support that I receive from my mother, Anna May Mazurek, my brother and sister-in-law, Fred and Sue Mazurek, and my sister, Christine Warmuth, whose famous words to me "Just get out there and do it" have been a key to many of my successful endeavors. I would also like to thank my wonderful colleagues and staff at The Ohio State University for their support, understanding, and ongoing commitment to our projects and their roles throughout this process. Finally, I would like to acknowledge the team at Wolters Kluwer for their assistance with and dedication to keeping this project on track.

Bernadette Mazurek Melnyk

Over the past 15 years, I have met so many wonderful healthcare providers who are kindred spirits and have the same goal that I do—to do whatever it takes to achieve best outcomes for patients who need our care. I feel so very blessed. As all of us—students, clinicians, clinical educators, faculty, and researchers—choose to adopt the evidence-based practice paradigm as our foundation for healthcare decisions, we will meet that goal! Thank you for demonstrating that ownership of practice is the key to healthcare transformation. In addition, I want to express my heartfelt thanks to each of you who personally have shared encouraging words with me about the value of our work to advance best practice in health care and how it has helped you make a difference in patients' lives and health experiences. Thank you for actualizing the dream of transforming health care, one client–clinician relationship at a time. As I reflect on this dream, I thank you, Bern, for the wonderful privilege I have had to work with you for over 25 years. Thank you for helping me grow and achieve goals that I may have not pursued without your push—I very much appreciate your mentoring and partnership!

Further reflection has led me to consider that with every edition of this book, I am amazed at how blessed I am to have the support of my precious family and friends. Every day, when I see my sweet, growing-up girls, I am inspired again to strive to achieve the goals of evidence-based care as a standard. Thank you Rachael and Ruth for your gift of love and laughter that you give Mom every day! Similarly, my mother, Virginia (Grandginny), has had experiences in health care as an older old adult (now 83) that have compelled me to consider the importance of advocating for evidence-based consumers. Thank you, Mom, for the many long talks and words of encouragement and being an example! Also, my brother, John, and his family, Angela, Ashton, and Aubrey, have enriched my life with their talents, particularly in music—thank you!—and have also spurred on my work toward best practice through their healthcare experiences. It is likely that all of us could speak to some good or some not-so-good healthcare encounters that serve as inspiration for our commitment to excellence in care. I am grateful to each of you reading this book who will take the knowledge contained in its pages and make it come alive in your work.

To those of you who have prayed for me during this writing adventure—thank you so very much! To my wonderful husband, Wayne, who consistently offers perspective and balance that are so important

xxii

to me—I can find no language that conveys how much I value your presence in my life! Finally, as I reflect on my lifework and the importance of improving healthcare outcomes through sustainable evidence-based practice, I am mindful of how important my gracious Savior and Friend's work has been in me, for which I am eternally grateful.

Publishing a book takes a team of dedicated professionals, much like a healthcare team, each with a unique role that is critical to the book's success. I am grateful to the Wolters Kluwer team with whom we have had the privilege to work. They have helped us live our dream. Finally, I cannot say enough "thank yous" to the many wonderful contributors to this work and the common goal that binds us together—improving health care. I am very grateful for their investment throughout the writing of the third edition of *Evidence-Based Practice in Nursing and Healthcare!*

Ellen Fineout-Overholt

Contents

UNIT 4 Creating and Sustaining a Culture and Environment for Evidence-Based Practice

UNIT 5 Step Six: Disseminating Evidence and Evidence-Based Practice Implementation Outcomes

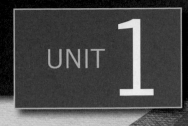

Steps Zero, One, Two: Getting Started

To accomplish great things, we must not only act but also dream; not only plan, but also believe.

—Anatole France

Chapter 1

Making the Case for Evidence-Based Practice and Cultivating a Spirit of Inquiry

Bernadette Mazurek Melnyk and Ellen Fineout-Overholt

It is now widely recognized throughout the globe that **evidence-based practice (EBP)** is key to delivering the highest quality of healthcare and ensuring the best patient outcomes at the lowest costs. Findings from numerous studies have indicated that an evidence-based approach to practice versus the implementation of clinical care that is steeped in tradition or based upon outdated policies results in a multitude of improved health, safety, and cost outcomes, including a decrease in patient morbidity and mortality (McGinty & Anderson, 2008; Williams, 2004). The goal of improving healthcare through enhancing the experience of care, improving the health of populations, and reducing per capita costs of healthcare has become known as the *Triple Aim*, which is the major focus of current efforts by healthcare systems across the United States (U.S.) (Berwick, Nolan, & Whittington, 2008). When clinicians know how to use the EBP process to implement the best care and when patients are confident that their healthcare providers are using evidence-based care, optimal outcomes are achieved for all.

Although there is an explosion of scientific evidence available to guide clinical practice, the implementation of evidence-based care by health professionals is typically not the norm in many healthcare systems across the U.S. and globe. However, when healthcare providers are asked whether they would personally like to receive evidence-based care if they found themselves in a patient role, the answer is resoundingly "yes!" For example:

- If your child was in a motor vehicle accident and sustained a severe head injury, would you want his neurologist to know and use the most effective, empirically supported treatment established from **randomized controlled trials (RCTs)** to decrease his intracranial pressure and prevent death?
- If your mother was diagnosed with Alzheimer's disease, would you want her nurse practitioner to give you information about how other family caregivers of patients with this disease have coped with the illness, based on evidence from well-designed qualitative and/or descriptive studies?
- If you were diagnosed with colon cancer today and were faced with the decision about what combination of chemotherapy agents to choose, would you want your oncologist to share with you the best and latest evidence regarding the risks and benefits of each therapeutic agent as generated from prior clinical trials with other similar cancer patients?

DEFINITION AND EVOLUTION OF EVIDENCE-BASED PRACTICE

In 2000, Sackett, Straus, Richardson, Rosenberg, and Haynes defined EBP as the conscientious use of current best evidence in making decisions about patient care. Since then, the definition of EBP has been broadened in scope and referred to as a lifelong problem-solving approach to clinical practice that integrates

- A systematic search for as well as critical appraisal and synthesis of the most relevant and best research (i.e., **external evidence**) to answer a burning clinical question
- One's own **clinical expertise**, which includes **internal evidence** generated from outcomes management or quality improvement projects, a thorough patient assessment, and evaluation and use of available resources necessary to achieve desired patient outcomes
- Patient preferences and values (Figure 1.1)

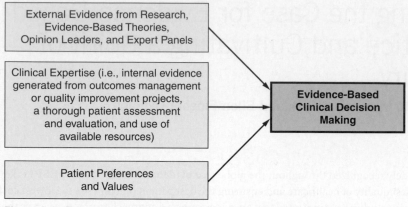

Figure 1.1: The components of EBP.

Unlike **research utilization,** which has been frequently operationalized as the use of knowledge typically based on a single study, EBP takes into consideration a synthesis of evidence from multiple studies and combines it with the expertise of the practitioner as well as patient preferences and values (Melnyk & Fineout-Overholt, 2011).

WHAT IS EVIDENCE?

Evidence is a collection of facts that are believed to be true. **External evidence** is generated through rigorous research (e.g., **RCTs** or **cohort studies**) and is intended to be generalized to and used in other settings. An important question when implementing external evidence from research is whether clinicians can achieve results in their own clinical practices that are similar to those derived from a body of evidence (i.e., Can the findings from research be translated to the real-world clinical setting?). This question of transferability is why measurement of key outcomes is still necessary when implementing practice changes based on evidence. In contrast, **internal evidence** is typically generated through practice initiatives, such as **outcomes management** or **quality improvement projects** that use internal evidence from patient data in an organization to improve clinical care. Researchers generate new knowledge through rigorous research (i.e., external evidence), and EBP provides clinicians the process and tools to translate the evidence into clinical practice and integrate it with internal evidence to improve the quality of healthcare and patient outcomes.

Unfortunately, there are many interventions (i.e., treatments) with substantial empirical evidence to support their use in clinical practice to improve patient outcomes that are not routinely used. For example, findings from a series of RCTs testing the efficacy of the COPE (Creating Opportunities for Parent Empowerment) Program for parents of critically ill/hospitalized and premature infants support that when parents receive COPE (i.e., an educational–behavioral skills-building intervention that is delivered by clinicians to parents at the point of care through a series of brief CDs, written information, and activity workbooks) versus an attention control program, COPE parents: (a) report less stress, anxiety, and depressive symptoms during hospitalization; (b) participate more in their children's care; (c) interact in more developmentally sensitive ways; and (d) report less depression and posttraumatic stress disorder symptoms up to a year following their children's discharge from the hospital (Melnyk, 1994; Melnyk et al., 2004, 2006; Melnyk & Feinstein, 2009). In addition, the premature infants and children of parents who receive COPE versus those whose parents who receive an attention control program have better behavioral and developmental outcomes as well as shorter hospital stays, which could result in billions of dollars of healthcare savings for the U.S. healthcare system if the program is routinely implemented by hospitals (Melnyk et al., 2006; Melnyk & Feinstein, 2009). Despite this strong body of evidence, COPE is not standard of practice in many hospitals throughout the nation.

In contrast, there are many practices that are being implemented in healthcare that have no or little evidence to support their use (e.g., double-checking pediatric medications, routine assessment of vital signs every 2 or 4 hours in hospitalized patients, use of a plastic tongue patch for weight loss). Unless we know what interventions are most effective for a variety of populations through the generation of evidence from research and practice data (e.g., outcomes management, quality improvement projects) and how to rapidly translate this evidence into clinical practice through EBP, substantial sustainable improvement in the quality and safety of care received by U.S. residents is not likely (Melnyk, 2012; Shortell, Rundall, & Hsu, 2007).

COMPONENTS OF EVIDENCE-BASED PRACTICE

Although evidence from **systematic reviews** of RCTs has been regarded as the strongest level of evidence (i.e., Level 1 evidence) on which to base practice decisions about treatments to achieve a desired outcome, evidence from descriptive and qualitative studies as well as from opinion leaders should be factored into clinical decisions when RCTs are not available. **Evidence-based theories** (i.e., theories that are empirically supported through well-designed studies) also should be included as evidence. In addition, patient preferences, values, and concerns should be incorporated into the evidence-based approach to decision making along with a clinician's expertise, which includes (a) clinical judgment (i.e., the ability to think about, understand, and use research evidence; the ability to assess a patient's condition through subjective history taking, thorough physical examination findings, and laboratory reports), (b) internal evidence generated from quality improvement or outcomes management projects, (c) clinical reasoning (i.e., the ability to apply the above information to a clinical issue), and (d) evaluation and use of available healthcare resources needed to implement the chosen treatment(s) and achieve the expected outcome (Figure 1.2).

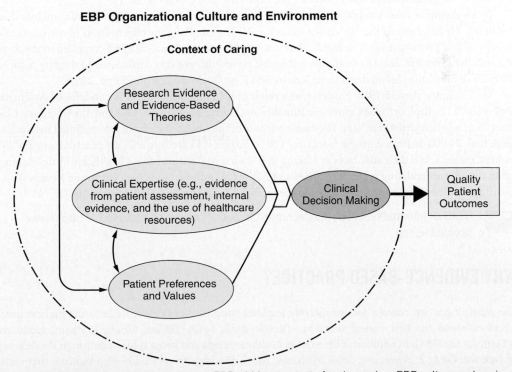

Figure 1.2: The merging of science and art: EBP within a context of caring and an EBP culture and environment results in the highest quality of healthcare and patient outcomes. © Melnyk & Fineout-Overholt, 2003.

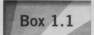

Box 1.1   Rule of Thumb for Determining Whether a Practice Change Should be Made

The level of the evidence + quality of the evidence = strength of the evidence →
Confidence to act upon the evidence and change practice!

Clinicians often ask how much and what type of evidence is needed to change practice. A good rule of thumb to answer this question is that there needs to be strong enough evidence to make a practice change. Specifically, the level of evidence plus the quality of evidence equals the strength of the evidence, which provides clinicians the confidence that is needed to change clinical practice (Box 1.1).

ORIGINS OF THE EVIDENCE-BASED PRACTICE MOVEMENT

The EBP movement was founded by Dr. Archie Cochrane, a British epidemiologist, who struggled with the efficacy (effectiveness) of healthcare and challenged the public to pay only for care that had been empirically supported as effective (Enkin, 1992). In 1972, Cochrane published a landmark book that criticized the medical profession for not providing rigorous reviews of evidence so that policy-makers and organizations could make the best decisions about healthcare. Cochrane was a strong proponent of using evidence from RCTs because he believed that this was the strongest evidence on which to base clinical practice treatment decisions. He asserted that reviews of research evidence across all specialty areas need to be prepared systematically through a rigorous process and that they should be maintained to consider the generation of new evidence (The Cochrane Collaboration, 2001).

In an exemplar case, Cochrane noted that thousands of low-birth-weight premature infants died needlessly. He emphasized that the results of several RCTs supporting the effectiveness of corticosteroid therapy to halt premature labor in high-risk women had never been analyzed and compiled in the form of a systematic review. The data from that systematic review showed that corticosteroid therapy reduced the odds of premature infant death from 50% to 30% (The Cochrane Collaboration, 2001).

Dr. Cochrane died in 1988. However, as a result of his influence and call for updates of systematic reviews of RCTs, the Cochrane Center was launched in Oxford, England, in 1992, and The Cochrane Collaboration was founded a year later. The major purpose of the Collaboration, an international network of more than 31,000 dedicated people from over 120 countries, is to assist healthcare practitioners, policy-makers, patients, and their advocates in making well-informed decisions about healthcare by developing, maintaining, and updating systematic reviews of healthcare interventions (i.e., Cochrane Reviews) and ensuring that these reviews are accessible to the public (The Cochrane Collaboration, 2001).

 Further information about the Cochrane Collaboration can be accessed at http://www .cochrane.org/

WHY EVIDENCE-BASED PRACTICE?

The most important reasons for consistently implementing EBP are that it leads to the highest quality of care and the best patient outcomes (Reigle et al., 2008; Talsma, Grady, Feetham, Heinrich, & Steinwachs, 2008). In addition, EBP reduces healthcare costs and geographic variation in the delivery of care (McGinty & Anderson, 2008; Williams, 2004). Findings from studies also indicate that clinicians report feeling more empowered and satisfied in their roles when they engage in EBP (Maljanian, Caramanica, Taylor, MacRae, & Beland, 2002; Strout, 2005). With recent reports of pervasive "burnout" among healthcare professionals and the pressure that many influential healthcare organizations exert on clinicians to deliver high-quality, safe care under increasingly heavy patient loads, the use and teaching of EBP may be key not only to providing outstanding care to patients and saving healthcare dollars, but also to reducing the escalating turnover rate in certain healthcare professions (Melnyk, Fineout-Overholt, Giggleman, & Cruz, 2010).

Despite the multitude of positive outcomes associated with EBP and the strong desire of clinicians to be the recipient of evidence-based care, an alarming number of healthcare providers do not consistently implement EBP or follow evidence-based clinical practice guidelines (Melnyk, Grossman, et al., 2012; Vlada et al., 2013). Findings from a survey to assess nurses' readiness to engage in EBP conducted by the Nursing Informatics Expert Panel of the American Academy of Nursing with a nationwide sample of 1,097 randomly selected registered nurses indicated that (a) almost half were not familiar with the term *evidence-based practice*, (b) more than half reported that they did not believe their colleagues use research findings in practice, (c) only 27% of the respondents had been taught how to use electronic databases, (d) most did not search information databases (e.g., Medline and CINAHL) to gather practice information, and (e) those who did search these resources did not believe they had adequate searching skills (Pravikoff, Pierce, & Tanner, 2005). Although a more recent national survey of more than 1,000 randomly selected nurses from the American Nurses Association showed improvement in the valuing of EBP, major barriers that were identified in the earlier survey continue to be reported by nurses, including time, organizational culture, and lack of EBP knowledge and skills (Melnyk, Fineout-Overholt, Gallagher-Ford, & Kaplan, 2012). In addition, nurses in this latest survey reported that, in addition to peer and physician resistance, a major barrier for implementation of EBP is nurse leader/manager resistance (Melnyk, Fineout-overholt, Gallagher-Ford et al., 2012).

On a daily basis, nurse practitioners, nurses, physicians, pharmacists, and other healthcare professionals seek answers to numerous clinical questions (e.g., In postoperative surgical patients, how does relaxation breathing compared to cognitive-behavioral skills building affect anxiety? In adults with dementia, how does a warm bath compared to music therapy improve sleep? In depressed adolescents, how does cognitive-behavioral therapy combined with Prozac compared to Prozac alone reduce depressive symptoms?). An evidence-based approach to care allows healthcare providers to access the best evidence to answer these pressing clinical questions in a timely fashion and to translate that evidence into clinical practice to improve patient care and outcomes.

Without current best evidence, practice is rapidly outdated, often to the detriment of patients. As a classic example, for years, pediatric primary care providers advised parents to place their infants in a prone position while sleeping, with the underlying reasoning that this is the best position to prevent aspiration in the event of vomiting. With evidence indicating that prone positioning increases the risk of sudden infant death syndrome (SIDS), the American Academy of Pediatrics (AAP) released a clinical practice guideline recommending a supine position for infant sleep that resulted in a decline in infant mortality caused by SIDS (AAP, 2000). As a second example, despite strong evidence that the use of beta-blockers following an acute myocardial infarction reduces morbidity and mortality, these medications are considerably underused in older adults in lieu of administering calcium channel blockers (Slutsky, 2003). Further, another recent study indicated adherence to evidence-based guidelines in the treatment of severe acute pancreatitis is poor (Vlada et al., 2013). Therefore, the critical question that all healthcare providers need to ask themselves is: Can we continue to implement practices that are not based on sound evidence and, if so, at what cost (e.g., physical, emotional, and financial) to our patients and their family members?

Even if healthcare professionals answer this question negatively and remain resistant to implementing EBP, the time has come when third-party payers will provide reimbursement only for healthcare practices whose effectiveness is supported by scientific evidence (i.e., pay for performance). Furthermore, hospitals are now being denied payment for patient complications that develop when evidence-based guidelines are not being followed. In addition to pressure from third-party payers, a growing number of patients and family members are seeking the latest evidence posted on websites about the most effective treatments for their health conditions. This is likely to exert even greater pressure on healthcare providers to provide the most up-to-date practices and health-related information. Therefore, despite continued resistance from some clinicians who are skeptical of or who refuse to learn EBP, the EBP movement continues to forge ahead with full steam.

Another important reason that clinicians must include the latest evidence in their daily decision making is that evidence evolves on a continual basis. As a classic example, because of the release of findings from the Prempro arm of the Women's Health Initiative Study that was sponsored by the National Institutes of Health, the clinical trial on hormone replacement therapy (HRT) with Prempro was ceased early—after only 2.5 years—because the overall health risks (e.g., myocardial infarction, venous thromboembolism, and invasive breast cancer) of taking this combined estrogen/progestin HRT were found to be far greater than the benefits (e.g., prevention of osteoporosis and endometrial cancer). Compared with women taking a placebo, women who received Prempro had a 29% greater risk of coronary heart disease, a 41% higher rate of stroke, and a 26% increase in invasive breast cancer (Hendrix, 2002a). For years, practitioners prescribed long-term hormone therapy in the belief that it protected menopausal women from cardiovascular disease because many earlier studies supported this practice. However, there were studies that left some degree of uncertainty and prompted further investigation (i.e., the Prempro study) of what was the best practice for these women. As a result of the Women's Health Initiative Study, practice recommendations changed. The evolution of evidence in this case is a good example of the importance of basing practice on the latest, best evidence available and of engaging in a lifelong learning approach (i.e., EBP) about how to gather, generate, and apply evidence.

Another example is an RCT that was funded by the National Institutes of Health, which compared the use of the medication Metformin, standard care, and lifestyle changes (e.g., activity, diet, and weight loss) to prevent type 2 diabetes in high-risk individuals. The trial was stopped early because the evidence was so strong for the benefits of the lifestyle intervention. The intervention from this trial was translated into practice within a year by the Federally Qualified Health Centers participating in the Health Disparities Collaborative, a national effort to improve health outcomes for all medically underserved individuals (Talsma et al., 2008). This rapid transition of research findings into practice is what needs to become the norm instead of the rarity.

KEY INITIATIVES UNDERWAY TO ADVANCE EVIDENCE-BASED PRACTICE

The gap between the publishing of research evidence and its translation into practice to improve patient care often takes decades (Balas & Boren, 2000; Melnyk & Fineout-Overholt, 2011) and continues to be a major concern for healthcare organizations as well as federal agencies. In order to address this research–practice time gap, major initiatives such as the federal funding of EBP centers and the creation of formal task forces that critically appraise evidence in order to develop screening and management clinical practice guidelines have been established.

The Institute of Medicine's Roundtable on Evidence-Based Medicine helped to transform the manner in which evidence on clinical effectiveness is generated and used to improve healthcare and the health of Americans. The goal set by this Roundtable is that, by the year 2020, 90% of clinical decisions will be supported by accurate, timely, and up-to-date information that is based on the best available evidence (McClellan, McGinnis, Nabel, & Olsen, 2007). The Roundtable convened senior leadership from multiple sectors (e.g., patients, healthcare professionals, third-party payers, policy-makers, and researchers) to determine how evidence can be better generated and applied to improve the effectiveness and efficiency of healthcare in the U.S. (Institute of Medicine of the National Academies, n.d.). It stressed the need for better and timelier evidence concerning which interventions work best, for whom, and under what types of circumstances so that sound clinical decisions can be made. The Roundtable placed its emphasis on three areas:

1. accelerating the progress toward a learning healthcare system, in which evidence is applied and developed as a product of patient care;

2. generating evidence to support which healthcare strategies are most effective and produce the greatest value; and

3. improving public awareness and understanding about the nature of evidence, and its importance for their healthcare (Institute of Medicine of the National Academies, n.d.).

Among other key initiatives to advance EBP is the U.S. Preventive Services Task Force (USPSTF), which is an independent panel of 16 experts in primary care and prevention who systematically review the evidence of effectiveness and develop recommendations for clinical preventive services, including screening, counseling, and preventive medications. Emphasis is placed upon which preventive services should be incorporated by healthcare providers in primary care and for which populations. The USPSTF is sponsored by the Agency for Healthcare Research and Quality (AHRQ), and its recommendations are considered the **gold standard** for clinical preventive services (AHRQ, 2008). EBP centers, funded by AHRQ, conduct systematic reviews for the USPSTF and are the basis upon which it makes its recommendations. The USPSTF reviews the evidence presented by the EBP centers and estimates the magnitude of benefits and harms for each preventive service. Consensus about the net benefit for each preventive service is garnered, and the USPSTF then issues a recommendation for clinical practice. If there is insufficient evidence on a particular topic, the USPSTF recommends a research agenda for primary care for the generation of evidence needed to guide practice (Melnyk, Grossman et al., 2012). The USPSTF (2008) produces an annual *Guide to Clinical Preventive Services* that includes its recommendations on screening (e.g., breast cancer screening, visual screening, colon screening, depression screening), counseling, and preventive medication topics along with clinical considerations for each topic. This guide provides general practitioners, internists, pediatricians, nurse practitioners, nurses, and family practitioners with an authoritative source for evidence to make decisions about the delivery of preventive services in primary care.

An app, the Electronic Preventive Services Selector (ePSS), also is available for free to help healthcare providers implement the USPSTF recommendations at https://itunes.apple.com/us/app/ahrq-epss/id311852560?mt=8

The current *Guide to Clinical Preventive Services* can be downloaded free of charge from **http://www.ahrq.gov/clinic/pocketgd.htm**

Similar to the USPSTF, a similar panel of national experts uses a rigorous systematic review process to determine the best programs and policies to prevent disease in communities. Systemic reviews by this panel answer the following questions: (a) Which program and policy interventions have been proven effective? (b) Are there effective interventions that are right for my community? and (c) What might effective interventions cost and what is the likely return on investment? These evidence-based recommendations for communities are available in a free evidence-based resource entitled *The Guide to Community Preventive Services* (http://www.thecommunityguide.org/index.html).

Another recently funded federal initiative is The Patient-Centered Outcomes Research Institute (PCORI), which is authorized by Congress to conduct research to provide information about the best available evidence to help patients and their healthcare providers make more informed decisions. PCORI's studies are intended to provide patients with a better understanding of the prevention, treatment and care options available, and the science that supports those options. See http://pcori.org/

The Magnet Recognition Program by the American Nurses Credentialing Center is also facilitating the advancement of EBP in hospitals throughout the U.S. The program was started in order to recognize healthcare institutions that promote excellence in nursing practice. Magnet-designated hospitals reflect a high quality of care. The program evaluates quality indicators and standards of nursing practice as defined in the American Nurses Association's (2004) *Scope and Standards for Nurse Administrators*. Conducting research and using EBP are critical for attaining Magnet status (Reigle et al., 2008). Hospitals are appraised on evidence-based quality indicators, which are referred to as Forces of Magnetism. The Magnet program is based on a model with five key components: (1) transformational leadership; (2) structural empowerment; (3) exemplary professional practice; (4) new knowledge, innovation, and improvements, which emphasize new models of care, application of existing evidence, new evidence, and visible contributions to the science of nursing; and (5) empirical quality results, which focus on measuring outcomes to demonstrate the benefits of high-quality care (American Nurses Credentialing Center, 2008).

THE STEPS OF EVIDENCE-BASED PRACTICE

The seven critical steps of EBP are summarized in Box 1.2 and described in more detail in this section.

Step 0: Cultivate a Spirit of Inquiry

Before embarking on the well-known steps of EBP, it is critical to cultivate a **spirit of inquiry** (i.e., a consistently questioning attitude toward practice) so that clinicians are comfortable with and excited about asking questions regarding their patients' care as well as challenging current institutional or unit-based practices. Without a culture and ecosystem or environment that is supportive of a spirit of inquiry and EBP, individual and organizational EBP change efforts are not likely to succeed and sustain (Melnyk, 2012; Rycroft-Malone, 2008). A culture that fosters EBP promotes this spirit of inquiry and makes it visible to clinicians by embedding it in its philosophy and mission of the institution.

Key elements of an EBP culture and environment include:

- A spirit of inquiry where all health professionals are encouraged to question their current practices
- A philosophy, mission, clinical promotion system, and evaluation process that incorporate EBP and EBP competencies
- A cadre of EBP mentors who have in-depth knowledge and skills in EBP, mentor others, and overcome barriers to individual and organizational change
- An infrastructure that provides tools to enhance EBP (e.g., computers for searching at the point of care, access to key databases and librarians, ongoing EBP educational and skills-building sessions, EBP rounds and journal clubs)
- Administrative support and leadership that values and models EBP as well as provides the needed resources to sustain it
- Regular recognition of individuals and groups who consistently implement EBP

Step 1: Formulate the Burning Clinical PICOT Question

In step 1 of EBP, clinical questions are asked in **PICOT format** (i.e., *P*atient population, *I*ntervention or *I*ssue of interest, *C*omparison intervention or group, *O*utcome, and *T*ime frame) to yield the most relevant and best evidence. For example, a well-designed PICOT question would be: In teenagers (the patient population), how does cognitive-behavioral skills building (the experimental intervention)

| **Box 1.2** | The Steps of the EBP Process |

0. Cultivate a spirit of inquiry within an EBP culture and environment.
1. Ask the burning clinical question in PICOT format.
2. Search for and collect the most relevant best evidence.
3. Critically appraise the evidence (i.e., rapid critical appraisal, evaluation, and synthesis).
4. Integrate the best evidence with one's clinical expertise and patient preferences and values in making a practice decision or change.
5. Evaluate outcomes of the practice decision or change based on evidence.
6. Disseminate the outcomes of the EBP decision or change.

compared to yoga (the comparison intervention) affect anxiety (the outcome) after 6 weeks of treatment (the time frame)? When questions are asked in a PICOT format, it results in an effective search that yields the best, relevant information and saves an inordinate amount of time (Stillwell, Fineout-Overholt, Melnyk, & Williamson, 2010). In contrast, an inappropriately formed question (e.g., What is the best type of intervention to use with teenagers who are anxious?) would lead to a search outcome that would likely include hundreds of non-usable abstracts and irrelevant information.

For other clinical questions that are not intervention focused, the meaning of the letter *I* can be "issue of interest" instead of "intervention." An example of a nonintervention PICOT question would be: How do new mothers who have breast-related complications perceive their ability to breast-feed past the first 3 months after their infants' birth? In this question, the population is new breast-feeding mothers, the issue of interest is breast-feeding complications, there is no appropriate comparison group, the outcome is their perception of their ability to continue breast-feeding, and the time is the 3 months after their infants' birth.

When a clinical problem generates multiple clinical questions, priority should be given to those questions with the most important consequences or those that occur most frequently (i.e., those clinical problems that occur in high volume and/or those that carry high risk for negative outcomes to the patient). For example, nurses and physicians on a surgical unit routinely encounter the question: In postoperative adult patients, how does morphine compared to hydromorphone affect pain relief? Another question might be: In postoperative patients, how does daily walking compared to no daily walking prevent pressure sores? The clinical priority would be answering the question of pain relief first, as pain is a daily occurrence in this population, versus putting a priority on seeking an answer to the second question because pressure ulcers rarely occur in postoperative adult patients. Chapter 2 provides more in-depth information about formulating PICOT questions.

Step 2: Search for the Best Evidence

The search for best evidence should first begin by considering the elements of the PICOT question. Each of the **keywords** from the PICOT question should be used to begin the search. The type of study that would provide the best answer to an intervention or treatment question would be systematic reviews or meta-analyses, which are regarded as the strongest level of evidence on which to base treatment decisions (Guyatt & Rennie, 2002). There are different levels of evidence for each kind of PICOT question (see Chapter 2 for more in-depth discussion). Although there are many hierarchies of evidence available in the literature to answer intervention PICOT questions (e.g., Guyatt & Rennie, 2002; Harris et al., 2001), we have chosen to present a hierarchy of evidence to address these questions that encompasses a broad range of evidence, including systematic reviews of qualitative evidence, also referred to as meta-syntheses (Box 1.3).

Box 1.3	Rating System for the Hierarchy of Evidence for Intervention/Treatment Questions

Level I: Evidence from a systematic review or meta-analysis of all relevant RCTs
Level II: Evidence obtained from well-designed RCTs
Level III: Evidence obtained from well-designed controlled trials without randomization
Level IV: Evidence from well-designed case–control and cohort studies
Level V: Evidence from systematic reviews of descriptive and qualitative studies
Level VI: Evidence from single descriptive or qualitative studies
Level VII: Evidence from the opinion of authorities and/or reports of expert committees

Modified from Guyatt, G., & Rennie, D. (2002). Users' guides to the medical literature. Chicago, IL: American Medical Association; Harris, R. P., Hefland, M., Woolf, S. H., Lohr, K. N., Mulrow, C. D., Teutsch, S. M., & Atkins, D. (2001). Current methods of the U.S. Preventive Services Task Force: A review of the process. *American Journal of Preventive Medicine, 20,* 21–35.

A **systematic review** is a summary of evidence on a particular topic, typically conducted by an expert or expert panel that uses a rigorous process for identifying, appraising, and synthesizing studies to answer a specific clinical question. Conclusions are then drawn about the data gathered through this process (e.g., In adult women with arthritis, how does massage compared to pharmacologic agents reduce pain after 2 weeks of treatment? In women, what factors predict heart disease in older adulthood?). Using a rigorous process of well-defined, preset criteria to select studies for inclusion in the review as well as stringent criteria to assess quality, bias is overcome and results are more credible. Population health stands a better chance for improvement when there is effective integration of scientific evidence through systematic reviews that are made available to influence policy-makers' decisions (Sweet & Moynihan, 2007).

Many systematic reviews incorporate quantitative methods to summarize the results from multiple studies. These reviews are called **meta-analyses**. A meta-analysis generates an overall summary statistic that represents the effect of the intervention across multiple studies. Because a meta-analysis can combine the samples of each study included in the review to create one larger study, the summary statistic is more precise than the individual findings from any one of the contributing studies alone (Ciliska, Cullum, & Marks, 2001). Thus, systematic reviews and meta-analyses yield the strongest level of evidence on which to base practice decisions. Caution must be used when searching for systematic reviews as some evidence reviews or narrative reviews may be labeled systematic reviews; however, they lack the rigorous process that is required of true systematic reviews (Fineout-Overholt, O'Mathúna, & Kent, 2008; Newhouse, 2008). Although studies are compared and contrasted in narrative and integrative reviews, a rigorous methodology with explicit criteria for reviewing the studies is often not used, and a summary statistic is not generated. Therefore, conclusions and recommendations by authors of narrative and integrative reviews may be biased.

In addition to the Cochrane Database of Systematic Reviews, the journals *Worldviews on Evidence-Based Nursing* and *Nursing Research* frequently provide systematic reviews to guide nursing practice across many topic areas. More information on *Worldviews* and *Nursing Research* can be found at **http://onlinelibrary.wiley.com/journal/10.1111/ (ISSN)1741-6787** and **http://www.nursingresearchonline.com/**

Evidence-based clinical practice guidelines are specific practice recommendations grouped together that have been derived from a methodologically rigorous review of the best evidence on a specific topic. Guidelines usually do not answer a single specific question, but rather a group of questions about care. As such, they have tremendous potential as tools for clinicians to improve the quality of care, the process of care, and patient outcomes as well as reduce variation in care and unnecessary healthcare expenditures (Fein & Corrato, 2008). The National Guideline Clearinghouse (visit http://www.guideline.gov) provides a mechanism to access detailed information on clinical practice guidelines for healthcare professionals, healthcare systems, and the public. The purpose of the National Guideline Clearinghouse is to further the dissemination and use of the guidelines. Examples of two guidelines housed at the National Guideline Clearinghouse include

◆ *Screening for coronary heart disease with electrocardiography: U.S. Preventive Services Task Force recommendation statement (Revised, 2012)*
◆ *Recommendations for prevention and control of influenza in children, 2011–2012*

It is important to note the latest publication date of clinical practice guidelines, as many guidelines need updating so that the latest evidence is included in making practice recommendations. It is also important to note the process through which the guidelines were created, as there are many guidelines that have been created by professional organizations that have not followed rigorous processes for development (e.g., systematic reviews) (Melnyk, Grossman et al., 2012). Although clinical practice guidelines have tremendous potential to improve the quality of care and outcomes for patients as well as reduce healthcare variation and costs, their success depends on a highly rigorous guideline development process and the incorporation of the latest best evidence. In addition, guideline success depends on implementation by healthcare providers (Fein & Corrato, 2008). More information about guideline development and implementation can be found in Chapter 8.

 A toolkit to enhance the use of clinical practice guidelines is available from the Registered Nurses' Association of Ontario and can be downloaded from its website at **http://ltctoolkit.rnao.ca**

If syntheses (e.g., systematic reviews, meta-analyses) are not available to answer a clinical practice treatment question, the next step should be a search for original RCTs that are found in databases such as MEDLINE or CINAHL (Cumulative Index of Nursing and Allied Health Literature). If RCTs are not available, the search process should then include other types of studies that generate evidence to guide clinical decision making (e.g., nonrandomized, descriptive, or qualitative studies). Chapter 3 contains more detailed information on searching for evidence.

Step 3: Critical Appraisal of Evidence

Step 3 in the EBP process is vital, in that it involves critical appraisal of the evidence obtained from the search process. Although healthcare professionals may view critical appraisal as an exhaustive, time-consuming process, the first steps of critical appraisal can be efficiently accomplished by answering three key questions as part of a rapid critical appraisal process in which studies are evaluated for their validity, reliability, and applicability to answer the posed clinical question (summarized in Box 1.4):

1. **Are the results of the study valid? (Validity)** That is, are the results as close to the truth as possible? Did the researchers conduct the study using the best research methods possible? For example, in intervention trials, it would be important to determine whether the subjects were **randomly assigned** to treatment or control groups and whether they were equal on key characteristics prior to the treatment.
2. **What are the results? (Reliability)** For example, in an intervention trial, this includes (a) whether the intervention worked, (b) how large a treatment effect was obtained, and (c) whether clinicians could expect similar results if they implemented the intervention in their own clinical practice setting (i.e., the preciseness of the intervention effect). In qualitative studies, this includes evaluating whether the research approach fits the purpose of the study, along with evaluating other aspects of the study.
3. **Will the results help me in caring for my patients? (Applicability)** This third critical appraisal question includes asking whether (a) the subjects in the study are similar to the patients for whom care is being delivered, (b) the benefits are greater than the risks of treatment (i.e., potential for harm), (c) the treatment is feasible to implement in the practice setting, and (d) the patient desires the treatment.

The answers to these questions ensure relevance and transferability of the evidence to the specific population for whom the clinician provides care. For example, if a systematic review provided evidence to support the positive effects of using distraction to alleviate pain in postsurgical patients between the ages of 20 and 40 years, those same results may not be relevant for postsurgical patients who are 65 years or older.

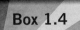 **Box 1.4**   Key General Critical Appraisal Questions

1. Are the results of the study valid? (Validity)
2. What are the results? (Reliability)
3. Will the results help me in caring for my patients? (Applicability)

In addition, even if an RCT supported the effectiveness of a specific intervention with a patient population, careful consideration of the risks and benefits of that intervention must be done before its implementation. When critically appraising a body of evidence to guide practice decisions, it is important not only to conduct rapid critical appraisal of the studies found in the search but also to evaluate all of the studies in the form of an evidence synthesis so that it can be determined whether the findings from the studies are in agreement or disagreement. A synthesis of the studies' findings is important in order to draw a conclusion about the body of evidence on a particular clinical issue. Unit 2 in this book contains in-depth information on critical appraisal of all types of evidence, from expert opinion and qualitative studies to RCTs and systematic reviews.

Step 4: Integrate the Evidence With Clinical Expertise and Patient Preferences to Make the Best Clinical Decision

The next key step in EBP is integrating the best evidence found from the literature with the healthcare provider's expertise and patient preferences and values to implement a decision. Consumers of healthcare services want to participate in the clinical decision-making process, and it is the ethical responsibility of the healthcare provider to involve patients in treatment decisions (Melnyk & Fineout-Overholt, 2006). Even if the evidence from a rigorous search and critical appraisal strongly supports that a certain treatment is beneficial (e.g., HRT to prevent osteoporosis in a very high-risk woman), a discussion with the patient may reveal her intense fear of developing breast cancer while taking HRT or other reasons that the treatment is not acceptable. Moreover, as part of the history-taking process or physical examination, a comorbidity or contraindication may be found that increases the risks of HRT (e.g., prior history of stroke). Therefore, despite compelling evidence to support the benefits of HRT in preventing osteoporosis in high-risk women, a decision against its use may be made after a thorough assessment of the individual patient and a discussion of the risks and benefits of treatment.

Similarly, a clinician's assessment of healthcare resources that are available to implement a treatment decision is a critical part of the EBP decision-making process. For example, on follow-up evaluation, a clinician notes that the first-line treatment of acute otitis media in a 3-year-old patient was not effective. The latest evidence indicates that antibiotic A has greater efficacy than antibiotic B as the second-line treatment of acute otitis media in young children. However, because antibiotic A is far more expensive than antibiotic B and the family of the child does not have prescription insurance coverage, the practitioner and parents together may decide to use the less expensive antibiotic to treat the child's unresolved ear infection.

Step 5: Evaluate the Outcomes of the Practice Change Based on Evidence

Step 5 in EBP is evaluating the evidence-based initiative in terms of how the change affected patient outcomes or how effective the clinical decision was with a particular patient or practice setting. This type of evaluation is essential in determining whether the change based on evidence resulted in the expected outcomes when implemented in the real-world clinical practice setting. Measurement of outcomes, especially "so-what" outcomes that are important to today's healthcare system (e.g., length of stay, readmission rates, patient complications turnover of staff, costs), is important to determine and document the impact of the EBP change on healthcare quality and/or patient outcomes (Melnyk & Morrison-Beedy, 2012). If a change in practice based on evidence did not produce the same findings as demonstrated in rigorous research, clinicians should ask themselves a variety of questions (e.g., Was the intervention administered in exactly the same way that it was delivered in the study? Were the patients in the clinical setting similar to those in the studies?). Chapter 10 contains information on how to evaluate outcomes of practice changes based on evidence. See Figure 1.3 for the key steps of EBP to improve quality healthcare.

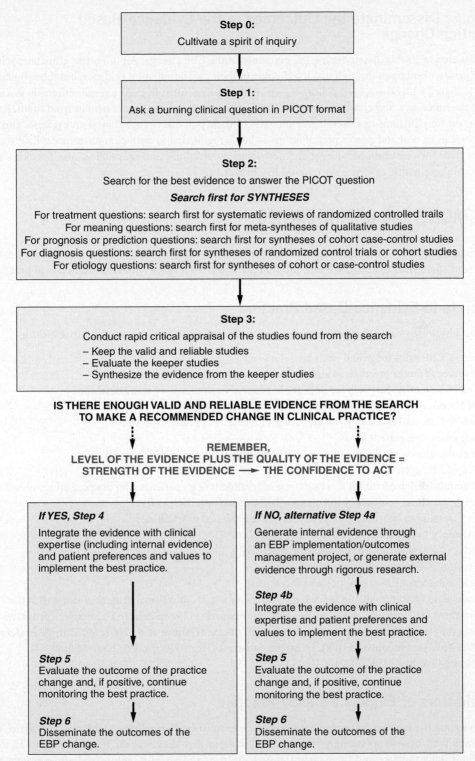

Figure 1.3: Steps of the EBP process leading to high-quality healthcare and best patient outcomes. © Melnyk & Fineout-Overholt, 2009.

Step 6: Disseminate the Outcomes of the Evidence-Based Practice Change

The last step in EBP is disseminating the outcomes of the EBP change. All too often, clinicians achieve many positive outcomes through making changes in their care based upon evidence, but those outcomes are not shared with others, even colleagues within their same institution. As a result, others do not learn about the outcomes, and clinicians as well as patients in other settings do not benefit from them. It is so important for clinicians to disseminate outcomes of their practice changes based on evidence through such venues as oral and poster presentations at local, regional, and national conferences; EBP rounds within their own institutions; journal and newsletter publications; and lay publications. Specific strategies for disseminating evidence are covered in Chapter 18.

OBSTACLES AND OPPORTUNITIES

Healthcare providers are struggling to deliver evidence-based care while managing demanding patient loads and attempting to keep pace with the volume of journal articles related to their clinical practices.

Barriers to Evidence-Based Practice

Nurses, physicians, and other health professionals cite a number of barriers to EBP that include

- Lack of EBP knowledge and skills
- Misperceptions or negative attitudes about research and evidence-based care
- Lack of belief that EBP will result in more positive outcomes than traditional care
- Voluminous amounts of information in professional journals
- Lack of time and resources to search for and critically appraise evidence
- Overwhelming patient loads
- Organizational constraints, such as lack of administrative support or incentives
- Lack of EBP mentors
- Demands from patients for a certain type of treatment (e.g., patients who demand antibiotics for their viral upper respiratory infections when they are not indicated)
- Peer pressure to continue with practices that are steeped in tradition
- Resistance to change
- Lack of consequences for not implementing EBP
- Peer and leader/manager resistance
- Lack of autonomy over practice and incentives
- Inadequate EBP content and behavioral skills building in educational programs along with the continued teaching of how to conduct rigorous research in baccalaureate and master's programs instead of teaching an evidence-based approach to care (Hannes et al., 2007; McGinty & Anderson, 2008; Melnyk, Fineout-Overholt, Feinstein, Sadler, & Green-Hernandez, 2008; Melnyk, Fineout-Overholt et al., 2012).

Facilitators of Evidence-Based Practice

To overcome the barriers in implementing EBP, there must be champions at all levels of practice (i.e., clinicians who believe so strongly in the EBP paradigm that they will do what it takes to facilitate it in their daily practice and their organizational culture) and an EBP culture and environment with mechanisms to support the cause (Fein & Corrato, 2008; Melnyk, 2012). For healthcare professionals to advance the use of EBP, misconceptions about how to implement practice based on the best available evidence need to be corrected, and knowledge and skills in this area must be enhanced. It must also be realized that changing behavior is complex and influenced by multiple factors, including beliefs, attitudes, resources, and the availability of evidence to change practice (McGinty & Anderson, 2008).

Facilitating conditions that have been found to enhance EBP include

- Support and encouragement from leadership/administration that foster a culture for EBP
- Time to critically appraise studies and implement their findings
- Research reports that are clearly written
- Evidence-based practice mentors who have excellent EBP skills as well as knowledge and proficiency in individual and organizational change strategies (Melnyk, 2007; Newhouse, Dearholt, Poe, Pugh, & White, 2007)
- Proper tools to assist with EBP at the point of care (e.g., computers dedicated to EBP; computer-based educational programs; Hart et al., 2008)
- Clinical promotion systems that incorporate EBP competencies for advancement (Newhouse et al., 2007)
- Evidence-based clinical practice policies and procedures (Oman, Duran, & Fink, 2008)
- Journal clubs and EBP rounds

OVERCOMING BARRIERS TO EVIDENCE-BASED PRACTICE

For evidence-based care to become the gold standard of practice, EBP barriers must be overcome. Federal agencies, healthcare organizations and systems, health insurers, policy-makers, and regulatory bodies must advocate for and require its use. Funding agencies must continue to establish translational research (i.e., how findings from research can best be transported into clinical practice to improve care and patient outcomes) as a high priority. Interdisciplinary professionals must work together in a collaborative team spirit to advance EBP. In addition, healthcare organizations must build a culture and environment of EBP and devise clinical promotion ladders that incorporate its use.

As an initial step, barriers and facilitators to EBP along with organizational culture and readiness for system-wide implementation of EBP must be assessed within an organization. Surveys or focus groups should first be conducted with healthcare providers to assess their baseline knowledge, beliefs, and behaviors regarding EBP (Melnyk, Fineout-Overholt, & Mays, 2008). Objective documentation of the status of EBP is essential to demonstrate a change in outcomes, even when there is a subjective consensus of the leaders regarding the state of EBP in their agency. An additional benefit of conducting surveys or focus groups at the outset of any new EBP initiative is that research shows that these strategies also are effective in raising awareness and stimulating a change to evidence-based care (Jolley, 2002).

As part of the survey or focus group, clinicians should be asked about their baseline knowledge of EBP as well as to what extent they believe that implementing EBP will result in improved care and better patient outcomes. This is a critical question because knowledge alone usually does not change behavior. Although healthcare providers must possess basic knowledge and skills about EBP, it is critical for them to believe that EBP will produce better outcomes in order for changes in their practices to occur (Melnyk, Fineout-Overholt, & Mays, 2008).

....
Belief at the beginning of any successful undertaking is the one ingredient that will ensure success.
—William James
....

Healthcare providers who do not believe that EBP results in improved care and patient outcomes need to be exposed to real-case scenarios in which evidence-based care resulted in better outcomes than care that was steeped in traditional practices. For example, many primary care providers continue to prescribe antidepressants as the sole treatment for depressed adolescents when RCTs have indicated that medication in combination with cognitive-behavioral therapy is better than medication alone in reducing depressive symptoms (Brent et al., 2008; Melnyk & Jensen, 2013). In addition, although rigorous systematic reviews of the effectiveness of metered-dose inhalers (MDIs) versus nebulizers in administering bronchodilators to children with asthma have indicated that MDIs are just as effective with fewer side effects, less emergency room time, and less hospital admission, nebulizers continue to be the preferred route of administration in many emergency rooms (Mason, Roberts, Yard, & Partridge, 2008).

Correcting Misperceptions

Because misperceptions about EBP constitute another barrier to its implementation, clarifying these perceptions and teaching the basics of EBP are critical to advancing evidence-based care. For example, many practitioners believe that searching for and critically appraising research articles is an overwhelming, time-consuming process. However, practitioners who have this belief frequently have not had exposure to databases such as the Cochrane Library and the National Guideline Clearinghouse, which can provide them with quick, easily retrievable systematic reviews and evidence-based guidelines to inform their practices. In addition, because many educational curricula continue to teach the in-depth critique of a single study versus time-efficient approaches to the gathering and critical appraisal of a body of empirical studies, clinicians may have the misperception that the EBP process is not feasible in the context of their current practice environments. Therefore, the basics of EBP (e.g., how to formulate a searchable question that will yield the best evidence, how to search for and rapidly critically appraise studies, how to synthesize the evidence) must be taught first in order to create baseline knowledge and skills.

The teaching of EBP can and should be accomplished with multiple strategies, including continuing education conferences with skills-building activities; interactive workshops; and dissemination of educational materials, such as journal articles, textbooks, and informational handouts (Davies, 2002). The best learning method incorporates the teaching of didactic information with interactive behavioral skills. Therefore, creating opportunities for clinicians to practice the skills that they are learning about in didactic sessions is superior to didactic sessions alone.

More detailed information about teaching EBP can be found in Chapters 16 and 17. Moreover, three active EBP centers housed in nursing college and schools in the U.S. can serve as resources for the teaching and implementation of EBP.

1. The Academic Center for Evidence-Based Nursing (ACE) at the University of Texas Health Science Center at San Antonio http://www.acestar.uthscsa.edu/
2. The Center for Transdisciplinary Evidence-based Practice at The Ohio State University http://www.nursing.osu.edu/sections/ctep/
3. The Sara Cole Hirsch Institute for Best Nursing Practice Based on Evidence at Case Western Reserve School of Nursing http://fpb.case.edu/Centers/Hirsh/

Both ACE and CTEP offer national and international EBP continuing education conferences for nurses and other interdisciplinary healthcare professionals, some of which have been funded by AHRQ. Preconference interactive workshops are also held in conjunction with ACE's and CTEP's conferences. The CTEP workshops focus on such topics as the foundations of EBP, implementing and sustaining EBP in healthcare systems, and teaching EBP. The Academic Center for Evidence-Based Nursing preconference workshops have varied in their focus from teaching EBP to systematic reviews. The CTEP also offers EBP mentorship immersion programs for clinicians and faculty along with an online EBP fellowship program. In addition, the Academic Center for Evidence-Based Nursing has a summer institute that offers academic and continuing education opportunities for those interested in learning more about EBP.

Centers for EBP have also been established internationally in countries such as Australia, New Zealand, Hong Kong, Germany, the United Kingdom, and Canada. The mission of most of these centers is to educate clinicians through workshops or formal courses on EBP or to conduct systematic reviews.

Other reputable sources of information about EBP are from abstraction journals, such as *Evidence-Based Medicine, Evidence-Based Nursing, Evidence-Based Mental Health*, and *Evidence-Based Health Policy & Management*. These are other mechanisms through which professionals can find evidence to guide their practice. These journals summarize high-quality studies that have important clinical implications and provide a commentary by an expert in the field. The commentary addresses strengths and limitations of the research reviewed.

Questioning Clinical Practices, Changing Practice With Evidence, and Evaluating Impact

Never stop questioning!
—Susan L. Hendrix

After basic EBP knowledge and skills are attained, it is important for healthcare professionals to ask questions about their current clinical practices (e.g., In neonates, how does the use of pacifiers compared to no pacifiers reduce pain during intrusive procedures? In adult surgical patients, how does heparin compared to antiembolic stockings prevent deep vein thrombosis within the first 2 months after surgery?). Efforts also should be made to prioritize practice problems within an organization or practice setting. One strategy for prioritizing practice problems is described by Rosenfeld et al. (2000), who conducted a survey and focus groups with nurses in a large academic health center to develop specific action plans around particular patient problems. Once high-priority areas were recognized, it was helpful to identify colleagues who had an interest in the same clinical question so that a collaboration could be formed to search for and critically appraise the evidence found. The results of this search and appraisal could be shared with colleagues through a variety of mechanisms (e.g., journal clubs, EBP practice rounds, or informational handouts). If a current practice guideline does not exist, one can be developed and implemented. However, guideline development is a rigorous endeavor, and adequate time must be allotted for the individuals who will complete the work (Davies, 2002). Useful processes for developing and implementing clinical practice guidelines are described in Chapter 8. To complete the EBP process, evaluation of the key outcomes of evidence implementation is essential to determine its effects on the process and outcomes of care.

Change to EBP within an organization or practice requires a clear vision, a written strategic plan, a culture and environment in which EBP is valued and expected, and persistence to make it happen. In addition, the chance to succeed in making a change to EBP and sustaining it will be greater where there is administrative support, encouragement and recognition, EBP mentors, expectations for EBP as contained in clinical promotion criteria and evaluations, inter-professional collaboration, and allocated resources. It is often best to start with a small evidence-based change with high impact, especially when there is skepticism about EBP and elevated levels of stress or complacency within a system, rather than to expect a complete change to EBP to happen within a short period of time. For example, finding a mechanism for routinely discussing evidence-based literature, such as journal clubs or EBP rounds that can spark interest and enhance "buy-in" from colleagues and administration, may be a wonderful start to facilitating a change to EBP.

I don't think there is any other quality so essential to success of any kind as the quality of perseverance. It overcomes almost everything, even nature.
—John D. Rockefeller

Further information about how to infuse EBP into clinical settings is provided in Chapters 9, 11, 13, and 14, which review a variety of specific EBP strategies and implementation models. In addition, Chapter 14 outlines assessment strategies for determining an organization's stage of change. It also provides multiple suggestions for motivating a vision for change to best practice, based primarily on evidence-based organizational change principles. For case examples on how evidence-based care can positively impact patient outcomes, see the section at the end of each unit titled Making EBP Real World: A Success Story. These case examples highlight how EBP can improve both the process and outcomes of patient care. Countless examples similar to these can be found in the literature. Evidence-based success stories stem from first asking compelling clinical questions, which emphasizes the need to cultivate a never-ending spirit of inquiry within our colleagues, our students, and ourselves. These case examples, along with the Women's Health Study, teach a valuable lesson: Never stop questioning because providers need to take evidence-based responsibility for clinical decisions and stay up to date with data that can further support or dramatically change their practice standards (Hendrix, 2002b). Once that spirit of inquiry is cultivated within us and our clinical settings, the journey toward a change to EBP will begin.

We have come to a time when the credibility of the health professions will be judged by which of its practices are based on the best and latest evidence from sound scientific studies in combination with clinical expertise, astute assessment, and respect for patient values and preferences. The chance to influence health policy also rests on the ability to provide policy-makers with the best evidence on which to make important decisions. However, it is important to remember that high-quality healthcare also depends on the ability to deliver EBP within a context of caring, which is the merging of science and art.

For EBP to evolve more quickly, commitments to advancing evidence-based care must be made by individuals, leaders, and organizations. Basic and graduate professional programs must teach the value and processes of EBP, leveled appropriately (see Chapter 15). Doctor of Philosophy (PhD) programs must prepare researchers and leaders who advance EBP through the generation of new knowledge from research to support the most effective practices, as well as the testing of established and new models of EBP implementation so that it can be determined which models are most effective on both staff and patient outcomes. Doctor of Nursing Practice (DNP) programs must prepare advanced practice nurses who are the best translators of evidence generated from research into clinical practice to improve care and outcomes (Melnyk, 2013). Researchers and practitioners across disciplines must also unite to produce evidence on the effectiveness of numerous practices and to answer high-priority, compelling clinical questions, as well as to determine how best those initiatives or interventions can be best translated into practice.

The time has come for practitioners from all healthcare professions to embrace EBP and quickly move from practices that are steeped in tradition or based on outdated policies to those that are supported by sound evidence from well-designed studies. In doing so, patients, healthcare professionals, and healthcare systems will be able to place more confidence in the care that is being delivered and know that the best outcomes for patients and their families are being achieved.

....

Knowing is not enough; We must apply. Willing is not enough; We must do.
—Goethe

....

EBP FAST FACTS

- ◆ Research supports that EBP improves healthcare quality and safety, patient outcomes, and healthcare costs.
- ◆ Evidence-based practice is a problem-solving approach to the delivery of healthcare that integrates the best evidence from research with a clinician's expertise, including internal evidence from patient data, and a patient's preferences and values.
- ◆ The level of evidence plus the quality of that evidence will determine whether a practice change should be made.
- ◆ Without EBP, it often takes decades to translate findings from research into real-world clinical practice settings.
- ◆ There are seven steps to EBP, which should be consistently implemented by clinicians to improve healthcare quality and patient outcomes (see Box 1.2).
- ◆ An EBP culture and environment must be created within an organization for EBP to sustain.

References

Agency for Healthcare Research and Quality. (2008). *U.S. Preventive Services Task Force.* Retrieved July 15, 2008, from http://www.ahrq.gov/clinic/USpstfix.htm

American Academy of Pediatrics. (2000). *Changing concepts of sudden infant death syndrome: Implications for infant sleeping environment and sleep position.* Elk Grove Village, IL: American Academy of Pediatrics.

American Nurses Association. (2004). *Scope and standards for nurse administrators.* Silver Spring, MD: Author.

American Nurses Credentialing Center. (2008). *Magnet model components and sources of evidence.* Silver Spring, MD: American Nurses Credentialing Center.

Balas, E. A., & Boren, S. A. (2000). *Managing clinical knowledge for healthcare improvements.* Germany: Schattauer Publishing Company.

Berwick, D.M., Nolan, T.W., & Whittington, J. (2008). The triple aim: Care, health and cost. *Health Affairs, 27*(3), 759–769.

Brent, D., Emslie, G., Clarke, G., Wagner, K. D., Asarnow, J. R., Keller, M., … Zelazny, J. (2008). Switching to another SSRI or to venlafaxine with or without cognitive behavioral therapy for adolescents with SSRI-resistant depression: The TORDIA randomized controlled trial. *JAMA, 299*(8), 901–913.

Ciliska, D., Cullum, N., & Marks, S. (2001). Evaluation of systematic reviews of treatment or prevention interventions. *Evidence-Based Nursing, 4,* 100–104.

Cochrane, A. L. (1972). *Effectiveness and efficiency: Random reflections on health services.* London: Nuffield Provincial Hospitals Trust.

Davies, B. L. (2002). Sources and models for moving research evidence into clinical practice. *Journal of Obstetric, Gynecologic, and Neonatal Nursing, 31,* 558–562.

Enkin, M. (1992). Current overviews of research evidence from controlled trials in midwifery obstetrics. *Journal of the Society of Obstetricians and Gynecologists of Canada, 9,* 23–33.

Fein, I. A., & Corrato, R. R. (2008). Clinical practice guidelines: Culture eats strategy for breakfast, lunch, and dinner. *Critical Care Medicine, 36*(4), 1360–1361.

Fineout-Overholt, E., O'Mathúna, D. P., & Kent, B. (2008). How systematic reviews can foster evidence-based clinical decisions. *Worldviews on Evidence-Based Nursing, 5*(1), 45–48.

Guyatt, G., & Rennie, D. (2002). *Users' guides to the medical literature.* Chicago, IL: American Medical Association.

Hannes, K., Vandersmissen, J., De Blaeser, L., Peeters, G., Goedhuys, J., & Aertgeerts, B. (2007). Barriers to evidence-based nursing: A focus group study. *Journal of Advanced Nursing, 60*(2), 162–171.

Harris, R. P., Hefland, M., Woolf, S. H., Lohr, K. N., Mulrow, C. D., Teutsch, S. M., & Atkins, D. (2001). Current methods of the U.S. Preventive Services Task Force: A review of the process. *American Journal of Preventive Medicine, 20,* 21–35.

Hart, P., Eaten, L., Buckner, M., Morrow, B. N., Barrett, D. T., Fraser, D. D., … Sharrer, R. L. (2008). Effectiveness of a computer-based educational program on nurses' knowledge, attitude, and skill level related to evidence-based practice. *Worldviews on Evidence-Based Nursing, 5*(2), 78–84.

Hendrix, S. L. (2002a). Implications of the women's health initiative. *A Supplement to the Female Patient, November,* 3–8.

Hendrix, S. L. (2002b). Summarizing the evidence. *A Supplement to the Female Patient, November,* 32–34.

Institute of Medicine of the National Academies. (n.d.). *Roundtable on evidence-based medicine.* Retrieved July 15, 2008, from http://www.iom.edu/CMS/28312/RT-EBM.aspx

Jolley, S. (2002). Raising research awareness: A strategy for nurses. *Nursing Standard, 16*(33), 33–39.

Maljanian, R., Caramanica, L., Taylor, S. K., MacRae, J. B., & Beland, D. K. (2002). Evidence-based nursing practice, Part 2: Building skills through research roundtables. *Journal of Nursing Administration, 32*(2), 85–90.

Mason, N., Roberts, N., Yard, N., & Partridge, M. R. (2008). Nebulisers or spacers for the administration of bronchodilators to those with asthma attending emergency departments? *Respiratory Medicine, 102*(7), 993–998.

McClellan, M. B., McGinnis, M., Nabel, E. G., & Olsen, L. M. (2007). *Evidence-based medicine and the changing nature of healthcare.* Washington, DC: The National Academies Press.

McGinty, J., & Anderson, G. (2008). Predictors of physician compliance with American Heart Association Guidelines for acute myocardial infarction. *Critical Care Nursing Quarterly, 31*(2), 161–172.

Melnyk, B. M. (1994). Coping with unplanned childhood hospitalization: Effects of informational interventions on mothers and children. *Nursing Research, 43,* 50–55.

Melnyk, B. M. (2007). The evidence-based practice mentor: A promising strategy for implementing and sustaining EBP in healthcare systems. *Worldviews on Evidence-Based Nursing, 4*(3), 123–125.

Melnyk, B. M. (2012). Achieving a high-reliability organization through implementation of the ARCC model for systemwide sustainability of evidence-based practice. *Nursing Administration Quarterly, 36*(2), 127–135.

Melnyk, B. M. (2013). Distinguishing the preparation and roles of the PhD and DNP graduate: National implications for academic curricula and healthcare systems. *Journal of Nursing Education, 52*(8), 442–448.

Melnyk, B. M., Alpert-Gillis, L., Feinstein, N. F., Crean, H., Johnson, J., Fairbanks, E., ... Corbo-Richert, B. (2004). Creating opportunities for parent empowerment (COPE): Program effects on the mental health/coping outcomes of critically ill young children and their mothers. *Pediatrics, 113*(6), 597–607 (electronic pages).

Melnyk, B. M., & Feinstein, N. (2009). Reducing hospital expenditures with the COPE (Creating Opportunities for Parent Empowerment) program for parents and premature infants: An analysis of direct healthcare neonatal intensive care unit costs and savings. *Nursing Administrative Quarterly, 33*(1), 32–37.

Melnyk, B. M., Feinstein, N. F., Alpert-Gillis, L., Fairbanks, E., Crean, H. F., Sinkin, R., ... Gross, S. J. (2006). Reducing premature infants' length of stay and improving parents' mental health outcomes with the COPE NICU program: A randomized clinical trial. *Pediatrics, 118*(5), 1414–1427.

Melnyk, B. M., & Fineout-Overholt, E. (2006). Consumer preferences and values as an integral key to evidence-based practice. *Nursing Administration Quarterly, 30*(1), 123–127.

Melnyk, B. M., & Fineout-Overholt, E. (2011). *Evidence-based practice in nursing & healthcare. A guide to best practice.* Philadelphia: Wolters Kluwer/Lippincott Williams & Wilkins.

Melnyk, B. M., Fineout-Overholt, E., Feinstein, N. F., Sadler, L. S., & Green-Hernandez, C. (2008). Nurse practitioner educators' perceived knowledge, beliefs, and teaching strategies. *Journal of Professional Nursing, 24*(1), 7–13.

Melnyk, B. M., Fineout-Overholt, E., Gallagher-Ford, L., & Kaplan, L. (2012). The state of evidence-based practice in US nurses: Critical implications for nurse leaders and educators. *Journal of Nursing Administration, 42*(9), 410–417.

Melnyk, B. M., Fineout-Overholt, E., Giggleman, M., & Cruz, R. (2010). Correlates among cognitive beliefs, EBP implementation, organizational culture, cohesion and job satisfaction in evidence-based practice mentors from a community hospital system. *Nursing Outlook, 58*(6), 301–308.

Melnyk, B. M., Fineout-Overholt, E., & Mays, M. (2008). The evidence-based practice beliefs and implementation scales: Psychometric properties of two new instruments. *Worldviews on Evidence-Based Nursing, 5*(4), 208–216.

Melnyk, B. M., Grossman, D. C., Chou, R., Mabry-Hernandez, I., Nicholson, W., Dewitt, T. G., ... US Preventive Services Task Force. (2012). USPSTF perspective on evidence-based preventive recommendations for children. *Pediatrics, 130*(2), 399–407.

Melnyk, B. M., & Jensen, Z. (2013). *A practical guide to child and adolescent mental health screening, early intervention and health promotion.* New York: NAPNAP.

Melnyk, B. M. & Morrison-Beedy, D. (2012). Setting the stage for intervention research: The "so what," "what exists" and "what's next" factors. In B. M. Melnyk & D. Morrison-Beedy (Eds.), *Designing, conducting, analyzing and funding intervention research. A practical guide for success.* New York, NY: Springer Publishing Company.

Newhouse, R. P. (2008). Evidence synthesis: The good, the bad, and the ugly. *Journal of Nursing Administration, 38*(3), 107–111.

Newhouse, R. P., Dearholt, S., Poe, S., Pugh, L., & White, K. M. (2007). Organizational change strategies for evidence-based practice. *Journal of Nursing Administration, 37*(12), 552–557.

Oman, K. S., Duran, C., & Fink, R. (2008). Evidence-based policy and procedures: An algorithm for success. *Journal of Nursing Administration, 38*(1), 47–51.

Pravikoff, D. S., Tanner, A. & Pierce, S. T. (2005). Evidence-based practice readiness study supported by academy nursing informatics expert panel. *Nursing Outlook, 53*, 49–50.

Reigle, B. S., Stevens, K. R., Belcher, J. V., Huth, M. M., McGuire, E., Mals, D., & Volz, T. (2008). Evidence-based practice and the road to Magnet status. *Journal of Nursing Administration, 38*(2), 97–102.

Rosenfeld, P., Duthie, E., Bier, J., Bowar-Ferres, S., Fulmer, T., Iervolino, L., ... Roncoli, M. (2000). Engaging staff nurses in evidence-based research to identify nursing practice problems and solutions. *Applied Nursing Research, 13*, 197–203.

Rycroft-Malone, J. (2008). Evidence-informed practice: From individual to context. *Journal of Nursing Management, 16*(4), 404–408.

Sackett, D. L., Straus, S. E., Richardson, W. S., Rosenberg, W., & Haynes, R. B. (2000). *Evidence-based medicine: How to practice and teach EBM.* London: Churchill Livingstone.

Shortell, S. M., Rundall, T. G., & Hsu, J. (2007). Improving patient care by linking evidence-based medicine and evidence-based management. *JAMA, 298*(6), 673–676.

Slutsky, J. (2003). *Clinical guidelines: Building blocks for effective chronic illness care. Slide presentation at web-assisted audio conference, "Causes of and Potential Solutions to the High Cost of Healthcare."* Rockville, MD: AHRQ.

Stillwell, S. B., Fineout-Overholt, E., Melnyk, B. M., & Williamson, K. M. (2010). Evidence-based practice, step by step: Asking the clinical question: A key step in evidence-based practice. *American Journal of Nursing, 110*(3), 58–61.

Strout, T. D. (2005). Curiosity and reflective thinking: Renewal of the spirit. In Clinical scholars at the bedside: An EBP mentorship model for today [Electronic version]. *Excellence in Nursing Knowledge.* Indianapolis, IN: Sigma Theta Tau International.

Sweet, M., & Moynihan, R. (2007). *Improving population health: The uses of systematic reviews*. New York, NY: Milbank Memorial Fund.

Talsma, A., Grady, P. A., Feetham, S., Heinrich, J., & Steinwachs, D. M. (2008). The perfect storm: Patient safety and nursing shortages within the context of health policy and evidence-based practice. *Nursing Research, 57*(1 Suppl), S15–S21.

The Cochrane Collaboration. (2001). *The Cochrane Collaboration—Informational leaflets*. Retrieved January 22, 2002, from http://www.cochrane.org/cochrane/cc-broch.htm#cc

U.S. Preventive Services Task Force. (2008). *Guide to clinical preventive services, 2008*. Rockville, MD: Agency for Healthcare Research and Quality. Available at http://www.ahrq.gov/clinic/pocketgd.htm

Vlada, A. C., Schmit, B., Perry, A., Trevino, J. G., Behms, K. E., & Hughes, S. J. (2013). Failure to follow evidence-based best practice guidelines in the treatment of severe acute pancreatitis. *HPB (Oxford), 15*(10), 822–827.

Williams, D. O. (2004). Treatment delayed is treatment denied. *Circulation, 109*, 1806–1808.

Chapter 2
Asking Compelling, Clinical Questions

Ellen Fineout-Overholt and Susan B. Stillwell

A prudent question is one-half of wisdom.

—Francis Bacon

Seeking and using health information has changed over the past several decades, not only for healthcare professionals (e.g., the Internet; electronic health records with evidence-based clinical decision support systems; Ferran-Ferrer, Minguillón, & Pérez-Montoro, 2013) but also for patients, who are motivated to access health information via the web (Shaikh & Shaikh, 2012). Over the past few years, significant strides have been made to make digital health information even more readily available, thus leading to informed clinical decisions that are evidence based (Institute of Medicine, 2011). In addition, growing complexity of patient illness has required practitioners to become increasingly more proficient at obtaining information they need *when* they need it. Access to reliable information is necessary to this endeavor (Kosteniuk, Morgan, & D'Arcy, 2013) as well as clinicians definitively identifying what they want to know and what they need to access (Fineout-Overholt & Johnston, 2005; Melnyk, Fineout-Overholt, Stillwell, & Williamson, 2010). Additionally, resources (e.g., computers, databases, and libraries) have to be in place to ensure that practitioners can retrieve needed information so that they can perform the best patient care possible. Not all practice environments have or allow unrestricted access to these resources. There are many variables that influence whether a practitioner has the capacity to gather information quickly (e.g., financial ability to purchase a computer, availability of Internet service providers); however, every clinician must be able to articulate the clinical issue in such a way that it maximizes the information obtained with the least amount of time investment. Hence, the first step in getting to the right information is to determine the "real" clinical issue and describe it in an answerable fashion, that is, a searchable, answerable question. However, skill level in formulating an answerable question can be a barrier to getting the best evidence to apply to practice (Gray, 2010; Green & Ruff, 2005; Rice, 2010). This chapter provides practitioners with strategies to hone skills in formulating a clinical question to clarify the clinical issue and to minimize the time spent in searching for relevant, valid evidence to answer it.

A NEEDLE IN A HAYSTACK: FINDING THE RIGHT INFORMATION AT THE RIGHT TIME

The key to successful patient care for any healthcare professional is to stay informed and as up to date as possible on the latest best practices. *External* pressure to be up to date on clinical issues increasingly comes from patients, employers, certifying organizations, insurers, and healthcare reform (Centers for Medicare & Medicaid Services, 2006; Greiner & Knebel, 2003; Rice, 2010). The clinician's personal desire to provide the best, most up-to-date care possible along with expectations from healthcare consumers that practice will be based on the latest and best evidence fosters evidence-based practice (EBP). However, the desire to gather the right information in the right way at the right time is not sufficient. Practical, lifelong learning skills (e.g., asking focused questions, learning to search efficiently) are required to negotiate the information-rich environment that every clinician encounters. With the amount of information that clinicians have at their disposal today, finding the right information at the right time is much like weeding through the haystack to find the proverbial needle. If one has any hope of finding the needle, there must be some sense of the needle's characteristics (i.e., a clear understanding of what is the clinical issue). Clinical questions arise from inquiry. Clinicians notice that there is something curious in the clinical environment that they then formulate into a question, or a patient or layperson may foster the question. Whoever initiates the question, it is important to carefully consider how to ask it so that it is reasonable to answer. Formulating the clinical question is much like identifying the characteristics of the needle. Question components guide the searching strategies undertaken to find answers. Yet, clinicians are not always equipped to formulate searchable questions (Melnyk, Fineout-Overholt, Feinstein, Sadler & Green-Hernandez, 2008), which often can result in irrelevant results and inefficient use of clinicians' time (Rice, 2010). Once the needle's characteristics are well understood (i.e., the PICOT question), knowing how to sift through the haystack (i.e., the evidence) becomes easier (see Chapter 3 for searching strategies).

Huang, Lin, and Demnar-Fushman (2006) found in a study examining the utility of asking clinical questions in **PICOT format** (i.e., *P*: population of interest; *I*: intervention or issue of interest; *C*: comparison of interest; *O*: outcome expected; and *T*: time for the intervention to achieve the outcome) that when clinicians asked clinical questions for their patient's clinical issues, their format almost always fell short of addressing all the aspects needed to clearly identify the clinical issue. Two of 59 questions contained an intervention (*I*) and outcome (*O*), but no other components (*P*, *C*, or *T*), although these aspects were appropriate. Currie et al. (2003) indicated that approximately two thirds of clinicians' questions are either not pursued or answers are not found even though pursued. However, if properly formulated, the question could lead to a more effective search. Price and Christenson (2013) concur with these researchers' findings, indicating that getting the question right determines the success of the entire EBP process. In addition, in a randomized controlled trial (RCT) examining the effect of a consulting service that provides up-to-date information to clinicians, Mulvaney et al. (2008) found that such a knowledge broker improves the use of evidence and subsequent care and outcomes. However, without having a well-built question to communicate what clinicians genuinely want to know, efforts to search for or provide appraised evidence will likely be less than profitable. Hoogendam, de Vries Robbé, and Overbeke (2012) determined that the **PICO(T) format** was not helpful in guiding efficient searches; however, their report did not indicate how they measured proficiency of participants in writing PICOT questions or how they were taught about their formulation. Learning how to properly formulate a clinical question is essential to a successful search and to effectively begin the EBP process.

The Haystack: Too Much Information

Although there is a plethora of information available and increasingly new modalities to access it, news of clinical advances can diffuse rather slowly through the literature. Additionally, only a small percentage of clinicians access and use the information in a timely fashion (Cobban, Edgington, & Clovis, 2008; Estabrooks, O'Leary, Ricker, & Humphrey, 2003; MacIntosh-Murray & Choo, 2005; McCloskey, 2008; Melnyk, Fineout-Overholt, Gallagher-Ford, & Kaplan, 2012; Pravikoff, Tanner, & Pierce, 2005). Clinicians are challenged with the task of effectively, proactively, and rapidly sifting through the haystack of scientific information to find the right needle full of the best applicable information for a patient or practice. Scott, Estabrooks, Allen, and Pollock (2008) found that uncertainty in clinicians' work environment promoted a disregard for research as relevant to practice. In a 2012 study of over 1,000 nurses, Melnyk and colleagues reinforced these researchers' finding with their participants indicating that lack of access to information was one of the top five deterrents to implementing EBP in daily practice. To reduce uncertainty and facilitate getting the right information at the right time, EBP emphasizes first asking a well-built question, then searching the literature for an answer to the question. This will better prepare all clinicians to actively discuss the best available evidence with colleagues and their patients.

The EBP process focuses on incorporating good information-seeking habits into a daily routine. Pravikoff et al. (2005) indicated that not all nurses were engaged in daily information seeking, supporting the notion that, in a busy clinical setting, there is seldom time to seek out information, which was reinforced in the study by Melnyk et al. (2012). The purchase of a good medical text and regular perusal of the top journals in a specialty were once considered adequate for keeping up with new information, but scientific information is expanding faster than anyone could have foreseen. The result is that significant clinical advances occur so rapidly that they can easily be overlooked. Reading every issue of the top three or four journals in a particular field from cover to cover does not guarantee that clinicians' professional and clinical knowledge is current. With the increase in biomedical knowledge (especially information about clinical advances), it is clear that the traditional notion of "keeping up with the literature" is no longer practical. Before the knowledge explosion as we know it today, Haynes (1993) indicated that a clinician would have to read 17–19 journal articles a day, 365 days a year to remain current. This compels every clinician to move toward an emphasis on more proactive information-seeking skills, starting with formulating an answerable, patient-specific question.

Digitization and the Internet have improved accessibility to information, regardless of space and time; however, these innovations have not resolved the issue of finding the right information at the right time. It is important to become friendly with and proficient at utilizing information technology, including the Internet and other electronic information resources, which means that clinicians must be skilled in using a computer. Access to computers at the point of care is also essential. The information needed cannot be obtained if the clinician has to leave the unit or seek an office to locate a computer to retrieve evidence. Proficient use and access to computers are essential to EBP and best practice. In addition, other barriers described by nurses and other healthcare professionals to getting the right information at the right time include (a) access to information, (b) a low comfort level with library and search techniques, (c) access to electronic resources, and (d) a lack of time to search for the best evidence (Melnyk & Fineout-Overholt, 2002; Melnyk, Fineout-Overholt, Gallagher-Ford & Kaplan, 2012; Pravikoff et al., 2005; Sackett, Straus, Richardson, Rosenberg, & Haynes, 2000). Skills in clinical question formulation lead to an efficient search process. Other barriers to finding the necessary evidence to improve patient outcomes can be adequately addressed through clinicians first learning to ask a searchable, answerable question.

....
The important thing is not to stop questioning.
—Albert Einstein
....

ASKING SEARCHABLE, ANSWERABLE QUESTIONS

Finding the right information in a timely way amidst an overwhelming amount of information is imperative. The first step to accomplish this goal is to formulate the clinical issue into a searchable, answerable question. It is important to distinguish between the two types of questions that clinicians might ask—background questions and foreground questions.

Background Questions

Background questions are those that need to be answered as a foundation for asking the searchable, answerable **foreground question** (Fineout-Overholt & Johnston, 2005; Stillwell, Fineout-Overholt, Melnyk, & Williamson, 2010; Straus, Richardson, Glasziou, et al., 2005). Background questions are those that ask for general information about a clinical issue. This type of question usually has two components: the starting place of the question (e.g., what, where, when, why, and how) and the outcome of interest (e.g., the clinical diagnosis). An example of a background question is: How does the drug acetaminophen work to affect fever? The answer to this question can be found in a drug pharmacokinetics text. Another example of a background question is: How does hemodynamics differ with positioning? This answer can be found in textbooks as well.

Often, background questions are far broader in scope than foreground questions. Clinicians often want to know the best method to prevent a clinically undesirable outcome. For example: What is the best method to prevent pressure ulcers during hospitalization? This question will lead to a foreground question, but background knowledge is necessary before the foreground question can be asked. In this example, the clinician must know what methods of pressure ulcer prevention are being used. Generally, this information comes from knowledge of what is being used in clinicians' practices and what viable alternatives are available to improve patient outcomes, or it may come from descriptive research, such as survey research. Once the methods most supported are identified, clinicians can formulate the foreground question, compare the two most effective methods of pressure ulcer prevention, and ask: Which one will work best in my population? If a clinician does not realize that the question at hand is a background question, time may be lost in searching for an answer in the wrong haystack (e.g., electronic evidence databases versus a textbook).

Foreground Questions

Foreground questions are those that can be answered from scientific evidence about diagnosing, treating, or assisting patients in understanding their prognosis. These questions focus on specific knowledge. In the first two background question examples, the subsequent foreground questions could be: In children, how does acetaminophen compared to ibuprofen affect fever? And: In patients with acute respiratory distress syndrome, how does the prone position compared to the supine position affect hemodynamic readings? The first question builds on the background knowledge of how acetaminophen works but can be answered only by a study that compares the two listed medications. The second question requires the knowledge of how positioning changes hemodynamics (i.e., the background question), but the two types of positioning must be compared in a specific population of patients to answer it. The foreground question generated from the third background question example could be: In patients at risk for pressure ulcers, how do pressure mattresses compare to pressure overlays affect the incidence of pressure ulcers? The answer provided by the evidence would indicate whether pressure mattresses or overlays are more effective in preventing pressure ulcers. The most effective method will become the standard of care. Recognizing the difference between the two types of questions is the challenge.

Straus, Richardson, Glasziou, and Haynes (2011) stated that a novice may need to ask primarily background questions. As one gains experience, the background knowledge grows, and the focus changes to foreground questions. Although background questions are essential and must be asked, it is the foreground questions that are the searchable, answerable questions and the focus of this chapter.

Clinical Inquiry and Uncertainty in Generating Clinical Questions

Where clinical questions come from (i.e., their origin) is an important consideration. On a daily basis, most clinicians encounter situations for which they do not have all the information they need (i.e., uncertainty) to care for their patients as they would like (Kahmi, 2011; Nelson, 2011; Scott et al., 2008). The role of uncertainty is to spawn **clinical inquiry**. Clinical inquiry can be defined as a process in which clinicians gather data together using narrowly defined clinical parameters to appraise the available choices of treatment for the purpose of finding the most appropriate choice of action (Horowitz, Singer, Makuch, & Viscoli, 1996).

Clinical inquiry must be cultivated in the work environment. To foster clinical inquiry, one must have a level of comfort with uncertainty. Uncertainty is the inability to predict what an experience will mean or what outcome will occur when encountering ambiguity (Cranley, Doran, Tourangeau, Kushniruk, & Nagle, 2009; Scott et al., 2008). Although uncertainty may be uncomfortable, uncertainty is imperative to good practice (Kamil, 2011) and to developing focused foreground questions (Nelson, 2011).

Clinicians live in a rather uncertain world. What works for one patient may not work for another patient or the same patient in a different setting. The latest product on the market claims that it is the solution to wound healing, but is it? Collaborating partners in caring for complex patients have their own ways of providing care. Formulating clinical questions in a structured, specific way, such as with PICOT formatting, assists the clinician in finding the right evidence to answer those questions and to decrease uncertainty. This approach to asking clinical questions facilitates a well-constructed search.

Price and Christenson (2013) indicated that the PICOT question is the key to the entire EBP process. Success with PICOT question formation fosters further clinical inquiry.

Clinical circumstances, such as interpretation of patient assessment data (e.g., clinical findings from a physical examination or laboratory data), a desire to determine the most likely cause of the patient's problem among the many it could be (i.e., differential diagnosis), or simply wanting to improve one's clinical skills in a specific area, can prompt five types of questions. The five types of foreground questions are

1. intervention questions that ask what intervention most effectively leads to an outcome;
2. prognosis/prediction questions that ask what indicators are most predictive of or carry the most associated risk for an outcome;
3. diagnosis questions that ask what mechanism or test most accurately diagnoses an outcome;
4. etiology questions that ask to what extent a factor, process, or condition is highly associated with an outcome, usually an undesirable outcome; and
5. meaning questions that ask how an experience influences an outcome, the scope of a phenomenon, or perhaps the influence of culture on health care.

Whatever the reason for the question, the components of the question need to be considered and formulated carefully to efficiently find relevant evidence to answer the question.

Posing the Question Using PICOT

Focused foreground questions are essential to judiciously finding the right evidence to answer them (Schardt, Adams, Owens, Keitz, & Fontelo, 2007). Foreground questions should be posed using PICOT format. Thoughtful consideration of each PICOT component can provide a clearly articulated question. Using a consistent approach to writing the PICOT question assists the clinician to systematically identify the clinical issue (Stillwell et al., 2010). Table 2.1 provides a quick overview of the PICOT question components. Well-built, focused clinical questions drive the subsequent steps of the EBP process (O'Connor, Green, & Higgins, 2011).

Table 2.1   PICOT: Components of an Answerable, Searchable Question

PICOT	
Patient population/disease	The patient population or disease of interest, for example: • Age • Gender • Ethnicity • With certain disorder (e.g., hepatitis)
Intervention or issue of interest	The intervention or range of interventions of interest, for example: • Therapy • Exposure to disease • Prognostic factor A • Risk behavior (e.g., smoking)

Comparison intervention or issue of interest	What you want to compare the intervention or issue against, for example:
	• Alternative therapy, placebo, or no intervention/therapy
	• No disease
	• Prognostic factor B
	• Absence of risk factor (e.g., nonsmoking)
Outcome	Outcome of interest, for example:
	• Outcome expected from therapy (e.g., pressure ulcers)
	• Risk of disease
	• Accuracy of diagnosis
	• Rate of occurrence of adverse outcome (e.g., death)
Time	The time involved to demonstrate an outcome, for example:
	• The time it takes for the intervention to achieve the outcome
	• The time over which populations are observed for the outcome (e.g., quality of life) to occur, given a certain condition (e.g., prostate cancer)

The patient population (*P*) may seem easy to identify. However, without explicit description of who the population is, the clinician can get off on the wrong foot in searching. The *Cochrane Handbook for Systematic Reviews of Interventions* (O'Connor et al., 2011) suggests careful consideration of the patient and the setting of interest. Limiting the population to those in a certain age group or other special subgroups (e.g., young adult females with lung cancer) is a good idea if there is a valid reason for doing so. Arbitrary designations for the patient population will not assist the clinician in retrieving the most relevant evidence.

The intervention or issue of interest (*I*) may include but is not limited to any exposure, treatment, diagnostic test, or predictor/prognostic factor, or it may be an issue that the clinician is interested in, such as fibromyalgia or a new diagnosis of cancer. The more specifically the intervention or issue of interest is defined, the more focused the search will be.

The comparison (*C*) needs special consideration as it is sometimes appropriate to include in a question and at other times does not need to be included. If the "*I*" is an intervention, the comparison can be a true control, such as a placebo, or another treatment, which is sometimes the usual standard of care. For example, a clinician wants to ask the question, in disabled, older adult patients (*P*), how does the use of level-access showers (*I*) compared to bed bathing (*C*) affect patient hygiene (*O*)? The intervention of interest is level-access showers, and the comparison is the usual care of bed bathing. In a meaning question, the "*I*" is an issue of interest. For example, a meaning question may be: How do parents (*P*) with children who have been newly diagnosed with cancer (*I*) perceive their parent role (*O*) within the first month after diagnosis (*T*)? In this question, there is no appropriate comparison to the issue of interest, and "*C*" is not found in the question.

The outcome (*O*) in the intervention example above is patient hygiene and the outcome of the meaning question above is the parental role. Specifically identifying the outcome (*O*) in a question enables the searcher to find evidence that examined the same outcome variable, although the variable may be measured in various ways.

In some questions, there may be more than one outcome of interest found in a study, but all of these outcomes fall under one umbrella. For example, the question may be: In preschool-age children, how does a flavored electrolyte drink compared to water alone affect symptoms of dry mouth, tachycardia, fever, and irritability? Instead of formulating the question this way, it may be better to use the umbrella term *dehydration* for all these symptoms that are listed; however, clinicians would keep in mind each of the outcomes that they desired to see change. The question would then be: In preschool-age children, how does a flavored electrolyte drink compared to water alone affect dehydration (e.g., dry mouth, tachycardia, fever, irritability)? Specifying the outcome will assist the clinician in focusing the search for relevant evidence.

Considering whether or not a time frame (*T*) is associated with the outcome is also part of asking a PICOT question. For example: In family members who have a relative undergoing cardiopulmonary resuscitation (*P*), how does presence during the resuscitation (*I*) compared to no presence (*C*) affect family anxiety (*O*) during the resuscitation period (*T*)? In the intervention example given earlier, there is no specific time identified for bathing or showering to achieve patient hygiene because it is immediately upon completion of these interventions. Although this is understood, it would not be incorrect to use "immediately after intervention" as the "*T*" for this question. However, for the meaning question example, it would be important to consider that the first month after diagnosis may be a critical time for parental role to be actualized for this population; therefore, it is essential to include a specific time in the question. To answer this meaning question, studies would be sought that collected data to evaluate parental role for a period of a month after diagnosis; studies with evaluation of parental role within less than 1 month would not be acceptable to answer the question. Time (*T*) and comparison (*C*) are not always appropriate for every question; however, population (*P*), intervention or issue of interest (*I*), and outcome (*O*) must always be present.

Three Ps of Proficient Questioning: Practice, Practice, Practice

The best way to become proficient in formulating searchable, answerable questions is to practice. This section includes five clinical scenarios that offer you the opportunity to practice formulating a searchable, answerable question. Read each scenario and try to formulate the question using the appropriate template for the type of question required (see Box 2.1 for a list of all question types and templates). Templates are guides and are designed to assist you in formulating each question and ensure that components of the question (i.e., PICOT) are not missed. Once you craft your questions, read the paragraphs that follow for help in determining the success of your question formulation.

Box 2.1	Question Templates for Asking PICOT Questions

Intervention
In _____ (*P*), how does _____ (*I*) compared to _____ (*C*) affect _____ (*O*) within _____ (*T*)?

Prognosis/Prediction
In _____ (*P*), how does _____ (*I*) compared to _____ (*C*) influence/predict _____ (*O*) over _____ (*T*)?

Diagnosis or Diagnostic Test
In _____ (*P*) are/is _____ (*I*) compared to _____ (*C*) more accurate in diagnosing _____ (*O*)?

Etiology
Are _____ (*P*), who have _____ (*I*) compared to those without _____ (*C*) at _____ risk for/of _____ (*O*) over _____ (*T*)?

Meaning
How do _____ (*P*) with _____ (*I*) perceive _____ (*O*) during _____ (*T*)?

Clinical Scenario 2.1

Intervention Example

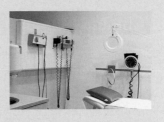

Glenda, a 45-year-old Caucasian woman, 5′6″ weighing 250 pounds, presented to her primary care provider (PCP) with complaints of malaise and "pressure in her head." The physical examination revealed that she was hypertensive (blood pressure 160/98).

Her PCP discussed putting her on an angiotensin-converting-enzyme (ACE) inhibitor for 6 months; however, Glenda wanted to try exercise and dietary alterations to promote weight loss as she had heard on the evening news that for every 10 pounds of weight loss, blood pressure was reduced by 5 mm Hg. You want to make sure that Glenda is safe, so you inform her that you are going to do a little homework to find out the latest evidence.

Clinical Scenario 2.1 is about an intervention. Given the suggested format below for an intervention question, fill in the blanks with information from the clinical scenario.

In _____ (**P**), how does _____ (**I**) compared to _____ (**C**) affect _____ (**O**) within _____ (**T**)?

_____

Remember that a well-formulated question is the key to a successful search. The question could be: In middle-aged Caucasian obese females (BME > 30 kg/m^2) (**P**), how does weight loss (**I**) compared to daily administration of ACE inhibitors (**C**) affect blood pressure (**O**) over 6 months (**T**)? A more general background question might read: In overweight women, what is the best method for reducing high blood pressure? Background knowledge would be necessary to know what effective methods were available for reducing blood pressure in this population. Intervention questions are about what clinicians do; therefore, it is important to be able to determine the *best* intervention to achieve an outcome. Once the question has been answered with confidence (i.e., well-done studies agree on the best intervention to achieve the outcome), the next step would be establishing that intervention as the standard of care.

In this example, the patient's concern has to do with her motivation to lose weight and her prior experience with a family member who did not have successful results with ACE inhibitors. She is asking the clinician to provide her with information about how successful she can be with what she prefers to engage versus what may be the accepted practice. Therefore, the "**I**" is the intervention that is most desired (e.g., weight loss) and the "**C**" is often what is the current standard of care or usual practice (e.g., ACE inhibitors).

The evidence to answer this type of question requires substantiated cause-and-effect relationships. The research design that best provides this information is an RCT. An RCT is defined as having three key elements: (1) an intervention or treatment group that receives the intervention, (2) a comparison or control group that has a comparison or control intervention, and (3) random assignment to either group (i.e., assignment of patients to either the experimental or comparison/control group by using chance, such as a flip of a coin). The groups are evaluated on whether or not an expected outcome is achieved. In the example, we would look for studies that had a defined sample (e.g., overweight women) with common characteristics (e.g., BME > 30 kg/m^2) that were randomly assigned to the intervention (i.e., weight loss program) and the comparison (i.e., daily ACE inhibitors) and evaluated if the desired outcome was achieved (i.e., reduction in

(continued)

Clinical Scenario 2.1 (continued)

blood pressure values). Ideally, we would search for a synthesis, or compilation of studies, that compared how daily administration of ACE inhibitors and weight loss affected blood pressure. A synthesis of these RCTs is considered Level 1 evidence to answer this type of question.

Keep in mind that syntheses are always Level 1 evidence, no matter what kind of question you may be asking. Table 2.2 provides an example of a clinical question and the levels of evidence that would answer that question. The Level 1 evidence is listed first. If well done (i.e., bias is minimized through rigorous research methods), this is the type of research that would give us the valid information that would enable us to have confidence in using the findings in clinical practice. With each drop in the level of evidence and/or drop in quality of the evidence, the confidence in using the findings drops. Hence, it is always the best idea to search for Level 1 evidence first. It is important to keep in mind that the type of clinical question will indicate the study design that would be synthesized as Level 1 evidence for that question (e.g., intervention questions require a synthesis of RCTs as Level 1 evidence).

In the desired RCTs found in our example, the blood pressure values for both groups would be evaluated after they received either what is called the experimental intervention (i.e., weight loss) or the comparison intervention (i.e., ACE inhibitor). It is important that the evaluation of the outcome occurs after the individuals receive the intervention; otherwise, causality is in question. Also, it is important that all other factors (e.g., age, comorbidities, genetic predisposition to high blood pressure) that may influence the outcome (e.g., blood pressure) be considered and key factors be accounted for (i.e., data collected about these factors, also called controlled for—one of the reasons for the name randomized *controlled* trial). When these factors are controlled for, and if it is shown that weight loss does just as good a job as or a better job than ACE inhibitors in reducing blood pressure, clinicians can confidently prescribe weight loss as an alternative intervention to manage high blood pressure for those who prefer it.

Table 2.2 **Examples of Different Types of Clinical Questions Using PICOT Format and the Hierarchy Indicating the Best Type of Evidence to Answer the Given Question**

Questions	Levels of Evidence to Answer This Type of Question
Intervention: In patients living in a long-term care facility who are at risk for pressure ulcers (*P*), how does a pressure ulcer prevention program (*I*) compared to the standard of care (e.g., turning every 2 hours) (*C*) affect signs of emerging pressure ulcers (*O*)?	1. Systematic review/meta-analysis (i.e., synthesis) of randomized controlled trials (RCTs) 2. RCTs 3. Non-RCTs 4. Cohort study or case–control studies 5. Meta-synthesis of qualitative or descriptive studies
OR	6. Qualitative or descriptive single studies
Diagnosis or diagnostic test: In patients with suspected deep vein thrombosis (*P*) is d-dimer assay (*I*) compared to ultrasound (*C*) more accurate in diagnosing deep vein thrombosis (*O*)?	7. Expert opinion

Prognosis/prediction: In patients who have a family history of obesity (BME > 30 kg/m²) (***P***), how does dietary carbohydrate intake (***I***) predict healthy weight maintenance (BME < 25 kg/m²) (***O***) over 6 mo (***T***)?

OR

Etiology: Are fair-skinned women (***P***) who have prolonged unprotected UV ray exposure (>1 h) (***I***) compared to darker-skinned women without prolonged unprotected UV ray exposure (***C***) at increased risk of melanoma (***O***)?

Meaning: How do middle-aged women (***P***) with fibromyalgia (***I***) perceive loss of motor function (***O***)?

1. Synthesis of cohort study or case–control studies
2. Single cohort study or case–control studies
3. Meta-synthesis of qualitative or descriptive studies
4. Single qualitative or descriptive studies
5. Expert opinion

1. Meta-synthesis of qualitative studies
2. Single qualitative studies
3. Synthesis of descriptive studies
4. Single descriptive studies
5. Expert opinion

Clinical Scenario 2.2

Prognosis Example

Shawn is a 63-year-old man who has been diagnosed with prostate cancer. He has been married to his wife, Laura, for 40 years and is greatly concerned about his ability to be physically intimate with her should he pursue surgery as a treatment method. He mentions

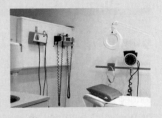

that he is most interested in living his life fully with as much normality as he can for as long as he can. He comes to you requesting information about whether or not having surgery will be the best plan for him.

Clinical Scenario 2.2 concerns prognosis. The following is the format for prognosis questions. Fill in the blanks with information from the clinical scenario.

In _____ (***P***), how does _____ (***I***) compared to _____(***C***) influence or predict _____ (***O***)?

The prognosis/prediction question for this example could read: In older adult patients with prostate cancer (***P***), how does choosing to undergo surgery (***I***) compared to choosing not to undergo surgery (***C***) influence lifespan and quality of life (***O***)? Prognosis/prediction questions assist the clinician in estimating a patient's clinical course across time. This type of question allows inference about the likelihood that certain outcomes will occur. Clinical issues that may lend themselves to be addressed with a prognosis/predictive question could involve patients' choices and future outcomes. The difference in prognosis or prediction questions and intervention questions is that the conditions (***I*** and ***C***) cannot be randomized due to the potential for harm (i.e., this would be unethical). In these questions, the "***I***" is the issue of interest (e.g., choice to have surgery) and the "***C***" is the counter to the issue of interest (i.e., the negative case) (e.g., choice not to have surgery).

(continued)

Clinical Scenario 2.2   (*continued*)

This is an important distinction for prognosis/predictive questions. Therefore, an answer to a prognosis/prediction question would require a study that examined a group of people with an identified condition (e.g., prostate cancer) that self-selected the issue of interest and counter issue (e.g., choosing surgery or not) and were observed over time to evaluate the likelihood of an outcome occurring or not. In the example, we would look for studies that followed a group of older adults with prostate cancer (a *cohort*) who chose to have surgery (*I*) or not (*C*) and then evaluated how the older adults reported their quality of life and how long they lived. This is called a *cohort study*. A single cohort study (i.e., not a synthesis) would be considered Level 2 evidence for prognosis/prediction questions (see Table 2.2). If there was a synthesis of cohort studies examining older adults with prostate cancer who had surgery or not and their relationship between their choice and their quality of life and how long they lived, then that would be Level 1 evidence. Case–control studies, further discussed in Chapter 5, are another study design that can be used to answer this kind of question.

Clinical Scenario 2.3

Diagnosis Example

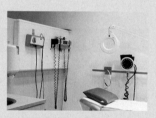

Brenda, a 33-year-old woman who is gravida 2 para 1 and in her sixth month of pregnancy, tells you that her right side is extremely tender and she feels rather nauseous, which is new for her. Her pregnancy is high risk and she has been on bed rest for 3 weeks to prevent preterm labor. You are suspicious of appendicitis, but upon ultrasound you are not sure. You consider getting a computed tomography (CT) scan to confirm your diagnosis; however, you are not sure of the benefits of its accuracy in comparison with its risks.

Clinical Scenario 2.3 is about diagnosis. Given the format for diagnosis questions, fill in the blanks with information from the clinical scenario.

In _____ (*P*) are/is _____ (*I*) compared to _____ (*C*) more accurate in diagnosing _____ (*O*)?

Questions about diagnosis are focused on determining how reliable a test is for clinical practice (i.e., the test will correctly identify the outcome each time it is used). Risks of the test, likelihood of misdiagnosis of a high-risk outcome, and cost of the test are some of the considerations for how such questions would be answered. Benefit of the test to patients is the overall goal of these kinds of questions. In the clinical example, the question could read: In pregnant women with suspected appendicitis (*P*), is ultrasound followed by CT (*I*) compared to ultrasound alone (*C*) more accurate in diagnosing appendicitis (*O*)?

The evidence to answer this type of question requires substantiated certainty that the diagnostic test will reliably provide a true positive (i.e., the outcome does exist and is diagnosed accurately by the test) or true negative (i.e., the outcome does not exist and is accurately diagnosed as such by the test). The research design that best provides this information (Level 1) is a synthesis of RCTs; this design involves groups that randomly (i.e., by chance) receive a diagnostic test and a comparison diagnostic test and are then evaluated based on the presence or absence of the expected outcome (i.e., diagnosis). Sometimes, however, it would be unethical to randomly assign a diagnostic test to some patients and not others because the risks for the diagnostic test or misdiagnosing the outcome are too high. In this situation, the best research design to answer the question would be a cohort study (see Table 2.2). This is the case in the example, as a CT scan would expose the fetus to considerable radiation. Therefore, we would look for studies that had a defined sample of pregnant women with suspected appendicitis who had the intervention (e.g., ultrasound with follow-up CT) or the comparison (e.g., ultrasound alone) as a matter of course. Most commonly, the comparison is the test considered to be the gold standard for the industry. The outcome would be determined by actual documentation of appendicitis in these women.

Clinical Scenario 2.4

Etiology Example

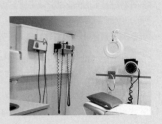

A 40-year-old woman with asthma comes to the clinic for her regularly scheduled physical examination. She has been listening to the radio and an expert indicated that beta-adrenergic agonists may help her manage her asthma. However, she is apprehensive since she had a friend who died after using this type of medication. She would like to know if this is likely to happen to her if she includes this medication in her asthma management plan.

Clinical Scenario 2.4 is an etiology scenario. Given the format for etiology questions, fill in the blanks with information from the clinical scenario.

Are _____ (**P**), who have _____ (**I**) compared to those without _____ (**C**) at _____ risk for/of _____ (**O**) over _____ (**T**)?

_____

In the example, the question could read: Are adult patients with asthma (**P**), who have beta-adrenergic agonists prescribed (**I**) compared to those without prescribed beta-adrenergic agonists (**C**) at increased risk for death (**O**)? In this case, the "**T**" would not be necessary.

Etiology questions help clinicians to address potential causality and harm. These questions can be answered by cohort or case–control studies that indicate what outcomes may occur in groups over time; however, it requires an abundance of longitudinal studies that consistently demonstrate these relationships for there to be confidence in the potential causality. For example, it is commonly believed that smoking causes lung cancer; however, there are people who defy this conviction by smoking all of their adult lives and yet have no diagnosis of lung cancer. Potential causality from case–control or cohort studies must be carefully interpreted. RCTs are the only design that establishes with confidence a cause-and-effect relationship between an intervention and an outcome. However, the difference in an etiology/harm question and an intervention question is that the conditions (*I* and *C*) cannot be randomized due to the potential for harm—which is often the reason for the question.

In the clinical scenario, potential for harm is the focus of the question. It is important to know the harm associated with an intervention. As always, it is preferable to search for syntheses first. To answer this type of question, the desired research design would be cohort or case–control studies in

(continued)

Clinical Scenario 2.4 (*continued*)

which groups of people with a given condition (e.g., asthma) were prescribed either the intervention of interest (i.e., *I*, e.g., beta-adrenergic agonists) or the comparison of interest (e.g., no beta-adrenergic agonists) by their healthcare providers and were observed over time to evaluate the likelihood of a suspected outcome (e.g., death) (see Table 2.2). In the example, we would look for studies that followed a group of adults with asthma that took beta-adrenergic agonists and adults with asthma that did not take beta-adrenergic agonists and determine the number of deaths in each group.

Clinical Scenario 2.5

Meaning Example

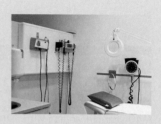

You are caring for Jim, a 68-year-old man, who has been in the intensive care unit (ICU) for 3 weeks. He is now extremely tenuous and could go into cardiac arrest at any moment. Your patient is ventilated; he is on several intravenously infused medications to maximize his cardiac function, and has continuous monitoring of heart rhythm, blood pressure, and oxygenation. Jim's daughter is very involved in her dad's care. She asks many questions about how his care is progressing and wants to be informed of any nuances. She raises a question about whether or not she would be welcome to be present should her dad go into cardiac arrest and have to be resuscitated. The healthcare team is adamantly opposed to her presence. She tells you it would be important to her dad and to her to be together during such a difficult situation, and she cannot understand the perspective of the healthcare team. To facilitate the best outcomes for your patient and his daughter, you determine to find evidence to inform decision making.

Clinical Scenario 2.5 is about meaning. The following is the format for meaning questions. Fill in the blanks with the information from the clinical scenario.

How do _____ (*P*) with _____ (*I*) perceive _____ (*O*) during _____ (*T*)?

_____

In this example, the question could read: How do family members (*P*) with a critically ill relative who is being resuscitated (*I*) perceive healthcare providers' responses to their presence (*O*) during the resuscitation (*T*)?

This question is remarkably different from the others that we have discussed. You may notice that a "*C*" is not present in this question. It is not required as there is no comparison to their family members' resuscitation (*I*) in regard to the healthcare providers' perceptions (*O*). The emphasis is on how the family members experience the resuscitation of their family member, particularly in regard to the healthcare providers' responses to their presence during the resuscitation. The best evidence to answer this type of question would be qualitative research. A synthesis of qualitative studies would be considered Level 1 evidence (see Table 2.2). Research designs such as an RCT, cohort, or case–control would not be able to provide the data required to answer this question. Therefore, we would look for qualitative studies, such as a phenomenological study (see Chapter 6), to answer this question.

All of these examples and templates are intended for practice. There may be various ways in which to ask a certain type of question; however, all the appropriate components must be present in the question. Clinicians, whether novice or expert, who use the PICOT format to construct a clinical question ensure that no component is missed and increase the likelihood that the question is answered (Huang et al., 2006; Price & Christenson, 2013). Consider your clinical scenario and try to identify the PICOT components specifically. Then formulate the question in a complete sentence. Carefully consider which template may work for the clinical situation driving your question, as it is not wise to try to form cookie-cutter questions (e.g., applying the intervention template to every situation), because some important component(s) most assuredly will be missed.

When evaluating the appropriateness of each question that arises from clinical issues you are most concerned about, consider the harm, cost, feasibility, and availability of the intervention, diagnostic test, or condition, as these can preclude the ability to apply the evidence to clinical practice. These issues also influence ethical considerations for implementing the best evidence (see Chapter 22).

WHY WORK HARD AT FORMULATING THE CLINICAL QUESTION?

It is important to note that a clinical question is not a research question. These questions differ primarily in their approach to the evidence in the literature. Research questions are directional and bring with them a sense of expectation of what will be found in the literature. Researchers have a vested interest in the intervention working. In contrast, clinical questions come with no expectations of what will be found in the literature. These questions ask about how an issue or intervention affects an outcome, which could be positive, negative, or neutral (i.e., no effect). Furthermore, well-formulated clinical questions guide clinicians away from searches that result in incorrect, too much, or irrelevant information.

Honing one's skills in formulating a well-built question can provide confidence that the clinical issue is well defined and the search will be more successful and timely. From their vast experience, Straus et al. (2011) identified that formulating a searchable, answerable question is the most difficult step in the EBP process. However, they also suggested several other benefits from constructing good questions, including clearly communicating patient information with colleagues, helping learners more clearly understand content taught, and furthering the initiative to become better clinicians through the positive experience of asking a good question, finding the best evidence, and making a difference. Various web-based resources can assist you in further understanding of how to formulate a searchable, answerable question.

 Find web-based information on formulating searchable, answerable questions at the following websites:

◆ Centre for Evidence-Based Medicine University of Toronto: **http://www.cebm.utoronto .ca/practise/formulate**
◆ The Center for Transdisciplinary Evidence-Based Practice at The Ohio State University: **http://nursing.osu.edu/sections/ctep/ctep-5-day-evidence-based-practice-immersion .html**
  ◆ Studentbmj.com: International Medical Student's Journal: **http://www.studentbmj.com/ back_issues/0902/education/313.html**

Formulating a well-built question is worth the time and effort it takes. It is step 1—and as some have said, the most challenging—toward providing evidence-based care to patients (Schlosser, Koul, & Costello, 2007; Straus et al., 2011).

....

Reason and free inquiry are the only effectual agents against error.
—Thomas Jefferson

....

EBP FAST FACTS

- ◆ **Background questions** contain a starting place of the question (e.g., what, where, when, why, and how) and an outcome of interest. These questions ask for general information about the clinical issue.
- ◆ **Foreground questions** focus on specific information and contain the PICOT elements, for example, "*P*": population of interest, "*I*": intervention or area of interest, "*C*": comparison intervention or area of interest, "*O*": outcome of interest, and "*T*": time it takes for the intervention or issue to achieve the outcome.
- ◆ Essential elements of a PICOT question include a "*P*," "*I*," and "*O*." The "*C*" or "*T*" may not always be appropriate for a clinical question. The "*C*," comparison, in PICOT questions is generally the usual standard of care.
- ◆ The purpose of the PICOT question is to hone the clinical issue and to guide the search of databases to locate the evidence to answer the clinical question.
- ◆ The type of PICOT question guides the desired research design search to best answer the question.

References

Centers for Medicare & Medicaid Services. (2006). *Post-acute care reform plan*. Retrieved July 8, 2008, from http://www.cms.hhs.gov/SNFPPS/Downloads/pac_reform_plan_2006.pdf

Cobban, S. J., Edgington, E. M., & Clovis, J. B. (2008). Moving research knowledge into dental hygiene practice. *Journal of Dental Hygiene, 82,* 21.

Cranley, L., Doran, D., Tourangeau, A., Kushniruk, A., & Nagle, L. (2009). Nurses' uncertainty in decision-making: A literature review. *Worldviews on Evidence-Based Nursing, 6*(1), 3–15.

Currie, L. M., Graham, M., Allen, M., Bakken, S., Patel, V., & Cimino, J. J. (2003). Clinical information needs in context: An observational study of clinicians while using a clinical information system. *American Medical Informatics Association Annual Symposium Proceedings/AMIA Symposium,* 190–194.

Estabrooks, C., O'Leary, K., Ricker, K., & Humphrey, C. (2003). The internet and access to evidence: How are nurses positioned? *Journal of Advanced Nursing, 42,* 73–81.

Ferran-Ferrer, N., Minguillón, J., & Pérez-Montoro, M. (2013). Key factors in the transfer of information-related competencies between academic, workplace, and daily life contexts. *Journal of the American Society for Information Science and Technology, 64*(6), 1112–1121.

Fineout-Overholt, E., & Johnston, L. (2005). Teaching EBP: Asking searchable, answerable clinical questions. *Worldviews on Evidence-Based Nursing, 2*(3), 157–160.

Gray, G. E. (2010). Asking answerable questions. In C. B. Taylor (Ed.), *How to practice evidence-based psychiatry: Basic principles and case studies* (pp. 17–19). Arlington, VA: American Psychiatric Publishing.

Green, M. L., & Ruff, T. R. (2005). Why do residents fail to answer their clinical questions? A qualitative study of barriers to practicing evidence-based medicine. *Academic Medicine, 80,* 176–182.

Greiner, A., & Knebel, E. (2003). *Health professions education: A bridge to quality*. Washington, DC: Institute of Medicine & National Academy Press.

Haynes, R. (1993). Where's the meat in clinical journals? *ACP Journal Club, 119,* A23–A24.

Hoogendam, A., de Vries Robbé, P., & Overbeke, A. J. (2012). Comparing patient characteristics, type of intervention, control, and outcome (PICO) queries with unguided searching: A randomized controlled crossover trial. *Journal Medical Library Association, 100*(2), 120–126.

Horowitz, R., Singer, B., Makuch, R., & Viscoli, C. (1996). Can treatment that is helpful on average be harmful to some patients? A study of the conflicting information needs of clinical inquiry and drug regulation. *Journal of Clinical Epidemiology, 49,* 395–400.

Huang, X., Lin, J., & Demnar-Fushman, D. (2006). Evaluation of PICO as a knowledge representation for clinical questions. *American Medical Informatics Association Proceedings,* 359–363.

Institute of Medicine. (2011). *Digital infrastructure for the learning health system: The foundation for continuous improvement in health and health care—Workshop series summary*. Washington, DC; The National Academies Press.

Kamhi. A. (2011). Balancing certainty and uncertainty in clinical practice. *Language, Speech and Hearing Services in Schools, 42,* 88–93.

Kosteniuk, J. G., Morgan, D. G., & D'Arcy, C. K. (2013). Use and perceptions of information among family physicians: Sources considered accessible, relevant, and reliable. *Journal of the Medical Library Association, 101*(1), 32–37.

MacIntosh-Murray, A., & Choo, C. W. (2005). Information behavior in the context of improving patient safety. *Journal of the American Society of Information Science & Technology, 56,* 1332–1345.

McCloskey, D. J. (2008). Nurses' perceptions of research utilization in a corporate health care system. *Journal of Nursing Scholarship, 40,* 39–45.

Melnyk, B. M., & Fineout-Overholt, E. (2002). Putting research into practice. *Reflections on Nursing Leadership, 28*(2), 22–25, 45.

Melnyk, B. M., Fineout-Overholt, E., Gallagher-Ford, L., & Kaplan, L. (2012). The state of evidence-based practice in US nurses: Critical implications for nurse leaders and educators. *Journal of Nursing Administration, 42*(9), 410–417.

Melnyk, B. M., Fineout-Overholt, E., Stillwell, S. B., & Williamson, K. M. (2010). Evidence-based practice: step by step: The seven steps of evidence-based practice. *American Journal of Nursing, 110*(1), 51–53.

Mulvaney, S., Bickman, L., Giuse, N., Lambert, E., Sathe, N., & Jerome, R. (2008). A randomized effectiveness trial of a clinical informatics consult service: Impact on evidence-based decision-making and knowledge implementation. *Journal of the American Medical Informatics Association, 15,* 203–211.

Nelson, N. (2011). Questions About certainty and uncertainty in clinical practice. *Language, Speech and Hearing Services in Schools, 42,* 81–87.

O'Connor, D., Green, S., & Higgins, J. (2011). *Handbook for systematic reviews of interventions;* Chapter 5 Defining the review question and developing criteria for including studies. Retrieved August 26, 2013, from http://handbook.cochrane.org

Pravikoff, D., Tanner, A., & Pierce, S. (2005). Readiness of U.S. nurses for evidence-based practice. *American Journal of Nursing, 105,* 40–50.

Price, C. & Christenson, R. (2013). Ask the right question: A critical step for practicing evidence-based laboratory medicine. *Annals of Clinical Biochemistry, 50*(4), 306–314.

Rice, M. J. (2010) Evidence-based practice problems: Form and Focus. *Journal of the American Psychiatric Nurses Association, 16*(5), 307–314.

Sackett, D. L., Straus, S. E., Richardson, W. S., Rosenberg, W., & Haynes, R. B. (2000). *Evidence-based medicine: How to practice and teach EBM.* Edinburgh: Churchill Livingston.

Schardt, C., Adams, M. B., Owens, T., Keitz, S., & Fontelo, P. (2007). Utilization of the PICO framework to improve searching PubMed for clinical questions. *BMC Medical Informatics and Decision Making, 7*(16), 1–6.

Schlosser, R., Koul, R., & Costello, J. (2007). Asking well-built questions for evidence-based practice in augmentative and alternative communication. *Journal of Communication Disorders, 40,* 225–238.

Scott, S., Estabrooks, C., Allen, M., & Pollock, C. (2008). A context of uncertainty: How context shapes nurses' research utilization behaviors. *Qualitative Health Research, 18,* 347–357.

Shaikh, M. H., & Shaikh, M. A. (2012). A prelude stride in praxis & usages of healthcare informatics. *International Journal of Computer Sciences Issues, 9*(6), 85–89.

Stillwell, S. B., Fineout-Overholt, E., Melnyk, B. M., & Williamson, K. (2010). Evidence-based practice, step by step: Asking the clinical question: A key step in evidence-based practice. *American Journal of Nursing, 110*(3), 58–61.

Straus, S. E., Richardson, W. S., Glasziou, P., & Haynes, R. B. (2005). *Evidence-based medicine: How to teach and practice EBM* (3rd ed.). Edinburgh: Churchill Livingston.

Straus, S. E., Richardson, W. S., Glasziou, P., & Haynes, R. B. (2011). *Evidence-based medicine: How to teach and practice it* (4th ed.). Edinburgh: Churchill Livingston.

Chapter 3
Finding Relevant Evidence to Answer Clinical Questions

Tami A. Hartzell, Ellen Fineout-Overholt, Sheila Hofstetter, and Elizabeth Ponder

Searching is half the fun: life is much more manageable when thought of as a scavenger hunt as opposed to a surprise party.

—Jimmy Buffett

In any clinical setting, there are numerous information resources (e.g., journal literature, practice-based data, patient information, textbooks) to answer a variety of questions about how to improve patient care or update clinical procedures and protocols. For example, a patient in the medical intensive care unit (ICU) is being treated for refractory atrial fibrillation without much success. After exhausting a range of treatment options, a collaborating clinician remembers hearing that clonidine, a well-known antihypertensive medication, has been used successfully elsewhere and wonders whether it would work with this patient. With the delays in treatment success, the patient has become more concerned as treatments fail. The patient asks whether listening to music might reduce her anxiety. While other members of the healthcare team find out about the use of clonidine, you notice that the patient always has an iTouch at her side and wonder if music may help. With this inquiry, you formulate the following PICOT question to address the patient's anxiety: In adult ICU patients undergoing difficult treatment plans (P), how does listening to music (I) compared to quiet (C) affect anxiety (O) while clinicians consider a plan of care (T)? Using the PICOT question as a guide, you conduct a systematic, efficient, and thorough search for evidence to answer the clinical question (Stillwell, Fineout-Overholt, Melnyk, & Williamson, 2010). You find several recent **randomized controlled trials** (RCTs) that report positive benefits of music therapy, including reducing anxiety. You share the evidence with the healthcare team, ask the music therapist for additional music, and initiate music therapy for your patient.

Finding the right information to answer a given question often requires using more than one resource (Table 3.1). When clinicians explore only one resource and find no evidence, they may incorrectly conclude that there is no evidence to answer their question. For example, if clinicians are searching for RCTs to answer a clinical question and only search a web-based search engine (e.g., Yahoo! or Google), they may not find any recent trials. Instead, they may find a case study that is presented in a journal. The temptation may be to ignore the case study and, since no RCTs can be found, conclude that there is no evidence to answer the question; however, to discard a case study would be inadvisable. While the case study may not be able to answer the clinical question fully or indicate a practice change, a case study can inform clinical care. When searching for answers to clinical questions, all evidence should be considered; however, caution must be used when deciding about practice changes that are based solely on evidence that may have substantial bias (e.g., case studies). Table 3.2 contains categories of clinical questions and the corresponding type of evidence that would best answer the question.

Since it is important to quickly find answers to clinical questions, searching for evidence that has already been appraised for the quality of the study methodology and the reliability of its findings is desirable. This pre-appraised literature can range from integrative **systematic reviews** to **meta-analyses** (see Chapter 5) and **meta-syntheses** (see Chapter 6) to synopses of single studies. By using pre-appraised literature, clinicians can cut down on the amount of time they spend in determining whether they have reliable information, which reduces the time between finding suitable evidence and providing appropriate care. Systematic reviews are the type of pre-appraised syntheses of studies that form the heart of evidence-based practice (EBP) (Stevens, 2001). However, there is often not enough quality research to

Table 3.1   **Sources of External Evidence**

Resource	Free or Subscription Required[a]	Document Types	Search Method
ACP Journal Club	Individual (ACP members receive web access as benefit of membership)	Synopses of single studies and reviews Expert clinical commentary FT	KW KP
BMJ Clinical Evidence	Individual	Summaries of evidence with recommendations Clinical commentary FT	KW Disease condition (e.g., diabetes) Category (e.g., gastrointestinal)
CINAHL		Journal article citation and abstract of primary studies, reviews, and synopses FT (with FT subscription)	KW KP TI SH (i.e., CINAHL Headings)
Cochrane Databases	Individual Free website access with restricted content Pay-per-view options	CDSR—FT systematic review DARE—citation and abstract summary of systematic review not completed by Cochrane CENTRAL—citation and abstract of clinical trials *Note:* Three of the five Cochrane databases are described here	KW SH (i.e., MeSH if you know the heading)
Dynamed		Summaries of evidence FT	KW Topic
EMBASE		Journal article citation and abstract of primary studies, reviews, and synopses Conference coverage	KW KP TI SH
Essential Evidence Plus	Individual	POEMs (Patient Oriented Evidence that Matters) synopses of evidence Clinical practice guidelines and guideline summaries FT	KW Topic
Evidence-Based Nursing	Individual	Synopses of single studies and reviews Expert clinical commentary FT	KW KP

(continued)

Table 3.1   **Sources of External Evidence** (continued)

Resource	Free or Subscription Required[a]	Document Types	Search Method
Joanna Briggs Institute EBP Database		Evidence-based recommended practices Evidence summaries Best Practice Information Sheets Systematic reviews Consumer Information Sheets	KW KP TI SH (MeSH) HW FT
MEDLINE	Free via PubMed Available as subscription from other vendors	Journal article citation and abstract of primary studies, reviews, and synopses FT (varies on PubMed; other vendors with FT subscription)	KW KP TI SH Clinical queries
National Guideline Clearinghouse	Free	Clinical practice guidelines Syntheses of selected guidelines FT	KW Category
National Institute for Health and Care Excellence	Free	Guidelines Standards Guidance Technology appraisals	KW KP TI Categories
PIER Physician's Information and Education Resource	Individual	Summaries of evidence for point-of-care issues in internal medicine FT	KW Topic Organ system
PsycINFO		Journal article citation and abstract of primary studies, reviews, and synopses FT (with FT subscription)	KW KP TI SH
Registered Nurses Association of Ontario	Free	Guidelines	KW Topic
Scottish Intercollegiate Guideline Network	Free	Guidelines	SH
Trip	Free	Journal article citation and abstract of primary studies, reviews, and synopses Guidelines Linkout to FT	KW KP TI Pico search builder Proximity
UpToDate	Individual[a]	Summaries of evidence	KW KP

[a]Institutional subscription is implied; separate listing if individual subscription available.
SH, subject heading; FT, full text; KW, keyword; KP, key phrase; TI, title.

Table 3.2   **Types of Studies to Answer Clinical Questions**

Examples of Clinical Questions	Best Evidence Design to Answer the Question
In patients with acute respiratory distress syndrome, how effective is prone positioning on weaning parameters compared to supine positioning?	Systematic reviews and meta-analyses Single RCTs
In pregnant women, how does prenatal care compared to no prenatal care affect a healthy delivery and a healthy baby?	Well-controlled, nonrandomized experimental studies
How do spouses with a loved one who has Alzheimer's disease perceive their ability to provide care?	Qualitative
What are the coping mechanisms of parents who have lost a child to AIDS?	Descriptive studies
What are the national standards for the prevention and management of wandering in patients with Alzheimer's disease who live in long-term care facilities?	Evidence-based clinical practice guidelines
	Opinion reports of experts and professional organizations

address all clinical issues with a synthesis; sometimes there may only be a handful of primary studies that exist. To facilitate finding this small number of studies, clinicians need to search more than one source when looking for evidence to answer a clinical question.

Systematic reviews (not a narrative review, see Chapter 5), primary studies, and guidelines may contain the answers—the question is how to efficiently and effectively find them. Often the process may seem like finding the proverbial needle in a haystack. In order to ensure that reliable evidence is found, clinicians must move beyond beginning search techniques (e.g., using only one resource instead of multiple resources) toward using available tools (resources and techniques) that help them find the needle in the haystack, the most essential evidence to answer their clinical question.

TOOLS FOR FINDING THE NEEDLE IN THE HAYSTACK

Given the consistent need for current information in health care, frequently updated databases that hold the latest studies reported in journals are the best choices for finding relevant evidence to answer compelling clinical questions (see Clinical Scenario 3.1).

The use of a standardized format, such as PICOT (Richardson, Wilson, Nishikawa, & Hayword, 1995) (see Chapter 2), to guide and clarify the important elements of the question is an essential first step toward finding the right information to answer the question. Generally, PICOT questions are expressed in everyday clinical terminology. Often, in searching for the best evidence to answer a PICOT question, clinicians encounter databases that have their own specific database language that helps eliminate or minimize searching errors such as spelling or missing a synonym of a keyword. Learning how to properly navigate through different databases will increase a clinician's ability to find relevant evidence. Novices to this type of searching are wise to consult a healthcare librarian who can assist them in this process. Many hospitals employ healthcare librarians who are able to help clinicians find their needle in the haystack either through one-on-one training or by searching on behalf of the clinician. If you are in an academic setting, you may have many healthcare librarians available for a consult.

Clinical Scenario 3.1

A 45-year-old mother of three has been newly diagnosed with asthma. She tells you that her friend who has asthma takes a medication that is long acting. She wonders why the one she has been prescribed is short acting. She asks you about whether there is support for Salbutamol, the short-acting medication she has been prescribed. You search the literature to help her with the answer. The PICOT question for the search is as follows: In adults with asthma (P), how does Salbutamol (I) compared to Salmeterol, a long-acting medication (C), affect asthma symptoms (O)?

Upon searching the Cochrane Database of Systematic Reviews (CDSR), you find two systematic reviews that recommend the longer-acting medication for patients who need therapy beyond an inhaled corticosteroid (Tee et al., 2007; Walters, Walters, & Gibson, 2002). In an effort to find more information, you decide to search the National Guideline Clearinghouse (NGC) to look for an evidence-based guideline on asthma management since longer-acting medications are used for asthma maintenance. The search reveals 11 guidelines for asthma management. One guideline is helpful to you as a healthcare provider (Scottish Intercollegiate Guidelines Network, 2012) because it contains a recommendation that addresses your clinical question. On the basis of the two systematic reviews (Level I evidence) that support the recommendation in the guideline, you discuss the plan of care and the patient's concerns with the healthcare team.

After formulating a well-built PICOT question, your next step is to determine the source most likely to contain the best evidence. Clinicians need **peer-reviewed** research to answer their questions, and most often the source of that evidence will be a database of published studies. These databases contain references to the healthcare literature, including conference proceedings, books, or journal publications. Although these databases may be discipline specific (i.e., allied health, nursing, medicine, psychology), clinicians need to choose the right databases that will help them get to the evidence that can answer their question. Knowing how to systematically search these databases is essential to a quick, successful retrieval of answers to a clinical question.

There are additional resources that offer busy clinicians best available evidence. While these resources save time, clinicians need to know how the appraisal process was performed to ensure that the pre-appraised evidence is trustworthy. For example, one resource a clinician might use would be a critically appraised topic (CAT). While some CATs are well done and reliable, others may not be. One example of a CAT would be the evidence posted by BestBets (**B**est **E**vidence **T**opics): http://bestbets. org/. Knowledge of the PICOT question, the best type of evidence to answer it, and **critical appraisal** are essential for clinicians to know which of these resources (i.e., the haystack) is the best to search for the desired information.

Tool 1: Sources of External Evidence—Description of the Haystack

Answers to clinical questions may be found in a variety of resources, ranging from practice data found in the healthcare record (i.e., **internal evidence**) to research articles in journals (i.e., **external evidence**), all of which have been moving from print to digital format. The transition of evidence to electronic format has enabled the clinician to gain more immediate access to external evidence through the use of point-of-care tools which integrate almost seamlessly into the electronic medical. These resources contain timely clinical topic summaries and are designed to provide both background information and the best available external evidence to improve patient care.

Types of Evidence Resources

Textbooks. Healthcare professionals can consult a good textbook to refresh or gain new knowledge. This background information may be all that is necessary in certain situations (see Chapter 2). At other times consulting a textbook may help the clinician to better understand the context for the PICOT question they are asking. Once clinicians have gathered their background information, they can begin to formulate their PICOT questions. When clinicians are trying to answer a specific question that requires more specialized knowledge (i.e., PICOT), textbooks are insufficient because the information may be incomplete or out of date. At this point, clinicians need to seek out research studies to answer their foreground (PICOT) questions (see Chapter 2).

Journals. A journal article is the typical source from which to find an answer to a foreground question (see Chapter 2), if one is to be found. The journal literature is an entry point; the place where all new ideas first enter the healthcare knowledge base and where clinicians first go to look for answers to their clinical questions. Journals contain a number of publication types, including systematic reviews, article synopses, research articles, narrative reviews, discussion articles, news items, editorials, and letters to the editor (listed from most to least useful in answering foreground questions).

Consolidated Resources and Beyond. Haynes (2007) characterized and organized this new genre of information resources in a pyramid framework (Figure 3.1). A simplified version of this pyramid is presented in Figure 3.1. The pyramid is a hierarchy where the most valid, least biased evidence is at the top. The pyramid's base contains original research articles and forms the foundation upon which the rest of the pyramid is built. Databases where these original research articles are indexed [e.g., MEDLINE® or the Cumulated Index to Nursing and Allied Health Literature (CINAHL)] are the gateways for finding this **body of evidence**. These databases contain the largest number and widest variation of articles reporting on clinical research. Clinicians who look for evidence within the base of the pyramid need specialized knowledge and skill both in finding the evidence and in appraising the worth of the evidence (Lefebvre, Manheimer, & Glanville, 2011a).

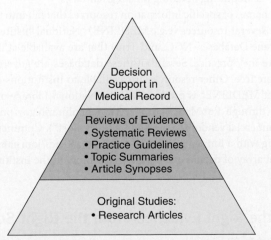

Figure 3.1: Pyramid framework for making evidence-based decisions (Adapted from Haynes, B. [2007]. Of studies, syntheses, synopses, summaries, and systems: The "5S" evolution of information services for evidence-based healthcare decisions. *Evidence-Based Nursing, 10*(1), 6–7.)

The next level of the pyramid, *Reviews of Evidence*, contains pre-appraised literature, which, when done well, may be considered one of the needles in the evidence haystack. New consolidated resources (e.g., Clinical Evidence, Dynamed™, Essential Evidence Plus, First Consult) have been designed to answer both background and foreground questions. They include comprehensive disease summaries, some as extensive as the equivalent of 40 print pages, that are formatted with sections and subcategories that are easily expanded. These summaries include hyperlinks to electronic journal articles or practice guidelines. They combine a textbook-like resource with easy access to the evidence contained in the journal literature—a format that is easy for busy clinicians to use. These resources can contain many types of evidence, ranging from systematic reviews, **clinical practice guidelines**, **health topic summaries**, to **article synopses**. Reviews within these resources are written by individuals or panels of experts who have evaluated the available evidence, determined its worth to practice, and made recommendations about how to apply it to a particular clinical issue. These resources are updated frequently. Guideline revisions frequently will trigger an update. While these sources of evidence are pre-appraised, it is important that clinicians understand the appraisal process used by each source of evidence to determine whether the information contained within them is reliable for clinical decision making. The appraisal process information is sometimes difficult to find. Terms like editorial policy or evidence-based methodology are frequently used to describe the appraisal process in the *About Us* section. Despite these vague terms, these resources can give the clinician an idea of the appraisal process that is used.

The pyramid's top layer, *Decision Support in Medical Record*, describes the ideal situation, a **clinical decision support system** integrated into the **electronic health record** (EHR). Here, data on a specific patient are automatically linked to the current best evidence available in the system that matches that patient's specific circumstances. Upon matching the evidence with patient data, the clinical decision support system assists clinicians with evidence-based interventions for that patient. This technology is important to healthcare decision making; therefore it is important to determine whether the information contained within these systems is evidence based or current (Haynes, 2007; Wright et al., 2011). Effective use of these resources requires that practitioners value the use of evidence in daily practice and have the knowledge and skills to use the given information.

The shape of the pyramid is significant in terms of the number of resources available. Although there are millions of original research articles on the bottom layer, the number of highly functioning computerized decision support systems is far fewer. The number of evidence reviews is somewhere in between. One reason for this disparity in resources is the time and money it takes to develop highly sophisticated EHR systems with integrated current evidence, systematic reviews, practice guidelines, summaries, and synopses—all requiring updating on a regular basis.

Table 3.1 includes the names of specific information resources that fall into the bottom two sections of the pyramid. There are several resources (e.g., MEDLINE®, National Institute for Health and Care Excellence [NICE], Cochrane Databases, NGC, and Trip) that are available at no cost to all healthcare providers, no matter where they practice. Several of these databases are government-sponsored databases, which is why they are free. Other resources are available to institutions through a subscription. It is important to note that MEDLINE® is produced by the National Library of Medicine (NLM) and is available free of charge through PubMed® (http://www.ncbi.nlm.nih.gov/pubmed) but can also be obtained for a cost via commercial vendors (e.g., Ovid®, EBSCOhost®). Commercial vendors offer their own search interfaces along with a limited number of **full-text** articles/journals. Each healthcare institution may have a different array of database offerings, depending on the institution size, professions it serves, and library budget.

Tool 2: Gathering the Right Evidence From the Right Source

Healthcare professionals, faculty, librarians, and students are all very busy in their roles and need reliable, efficient sources for evidence. The key is to know how to match the sources of evidence with the question to be answered.

Which Resource or Database Is a Good Match?

Reliable, accurate evidence is needed to reduce the risk, uncertainty, and time involved in clinical decision making that will lead to desired patient outcomes. With all of the resources potentially available to clinicians, the first step in finding answers to their clinical questions is to search for evidence in synthesized, pre-appraised resources (e.g., CDSR, Database of Reviews of Effects [DARE], American College of Physicians [ACP] Journal Club, and the journal, *Evidence-Based Nursing* [EBN]). See Table 3.1 for more information on these resources. Finding the evidence in full text (i.e., electronic copies of articles available online) can promote timely decision making. While there are open-source full-text articles available (i.e., no fee), a subscription is required to access most full-text journals (see Table 3.1). For example, in the CDSR, only an abstract of the systematic review can be obtained without a subscription. To obtain the full systematic review, a subscription is required or a fee may be paid per article.

For point-of-care decisions, clinicians may choose to consult one of the pre-appraised summaries or synopsized resources listed earlier. However, when making practice changes, it is important to either find a synthesis that has conducted an exhaustive search (i.e., found all that we know on the topic) or get as close to that as possible by searching multiple databases to try to ensure that studies are not missed. Searching subject-specific databases that index peer-reviewed research is the next step for finding best available evidence. For example, searching MEDLINE®, which contains thousands of articles in hundreds of journals that cut across disciplines, enables clinicians to find a large chunk of the evidence that exists on a topic. However, solely searching MEDLINE® would be a limitation, in that other databases index journals not covered in MEDLINE® and studies in those journals would not be discovered because the clinician didn't search another database; therefore key knowledge that might impact outcomes could be missed. Other healthcare databases to consider searching would be CINAHL and PsycINFO®.

Health care covers a wide range of topics. In addition, clinicians should think about which organizations or professional associations might produce evidence (e.g., guidelines, standards) and search their websites. Furthermore, if a question focuses on issues that are not indexed within the mainstream healthcare databases, a healthcare librarian can recommend other databases that can provide evidence to answer a PICOT question (e.g., Educational Resources Information Center [ERIC], Business Abstracts [ABI/INFORM], Computing Reviews, Social Sciences Citation Index® [SSCI], and Health Business Elite™).

When searches in indexed databases do not lead to sufficient quality evidence and clinicians wish to explore what other evidence is available, they may turn to web-based free resources such as Google to search for *grey literature*. Grey literature is unpublished evidence that has not been included in databases that clinicians routinely search. It may take the form of reports, unpublished drug trials, or unpublished conference proceedings. Grey literature can be elusive, so searching any web-based, nonindexed search engine, such as Google or Google Scholar, can provide value; however, caution should be used and careful evaluation of the evidence retrieved from these sources is required. Clinicians should follow an appraisal process to ensure the information is reliable. While major search engines may help clinicians get started in finding grey literature, much of this type of literature lies in the **deep web**, which is estimated to be 400 to 550 times larger than the surface web (Olson, 2013). Healthcare librarians are best able to navigate the deep web, and collaboration with the librarian is crucial when searching for grey literature. The Cochrane Collaboration attempts to seek out deep web resources and asserts that 10% of its citations come from grey literature (Lefebvre et al., 2011a).

Clinicians should keep in mind that Google may find older resources, and older resources may not be relevant for answering clinical questions. Also, many journals appear in Google Scholar, but may not be found while searching in Google. When choosing between Google and Google Scholar the busy clinician needs to keep in mind that Google Scholar searches across evidence that is found primarily in academic publications and will therefore find mostly peer-reviewed evidence (Younger, 2010). In a small study, Nourbakhsh and colleagues reported that using both PubMed® and Google Scholar could retrieve different evidence. Google Scholar tended to find more articles, and the articles it found were more likely to be classified as relevant, and were more likely to be written in journals with higher impact factors (Nourbakhsh, Nugent, Wang, Cevik, & Nugent, 2012). Web-based search engines, such as Google and

Google Scholar, are insufficient as sole sources of evidence, but using Google Scholar in conjunction with PubMed® and other databases may result in a clinician finding more evidence to answer their clinical question.

 For more on evaluating information on the Internet, visit:
http://www.lib.unc.edu/instruct/evaluate/

Final Key Resource for Finding Evidence: Collaboration With Healthcare Librarians

An essential step in achieving success is knowing the extent of one's resources. Collaboration with librarians who are knowledgeable about EBP is essential to get efficient answers to clinical questions. While all clinicians may not be expert searchers, each one should have the skills to be able to search and find their own answers as they have time and resources to do so. Librarians, with their specialized knowledge in the organization of information, can be helpful at any point in the search; however, librarians shine when clinicians have attempted to search multiple databases and other resources but do not find the evidence they seek. However, there are occasions when time is short and system infrastructures must be in place to facilitate finding evidence to answer the clinical question. Whenever possible, healthcare librarians need to be brought in early so that they are involved in the culture shift toward EBP. They are the knowledge brokers and knowledge miners of health care. Without their involvement in establishing an EBP culture, important pieces will be missed. Often librarians are able to find evidence to answer a clinical question when clinicians cannot. As you formulate your PICOT question, consider some advice and "take your librarian to lunch."

Get to know what resources are available in your organization to help you hone your searching skills. Take time to watch the short tutorials that most databases provide. Get to know your healthcare librarian and make sure you share your areas of interest so they can notify you about recent studies that come to their attention. This collaboration enables you to become aware of other evidence in real time. By staying current, you are able to respond more quickly when new evidence seems to suggest a practice change. Key aspects that contribute to clinician–librarian collaboration are dialogue, role delineation, and purpose. Talk about how PICOT questions are the drivers of searches. Discuss how keywords are a wonderful start to searching, but not sufficient to close the search. Explore the most effective way for clinicians to get the data now.

Currently, some healthcare professionals are finding evidence at the bedside. However, in 2020, it is expected that all healthcare professionals will be evidence-based clinicians, conducting rapid, efficient searches *at the bedside,* often in sources of evidence that will not be primary databases (IOM, 2009). For this to happen, collaboration between librarians and clinicians will be instrumental in exploring how to access information rapidly and efficiently. As information experts, librarians are partners with clinicians in achieving the mission of transforming health care from the inside out. The desired effect of the clinician–librarian collaboration is synergy that leads to consistent best practices by clinicians to achieve optimal outcomes for healthcare consumers.

Tool 3: Understanding Database Structure and Searching the Databases

When searching databases for evidence, clinicians need to be aware of features common to most databases. Understanding the structure and content of a particular information resource before attempting to search it is critical. Without this background, the search terms and strategies used may not **yield** the desired information, or the chosen database may not contain the information sought. It is important to note the fundamental difference between licensed databases, such as PubMed® or CINAHL, and search engines, such as Yahoo! or Google. Licensed databases list the journals they index, so it's easy for the searcher to know which journals they are searching in a given database. This decreases the likelihood of missing an important journal because the searcher knows from the start whether or not they are searching key journals. This transparency isn't available from Google or other search engines. The searcher may be searching the Internet, but has no idea what is being searched.

Types of Databases

Databases today are likely to contain records (i.e., article citations) as well as the full text of many types of documents. Records include the terms that were used to describe the content (subject headings) and other details. CINAHL, which indexes citations dealing with healthcare issues across multiple disciplines, and PsycINFO®, which indexes citations dealing with psychological, behavioral, and health sciences, are databases whose primary content is made up of records. Box 3.1 contains an example of a bibliographic record from MEDLINE®.

Full-text databases that contain whole articles or books, including the text, charts, graphs, and other illustrations are often referred to as *point-of-care* resources. These resources may be enhanced by supplemental data (i.e., in spreadsheets), by multimedia content, and/or by hypertext links to other articles and supporting references and frequently contain patient care recommendations supported by links to general patient care information, evidence-based articles, or guidelines. Examples of point-of-care resources would be Dynamed™ and Nursing Reference Center™. Examples of other full-text resources would be online journals or books (e.g., *Evidence-Based Nursing* or *Harrison's Online*) or systematic reviews (Cochrane Library).

Content of Databases

A clinician must be familiar with what databases and other information resources are available and what they contain before determining the value of searching it for answers to particular clinical questions. Databases can contain references to articles, the full text of the articles, entire books, dissertations, drug and pharmaceutical information, and other resources (e.g., news items, clinical calculators). To determine which databases to search, clinicians must consider the clinical question and which databases might contain relevant evidence. Evidence can come from multiple databases that primarily serve certain disciplines (e.g., nursing and allied health, medicine, biomedicine, psychology). However, searching only one database or only in one's discipline will limit clinicians in retrieving the best evidence to answer their questions.

Box 3.1   MEDLINE Example

Buteyko technique use to control asthma symptoms. [Review]
Austin G.
Nursing Times. 109(16):16-7, 2013 April 24–30.
[Case Reports. Journal Article. Review]
The Buteyko breathing technique is recommended in national guidance for control of asthma symptoms. This article explores the evidence base for the technique, outlines its main principles, and includes two cases studies.
   MeSH Heading
   *Asthma/nu [Nursing].
   *Asthma/th [Therapy].
   *Complementary Therapies/mt [Methods].
   Humans.
   Male.
   Middle Aged.
   *Respiratory Therapy/mt [Methods].

Searching Databases

To effectively find answers to questions, clinicians need to understand a few details about the databases they are searching, such as (1) Is the evidence current? (2) Will **subject headings** and/or keywords be more effective in getting to the best evidence quickly? (3) How frequently is the database updated?

Often clinicians wonder how many years back they should search. Although some consider searching back 5 years as sufficient, this may not be adequate to discover evidence that can address the clinical issue. While there is no rule for how far back to search for evidence, clinicians should search until they can confidently indicate that there is little or no evidence to answer their clinical question or they feel confident that the evidence they have found represents the body of evidence that exists. For example, Dr. Priscilla Worral of SUNY Upstate Health System, in a situation in which clinicians in the emergency department (ED) were using salt pork to prevent rebleeding from epistaxis, indicated that she had to search for articles back to the late 1800s to find relevant evidence to her clinical question (P.S. Worral, personal communication, 2001). To accomplish the goal of finding all that we know about a topic, the databases we use must include older evidence that has been published as well as the newer evidence. This enables clinicians to search over a large span of time to find the best answer to their question. For example, MEDLINE offers citations ranging from the late 1940s to the present.

Knowing that evidence is current is another consideration. Clinicians must be aware of the years covered in a database. The CDSR, for instance, always states the date of the most recent update. Other resources also require investigating how current they are. For example, online textbooks are updated much less frequently than point-of-care resources. Most point-of-care resources follow an update protocol which might dictate a yearly or biannual review. Additionally, point-of-care resources will be updated as soon as the reviewers become aware that guidelines or other resources have been revised. If there is no known date for evidence (e.g., Internet sources of evidence), it may be outdated, making it difficult for the clinician to determine its applicability.

Keyword, Title, and Subject Heading Searching

Searchers use three major search strategies across multiple databases and resources to increase the certainty that best evidence is not missed. These strategies rely on keyword searching, subject heading searching (also called controlled vocabulary, MESH®, descriptors, thesaurus), and title searching. Because each of the three major search strategies has strengths and weaknesses, all three are used in combination and when they are used together they provide high levels of certainty that best evidence is not missed (Table 3.3).

Before the search begins, the searcher formulates a PICOT research question. After formulation of the PICOT question, there are several approaches to the search. The Cochrane Handbook (2011) recommends that the search begins with the terms for the population (P) and intervention (I). Others recommend beginning with the outcome (O) and intervention (I) (Stillwell et al., 2010). All approaches recommend using as many synonyms for the keywords and related subject headings as possible, and to combine these synonym searches with "OR" (see the Try This example and the Application Case Study found on this book's companion website).

Keywords. The first major search strategy is KEYWORD searching. Keywords are generated from the PICOT question. Using keywords is the most common search strategy used across databases, search engines (e.g., Google), and other online resources. With this technique, searchers enter all appropriate keywords, including common terms, synonyms, acronyms, phrases, coined phrases, and brand names. Searchers scan the citations found with this search, continuing to note the alternate terms and synonyms that are found and use these terms as searching continues. Keyword searching will attempt to locate the keyword entered in the title, abstract, or other searchable fields in the digital record. The citations that are found will only be those records that contain the keyword(s) used in the search somewhere in the record. The strength of the keyword search strategy is that it provides a quick snapshot of how helpful the database is in finding relevant evidence to answer the PICOT question.

Table 3.3   **Strengths and Weakness of Three Search Strategies**

Search Strategies	Strengths	Weaknesses
Keyword Search	Provides quick snapshot of resource's relevance to PICOT question Identifies records when keyword appears with and without major relevancy Included in three most power search strategies	Misses studies when authors' choices of keywords differ Requires advanced search skills to quickly sort for relevancy among too many citations Requires combined subject headings search Requires all three strategies to achieve certainty nothing was missed
Subject Headings Search*	Provides quick snapshot of resources' relevance to PICOT question Retrieves only citations when topic is at least 25% relevant to topic Increases chances that best citations will not be missed when authors and searchers use different synonyms because of database Maps all synonyms to one assigned subject heading Retrieves citations searched using related and narrower MeSH terms associated with the searcher's MeSH Increases chances that MeSH's broader terms identifying fields, environments, settings, industries, can be combined with a very specific common keyword to target relevant citations. Included in the three most powerful search strategies	Not always assigned for every keyword (i.e., new cutting edge terminology, coined phrases, acronyms), may not yet be assigned MeSH®, nor be a successful match for auto mapping Requires combining three major search strategies to avoid missing something Not available across all major databases, search engines
Title Search	Provides quick snap shot to resources' relevance to topic Increases chances that keywords appearing in title are major topics Increases chances that the P & I are related as required for PICOT question Increases chances assigned subject headings are precise and best for a subject heading search Effective in quickly targeting highly relevant articles within all search strategies. Included in three most powerful search strategies	Misses studies when author's choices of title words differ Requires all three major strategies to achieve certainty nothing missed Not available across all major databases, search engines. Note: Google Scholar provides title search mode

The inherent challenge to keyword searching is that all synonyms, plurals, and alternate spellings of each keyword must be included in the search or evidence will be missed. For example, entering the keyword *behavior* will find any citations containing the word *behavior* in either the title or abstract of that citation. All records with the alternative spelling *behaviour* in the title or abstract would be missed. In addition, different spellings of singulars and plurals (e.g., *mouse* and *mice*) must be included or evidence will be missed.

Using keywords can be ambiguous and jargon-laden. Consider the following question: *Are people diagnosed with AIDS more likely to acquire pneumonia in the community than the elderly?* An example of a keyword search for this question might start with the word *AIDS.* This search would include articles on other types of aids, such as visual aids, aid to dependent children, and hearing aids. In addition, this search would retrieve only articles containing the word *AIDS.* Those articles that used *acquired immune deficiency syndrome* or *acquired immunodeficiency syndrome* would be potentially missed. Searching with keywords can be helpful, especially when no subject heading exists to adequately describe the topic searched. When a topic is so recent that there is likely to be very little available in the journal literature, using keywords may be the best way to find relevant evidence because subject heading for the topic is unlikely. For this reason, the importance of carefully formulating the PICOT question cannot be over-emphasized. Using any term(s) that will describe the PICOT components of the clinical question will assist in obtaining the best search in the shortest time.

Another weakness of the keyword strategy is that even though your keywords appear in the document's searchable fields, it does not mean that the article has these concepts as major topics. Also, the author may not have used the keywords you chose to search, so you may have missed best evidence. Yet another weakness with keyword searching is that you can potentially find a large yield (i.e., results). With only keyword searching, searchers may not have the skills to quickly target the most relevant results and can waste time scanning and sorting articles for relevance. This keyword approach weakness is mitigated when used in combination with two additional strategies, subject heading and title searching.

Subject Headings. The second major search strategy that can quickly identify articles to answer your clinical question is the SUBJECT HEADINGS search. An advanced searcher will utilize a standardized set of preselected terms known as subject headings in order to locate all material that is available on a particular topic. Subject headings may be referred to as controlled vocabulary, subject terms, thesaurus, descriptors, or taxonomies. The content of an article will determine which subject headings it falls under (e.g., fibromyalgia or fatigue). These subject headings are used to help the searcher find information on a particular topic, no matter what words the author may use to refer to a concept in the text. If a database incorporates subject headings with keyword searching, regardless of what words the author used in the article, when searchers type their words into the search box of the database the database "maps" or finds the subject headings that best match the keyword. Using subject headings, searchers can broaden their searches without having to consider every synonym for the chosen keyword. An example of subject headings is Medical Subject Headings (**MeSH**®), which is the set of terms used by the NLM to describe the content of articles indexed in MEDLINE®. If the MeSH® term *acquired immunodeficiency syndrome* was searched, all of these articles would contain information about it regardless of what terms the author(s) chose to use when writing, including HIV, HIV-positive, acquired immune deficiency syndrome, STI, STD, sexually transmitted disease, and sexually transmitted infection.

Many subject heading systems also have a hierarchical structure that helps the searcher retrieve the more specific terms that fall under a general term. In searching a general MeSH® term such as *heart diseases,* the PubMed® search engine automatically maps keywords to subject headings and retrieves every term that is listed under it in the hierarchical "tree structure." This search retrieves articles ranging from myocardial infarction to familial hypertrophic cardiomyopathy and everything in between—all at one time. Some search engines, rather than doing it automatically, offer the user the option of including or not including all of the specifics under a general term (e.g., Ovid presents the option to "explode" the subject heading, which means to include all the specific terms listed under a more general heading). Exploding the search term when using subject headings is recommended, though it may at times yield some irrelevant studies. When clinicians use the explode feature and retrieve irrelevant articles, they can eliminate many of them by setting appropriate limits and combining subject heading searches using the PICOT question as the guide. Some search systems enable the searcher to click on the subject heading and see the other narrower headings in the controlled vocabulary tree structure. This option helps the searcher create the most relevant search by making a decision about whether to explode terms in the search.

An example of the usefulness of the explode function is a search to find information on food poisoning. In MEDLINE®, the MeSH® term *food poisoning* is the broad subject heading that describes various types of food poisoning, including botulism, ciguatera poisoning, favism, mushroom poisoning, salmonella poisoning, and staphylococcal poisoning. Using this heading to initiate the search and then exploding it means that the name of each of those types of food poisoning is a part of the search without entering each one into the search strategy, saving valuable search time. In a PubMed® MeSH® search, the term you enter is automatically exploded. In the search, you have to instruct PubMed® NOT to explode the term.

Most large databases, such as MEDLINE®, CINAHL, and PsycINFO®, use subject headings to describe the content of the items they index. Most search engines will attempt to map the keyword entered in the search box to a subject heading. This assists the searcher in finding relevant evidence without needing to know the subject heading up front. For example, in most search engines, the term *Tylenol*™ is mapped to the generic term *acetaminophen*, as is the European term *paracetamol*, or any of the following that are acetaminophen types of pain relievers: *Tempra*®, *Panadol*®, and *Datril*®. As the system searches the subject heading *acetaminophen*, any article using the term *Tylenol*™ or any of the other words above will be retrieved because an indexer cataloged it under that heading, regardless of the term used in the article.

There is a caveat to subject headings searching: This mapping process may not be efficient with very current topics that have only recently entered the literature. In these cases, a subject heading likely is not available; therefore, keyword searching, using synonyms or variant forms of the word, may yield more relevant results. For example, the MeSH® term, *resistance training*, did not become a subject heading until 2009. The only way a searcher could retrieve relevant evidence was to use the keywords *weight training*, *strength training*, *weight bearing*, or additional keywords.

In some cases, **truncation** should be considered. Truncation uses special symbols in combination with words or word parts to enhance the likelihood of finding relevant studies. Truncation is usually indicated by a word or part of a word followed by an asterisk (*). In PubMed® and CINAHL, the asterisk is used to replace any number of letters at the end of the word. For example, in PubMed®, to truncate *adolescent*, one would use *adolescen** to retrieve *adolescent, adolescents,* or *adolescence*. Again, a librarian and the help section of individual databases can offer guidance to determine relevant search characters or symbols.

Some evidence-based resources do not have subject headings, or they rely on the searcher to be familiar with existing subject headings. For example, any of the Cochrane databases can be searched using MeSH® or keywords. To search using the MeSH® option, you have to know the MeSH® term you want to search. If you use MeSH® often, you may know the term you want to search and can easily make use of this feature. If you want to find the appropriate subject headings, you may search MeSH® independently through PubMed®. *A cautionary note:* don't rely on MeSH® alone when searching the Cochrane databases as you will exclude relevant, unique citations that are indexed in other databases whose records Cochrane includes. Nevertheless, keyword searching requires some creativity; the searcher must think of all the different ways that an author could have referred to a particular concept. To maximize your search, keep in mind the caveats about keyword searching that were described earlier in this chapter.

Title Search. The TITLE search is the final major search strategy. Searching your P, I, and O terms in the title increases the chance of finding relevant citations. The keyword is the mechanism for title searching and should not be attempted until you know the keywords that are most frequently used. The weakness of the title search is that if authors do not use your terms in their title, you could miss best evidence. Your vigilance at listing all the synonyms that an author could use for your PICOT question is essential to refining your search and increasing your certainty that best evidence is not missed.

Combining and Limiting Searches

In a focused search for a clinical topic using the PICOT question as the framework for the search, clinicians have the option to enter multiple concepts simultaneously into the search system. The disadvantage of this method is that there is no way to determine which concept has the most evidence available. To see how many **hits** (i.e., articles or studies that contain the searched word) that each term retrieves, clinicians can enter the terms from the PICOT question into the search box one at a time. By entering them one at a time, especially in very large databases (e.g., MEDLINE®, CINAHL), you can discover the number of hits for each individual term searched. For example, searching MEDLINE® for the keywords *Tylenol*™ and *pain* separately yielded 67 and 180,694 hits, respectively; however, when searching them together, *Tylenol*™ *AND pain*, the yield was 32. There is clearly more evidence about pain than Tylenol™. It is important to consider that out of a possible 67 studies, only 32 were found that contained both terms. To enter each PICOT term individually may not be possible with every search due to competing clinical priorities; however, it is the best method to fully understand what evidence exists to answer the clinical question.

When combining subject headings or keywords, the Boolean operators *AND* or *OR* are usually used. The *AND* operator is useful when attempting to link different concepts together (e.g., PICOT question). Using *AND* is appropriate when clinicians wish to narrow their search by having both of the combined terms required in the retrieved articles. Since *AND* is a restrictive word (i.e., both words must appear in the article), it will reduce the number of articles retrieved, which serves well with a finely honed PICOT question. Figure 3.2 illustrates the concept of the Boolean operator *AND*.

Conversely, the *OR* Boolean operator is generally used to expand a search as either one or both of the search terms will be included in the results list. When searching for concepts using synonyms, *OR* should be used. Figure 3.3 illustrates the concept of the Boolean operator *OR*. Each search system has its own unique way of combining terms. For example, one system may require typing in the word *AND* or *OR*, while another may offer the ease of clicking on a "combine" option and specifying the correct connector. Consulting the databases' help documents can assist in determining the unique ways to conduct a search using Boolean operators within that database.

Below is an example that illustrates the principle of combining search terms. A clinician begins to search for articles to answer the following diagnosis question:

In patients with suspected schizophrenia, is magnetic resonance imaging (MRI) compared with computed tomography (CT scan) more accurate in diagnosing schizophrenia?

The search would use the keywords *MRI*, *CT scan*, *schizophrenia*, and *diagnos**. The use of *diagnos** enables the searcher to capture diagnose, diagnosis, or diagnosing with one search term. If the use of

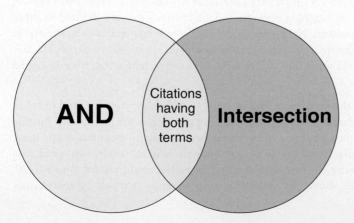

Figure 3.2: Boolean operator AND.

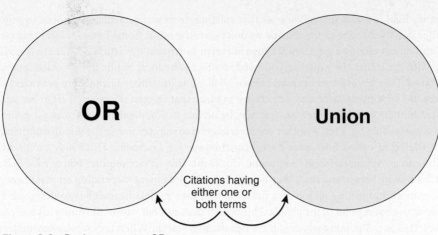

Figure 3.3: Boolean operator OR.

subject headings is an option, that would also be used. The terms *MRI* and *CT scan* would first be combined using the *AND* operator (*MRI* AND *CT scan* forming the first search statement (s1). Those results would then be combined with the terms *schizophrenia* (s2) and *diagnos** (s3) using *AND* (i.e., s1 and s2 and s3) because this search would theoretically yield the best answer to the question. However, if few results were found, the yield could be increased by using the Boolean OR (*MRI* OR *CT scan* MRI) forming the first search statement (s1). Those results would then be combined with the terms *schizophrenia* (s2) and *diagnosis* (s3) using the Boolean operator *AND* (i.e., s1 and s2 and s3). This search might provide some insight into the answer to the question; although, it won't answer it completely.

Different databases treat terms entered in the search box in different ways; therefore, use caution when searching various databases. While it is important to use the same keywords when searching in different databases and, as much as possible, the same approach, each database may require a slight variation to the search strategy. Some unique aspects of databases may not be evident. For example, PubMed® automatically puts *AND* (Boolean operator) between words, as does Google. Other search engines may look for the keywords entered together as a phrase first, while other search systems automatically put *OR* (Boolean operator) between the terms. Before searching a database, it will be helpful to take time to consult help documents to become familiar with how the database searches terms.

Limiting Searches. Since databases can be very large and even the best search strategies cannot retrieve only desired articles, often there are more citations retrieved than are relevant to a clinical question. The "limit" function is designed to help the searcher pare down a large list of citations to more relevant studies. Choosing the limit function leads one to a set of options for limiting the results by various parameters (e.g., study design [called publication type], language, human studies, publication year, age, gender, full text). For example, limiting the results of a search to a type of study design (e.g., RCTs or meta-analysis) can help the searcher know how many of the articles in that yield are higher-level evidence to answer the clinical question (see Chapter 2). Higher-level evidence helps the searcher answer the clinical question with relevant, stronger studies; thereby increasing confidence that the clinical outcome can be achieved.

Another limit option, full text, narrows the search to "e-documents" where the entire article is available electronically. The ease of limiting a search to full-text retrieval can be tempting; however, clinicians can miss evidence by limiting their search to only those articles where full text is readily available. Keep in mind that the answer to a clinical question comes from a body of evidence, not just a few articles; therefore, it is important that searchers seek all relevant articles to answer the clinical question.

Sometimes the full-text article is available, but the library does not have a subscription to the journal and the publisher will not grant access unless a fee is paid. If you don't want to pay the publisher for the article, find out if the library you are affiliated with can get a copy through *interlibrary loan*.

Interlibrary loan is a network of libraries that collaborate to supply articles or books to other libraries that either don't subscribe to the journal or don't own the book. Some libraries offer this service at no charge and others charge a fee. Contact your librarian to request the article or, if there is no librarian to partner with regarding the evidence you need, contact your local public library. Also, many local college libraries, state libraries, or hospital libraries will allow unaffiliated healthcare providers to use their resources. Be aware that there may be policies in place that restrict library staff from assisting unaffiliated users in their searches. Likewise, you may be unable to borrow their resources. Copying of articles is generally available for a fee. Another solution may be to register to use the document delivery service through the NLM called Loansome Doc.® Instructions for Loansome Doc® may be found at: http://www.nlm.nih.gov/pubs/factsheets/loansome_doc.html. This service requires you to establish a relationship with a nearby library and there may be a fee for each document, depending on that library's policies.

An important limiting option in a database that uses subject headings is to designate the subject headings as the main point of the article. This option does not fall within the limits list but can be found as the searcher is designating which subject headings to search. When indexers assign subject headings for MEDLINE®/PubMed, CINAHL, and PsycINFO®, they will index the subject headings as either a major or minor concept for each article. In the sample MEDLINE record in Box 3.1, the asterisk (*) beside some MeSH® terms indicates the subject headings the indexer considered to be the main points of the article. Many search systems permit the searcher to limit the search to articles where a particular concept is the main focus of the article. For example, Ovid provides the "focus" option to the right of the subject heading. Limiting a subject heading to the main point will increase the relevancy of the retrieved articles.

The final method for limiting the number of relevant citations is conducted when reviewing studies that might be appraised (i.e., after the search strategy in the database is complete), not within the search of the database. Before a search strategy is begun, clinicians identify specific conditions that will assist in determining which evidence they will keep (keepers) and which evidence they will discard once they have completed their search. These conditions are called **inclusion** and **exclusion criteria**. For example, an inclusion criterion may be that a sample for a study must be at least 50% female to make the studies useful to the clinician and be relevant to her population of patients. An exclusion criterion may be that clinicians will not accept studies that compare three different medications. The fifth part of the PICOT question—time—is often an inclusion or exclusion criterion. If a study does not follow patients long enough to establish the effect of the intervention, the study is not relevant. These criteria for acceptable studies may not always be met through the search strategy. Often, the abstract does not address all of the inclusion and exclusion criteria. The entire study may need to be obtained to determine whether it is a keeper. Establishing inclusion and exclusion criteria before starting a search allows the searcher to quickly identify the most relevant evidence to appraise.

Keepers: Managing Citations of Interest

Once a search is completed, each database will provide options for managing the "keeper" citations. Most databases provide methods for printing, saving, or e-mailing citations. Each database may also provide other specialized features for dealing with selected citations: PubMed® has the Clipboard, while EBSCOhost® uses folders. Databases may also allow users to set up individual accounts that offer customization of certain features or the ability to save desired settings. Familiarizing yourself with these options can spare you frustration and may save you a great deal of time. Collaborate with a librarian to learn about these time-saving options. Many databases provide "Help" documentation that can assist users in learning about these features.

Saving Searches: Why and How

Saving the search strategy or search history (i.e., how you went about the search) is necessary if you want to repeat the search or communicate the search to someone else. One way to capture the search details so that they can be replicated is to save the search history when you conduct the initial search.

Each search engine offers different mechanisms for saving a search. Let's take the example of updating a healthcare procedure. The initial in-depth search was completed, and relevant studies informed the recommendations in the current procedure. It is now time to update the procedure; however, without a saved search, the review group will have to start from scratch and may not choose the same approach (e.g., keywords, subject headings, and combinations) used by the original group. With a saved search, the review group simply follows the same strategy to determine what is new since the last revision of the procedure. It also gives the review group an opportunity to appropriately introduce new search terms that may need to be included. Consult the user guide or help section of any database to learn more about saving your search.

Another way to document the search strategy is to capture the strategy through a *screenshot*. A screenshot is a picture of the computer screen. When you capture your search this way, be sure that the search strategy is clear on your computer screen. The screen capture should include only the steps you took in your search, not the citations of articles. Most databases offer this option to searchers; it is frequently referred to as the search history. If you are unfamiliar with how to capture a screenshot, this is a perfect opportunity to use keywords to search your favorite web-based database to find out the steps for how to capture a screenshot. Once you have captured the screenshot(s) of your search, paste it into a document that you can save electronically and keep for later use.

Organizing Searches

Often there is a need to organize the evidence found, as the large number of articles retrieved can be overwhelming (Stillwell et al., 2010). Practitioners need to organize evidence in some way so that they may easily find the evidence through each step of their EBP journey. Reference management software (RMS) is one solution. Often referred to as citation managers, this software is designed to offer options that save, search, sort, share, and continuously add, delete, and organize promising citations. Some web-based examples include RefWorks and Endnote®. Many libraries provide this type of software for their users; therefore, readers should check with their library before purchasing any RMS software. If clinicians must select an RMS product, they need to compare purchase/subscription fees, features, ease of use, and speed. Approximate annual fees for individuals can range from $100 to $300 per year, depending upon vendor/desired features. In addition to subscription-based RMS, several open-source RMS options are Mendeley and Zotero, two free reference management tools that promote collaboration among researchers.

 Check out these free reference management software options!
Zotero: http://www.zotero.org Mendeley: http://www.mendeley.com

Practitioners can work with teams at multiple sites or their own institution using web-based RMS that is designed to import/export citations from all of the commonly searched databases as well as sort the citations by author, journal title, and keywords. Organizing the evidence in folders by clinical meaningfulness, specific PICOT concepts, or strength of evidence allows a clinician or team to add to and keep track of the relevant information they find and use. Through sharing citations with the team or organizing them for their own initiatives, clinicians can reduce the time invested in evidence retrieval and improve access to current information for the entire team.

Tool 4: Choosing the Right Database

Of the many databases that index healthcare literature, some are available through several vendors at a cost, some are free of charge, and some are available at least in part, both free of charge and through a vendor for a fee. As noted previously, MEDLINE® can be accessed free of charge through the NLM's PubMed® or obtained by subscription through other providers (e.g., Ovid). Table 3.1 contains information about access to some of these databases.

This chapter focuses primarily on the following databases:

- Cochrane Database
- NGC
- MEDLINE®
- Trip
- CINAHL
- Embase (**Excerpta Medica Online**)
- PsycINFO®

MEDLINE® and CINAHL are among the best-known comprehensive databases that contain much of the scientific knowledge base in health care. However, the amount of information in health care exceeds the capacity of either of these databases. In addition to MEDLINE® and CINAHL, there are other types of databases that provide more readily available information in summaries and synopses (e.g., UpToDate®, Clinical Evidence). Some of these databases are highly specialized, and their numbers are growing in response to clinicians' desire for quick access to evidence.

Cochrane Databases

Classified as an international not-for-profit organization, the Cochrane Collaboration represents the efforts of a global network of dedicated volunteer researchers, healthcare professionals, and consumers who prepare, maintain, and promote access to the Cochrane Library's six databases: (1) **CDSR**, (2) **DARE**, (3) **Cochrane Central Register of Controlled Trials (CENTRAL)**, (4) **Cochrane Methodology Register,** (5) **Health Technology Assessment**, and (6) **NHS Economic Evaluation Database**. There is also the Cochrane Nursing Care Field within the Cochrane Collaboration. The purpose of the nursing care field is to support the conduct, dissemination, and utilization of Cochrane systematic reviews in the field of nursing.

The Cochrane Handbook of Systematic Reviews of Interventions is a free, authoritative, online handbook that documents the process that should be used by clinicians who are conducting a systematic review. For searchers, it provides an entire section on how to search for studies to support EBP. The online handbook is available at www.cochrane-handbook.org.

Cochrane Database of Systematic Reviews. The Cochrane Library's gold standard database is the CDSR. It contains Cochrane full-text systematic reviews and should be searched first to answer intervention questions. Although the CDSR is a fairly small database, in part because systematic reviews are still relatively new and few, the CDSR contains a large number of valuable, synthesized (i.e., critically appraised, compiled, and integrated) RCTs. Unlike MEDLINE® (e.g., 16 million citations) and CINAHL (e.g., 3 million citations), the CDSR contains a few thousand citations and is limited to a single publication type—systematic reviews—including meta-analyses. A single word search in the MEDLINE® or CINAHL databases can easily result in thousands of hits. Because the CDSR is a small database, the broadest search is likely to retrieve only a small, manageable number of hits. This makes the database easy to search and the results easy to review. When reading the search results, the label "Review" refers to a completed Cochrane review and the label "Protocol" applies to Cochrane reviews that are in the initial stages of gathering and appraising evidence. It is helpful to know that protocols are in the pipeline; however, it can be disappointing not to find a full review. If a full Cochrane review is retrieved during a search, clinicians can save time because they do not need to conduct the critical appraisal and synthesis of primary studies, as that has already been done. However, clinicians need to critically appraise the systematic review itself. Chapter 5 contains more information on critically appraising systematic reviews.

Clinicians may access the citations (as well as abstracts of systematic reviews) free of charge at http://www.cochrane.org. A paid subscription allows searchers to view the full text of all reviews and protocols. On February 1, 2013, authors producing a systematic review could choose at the time of publication, one of two options for publishing their review: gold or green open access. Gold open access allows immediate access to the entire review if the authors agree to pay the publication charge fee. Green open access offers free access to the full review 12 months after publication. Beginning in February 2014, reviews that were published in the CDSR one year prior will be available full text. Systematic reviews published prior to February 1, 2013, will remain accessible by abstract only without a paid subscription. Check to see if your library has a subscription. If they don't have a subscription, another option is to access the full-text version of a review by paying for it separately (pay-per-view). This option is offered on each abstract summary page.

DARE Database. The DARE database is produced by the Centre for Reviews and Dissemination at the University of York, UK. The DARE database complements the CDSR by providing critical assessments of systematic reviews not produced by The Cochrane Collaboration.

CENTRAL Database. The CENTRAL database serves as the most comprehensive source of reports of controlled trials. As of January 2008, CENTRAL contains nearly 530,000 citations of controlled trials. Of these 310,000 were from MEDLINE, 50,000 were from EMBASE, and 170,000 from other sources including other databases and handsearching (Lefebvre, Manheimer, & Glanville, 2011a, 2011b, 2011c). For those clinicians without access to EMBASE or other resources, including grey literature, but who have access to CENTRAL, this means access to trials to which they may not have otherwise.

 The databases produced by The Cochrane Collaboration can be accessed via **http://www .cochrane.org**

National Guideline Clearinghouse
NGC is a free public resource for international evidence-based clinical practice guidelines. It is supported by the Agency for Healthcare Research and Quality (AHRQ) and the U.S. Department of Health and Human Services. NCG contains over 2,400 international evidence-based clinical practice guidelines. NCG informs clinicians on how the guidelines were developed and tested, and how they should be used (e.g., an algorithm). Guidelines have been developed by many professional associations, and they each describe a plan of care for a specific set of clinical circumstances involving a particular population. NGC uses many resources to identify current and relevant recommendations that make up the guideline (see Chapter 8) such as PubMed®, EMBASE, CINAHL, PsycINFO®, and the Emergency Care Research (ECRI) Institute. Links to the electronic version of the latest set of guidelines are provided when available. The best intervention guidelines are based on the rigorous scientific evidence obtained from systematic reviews or RCTs. Some guidelines are a consensus of expert opinion and, while they are not the strongest evidence, can still assist in decision making.

There are several reasons why clinicians should use the NCG. First, NCG has the ability to compare two or more guidelines side by side. This allows the clinician to directly compare all aspects of each guideline and, in this way, determine whether a PICOT question is answered by a single recommendation within the guideline. It should be noted that guidelines themselves do not address PICOT questions; however, recommendations within guidelines may. The proper approach to using a guideline to answer a PICOT question is to cite the supporting evidence of the recommendation that addresses the question.

Another benefit is a recently added feature to NGC that enables the clinician to create a matrix for guidelines by clinical specialty. Furthermore, there is a complete list of alphabetically arranged guidelines for clinicians who wish to locate guidelines published by a particular organization.

 The NGC can be found at **www.guideline.gov**

MEDLINE®
MEDLINE® is one of the world's largest searchable databases covering medicine, health, and the biomedical sciences. MEDLINE® is a premier database produced by the NLM and is available through PubMed® at no charge from any computer with internet access. The NLM also leases the MEDLINE®

data to vendors. These companies load the database into their own interface and sell subscriptions to their database. Ovid is one of several companies that do this. It is important to know that the original file of indexed citations is the same MEDLINE® product in PubMed® as in any of these other vendors' versions of the file. It contains citations from more than 5,600 worldwide journals in 39 languages, although its primary focus tends to be on North American journals. Coverage spans from 1946 to the present. MEDLINE® uses MeSH® to index articles and facilitate searches.

 The MEDLINE® database is available free of charge through PubMed® at http://www.ncbi .nlm.nih.gov/pubmed

Trip

Trip first came on the scene in 1997. Known then as the TRIP (Turning Research Into Practice) Database, it has continuously evolved into one of the leading clinical search engines for evidence-based content. While Trip is a commercial company, the cofounders assert that the business is run more like a not-for-profit company. Access to the website continues to be free. Trip loads the content of PubMed® every 2 weeks and loads secondary evidence such as summaries, synopses, and syntheses, once a month. The process for adding secondary content has been developed by the founders of the database and, over the years, users have suggested sources as well. Clinicians can find research evidence as well as other content (e.g., images, videos, patient information leaflets, educational courses, and news).

The first step to optimize the Trip search experience is to register. Registering enables the clinician to take advantage of other features such as automated searches and the ability to track CPD/CME (Continuing Professional Development/Continuing Medical Education).

Trip offers two search features that work independently of one another. For novice searchers, the PICO search box is the place to start. PICO offers four search boxes that follow the first four elements of a PICO question. This helps to focus the searcher. It is not necessary to enter a term for each element, but it would be wise for the searcher to use as many of the elements as possible for better results. The second search feature is the Advanced Search box. This enables the searcher to do proximity searching. Proximity searching, also referred to as adjacency searching, allows the searcher to find an exact phrase or to look for specific words occurring between 2, 3, 5, or 10 words apart from each other. An example of proximity searching for 5 words apart would be entering the term *chest congestion* and finding an article entitled *Chest ultrasound and hidden lung congestion in peritoneal dialysis patients*. The Advanced Search box also allows the searcher to limit words or phrases to the title.

The limits in the Trip database are found in the Refine Results menu on the right side of the webpage. It allows searchers to limit results to the type of content that will best answer their clinical question and to further limit by publication date or clinical area. Trip offers a rudimentary citation analysis feature, Important Papers, which lists the most linked-to papers from the results of the search. While new publications won't have many, if any, related citations within other works for research studies and articles that have been published for some time, it gives the searcher an idea of how many times the evidence has been cited by other researchers.

 Trip is available free of charge at http://www.tripdatabase.com

CINAHL

The CINAHL database is produced by EBSCOhost® and contains citations from many subject areas including nursing, biomedicine, and alternative/complementary medicine. CINAHL includes more than 2.7 million citations from over 3,000 journals from 1981 to the present as well as more than 70 full-text journals from 1992 to the present. Available through a library subscription, CINAHL retrieves content from journals, books, drug monographs, and dissertations, and includes images that are often difficult to locate in other databases. In addition to the base CINAHL subscription, EBSCOhost® also offers a more robust version of CINAHL in CINAHL Plus, which indexes more than 4,500 journals from 1937 to the present. Full-text versions of both CINAHL and CINAHL Plus are also available. The most recent version, CINAHL Complete, now indexes over 5,000 journals dating back to 1937 with more than 1,300 included in full text. CINAHL can be searched by keywords which retrieves the keyword in any of the indexed fields. The CINAHL database provides subject headings (CINAHL headings) that can be used instead of or in conjunction with keyword searching.

Searchers should be aware that checking the box for "suggest subject terms" will force a subject heading search. To enable keyword searching, choose your keywords at the bottom of the list of proposed subject headings. This will render a combined search of the chosen subject heading *and* your keywords. Video tutorials for searching are available through EBSCOhost's Youtube Channel at www .youtube.com/user/ebscopublishing/

 The CINAHL database is available at http://www.ebscohost.com/cinahl/

Embase

Embase provides comprehensive coverage of biomedicine, with a strong emphasis on drugs and pharmacology. There are over 22 million records from 1974 to the present, in 40 languages in EMBASE. Over 7,500 journals including all journals indexed by MEDLINE® and 2,000 unique journals are indexed. Embase is produced by the publishing company, Elsevier, Inc., and is only available by subscription.

 The EMBASE database is available at http://www.embase.com

PsycINFO®

PsycINFO® is a database produced by the American Psychological Association (APA) and includes scattered publications from 1597 to the present and comprehensive coverage from the late 1800s to the present. Available by subscription only, this database indexes literature in psychology, behavioral sciences, and mental health and contains more than 3.4 million citations. PyscINFO® includes citations to books and book chapters, comprising approximately 11% of the database. Dissertations can also be found within this database.

PsycINFO is available at http://www.apa.org/psycinfo/

Searching the literature can be both rewarding and challenging, primarily because the volume of healthcare literature is huge. The MEDLINE® database alone provides reference to more than 17 million citations; however, it cannot cover *all* worldwide healthcare journals. Searching multiple databases can increase the number of relevant articles found while searching. The databases discussed here impose organization on the chaos that is the journal literature. Each database offers coverage that is broad and sometimes overlapping. Knowing which databases to search first and for what information is necessary for a successful, efficient search.

> **Never give up, for that is just the place and time that the tide will turn.**
> **—Harriet Beecher Stowe**

A Unique Case: PubMed®

PubMed® is a broad database produced and maintained by the National Center for Biotechnology Information (NCBI) at the NLM. In 2010, this database contained more than 19 million citations to articles from more than 22 million journals published worldwide (NLM, 2005). PubMed® also covers many subject areas, including the biomedical sciences, nursing, dentistry, and pharmacy.

There are a couple of characteristics that make PubMed® unique. First, it is a completely free database; second, NLM, which has been indexing evidence since 1879, is committed to providing access to all evidence. At its web debut in 1997, the oldest citations contained in PubMed® were from 1966, but that has changed dramatically since 2003 when the first group of older citations (1.5 million citations dated 1953–1965) was added to the database. As of 2013, the oldest citations date back to 1945.

PubMed® is accessible at http://www.pubmed.gov. NCBI has made it possible for libraries to link their electronic and print serial holdings to citations in the database, making it easy for their clientele to access full-text articles they own through the PubMed® database and to identify which articles are available in print at the library. Any clinician affiliated with a library should check with that library to learn more about how to use PubMed® and access their full-text and print resources.

PubMed® provides access to the information that makes up the foundation and middle section of the Haynes (2007) Evidence Pyramid: original research studies and reviews of evidence. PubMed® also provides free online access to the MEDLINE® database. MEDLINE® citations in PubMed® are indexed with MeSH® terms. If searchers want to search only MEDLINE®, they can retrieve citations using MeSH® terms.

While MEDLINE® resides within the PubMed® database, PubMed® contains more citations than MEDLINE®. Citations that are in PubMed® but not in MEDLINE®—approximately 8%—are *not* indexed with MeSH® terms. To facilitate full use of the information in PubMed®, the NLM developed automatic term mapping, which searches the keywords entered in the search box and maps them to any appropriate MeSH® terms. This enables keywords to more effectively search *both* indexed and nonindexed citations in PubMed®. In addition, a particular logic has been built into automatic term mapping to make it even more effective. There are three steps to this process:

1. **MeSH® term:** Automatic term mapping first looks for a match between what is typed into the search box and a table of MeSH® terms. If there is a match with a MeSH® term, the MeSH® term plus the keyword will be used to run the search.
2. **Journal title:** If there is no match with a MeSH® term, what has been typed in the search box is next compared with a table of journal titles. If there is a match, the journal title is used to run the search.
3. **Author name:** If there is no match with either a MeSH® term or a journal title, the words in the search box are then compared with a table of author names. If there is a match, that author name is used to run the search.

Automatic term mapping begins with the words entered into the search box as a single unit. If it cannot find a match in any of the three tables, it will drop the word that is farthest to the right in the search string, look at the remaining words, and run through the three steps of automatic term mapping, looking for a match. If a match is found, then automatic term mapping will use the match (MeSH® term, journal title, or author name) plus the keyword as part of the search and return to process the term that was previously dropped (the term farthest to the right in the search string).

Box 3.2   # Details of PubMed Automatic Term Mapping for Breast Cancer

"breast neoplasms"[MeSH Terms] OR ("breast"[All Fields] AND "neoplasms"[All Fields]) OR "breast neoplasms"[All Fields] OR ("breast"[All Fields] AND "cancer"[All Fields]) OR "breast cancer"[All Fields]

◆ The "breast neoplasms"[MeSH Terms] portion of the search will retrieve relevant information from the indexed portion of the MEDLINE database, since breast cancer is not a MeSH term.
◆ The ("breast"[All Fields] AND "neoplasms"[All Fields]) OR "breast neoplasms" [All Fields] OR ("breast"[All Fields] AND "cancer"[All Fields]) OR "breast cancer"[All Fields] portion of the search will retrieve information from the nonindexed portion of the database.

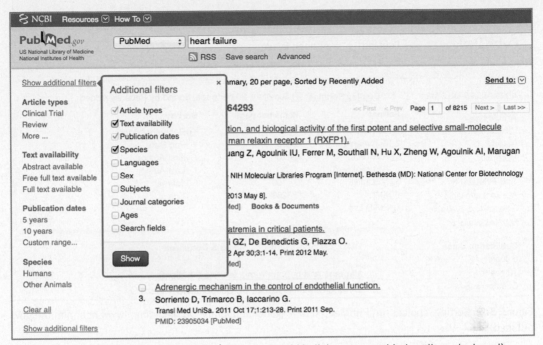

Figure 3.4: Filters in PubMed. (From National Library of Medicine, www.ncbi.nlm.nih.gov/pubmed)

An example of automatic term mapping is presented in Box 3.2. Using the following PICOT question, *How do women (P) diagnosed with breast cancer (I) perceive their own mortality (O)?* you begin with typing *breast cancer* as one of the search terms in the search box in PubMed® and run the search. To better understand the results, click on "Details," which shows how PubMed® used automatic term mapping to process the search.

Once a search has been run, PubMed® provides the option to further refine retrieval by using filters. Some of these filters are called limits in other databases. To access these filters, click on the Show Additional Filters located on the left of the page. Limiting to certain dates of publication, certain languages, human or animal studies, and types of publications (e.g., clinical trial, meta-analysis) are some of the options. Figure 3.4 shows some examples of the many filters that can be applied.

When reviewing search results in PubMed®, it is important to note that search results appear in the order in which they were added to the database. This means that the first citation is the citation that meets the search criteria and was most recently added to the database. To find the most recently published article, use the "Sort by Pub Date" option that can be found in the Display Settings dropdown menu (Figure 3.5).

The search strategy carefully designed using PICOT as a guide is entered into the search box in PubMed® and run. Appropriate limits are applied, and the results sorted. To further separate the citations of interest from others, PubMed® provides the Send To options (e.g., e-mail, clipboard; Figure 3.6).

This has been a brief introduction to PubMed®. Additional information on searching PubMed® can be found in:

◆ Tutorials: PubMed® home page under Using PubMed or directly from http://www.nlm.nih.gov/bsd/disted/pubmed.html
◆ PubMed Help: http://www.ncbi.nlm.nih.gov/books/NBK3827
◆ PubMed Quick Start Guide: http://www.ncbi.nlm.nih.gov/books/NBK3827/#pubmedhelp.PubMed_Quick_Start
◆ Healthcare librarians in your facility or in a partnering agency

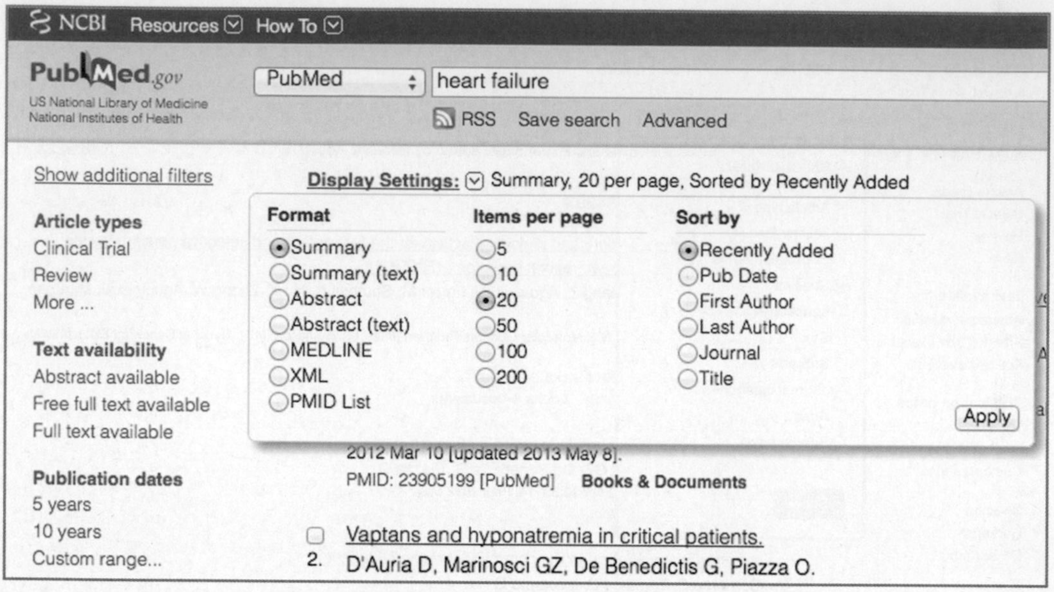

Figure 3.5: Sorting choices in PubMed. (From National Library of Medicine, www.ncbi.nlm.nih.gov/pubmed)

Tool 4: Help Finding the Needle: Specialized Search Functions

Many databases have specialized search functions to help busy clinicians find evidence as quickly as possible. This section discusses the specific search functions available in PubMed®, Ovid, and EBSCOhost® that can assist in finding relevant evidence quickly.

PubMed® Special Queries

PubMed® provides several filters for busy clinicians to quickly find the needle in their haystack. Clinicians may wish to explore two, Clinical Queries and Health Services Research Queries. Both are freely available and are easily accessed via the Clinical Queries or Topic-Specific Queries link under PubMed Tools on the PubMed® home page. These search filters were developed by Haynes and associates, and enable the busy clinician to single out specific clinical research areas they are interested in without refining their own search strategy further (PubMed®, 2013).

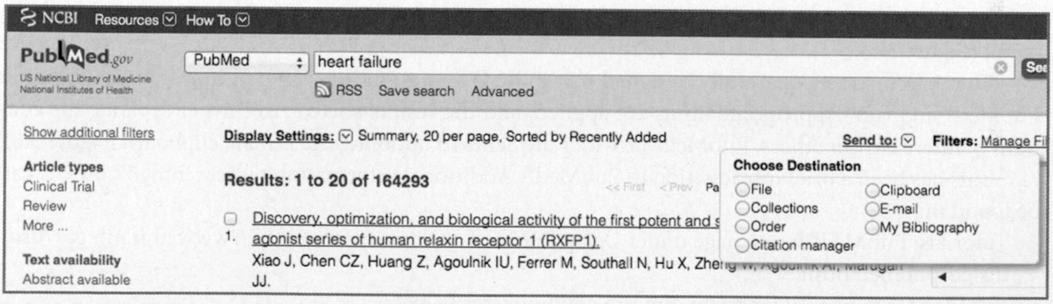

Figure 3.6: "Send to" options in PubMed. (From National Library of Medicine, www.ncbi.nlm.nih.gov/pubmed)

Clinical Queries. **Clinical Queries** provides two very useful search options: Clinical Study Category and Systematic Reviews. Search by Clinical Study Category provides a quick way to limit results to a specific study category. When using this feature, search terms are entered in the query box, the type of clinical question must be selected (etiology, diagnosis, therapy, prognosis, or clinical prediction guide), and the scope of the search is selected (broad or narrow), as shown in Figure 3.7 (see also Table 3.2).

When a search is run, PubMed® applies specific search filters to limit retrieval to the desired evidence. This means that PubMed® automatically adds terms to the search in order to find the type of evidence needed. A quick look at the Details box after running a search will show what terms were added. PubMed® also provides a link to the filter table that shows the different search filters and the terms associated with them.

Systematic reviews are retrieved automatically when you enter your keyword in the search box on the Clinical Query page (see Figure 3.7).

Health Services Research. **Health Services Research (HSR) Queries** is a search filter that finds PubMed® citations relating to healthcare quality or healthcare costs, e.g., Appropriateness, Process assessment, Outcomes assessment, Costs, Economics, Qualitative research, and Quality improvement. It was developed by the National Information Center on Health Services Research and Health Care Technology (NICHSR), and is accessed via the Topic-Specific Queries link under PubMed Tools on the PubMed® home page. Available study categories are displayed in Figure 3.8. If you find that you require this specialized filtering it is wise to consult a librarian for extra guidance.

 More information about PubMed® special queries can be found at **http://www.nlm.nih.gov/bsd/special_queries.html**

Clinical Queries in Ovid

Ovid Clinical Queries (OCQ) limits retrieval to best evidence and what Ovid refers to as clinically sound studies. To access OCQ, a searcher enters search statements in the main search box. Results are displayed on Ovid's main search page within Search History. To limit retrieved results, select Additional Limits to view Ovid's menu of limits. Find the Clinical Queries' dropdown menu and select the clinical query that best serves the purposes of your PICOT question.

S NCBI   Resources ⊘ How To ⊘   Sign in to NCB

PubMed Clinical Queries

Results of searches on this page are limited to specific clinical research areas. For comprehensive searches, use PubMed directly.

| heart failure   ⊗ | **Search** |

Clinical Study Categories   **Systematic Reviews**   **Medical Genetics**

Category: [Therapy   ⬍]   Topic: [All   ⬍]
Scope: [Etiology
           Diagnosis
           Therapy
           Prognosis
           Clinical prediction guides]

Results: 5 ~~of 5~~   **Results: 5 of 3559**   **Results: 5 of 8566**

Vaptans and hyponatremia in critical patients.   Exercise training undertaken by people within 12   Adult Cardiac Expression of the Activating
D'Auria D, Marinosci GZ, De Benedictis G, Piazza O.   months of lung resection for non-small cell lung   Transcription Factor 3, ATF3, Promotes Ventricular
Transl Med UniSa. 2012 May; 3:1-14. Epub 2012 Apr 30.   cancer.   Hypertrophy.
                                                   Cavalheri V, Tahirah F, Nonoyama M, Jenkins S, Hill K.   Koren L, Elhanani O, Kehat I, Hai T, Aronheim A.
Exercise training undertaken by people within 12   Cochrane Database Syst Rev. 2013 Jul 31; 7:CD009955.   PLoS One. 2013; 8(7):e68396. Epub 2013 Jul 3.
months of lung resection for non-small cell lung   Epub 2013 Jul 31.
cancer.   Barth syndrome.

Figure 3.7: Clinical study categories in PubMed®. (From National Library of Medicine, www.ncbi.nlm.nih.gov/pubmed)

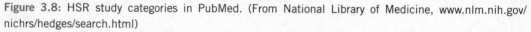

Figure 3.8: HSR study categories in PubMed. (From National Library of Medicine, www.nlm.nih.gov/nichrs/hedges/search.html)

The OCQ dropdown menu offers limits that retrieve clinically sound studies. Searchers select a query based on what the PICOT question is targeting (e.g., therapy, diagnosis, prognosis, reviews, clinical prediction guides, qualitative studies, etiology, costs, economics). Additionally, within each query, there are options to further refine the search. The refinement options include "Sensitive" (i.e., most relevant articles but probably some less relevant ones), "Specific" (i.e., mostly relevant articles but probably omitting a few), and "Optimized" (i.e., the combination of terms that optimizes the trade-off between sensitivity and specificity). Again, consult your healthcare librarian if you need help with using Ovid's clinical queries.

Evidence-Based Practice "Limiter" in CINAHL

Databases typically offer options for limiting search results to allow quick retrieval of the most relevant and focused citations. "Limiters" that are commonly offered allow you to narrow your citation search by options such as publication type, age groups, gender, clinical queries, language, peer reviewed, and full text. CINAHL provides an additional option within its Special Interest category of limits called Evidence-Based Practice. Selecting the EBP limiter allows you to narrow your results to articles from EBP journals, about EBP, research articles (including systematic reviews, clinical trials, meta-analyses, and so forth), and commentaries on research studies.

A Final Tool: Time and Money

Producing, maintaining, and making databases available is financially costly and time-consuming. Although computer technology has revolutionized the print industry and made it easier to transfer documents and information around the world in seconds, the task of producing databases still relies on people to make decisions about what to include and how to index it. Databases produced by government agencies, such as MEDLINE®, are produced with public money and are either very inexpensive or without cost to the searcher. The MEDLINE® database is available to anyone in the world who has access to the Internet through PubMed®. The data in MEDLINE® can be leased by vendors and placed in a variety of databases that will be accessed by healthcare providers, librarians, and others. Private organizations that produce biomedical databases, such as CINAHL or the CDSR, license their products. If there is no in-house library, it is worth the time and effort to locate libraries in the area and find out their access policies for these databases.

For clinicians to practice based on evidence, access to databases is essential. Costs for supporting databases include licensing fees, hardware, software, Internet access, and library staff to facilitate its use (if available). Institutions must make decisions about what databases to subscribe to, and these decisions may be based on the resources available. Not all healthcare providers have libraries in their facilities. In these situations, clinicians or departments can consult with partnering librarians about securing access to databases that they consider critical to evidence-based care.

Although there is a cost associated with searching databases for relevant evidence, regular searching for answers to clinical questions has been shown to save money. Researchers conducted an outcome-based, prospective study to measure the economic impact of MEDLINE® searches on the cost both to the patient and to the participating hospitals (Klein, Ross, Adams, & Gilbert, 1994). They found that searches conducted early (i.e., in the first half) in patients' hospital stays resulted in significantly lower cost to the patients and to the hospitals, as well as shorter lengths of stay. Almost 10 years later, a multisite study found that physicians, residents, and nurses who utilized library and information resources reported a 7% reduction in length of stay (Marshall et al., 2013).

Clinicians must remember the costs of both searching and obtaining relevant evidence, as well as the costs of not searching for and applying relevant evidence. Computerized retrieval of medical information is a fairly complex activity. It begins by considering the kind of information needed, creating an answerable PICOT question, planning and executing the search in appropriate databases, and analyzing the retrieved results.

> Do not go where the path may lead, go instead where there is no path and leave a trail.
> —Ralph Waldo Emerson

HOW TO KNOW YOU HAVE FOUND THE NEEDLE

Successfully searching for relevant evidence is as important as asking a well-built PICOT question. For clinicians to get the answers they need to provide the best care to their patients, they must choose appropriate databases; design an appropriate search strategy using keyword, title, and subject headings; use limits; and successfully navigate in the databases they are searching. In addition, clinicians must consider the cost of *not* searching for the best evidence. Commitment to finding valid, reliable evidence is the foundation for developing the skills that foster a sound search strategy which, in turn, helps to reduce frustration and save time. Box 3.3 contains the steps of an efficient search.

The key to knowing whether the needle has been found is to further evaluate the selected studies from a successfully executed search. This evaluation method is called *critical appraisal*, the next step in the EBP process (see Chapters 4–7). Some journals are dedicated to the pre-appraisal of existing literature. Most of these articles are not syntheses (e.g., systematic reviews), but rather critical appraisals of current single studies. For example, the journal *Evidence-Based Nursing* reviews over 50 journals and about 25,000 articles per year. They identify and publish approximately 96 reviews of articles (both quantitative and qualitative) annually. The *ACP Journal Club* is another publication dedicated to pre-appraised literature. More than 100 journals are scanned for evidence relevant to clinicians. Specific criteria are applied to the appraised articles, and the appraisals are published bimonthly in the journal.

Box 3.3 Steps to an Efficient Search to Answer a Clinical Question

◆ Begin with PICOT question—generates keywords.
◆ Establish inclusion/exclusion criteria *before* searching so that the studies that answer the question are easily identifiable. Apply these criteria after search strategy is complete.
◆ Use subject headings, when available.
◆ Expand the search using the explode option, if not automatic.
◆ Use available mechanisms to focus the search so that the topic of interest is the main point of the article.
◆ Combine the searches generated from the PICOT keywords that mapped onto subject headings, if the database does not automatically do this for you.
◆ Limit the *final* cohort of studies with meaningful limits, such as language, human, type of study, age, and gender.
◆ Organize studies in a meaningful way using reference management software.

These types of journals assist the clinician in reducing the time it takes from asking the question to applying valid evidence in clinical decision making.

....
Do what you can, with what you have, where you are.
—Theodore Roosevelt
....

NEXT STEPS

What can be done when a thorough search to answer a compelling clinical question yields either too little valid evidence to support confident practice change (i.e., inconclusive evidence) or no evidence? In most cases, clinicians are not in positions to do full-scale, multisite clinical trials to determine the answer to a clinical question, and the science may not be at the point to support such an investigation. However, determining what is effective in the clinician's own practice by implementing the best evidence available can generate internal evidence. In addition, generating external evidence by conducting smaller scale studies, either individually or with a team of researchers, is an option. Chapters 19 and 20 address how to generate evidence to answer clinical questions. However, the starting place for addressing any clinical issue is to gather and evaluate the existing evidence using strategies and methods described in this chapter.

EBP FAST FACTS

◆ Good searching starts with a well-formulated clinical question.
◆ Searching takes skills and practice (i.e., time).
◆ Searching all relevant databases is essential to find the body of evidence to answer a PICOT question.
◆ Although limiting to full text can be a useful tool to get a rapid return on a search, there may be relevant studies that are not captured in such a limited search.

- PubMed is a free database that uses automatic mapping for subject headings.
- Boolean connectors are AND (narrows search) and OR (expands search).
- There are three approaches to searching and should be used in this order: (1) keywords (from PICOT question); (2) subject headings; (3) title (if necessary).
- Title searches should be used when too much evidence is found.

References

British Thoracic Society, & Scottish Intercollegiate Guidelines Network. (2012). *British guideline on the management of asthma* (Revised ed.). Edinburgh, Scotland: Scottish Intercollegiate Guidelines Network.

Haynes, B. (2007). Of studies, syntheses, synopses, summaries, and systems: The "5S" evolution of information services for evidence-based healthcare decisions. *Evidence-Based Nursing, 10*(1), 6–7.

Institute of Medicine (US) Roundtable on Evidence-Based Medicine. Leadership Commitments to Improve Value in Healthcare: Finding Common Ground: Workshop Summary. Washington (DC): *National Academies Press (US)*; 2009.

Klein, M. S., Ross, F. V., Adams, D. L., & Gilbert, C. M. (1994). Effect of online literature searching on length of stay and patient care costs. *Academic Medicine, 69,* 489–495.

Lefebvre, C., Manheimer, E., & Glanville, J. (2011a). Chapter 6: Searching for studies. In J. P. T. Higgins & S. Green (Eds.), *Cochrane handbook for systematic reviews of interventions* (Version 5.1.0). Online: Cochrane Collaboration.

Lefebvre, C., Manheimer, E., & Glanville, J. (2011b). 6.2.1 Bibliographic databases. In J. P. T. Higgins & S. Green (Eds.), *Cochrane handbook for systematic reviews of interventions* (Version 5.1.0). Online: Cochrane Collaboration.

Lefebvre, C., Manheimer, E., & Glanville, J. (2011c). 6.2.1.8 Grey literature databases. In J. P. T. Higgins & S. Green (Eds.), *Cochrane handbook for systematic reviews of interventions* (Version 5.1.0). Online: Cochrane Collaboration.

Marshall, J. G., Sollenberger, J., Easterby-Gannett, S., Morgan, L., Klem, M. L., Cavanaugh, S. K., & Hunter, S. (2013). The value of library and information services in patient care: Results of a multisite study. *Journal of the Medical Library Association, 101*(1), 38–46. doi:10.3163/1536-5050.101.1.007

National Library of Medicine. (2013). *Fact sheet: PubMed®: MEDLINE® retrieval on the world wide web.* Retrieved April 26, 2013, from http://www.nlm.nih.gov/pubs/factsheets/pubmed.html

National Library of Medicine. (2005). *PubMed help [internet].* Bethesda (MD): National Center for Biotechnology Information (US) [updated March 25, 2014].

Nourbakhsh, E., Nugent, R., Wang, H., Cevik, C., & Nugent, K. (2012). Medical literature searches: A comparison of PubMed and Google scholar. *Health Information & Libraries Journal, 29*(3), 214–222. doi:10.1111/j.1471-1842.2012.00992.x

Olson, C. A. (2013). Using the grey literature to enhance research and practice in continuing education for health professionals. *Journal of Continuing Education in the Health Professions, 33*(1), 1–3. doi:10.1002/chp.21159

PubMed clinical queries. Retrieved April 14, 2013, from http://www.ncbi.nlm.nih.gov/pubmed/clinical

Richardson, W. S., Wilson, M. C., Nishikawa, J., & Hayword, R. S. (1995). The well-built clinical question: A key to evidence-based decisions, *ACP J Club, 123*(3), A12–A13.

Stevens, K. R. (2001). Systematic reviews: The heart of evidence-based practice. *AACN Clinical Issues: Advanced Practice in Acute and Critical Care, 12*(4), 529–538.

Stillwell, S. B., Fineout-Overholt, E., Melnyk, B. M., & Williamson, K. M. (2010). Evidence-based practice, step by step: Searching for the evidence. *American Journal of Nursing, 110*(5), 41–47. doi:10.1097/01.NAJ.0000372071.24134.7e

Tee, A., Koh, M. S., Gibson, P. G., Lasserson, T. J., Wilson, A., & Irving, L. B. (2007). Long-acting beta2-agonists versus theophylline for maintenance treatment of asthma. *Cochrane Database of Systematic Reviews, 3.* Art. No.: CD001281. doi:10.1002/14651858.CD001281.pub2

Walters, E. H., Walters, J. A. E., & Gibson, P. G. (2002). Regular treatment with long acting beta agonists versus daily regular treatment with short acting beta agonists in adults and children with stable asthma. *Cochrane Database of Systematic Reviews, 3.* Art. No.: CD003901. doi:10.1002/14651858.CD003901

Younger, P. (2010). Using Google scholar to conduct a literature search. *Nursing Standard, 24*(45), 40–46.

Wright A; Pang J; Feblowitz JC; Maloney FL; Wilcox AR; Ramelson HZ; Schneider LI; Bates DW (2011). A method and knowledge base for automated inference of patient problems from structured data in an electronic medical record. *Journal of the American Medical Informatics Association, 18*(6), 859–67.

Using Evidence-Based Practice to Reduce Catheter-Associated Urinary Tract Infections in a Long-Term Acute Care Facility

Tina L. Magers, MSN, RN-BC

Nursing Professional Development and Research Coordinator
Mississippi Baptist Health Systems
Jackson, Mississippi

Step 0: The Spirit of Inquiry Ignited

Long-term acute care hospitals (LTACHs) are particularly challenged with healthcare-associated infections due to their population experiencing complicated healthcare conditions and an average length of stay of greater than 25 days. Catheter-associated urinary tract infections (CAUTIs) are the most common hospital-associated infections. Approximately 25% of all hospitalized patients will experience a short-term urethral catheter (UC) (Gould et al., 2009). The most common mitigating factor in all patients with UC is the number of days catheterized. Multiple studies have described reminder systems that significantly reduced the number of catheter days (CDs), and excellent results have been achieved when a nurse-driven protocol is used to evaluate the necessity of continued urethral catheterization. A multidisciplinary team spearheaded by an evidence-based practice (EBP) mentor led an EBP change project to reduce CAUTIs, which were problematic, in the Mississippi Hospital for Restorative Care in Jackson, Mississippi. The team wondered what evidence existed that could inform a practice change to reduce CAUTIs in their institution. Stakeholders included the staff nurses, unit educator, nurse manager, and the medical director of the LTACH. Infection preventionists, accreditation director, and quality improvement staff also participated.

Step 1: The PICOT Question Formulated

In adult patients hospitalized in an LTACH (P), how does the use of a nurse-driven protocol for evaluating the appropriateness of short-term UC continuation or removal (I), compared to no protocol (C), affect the number of CDs (O_1) and CAUTI rates (O_2) over a 6-month postintervention period (T)?

Step 2: Search Strategy Conducted

Guided by the PICOT question, a systematic literature search was conducted. The databases searched included the Cumulative Index to Nursing and Allied Health Literature (CINAHL), Cochrane Database of Systematic Reviews (CDSR), Cochrane Central Register of Controlled Trials, the Database of Abstracts of Reviews of Effects (DARE), Ovid Clinical Queries, and PubMed. Keyword and controlled vocabulary searches included the following terms: *catheter-related; urinary catheterization; urinary tract infection, prevention, and control; catheter-associated,* limited to *urinary,* and *protocol.* Including hand searches, the search yielded over 69 background articles, 6 systematic reviews, 6 major guidelines, and 37 studies for rapid critical appraisal and synthesis.

Step 3: Critical Appraisal of the Evidence Performed

The purpose of rapid critical appraisal is to determine whether the literature identified in the search is "relevant, valid, reliable, and applicable to the clinical question" (Melnyk, Fineout-Overholt, Stillwell, & Williamson, 2010). In appraising the sources, the following were considered: the level of evidence, whether the studies and reviews were well conducted, and the degree to which each answered the clinical question (Fineout-Overholt, Melnyk, Stillwell, & Williamson, 2010a). Although no studies were found involving patients in LTACHs, the studies about patients in acute and critical care facilities were considered relevant to the clinical question because patients in such facilities require hospital-level care, though for shorter periods.

Through rapid critical appraisal, 14 individual studies and one systematic review were identified for synthesis. In order to organize these studies, an evaluation table was created, and synthesis tables were developed to clarify similarities and differences among the findings (Fineout-Overholt, Melnyk, Stillwell, & Williamson, 2010b). Levels of evidence ranged from level I, which represents the highest quality, seen in systematic reviews, to level VI, which characterizes descriptive studies (Fineout-Overholt et al., 2010a). The studies were a broad collection with seven international studies and eight from the United States, all published from 1999 to 2011. The samples aggregated to over 17,000 subjects. Fourteen of the 15 studies used a protocol to reduce device days and CAUTIs; however, no two studies used identical protocols. The body of evidence indicated a variety of independent variables with minimal risk and encouraged early removal of UCs to reduce CAUTI rates and CDs. All studies that reported CDs and/or CAUTI rates had results trending in the desired direction of reduction, and most showed statistically significant results (Apisarnthanarak et al., 2007; Benoist et al., 1999; Bruminhent, Keegan, Lakhani, Roberts, & Passalacqua, 2010; Crouzet et al., 2007; Elpern et al., 2009; Fuchs, Sexton, Thornlow, & Champagne, 2011; Goetz, Kedzuf, Wagener, & Muder, 1999; Hakvoort, Elberink, Vollebregt, Van der Ploeg, & Emanuel, 2004; Huang et al., 2004; Loeb et al., 2008; Meddings, Rogers, Macy, & Saint, 2010; Reilly et al., 2006; Rothfeld & Stickley, 2010; Saint, Kaulfman, Thompson, Rogers, & Chenoweth, 2005; Topal et al., 2005). These were the keeper studies that provided the body of evidence upon which to make an EBP change.

Step 4: Evidence Integrated With Clinical Expertise and Patient Preferences to Inform a Decision and Practice Change Implemented

The best patient outcomes result when a change in practice is based on the best evidence and combined with clinical expertise and patient preferences (Melnyk et al., 2010). Such integration involves team building, institutional approval, project planning, and implementation. Building a team with input from a wide range of stakeholders and gaining their trust lend valuable support to EBP projects and promote a culture that is supportive of future projects (Gallagher-Ford, Fineout-Overholt, Melnyk, & Stillwell, 2011).

The project team's role was established by defining the goals and purpose. Upon review of the external and internal evidence, the stakeholders agreed that the goal was to improve the quality of the care provided using best practice and their purpose was to design, implement, and evaluate an innovative approach based on the evidence to reduce CDs and CAUTIs by using a nurse-driven protocol. Based on the literature, a protocol was written listing eight criteria for the continuation of a short-term UC. During this phase of the project, it was important to collaborate with the physician medical director of the hospital and receive his support. The draft protocol was presented with the evidence to the medical executive committee of the hospital. It received final approval without difficulty. An institutional review board (IRB) application was written for approval of the EBP project and data collection. It gained approval as a minimal-risk project.

Project planning included designing the process for change in practice. Realizing that the key to reducing CAUTI risk was to compare their daily patient assessments with the eight appropriate indications for UC continuation, the nurses decided that the best way to promote consistent use of the protocol was to express the protocol in algorithm form. An education plan was designed and implemented by the staff nurses in small group inservices. The EBP mentor contributed written tools for nursing staff and the physicians including handouts and unit posters.

Step 5: Outcomes Evaluated

The evaluation of outcomes included finding data sources for device days and CAUTIs, which the infection preventionist provided to the team. The SPSS version 18 software was used to compare a baseline of 12 months to 6 months of postintervention data. The results demonstrated outcomes congruent with the evidence showing a significant reduction in CDs [↓ 26.1%; $P \leq 0.001$ (MD 3.43 days; 95% CI, 2.99 to 3.87)] and a clinically significant reduction in CAUTI rates [↓ 33%; $P = 0.486$ (MD 1.34 days; 95% CI, -1.74 to 4.44)]. The CDs reduced with statistical significance and the CAUTI rates reduced by 33%; however, this finding was not statistically significant. Our results indicated that CDs and CAUTIs were nurse-sensitive indicators that can be mitigated by nursing judgment and implementation of best practices based on the evidence.

Step 6: Project Outcomes Successfully Disseminated

The team disseminated the project and its outcomes to both internal and external audiences. Internally, reports were provided to the Nursing Quality Council, Nursing EBP and Research Council, Nursing Leadership Council, Organization Infection Control Committee, Clinical Improvement Committee, and unit staff through a communication fair. A final report was sent to the hospital IRB Committee. Externally, the project was presented at a local Sigma Theta Tau (STTI) Chapter, Region 8 STTI Conference, 2012 Nurse Manager Congress, and at the Ohio State University Center for Transdisciplinary Evidence-based Practice (CTEP) immersion workshop, *Evidence-Based Practice: Making It a Reality in Your Organization* (2012, 2013). In June 2013, a manuscript was published in the *American Journal of Nursing* (Magers, 2013).

References

Apisarnthanarak, A., Thongphubeth, K., Sirinvaravong, S., Kitkangvan, D., Yuekyen, C., Warachan, B., … Fraser, V. J. (2007). Effectiveness of multifaceted hospital-wide quality improvement programs featuring an intervention to remove unnecessary urinary catheters at a tertiary care center in Thailand. *Infection Control Hospital Epidemiology, 28*(7), 791–798.

Benoist, S., Panis, Y., Denet, C., Mauvais, F., Mariani, P., & Valleur, P. (1999). Optimal duration of urinary drainage after rectal resection: A randomized controlled trial. *Surgery, 125*(2), 135–141.

Bruminhent, J., Keegan, M., Lakhani, A., Roberts, I., & Passalacqua, J. (2010). Effectiveness of a simple intervention for prevention of catheter-associated urinary tract infections in a community teaching hospital. *American Journal of Infection Control, 38*, 689–693.

Crouzet, J., Bertrand, X., Venier, A. G., Badoz, C., Hussson, C., & Talon, D. (2007). Control of the duration of urinary catheterization: Impact on catheter-associated urinary tract infection. *Journal of Hospital Infection, 67*, 253–257.

Elpern, E., Killeen, K., Ketchem, A., Wiley, A., Patel, G., & Lateef, G. (2009). Reducing use of indwelling urinary catheters and associated urinary tract infections. *American Journal of Critical Care, 18*, 535–541. doi:10.4037/ajcc2009938

Fineout-Overholt, E., Melnyk, B. M., Stillwell, S. B., & Williamson, K. M. (2010a). Evidence-based practice: Step by step: Critical appraisal of the evidence: Part I. *American Journal of Nursing, 110*(7), 47–52.

Fineout-Overholt, E., Melnyk, B. M., Stillwell, S. B., & Williamson, K. M. (2010b). Evidence-based practice: Step by step: Critical appraisal of the evidence: Part II. *American Journal of Nursing, 110*(9), 41–48.

Fuchs, M., Sexton, D., Thornlow, D., & Champagne, M. (2011). Evaluation of an evidence-based nurse-driven checklist to prevent hospital-acquired catheter-associated urinary tract infections in intensive care units. *Journal of Nursing Care Quality, 26*, 101–109. doi:10.1097/NCQ.0b013e3181fb7847

Gallagher-Ford, L., Fineout-Overholt, E., Melnyk, B., & Stillwell, S. (2011). Evidence-based practice step by step: Implementing an evidence-based practice change. *American Journal of Nursing, 111*(3), 54–60.

Goetz, A. M., Kedzuf, S., Wagener, M., & Muder, R. R. (1999). Feedback to nursing staff as an intervention to reduce catheter-associated urinary tract infections. *American Journal of Infection Control, 27*, 402–404.

Gould, C., Umscheid, C., Agarwal, R., Kuntz, G., Peguess, D., & Centers for Disease Control and Prevention Healthcare Infection Control Practices Advisory Committee (HICPAC). (2009). *Guideline for prevention of catheter-associated urinary tract infections 2009*. Retrieved from http://www.cdc.gov/hicpac/pdf/CAUTI/CAUTIguideline2009final.pdf

Hakvoort, R. A., Elberink, R., Vollebregt, A., Van der Ploeg, I., & Emanuel, M. H. (2004). How long should urinary bladder catheterisation be continued after vaginal prolapse surgery? A randomized controlled trial comparing short term *versus* long term catheterisation after vaginal prolapse surgery. *British Journal of Obstetric Gynaecology, 111*, 828–830. doi:10.111/j.1471-0528.2004.00181.x

Huang, W. C., Wann, S. R., Lin, S. L., Kunin, C. M., Kung, M. H., Lin, C. H., ... Lin, T. W. (2004). Catheter-associated urinary tract infections in intensive care units can be reduced by prompting physicians to remove unnecessary catheters. *Infection Control and Hospital Epidemiology, 25*(11), 974–978.

Loeb, M., Hunt, D., O'Halloran, K., Carusone, S. C., Dafoe, N., & Walter, S. D. (2008). Stop orders to reduce inappropriate urinary catheterization in hospitalized patients: A randomized controlled trial. *Journal of General Internal Medicine, 23*(6), 816–820. doi:10.1007/s11606-008-0620-2

Magers, T. (2013). Using evidence-based practice to reduce catheter-associated urinary tract infections. *American Journal of Nursing, 113*(6), 34–42. doi:10.1097/01.NAJ.0000430923.07539.a7

Meddings, J., Rogers, M. A., Macy, M., & Saint, S. (2010). Systematic review and meta-analysis: Reminder systems to reduce catheter-associated urinary tract infections and urinary catheter use in hospitalized patients. *Clinical Infectious Disease, 51*(5), 550–560. doi:10.1086/655133

Melnyk, B. M., Fineout-Overholt, E., Stillwell, S. B., & Williamson, K. M. (2010). Evidence-based practice: Step by step: The seven steps of evidence-based practice. *American Journal of Nursing, 110*(1), 51–52.

Reilly, L., Sullivan, P., Ninni, S., Fochesto, D., Williams, K., & Fetherman, B. (2006). Reducing catheter device days in an intensive care unit: Using the evidence to change practice. *AACN Advanced Critical Care, 17*(3), 272–283.

Rothfeld, A. F., & Stickley, A. (2010). A program to limit urinary catheter use at an acute care hospital. *American Journal of Infection Control, 38*(7), 568–571. doi:10.1016/ajic.2009.12.017

Saint, S., Kaulfman, S. R., Thompson, M., Rogers, M. A., & Chenoweth, C. E. (2005). A reminder reduces urinary catheterization in hospitalized patients. *Joint Commission Journal on Quality and Patient Safety, 31*(8), 455–462.

Topal, J., Conklin, S., Camp, K., Morris, V., Balcezak, T., & Herbert, P. (2005). Prevention of nosocomial catheter-associated urinary tract infections through computerized feedback to physicians and a nurse-directed protocol. *American Journal of Medical Quality, 20*(3), 121–126. doi:10.1177/1062860605276074

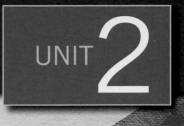

Step Three: Critically Appraising Evidence

Chapter 4
Critically Appraising Knowledge for Clinical Decision Making

Kathleen R. Stevens

> Knowledge, the object of Knowledge, and the Knower are the three factors which motivate action.
>
> —Friedrich von Schiller

In this unit, you will learn how to critically appraise quantitative and qualitative external evidence as well as integrate this evidence with patient preferences and your expertise. Chapter 4 provides an overview of foundational information that will help you maximize your learning in this unit.

Practitioners who want to know which actions to take in a given clinical situation are asking clinical questions. For example: (a) In adult surgical patients, how do videotaped preparation sessions compared to one-to-one counseling affect preoperative anxiety? and (b) In home-bound older adults, how does a fall prevention program compared to no fall prevention program affect the number of fall-related injuries? In an attempt to select the most effective action, each clinical decision made or action taken is based on knowledge. This knowledge may be derived from a variety of sources, such as research, theories, experience, tradition, trial and error, authority, or logical reasoning.

In addition to the knowledge gained from their clinical experiences, increasingly healthcare providers are compelled to create and use evidence from research to determine effective strategies for implementing system-based change to improve care processes and patient outcomes (IOM, 2011). Often, this array of knowledge and evidence is so diverse that clinicians are challenged to determine which action(s) will be the most effective in improving patient outcomes.

The critical appraisal of such evidence for decision making is one of the most valuable skills that the clinician can possess in today's healthcare environment. Distinguishing the best evidence from unreliable evidence and unbiased evidence from biased evidence lies at the root of the impact that clinicians' actions will have in producing their intended outcomes.

KNOWLEDGE SOURCES

The healthcare professions have made major inroads in identifying, understanding, and developing an array of knowledge sources that inform clinical decisions and actions. We now know that systematic inquiry in the form of research produces the most dependable knowledge upon which to base practice. In addition, practitioners' expertise and patients' choices and concerns must be taken into account in providing effective and efficient health care. Research, expertise, and client choices are all necessary evidence to integrate into decision making, but each alone is insufficient for best practice.

In the past, most clinical actions were based solely on logic, tradition, or conclusions drawn from keen observation (i.e., expertise). Although effective practices sometimes have evolved from these knowledge sources, the resulting practice has been successful less often than hoped for in reliably producing intended patient outcomes. Additionally, conclusions that are drawn solely from practitioner observations can be biased because such observations usually are not systematic. Similarly, non-evidence-based practices vary widely across caregivers and settings. The result is that, for a given health problem, a wide variety of clinical actions are taken without reliably producing the desired patient outcomes. That being said, the process for generating practice-based evidence (e.g., **quality improvement [QI] data or internal evidence**) has become increasingly rigorous and must be included in sources of knowledge for clinical decision making.

It is well recognized that systematic investigation (i.e., research) holds the promise of deepening our understanding of health phenomena, patients' responses to such phenomena, and the probable impact of clinical actions on resolving health problems. Following this realization, research evidence (i.e., **external evidence**) has become highly valued as the basis for clinical decisions.

The research utilization (RU) and evidenced-based practice (EBP) movements have escalated attention to the knowledge base of clinical care decisions and actions. In the mid-1970s, RU represented a rudimentary approach to using research as the prime knowledge source upon which to base practice. In the early stages of developing research-based practice when electronic sources of information were not readily available, RU approaches promoted using results from a single study as the basis for practice.

Several problems arise with this approach, particularly when more than one study on the same topic has been reported. Multiple studies can be difficult to summarize and may produce conflicting findings, and large and small studies may hold different conclusions. To improve the process of moving research knowledge into practice, mechanisms to enhance the external evidence produced through research have improved as well as more sophisticated and rigorous approaches for evaluating research have been developed. These approaches are largely embodied in the EBP paradigm.

....

What is important is to keep learning, to enjoy challenge, and to tolerate ambiguity. In the end there are no certain answers.
—Martina Horner

....

WEIGHING THE EVIDENCE

The EBP movement catapults the use of knowledge in clinical care to new heights of sophistication, rigor, and manageability. A key difference between the mandate to "apply research results in practice" and today's EBP paradigm is the acknowledgment of the relative weight and role of various knowledge sources as the bases for clinical decisions.

Best Practice and EBP

"Evidence" is now viewed and scrutinized from a clinical epidemiological perspective. This means that the practitioner takes into account the validity and reliability of the specific evidence when clinical recommendations are made (Fineout-Overholt, Melnyk, Stillwell, & Williamson, 2010a, 2010b, 2010c; Stevens, Abrams, Brazier, Fitzpatrick, & Lilford, 2001). The EBP approach addresses variation in ways of managing similar health problems and the deficit between scientific evidence and clinical practice. In other words, it makes clear the external evidence underlying effective practice (i.e., best practice) and specifies actions for addressing insufficient scientific evidence. In addition, EBP methods such as systematic reviews increase our ability to manage the ever-increasing volume of information produced in order to develop best practices. Indeed, systematic reviews are identified by QI experts as the key link between research and practice (IOM, 2008, 2011).

Best practice is not new to healthcare providers. For example, mandatory continuing education for licensure in many states is regulatory testimony to the value of staying abreast of new developments in health care. However, emphasis on best practice has shifted from keeping current through traditional continuing education to keeping current with the latest and best available evidence that has been critically appraised for quality and impact at the moment it is needed. Reliance on inexplicit or inferior knowledge sources (e.g., tradition or trial and error) is rapidly becoming unacceptable practice in today's quality-focused climate of health care. Rather, the focus is changing to replacing such practices with those based on a quality of knowledge that is said to include certainty and, therefore, predictability of outcome.

> **We don't receive wisdom; we must discover it for ourselves after a journey that no one can take for us or spare us.**
> **—Marcel Proust**

CERTAINTY AND KNOWLEDGE SOURCES

The goal of EBP is to use the highest quality of knowledge in providing care to produce the greatest positive impact on patients' health status and healthcare outcomes. This entails using the following knowledge sources for care:

- Valid research evidence as the primary basis of clinical decisions (i.e., external evidence)
- Clinical expertise to best use research by filling in gaps and combining it with practice-based evidence (i.e., internal evidence) to tailoring clinical actions for individual patients' contexts
- Patient choices and concerns for determining the acceptability of evidence-based care to the individual patient

In clinical decisions, the key criterion for quality of underlying knowledge is certainty. Certainty is the level of sureness that the clinical action will produce the intended or desired outcome. Because clinical actions are intended to assist patients in achieving a health goal, we can say with high certainty that what we do with patients is likely to move them toward that intended goal. To appraise certainty, the practitioner must first uncover the source of knowledge underlying the contemplated clinical action and then appraise the quality of that knowledge.

> **The intuitive mind is a sacred gift and the rational mind is a faithful servant.**
> **—Albert Einstein**

RATING STRENGTH OF THE SCIENTIFIC EVIDENCE

EBP experts have developed a number of taxonomies to rate varying levels of evidence as well as strength of evidence (i.e., the level of evidence plus the quality of evidence). These assessments of the strength of scientific evidence provide a mechanism to guide practitioners in evaluating research for its applicability to healthcare decision making. Most of these taxonomies or hierarchies of evidence are organized around various research designs. For example, when asking a question about interventions, many refer to the syntheses of randomized controlled trials (RCTs) as a research design of highest order, and most taxonomies include a full range of evidence, from systematic reviews of RCTs to expert opinions. However, simply leveling evidence is not sufficient for assessing quality or impact of evidence.

According to the Agency for Healthcare Research and Quality (AHRQ, 2002), grading the strength of a body of evidence should incorporate three domains: quality, quantity, and consistency. These are defined as follows:

- **Quality:** the extent to which a study's design, conduct, and analysis have minimized selection, measurement, and confounding biases (internal validity) (p. 19)

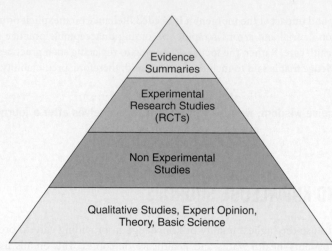

Figure 4.1: Strength of evidence rating pyramid. (© 2007 Stevens & Clutter. Used with permission.)

◆ **Quantity:** the number of studies that have evaluated the clinical issue, overall sample size across all studies, magnitude of the treatment effect, and strength from causality assessment for interventions, such as relative risk or odds ratio (p. 25)
◆ **Consistency:** whether investigations with both similar and different study designs report similar findings (requires numerous studies) (p. 25)

In an AHRQ study (2002) in which 109 resources for evaluating evidence were reviewed to determine whether they met the above criteria, 7 of 19 systems for reviewing evidence were judged to include all three domains. Four of the seven indicated that systematic reviews of a body of literature represented the highest level of evidence for interventions, and five of the seven included expert opinion as evidence. Box 1.3 presents a sample system to determine the level of evidence for intervention questions. The level combined with the quality of the evidence that is assessed through critical appraisal reflects the strength of evidence, which determines the impact. This is a key concept for clinicians to understand when applying external evidence to practice. Figure 4.1 illustrates a basic strength-of-evidence rating hierarchy for interventions (Stevens & Clutter, 2007). The higher the evidence is placed on the pyramid, the more confident the clinician can be that the intervention will cause the targeted health effect.

APPRAISING KNOWLEDGE SOURCES

Critical appraisal of evidence is a hallmark of EBP. Although critical appraisal is not new, it has become a core skill for those who plan to use evidence to support healthcare decisions (Stevens et al., 2001). The evolution of EBP from evidence-based medicine (EBM) has heavily influenced the current emphasis on critical appraisal of evidence. At times, EBP has been criticized as having a sole focus on appraisal of RCTs. However, EBM leaders did not intend for appraisal of RCTs to be the final point of critical appraisal. The *Cochrane Handbook for Systematic Reviews of Interventions* (Higgins & Green, 2011), the most highly developed methodological source for conducting systematic reviews, states that RCTs are the first focus of current systematic reviews; however, other evidence is reviewed when relevant, making explicit that the focus on RCTs is an interim situation (Box 4.1).

EBP methodologists are actively developing and using methods for systematically summarizing the evidence generated from a broad range of research approaches, including qualitative research. Evidence

---

Box 4.1	Randomized Controlled Trials and Systematic Reviews

Early on, the Cochrane Collaboration expressed through its colloquia and the *Cochrane Reviewers' Handbook*, an explanation of their focusing initial efforts on systematic reviews of RCTs: Such study designs are more likely to provide reliable information about "what works best" in comparing alternative forms of health care (Kunz, Vist, & Oxman, 2003). At the same time, the Collaboration highlighted the value of systematically reviewing other types of evidence, such as that generated by cohort studies, using the same principles that guide reviews of RCTs. "Although we focus mainly on systematic reviews of RCTs, we address issues specific to reviewing other types of evidence when this is relevant. Fuller guidance on such reviews is being developed." (Clarke & Oxman, 2003, no pagination)

---

from all health science disciplines and a broad array of healthcare topics, including nursing services, behavioral research, and preventive health, are available to answer clinical questions (Stevens, 2002).

The meaning of *evidence* is fully appreciated within the context of best practice, which includes the following (Stevens, 2002):

◆ Research evidence
◆ Clinical knowledge gained via the individual practitioner's experience
◆ Patients' and practitioners' preferences
◆ Basic principles from logic and theory

An important task in EBP is to identify which knowledge is to be considered as evidence for clinical decisions. The knowledge generated from quantitative and qualitative research, clinical judgment, and patient preferences forms the crucial foundation for practice. Depending on the particular source of knowledge, varying appraisal approaches can be used to determine its worth to practice. The chapters in Unit 2 describe appraisal approaches for the main types of evidence and knowledge to guide clinical practice:

◆ Evidence from quantitative research
◆ Evidence from qualitative research
◆ Clinical judgment
◆ Knowledge about patient concerns, choices, and values

The authors of the following chapters apply generic principles of evidence appraisal to the broad set of knowledge sources used in health care. The purpose of critically appraising these sources is to determine the certainty and applicability of knowledge, regardless of the source.

UNDERSTANDING INTERNAL EVIDENCE AND TRACKING OUTCOMES OF EVIDENCE-BASED PRACTICE

Evidence is a collection of facts that grounds one's belief that something is true. While external evidence is generated from rigorous research and is typically conducted to be used across clinical settings, internal evidence is that generated by outcomes management, QI, or EBP implementation projects. Unlike external evidence, the generation of internal evidence is intended to improve clinical practice and patient outcomes within the local setting where it is conducted (see Chapter 1).

A number of scientifically sound systems of quality indicators provide the foundational evidence for tracking quality of care over time. The value of such evidence is that impact of improvement in innovations can be traced, overall performance can be documented at regular intervals, and areas for improvement can be targeted for intervention. Several of these quality indicator systems offer opportunities for individual healthcare agencies to survey their own agencies and compare their results with national benchmarks (see Chapter 10). Three of these quality indicator systems that generate internal (i.e., practice-based) evidence are described in the following sections.

AGENCY FOR HEALTHCARE RESEARCH AND QUALITY NATIONAL HEALTHCARE QUALITY REPORT

A notable addition to national quality indicators in the United States (U.S.) is the AHRQ *National Healthcare Quality Report*. The purpose of the report is to track the state of healthcare quality for the nation on an annual basis. In terms of the number of measures and number of dimensions of quality, it is the most extensive ongoing examination of quality of care ever undertaken in the U.S. or in any major industrialized country worldwide (AHRQ, 2013).

This evidence is used as a gauge of improvement across the nation. These reports measure trends in effectiveness of care, patient safety, timeliness of care, patient centeredness, and efficiency of care. Through these surveys, clinicians can locate indices on quality measures, such as the percentage of heart attack patients who received recommended care when they reached the hospital or the percentage of children who received recommended vaccinations.

The first report, in 2004, found that high-quality health care is not yet a universal reality and that opportunities for preventive care are often missed, particularly opportunities in the management of chronic diseases in the U.S. Subsequent surveys have found both that healthcare quality is improving in small increments (about 1.5% to 2.3% improvement) and that more gains than losses are being made. Core measures of patient safety improvements reflect gains of only 1% (AHRQ, 2012). These national data as well as others described in the following sections can be helpful to organizations making clinical decisions. Best practice would be when these data are combined with external evidence supporting action to improve outcomes.

NATIONAL QUALITY FORUM

Other internal evidence useful in QI may be gleaned from a set of quality indicators that were developed by the National Quality Forum (NQF). The NQF is a not-for-profit membership organization created to develop and implement a national strategy for healthcare quality measurement and reporting. The NQF is regarded as a mechanism to bring about national change in the impact of healthcare quality on patient outcomes, workforce productivity, and healthcare costs. It seeks to promote a common approach to measuring healthcare quality and fostering system-wide capacity for QI (NQF, 2008).

Recently, the NQF endorsed a set of 15 consensus-based nursing standards for inpatient care. Known as the NQF-15, these measures represent processes and outcomes that are affected, provided, and/or influenced by nursing personnel. These factors and their structural proxies (e.g., skill mix and nurse staffing hours) are called *nursing-sensitive measures*. The NQF's endorsement of these measures marked a pivotal step in the efforts to increase the understanding of nurses' influence on inpatient hospital care and promote uniform metrics for use in internal QI and public reporting activities. The NQF-15 includes measures that examine nursing contributions to hospital care from three perspectives: patient-centered outcome measures (e.g., prevalence of pressure ulcers and inpatient falls), nursing-centered intervention measures (e.g., smoking cessation counseling), and system-centered measures (e.g., voluntary turnover and nursing care hours per patient day; NQF, 2008).

NATIONAL DATABASE OF NURSING QUALITY INDICATORS

In 1998, the National Database of Nursing Quality Indicators® (NDNQI®) was established by the American Nurses Association to facilitate continued indicator development and further our understanding of factors influencing the quality of nursing care. The NDNQI provides quarterly and annual reports on structure, process, and outcome indicators to evaluate nursing care at the unit level. The structure of nursing care is reflected by the supply, skill level, and education/certification of nursing staff. Process indicators reflect nursing care aspects such as assessment, intervention, and registered nurse job satisfaction. Outcome indicators reflect patient outcomes that are nursing-sensitive and improve if there is greater quantity or quality of nursing care, such as pressure ulcers, falls, and IV infiltrations. There is some overlap between NQF-15 and NDNQI as a result of the adoption of some of the NDNQI indicators into the NQF set. The NDNQI repository of nursing-sensitive indicators is used in further QI research.

COMBINING INTERNAL AND EXTERNAL EVIDENCE

At the core of local QI and generation of internal evidence is the planned effort to test a given change to determine its impact on the desired outcome. **The Plan-Do-Study-Act (PDSA) cycle** has become a widely adopted and effective approach to testing and learning about change on a small scale. In PDSA, a particular change is planned and implemented, results are observed (studied), and action is taken on what is learned. The PDSA cycle is considered a scientific method used in action-oriented learning (IHI, 2011; Speroff & O'Connor, 2004). The original approach is attributed to Deming and is based on repeated small trials, consideration of what has been learned, improvement, and retrial of the improvement. The PDSA cycle tests an idea by putting a planned change into effect on a temporary and small-trial basis and then learning from its impact. The approach suggests a conscious and rigorous testing of the new idea. (See Box 4.2 for the steps of the PDSA cycle.) Small-scale testing incrementally builds the knowledge about a change in a structured way. By learning from multiple small trials, the new idea can be advanced and implemented with a greater chance of success on a broad scale (IHI, 2010). Combining PDSA with external evidence that corroborates the practice change increases the effectiveness of the carefully evaluated outcome for sustained change.

Box 4.2   Four Stages of the PDSA Cycle

The four stages of the PDSA cycle include:
1. **PLAN:** Plan the change and observation.
2. **DO:** Try out the change on a small scale.
3. **STUDY:** Analyze the data and determine what was learned.
4. **ACT:** Refine the change, based on what was learned, and repeat the testing.

Finally, the action is based on the probability that the change will improve the outcome; however, without external evidence to support this improvement, the degree of certainty for any PDSA cannot be 100%.

OTHER QUALITY IMPROVEMENT INITIATIVES

New QI initiatives have put into play new expectations for generating evidence and sources and applications of evidence. The National Strategy for Quality Improvement in Health Care (DHHS, 2012) was established by the Department of Health and Human Services to serve as a blueprint across all sectors of the healthcare community—patients, providers, employers, health insurance companies, academic researchers, and all government levels—to prioritize QI efforts, share lessons, and measure collective success collective success. Success is targeted toward three aims: (1) improving the patient experience of care (including quality and satisfaction); (2) improving the health of populations; and (3) reducing the per capita cost of health care. With this national initiative comes the need to generate evidence about the effectiveness of improvement innovations in terms of the three aims as outcomes. National consensus on key quality measures is also evolving. Nurse scientists and their clinical partners will generate new evidence using these measures and the evidence will be suited for informing decisions about care and care delivery. In this new movement, *remaining current* will be an important challenge as the rapid-paced National Strategy achieves rapid-cycle testing of new healthcare delivery models and cost impact.

In the world of QI, practice-based evidence holds an important place. Such evidence detects the trends within a given setting so that improvement goals can be set against best practice. At the same time, a hybrid field of improvement science is emerging as a framework for research that focuses on healthcare delivery improvement. The goal of the field is to determine which improvement strategies work as we strive to assure safe and effective care (Stevens, 2013). In other words, the field generates evidence about EBP—how to process it and how to promote uptake and sustainment of it.

The importance of evidence on the topic of "integrating best practice into routine care" is suggested in the *Future of Nursing* report (IOM, 2010). This report recommends that, as best practices emerge, it is essential that all members of the healthcare team be actively involved in making QI changes. Together with members of other disciplines, nurses are called on to be leaders and active followers in contributing to these improvements at the individual level of care, as well as at the system level of care (IOM, 2010). Accountable leaders of integration of EBP will rely on results of improvement and implementation research to inform their improvement initiatives. The field is yet nascent; at the same time, nurses are leading in significant advances to produce the evidence needed for improvement (Stevens, 2009, 2012).

Another initiative affecting EBP is that of the Patient-Centered Outcomes Research Institute (PCORI). The stated mission of PCORI is as follows: "The Patient-Centered Outcomes Research Institute (PCORI) helps people make informed health care decisions, and improves health care delivery and outcomes, by producing and promoting high integrity, evidence-based information that comes from research guided by patients, caregivers and the broader health care community" (PCORI, 2013). The work of PCORI assures that new forms of evidence are entered into our decision making—that of the voice of the patient, family, and caregivers. In addition, patient-centered outcomes research results are formed in such a way that it is useful to these same stakeholders as they make informed healthcare decisions in assessing the value of various healthcare options and how well these meet their preferences.

OVERVIEWS OF FOLLOWING THREE CHAPTERS

Quantitative Evidence: Chapter 5

The nature of evidence produced through quantitative research varies according to the particular design utilized. Chapter 5, "Critically Appraising Quantitative Evidence for Clinical Decision Making," details the various types of quantitative research designs, including case studies, case–control studies, and cohort studies, as well as RCTs, and concludes with a discussion of systematic reviews. Distinctions among **narrative reviews**, **systematic reviews**, and **meta-analyses** are drawn. Helpful explanations about systematic reviews describe how data are combined across multiple research studies. Throughout, critical appraisal questions and hints are outlined.

Qualitative Evidence: Chapter 6

Given the original emphasis on RCTs (experimental research design) in EBP, some have inaccurately concluded that there is no role for qualitative evidence in EBP. Chapter 6, "Critically Appraising Qualitative Evidence for Clinical Decision Making," provides a compelling discussion on the ways in which qualitative research results answer clinical questions. The rich understanding of individual patients that emerges from qualitative research connects this evidence strongly to the elements of patient preferences and values—both important elements in implementation of EBP.

Patient Preferences and Values and Clinician Expertise in Evidence-Based Decision Making

Chapter 7, "Integration of Patient Preferences and Values and Clinician Expertise into Evidence-based Decision Making," outlines the roles of two important aspects of clinical care decision making: patient choices and concerns and clinical judgment. The discussion emphasizes patient preferences not only as perceptions of self and what is best but also as what gives meaning to a person's life. The role of clinical judgment emerges as the practitioner weaves together a narrative understanding of the patient's condition, which includes social and emotional aspects and historical facts. Clinical judgment is presented as a historical clinical understanding of an individual patient—as well as of psychosocial and biological sciences—that is to be combined with the evidence from scientific inquiry. The roles of clinical judgment, clinical expertise, and patient values, choices, and concerns are essential to evidence-based care.

Critical appraisal of evidence and knowledge used in clinical care is a requirement in professional practice. These chapters will provide a basis for understanding and applying the principles of evidence appraisal to improve health care.

....

Knowledge speaks, but wisdom listens
—Jimi Hendrix

....

EBP FAST FACTS

◆ External evidence is scientific research.
◆ Internal evidence is clinically generated data.
◆ The strength of the evidence is a combination of the level of evidence in a hierarchy and how well the research was conducted and reported.
◆ QI is distinct from evidence-based practice and research.
◆ Critical appraisal of evidence is imperative for EBP to thrive.

References

Agency for Healthcare Research and Quality. (2002). *Systems to rate the strength of scientific evidence*. (AHRQ Publication No. 02-E016). Rockville, MD: Author. Retrieved July 24, 2013, from http://archive.ahrq.gov/clinic/epcarch.htm

Agency for Healthcare Research and Quality. (2012). *National healthcare quality report: Acknowledgments*. Rockville, MD: Agency for Healthcare Research and Quality. Retrieved May 2013, from www.ahrq.gov/research/findings/nhqrdr/nhqr12/acknow.html

Agency for Healthcare Research and Quality. (2013). *National healthcare quality report 2012*. (AHRQ Publication No. 13-0002). Retrieved July 25, 2013, from www.ahrq.gov/research/findings/nhqrdr/index.html

Clarke, Mike, and A. D. Oxman. "Cochrane Reviewers' Handbook 4.1. 6 [updated January 2003]." *The Cochrane Library* 1 (2003).

Department of Health and Human Services (DHHS). (2012). *2012 Annual progress report to congress*. Washington, DC: National Strategy for Quality Improvement in Health Care, March 2011.

Fineout-Overholt, E., Melnyk, B. M., Stillwell, S. B., & Williamson, K. M. (2010a). Evidence-based practice, step by step: Critical appraisal of the evidence: Part III. *American Journal of Nursing, 111*(11), 43–51.

Fineout-Overholt, E., Melnyk, B. M., Stillwell, S. B., & Williamson, K. M. (2010b). Evidence-based practice, step by step: Critical appraisal of the evidence: Part II. *American Journal of Nursing, 110*(9), 41–48.

Fineout-Overholt, E., Melnyk, B. M., Stillwell, S. B., & Williamson, K. M. (2010c). Evidence-based practice step by step: Critical appraisal of the evidence: Part I. *American Journal of Nursing, 110*(7), 47–52.

Higgins, J. P. T., & Green, S. (Eds.). (2011). *Cochrane handbook for systematic reviews of interventions* Version 5.1.0 [updated March 2011]. The Cochrane Collaboration, 2011. Available from www.cochrane-handbook.org

Institute for Healthcare Improvement (IHI). (2010). *Plan-Do-Study-Act (PDSA)*. Retrieved from http://www .ihi.org/knowledge/Pages/HowtoImprove/default.aspx. Accessed July 25, 2013.

Institute for Healthcare Improvement (IHI). (2011). *Science of improvement: Testing changes.* Retrieved from http://www.ihi.org/knowledge/Pages/HowtoImprove/ScienceofImprovementTestingChanges.aspx. Accessed August 25, 2013.

Institute of Medicine (IOM). (2008). *Knowing what works in health care: A roadmap for the nation*. Washington, DC: National Academies Press.

Institute of Medicine (IOM). (2010). *The future of nursing: Focus on scope of practice* [Committee on the Robert Wood Johnson Foundation Initiative on the Future of Nursing]. Washington, DC: National Academies Press.

Institute of Medicine (IOM). (2011). *Finding what works in health care: Standards for systematic reviews.* [Committee on Standards for Systematic Reviews of Comparative Effective Research; Board on Health Care Services]. Washington, DC: National Academies Press.

Kunz, R., Vist, G., & Oxman, A. D. (2003). Randomisation to protect against selection bias in healthcare trials (Cochrane Methodology Review). In *Cochrane Library, 1*. Oxford: Update Software.

National Quality Forum (NQF). (2008). *About us*. Retrieved July 24, 2013, from http://www.qualityforum.org/about/

Patient-Centered Outcomes Research Institute (PCORI). (2013). *Mission and vision.* Retrieved from http://pcori.org/about-us/mission-and-vision/. Accessed July 24, 2013.

Speroff, T., & O'Connor, G. T. (2004). Study designs for PDSA quality improvement research. *Quality Management in Health Care, 13*(1), 17–32.

Stevens, A., Abrams, K., Brazier, J., Fitzpatrick, R., & Lilford, R. (Eds.). (2001). *The advanced handbook of methods in evidence based healthcare.* London: Sage Publications.

Stevens, KR & Clutter, PC. (2007). Research and the Mandate for Evidence-based Quality, and Patient Safety. In (M Mateo & K Kirchhoff, eds.) *Research for advanced practice nurses: from evidence to practice.* New York: Springer Publishing Co.

Stevens, K. R. (2002). The truth, the whole truth...about EBP and RCTs. *Journal of Nursing Administration, 32*(5), 232–233.

Stevens, K. R. (2009). *A research network for improvement science: The Improvement Science Research Network, 2009.* ($3.1 million NIH 1 RC2 NR011946-01). Retrieved from http://era.nih.gov/commons/

Stevens, K. R. (2012). Delivering on the promise of EBP. *Nursing Management, 3*(3), 19–21.

Stevens, K. R. (2013). *What is improvement science?* Retrieved from www.ISRN.net. Accessed July 25, 2013.

Chapter 5

Critically Appraising Quantitative Evidence for Clinical Decision Making

Dónal P. O'Mathúna and Ellen Fineout-Overholt

The reason most people never reach their goals is that they don't define them, or ever seriously consider them as believable or achievable. Winners can tell you where they are going, what they plan to do along the way, and who will be sharing the adventure with them.

—Denis Watley

This chapter provides keys to understanding different types of quantitative research. Engaging it is much like the young lumberjack who, on the first day of his first job, felled numerous trees with his handsaw. The foreman was so impressed with the young man that he provided a chain saw for the next day's work. At the end of the second day, the foreman was shocked to find out that the young lumberjack had only taken down one tree the entire day. When the foreman started up the chain saw, the lumberjack jumped back and said, "Is that thing supposed to sound that way?" All day long he had been using the chain saw as the tool he knew how to use—the handsaw. Clinicians will need to invest in learning to use the tool of research, which includes both quantitative and qualitative designs (Chapter 6). It will take some time and effort, but the rewards will be rich for both clinicians and the patients for whom they care.

Clinicians read healthcare literature for various reasons. Some do it solely in an attempt to keep up to date with the rapid changes in care delivery. Others may have a specific clinical interest and want to be aware of the current research results in their field. With the advent of the evidence-based practice (EBP) healthcare movement, clinicians are increasingly using research evidence to help them make informed decisions about how best to care for and communicate with patients to achieve the highest quality outcomes. EBP is no longer focused on medical decision making, but is taught and practiced within nursing, physiotherapy, dentistry, humanitarian health care, and many other fields of health and social care.

EBP involves integrating clinical expertise, patients' values and preferences, and the current best research evidence. However, few practitioners, if any, can keep up with all the research being published, even with various electronic tools currently available (Loher-Niederer, Maccora, & Ritz, 2013). With current competing priorities in healthcare settings, it is challenging to determine which studies are best for a busy practitioner to use for clinical decision making. In addition, researchers may propose various, sometimes contradictory, conclusions when studying the same or similar issues, making it quite challenging to determine which studies can be relied on. Even the usefulness of preappraised studies such as systematic reviews is sometimes difficult to discern.

As a result, an evidence-based practitioner must evaluate which evidence is most appropriate for any attempt to answer clinical questions. This requires the necessary skills to critically appraise the available studies to answer the question and then determine the strength of the evidence (i.e., the confidence to act) from the gestalt of all the studies (i.e., more than a summary of the studies). In **critical appraisal**, the research is evaluated for its strengths, limitations, and value/worth to practice (i.e., how well it informs clinician decision making to have an impact on outcomes). Clinicians cannot focus only on the flaws of the research, but must weigh the limitations with the strengths to determine a study's worth to practice. Appraising research is similar to how a jeweler appraises gemstones, weighing the characteristics of a diamond (e.g., clarity, color, carat, and cut) before declaring its worth (Fineout-Overholt, 2008).

First, it is important to determine the best match between the kind of question being asked and the research methodology available to answer that question (see Chapter 2, Table 2.2). Different levels of evidence are described in Chapter 2, and those levels will be referred to herein critically appraising different quantitative research methodologies.

This chapter begins with an overview of the general questions to ask in critically appraising quantitative evidence. These are essential for every clinician to successfully use the tool of research. This is followed by discussion of the Hierarchy of Evidence for intervention questions (levels of evidence), and a more detailed analysis of the specific questions to address in appraising quantitative evidence. These involve examining validity, reliability, and applicability. These sections will examine such issues as bias, confounding results, effect size, and confidence intervals (CIs). These appraisal principles will then be applied to different types of research designs: case studies, case–control studies, cohort studies, randomized controlled trials (RCTs), and systematic reviews. Each section describes the characteristics of each type of design and provides appraisal questions specific for that type of design. Each section concludes with a worked example in a clinical scenario entitled "What the Literature Says: Answering a Clinical Question." Readers are encouraged to read the material about the research design first (the instruction manual) and then read the application in a clinical scenario (see a demonstration of the tool).

PRELIMINARY QUESTIONS TO ASK IN A CRITICAL APPRAISAL

Quantitative research papers generally follow a convention when presenting results. This approach can assist with critical appraisal by identifying standard criteria by which each study should be appraised. Overview questions will be asked of each quantitative study (Box 5.1).

Why Was the Study Done?

A clear explanation of why the study was carried out (i.e., the purpose of the study) is crucial and should be stated succinctly in the report being critically appraised. This can be elaborated on in the aims of the study. The brief background literature presented in a study should identify the gap that this research was designed to fill. This provides the reader with an understanding of how the current research fits within the context of reported knowledge on the topic. Clear descriptions of how researchers conducted their statistical analyses assist the reader in evaluating the reliability and applicability of the study results and protect against data dredging.

What Is the Sample Size?

The study sample size should be sufficient to ensure reasonable confidence that the role of chance is minimized as a contributor to the results and that the true effect of the intervention will be

 Box 5.1 Overview Questions for Critical Appraisal of Quantitative Studies

◆ Why was the study done?
◆ What is the sample size?
◆ Are the measurements of major variables valid and reliable?
◆ How were the data analyzed?
◆ Were there any untoward events during the conduct of the study?
◆ How do the results fit with previous research in the area?
◆ What does this research mean for clinical practice?

demonstrated. Researchers should conduct an a priori (i.e., done before starting the study) calculation called a power analysis, which assists them in determining what the sample size should be in order to minimize findings that are based on chance. Two general types of errors can occur. **Type I errors** occur when researchers conclude from an experiment that a difference exists between interventions (i.e., false positives), when in reality there is no difference. Type II errors occur when there truly is a difference between interventions, but researchers conclude that one does not exist (i.e., false negatives) (Table 5.1). Power analyses help to minimize such errors, and should be reported in the methods section of the research report. If a power analysis is not reported, no assumptions can be made about the adequacy or inadequacy of the sample size for minimizing chance findings. Sometimes ethical, economic, and other practical considerations impact the sample size of a study. Careful consideration of how the sample size affects the validity of findings should be considered when appraising a study.

Are the Measurements of Major Variables Valid and Reliable?

The concepts of validity and reliability discussed regarding a study's results differ from the concepts of validity and reliability discussed in the measurement of outcomes. In this section of the chapter, the focus is on how well an instrument measures a concept (i.e., the accuracy and consistency of the measures). A valid instrument is one that measures what it is purported to measure. For example, an instrument that is expected to measure fear should indeed measure fear (and not anxiety, for example). A reliable instrument is one that is stable over time (i.e., it performs the same way each time responders answer the questions) and is composed of individual items or questions that consistently measure the same construct. Several statistical techniques can be applied to instrument results to determine their reliability (e.g., Cronbach's alpha).

Published research reports should discuss the validity and reliability of the outcome measures used in the study in the methods section. Investigators should address issues or concerns they have with the validity or reliability of their results in the discussion section of the research report. It is important for the critical appraiser to keep in mind that without valid and reliable measurement of outcomes, the study results are not clinically meaningful.

Table 5.1   Implications of Study Results Found by Chance

		Study Results	
		Researchers Found That the *Intervention Worked* (i.e., They Rejected the Null* Hypothesis)	Researchers Found That the *Intervention Did Not Work* Better Than the Comparison Intervention (i.e., They Accepted the Null* Hypothesis)
Reality options	True positive (statistically significant, $p < 0.05$)	On target finding	Oops-made a **Type II error** (false negative-said it did not work, when really it did)
	True negative (statistically significant, $p > 0.05$)	Oops—made a **Type I error** (false positive—said it did work when really it did not)	On target finding

*Null hypothesis: there is no difference between the intervention and comparison groups (the intervention did not work).

How Were the Data Analyzed?

Clinicians do not need to be familiar with a large number of complex approaches to statistical analysis. Even experts in statistics have challenges keeping up with current statistical techniques. Researchers reviewed articles published in the journal *Pediatrics* and found that readers who were very familiar with the 10 most common statistical concepts would still encounter unfamiliar statistical procedures in the journal's articles (Hellems, Gurka, & Hayden, 2007). The authors reported that an anonymous reviewer of their article commented, "I have never heard of some of these, and I teach this stuff!" Although challenging, clinicians need a general understanding of how to interpret some common statistical tests and the types of data that are appropriate for their use. For those new to critical appraisal, spotting common mistakes in statistics can be a great opportunity to learn the methods (Bono & Tornetta, 2006; Strasak, Zaman, Pfeiffer, Göbel, & Ulmer, 2007). Some common statistical errors include the following:

◆ *Focusing only on the* **p value**. Choosing a statistical test because it gives the answer for which the investigator had hoped (e.g., statistical significance) is ill-advised. A statistical test should be chosen on the basis of its appropriateness for the type of data collected. Authors should give clear justifications for using anything other than the most commonly used statistical tests.

◆ *Data dredging, or conducting a large number of analyses on the same data*. This can be problematic because the more analyses conducted, the more likely that a significant result will be found due only to chance.

◆ *Confusing statistical significance with clinical importance*. A small difference between large groups may be statistically significant, but be such a rare event that few will benefit from it. For example, if an intervention reduces blood pressure by 2 mm Hg, the finding might be statistically significant in a study with a large sample, but it would not be clinically meaningful. On the other hand, a large difference between small groups may not be statistically significant, but may make an important clinical difference.

◆ *Missing data*. Incomplete data are surprisingly common, and, when noted, should raise questions during critical appraisal. Researchers should indicate in their report how they addressed any incomplete data. If this issue is not addressed, the problem may be an oversight in the report, a restrictive word count from the publisher, or a poorly conducted study—all of which should be considered carefully. If the issue is an oversight in reporting or word count restriction, contacting the researcher is in order to discuss how missing data were addressed.

◆ *Selective reporting*. Inappropriately publishing only outcomes with statistically significant findings can lead to missing data. This can occur where only studies with positive findings are published—leading to publication bias—or where only positive outcomes within a study are published—leading to selective outcome reporting bias (Howland, 2011). Within a study, a flowchart is an efficient mechanism to account for all patients and show how the various groups progressed through the study. Figure 5.1 gives an example of how a flowchart visually summarizes the study design and how the numbers of subjects were used in the statistical analyses.

Were There Any Untoward Events During the Conduct of the Study?

During critical appraisal, it is important to understand how problems that arose during a study influenced the final results. These issues may be unpredictable and occur randomly or they may arise because of a flaw or flaws in the original study design. One such problem is loss to follow-up (i.e., study attrition), which results in missing data and introduction of bias. Research reports should provide explanations for all adverse events and withdrawals from the study and how those events affected the final results (supported by evidence regarding how those conclusions were reached).

How Do the Results Fit With Previous Research in the Area?

Except on rare occasions when researchers investigate completely new areas of interest, studies fit into a growing body of research evidence. A study report should begin with a **systematic review** of previous literature that substantiates why this study was conducted. In a study report, the evidence review is the

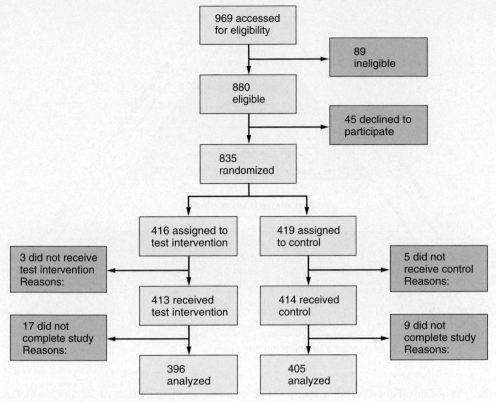

Figure 5.1: Study participants flowchart.

context in which the current research is meaningful. This review should provide confidence that the researchers took advantage of previous researchers' experiences (positive and negative) in conducting studies on this topic. In addition, the discussion section of the report should discuss the study findings in light of what is already known and how those findings complement or contradict previous work. In writing the report, the evidence review and discussion should be framed in such a way that the clinician will understand the purpose and context of the research.

What Does This Research Mean for Clinical Practice?

The point of critical appraisal of all research and subsequent evidence-based decision making in health care is to apply research findings to improve clinical practice outcomes. Therefore, asking what the research means for clinical practice is one of the most important questions to keep in mind during critical appraisal. Clinicians should look at the study population and ask whether the results can be extrapolated to the patients in *their* care.

While it is imperative that these general questions are asked of every study, it is also important to ask additional, design-specific appraisal questions to determine the worth of each study to clinical decision making. The following sections provide those design-specific questions.

HIERARCHY OF EVIDENCE

A **hierarchy of evidence** is the same as levels of evidence and provides guidance about the types of research studies, if well done, that are more likely to provide reliable answers to a specific clinical question (Figure 5.2). There are various hierarchies, or levels, of evidence; which hierarchy is appropriate depends

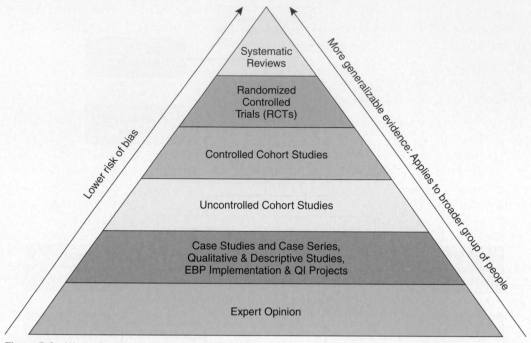

Figure 5.2: Hierarchy of evidence for intervention questions.

on the type of clinical question being asked. For intervention questions, the most appropriate hierarchy of evidence ranks quantitative research designs (e.g., a systematic review of **randomized controlled trials**) at the highest level of confidence compared with designs that give lower levels of confidence (e.g., descriptive studies). Other types of questions are best answered by other hierarchies.

The higher a methodology ranks in the hierarchy, the more likely the results accurately represent the actual situation and the more confidence clinicians can have that the intervention will produce the same health outcomes in similar patients for whom they care. An RCT is the best research design for providing information about cause-and-effect relationships. A systematic review of RCTs provides a compilation of what we know about a topic from multiple studies addressing the same research question, which ranks it higher in the hierarchy than a single RCT. A systematic review (i.e., a synthesis of these studies) of a large number of high-quality RCTs of similar design (i.e., have **homogeneity**) is the strongest and least-biased method to provide confidence that the intervention will consistently bring about a particular outcome (Fineout-Overholt, O'Mathúna, & Kent, 2008; Guyatt, Rennie, Meade, & Cook, 2008; Turner, Balmer, & Coverdale, 2013). Such systematic reviews have been called the "heart of evidence-based practice" (Stevens, 2001).

CRITICAL APPRAISAL PRINCIPLES OF QUANTITATIVE STUDIES

A search of the literature to answer a clinical question can be exasperating if it reveals multiple studies with findings that do not agree. It can be disappointing to find a new study where a promising intervention is found to be no more effective than a **placebo**, particularly when an earlier study reported that the same intervention was beneficial. (Placebos are pharmacologically inert substances [like a sugar pill] and will be discussed later in the chapter when examining RCTs.) Given the resulting confusion and uncertainty, it is reasonable for clinicians to wonder if external evidence (i.e., research) is really that helpful.

Ideally, all studies would be designed, conducted, and reported perfectly, but that is not likely. Research inherently has flaws in how it is designed, conducted, or reported; however, study results should not be dismissed or ignored on this basis alone. Given that all research is not perfect, users of research must learn to carefully evaluate research reports to determine their worth to practice through critical appraisal. The critical appraisal process hinges on three overarching questions that apply to any study (Verhagen, de Vet, de Bie, Boers, & van den Brandt, 2001):

1. Are the results of the study valid? (Validity)
2. What are the results? (Reliability)
3. Will the results help me in caring for my patients? (Applicability)

This process provides clinicians with the means to interpret the quality of studies and determine the applicability of the synthesis of multiple studies' results to their particular patients (Crombie, 1996; Sirriyeh, Lawton, Gardner, & Armitage, 2012; University College London, 2011).

When appraising quantitative studies, it is important to recognize the factors of validity and reliability that could influence the study findings. Study validity and reliability are determined by the quality of the study methodology. In addition, clinicians must discern how far from the true result the reported result may be (i.e., compare the study result with the outcome that can be replicated in practice [can I get what they got]). Since all studies have some flaws, the process of critical appraisal should assist the clinician in deciding whether a study is flawed to the point that it should be discounted as a source of evidence (i.e., the results cannot reliably be used in practice). Interpretation of results requires consideration of the **clinical significance** of the study findings (i.e., the impact of the findings clinically), as well as the **statistical significance** of the results (i.e., the results were not found by chance).

Are the Study Results Valid? (Validity)

The validity of a study refers to whether the results of the study were obtained via sound scientific methods. Bias and/or confounding variables may compromise the validity of the findings (Goodacre, 2008a). The less influence these factors have on a study, the more likely the results will be valid. Therefore, it is important to determine whether the study was conducted properly before being swayed by the results. Validity must be ascertained before the clinician can make an informed assessment of the size and precision of the effect(s) reported.

Bias

Bias is anything that distorts study findings in a systematic way and arises from the study methodology (Polit & Beck, 2007). Bias can be introduced at any point in a study. When critically appraising research, the clinician needs to be aware of possible sources of bias, which may vary with the study design. Every study requires careful examination regarding the different factors that influence the extent of potential bias in a study.

Selection Bias. An example of bias could be how participants are selected for inclusion into the different groups in an intervention study. This selection may occur in a way that inappropriately influences who ends up in the experimental group or comparison group. This is called selection bias and is reduced when researchers **randomly assign** participants to experimental and comparison groups. This is the "randomized" portion of the RCT, the classic experimental study. In an RCT, all other variables should be the same in each group (i.e., the groups should be homogenous). Differences in the outcomes should be attributable to the different interventions given to each group. A controlled trial in which researchers do not properly randomize participants to the study groups will likely have a different outcome when compared with one using the best randomization methods, as there is inherently more bias in poorly randomized studies (Kunz & Oxman, 1998). Other study designs (e.g., quasi-experimental, cohort, case studies) do not randomly allocate participants and risk introduction of selection bias into the research.

Figure 5.3 shows how participants could be selected for an experimental study. For example, researchers want to study the effect of 30 minutes of daily exercise in adults who are over 80 years of age. The ideal, but usually infeasible, sample to include in a study is the **reference population**; that is, those people in the past, present, and future to whom the study results can be generalized. In this case, the

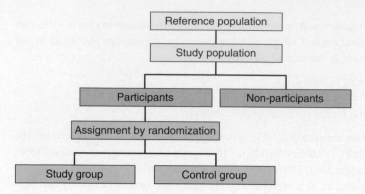

Figure 5.3: Experimental hierarchy.

reference population would be all those over 80 years of age. Given the difficulty of obtaining the reference population, researchers typically use a study population that they assume will be representative of the reference population (e.g., a random sample of older adults over 80 years of age who live in or within a 25-mile radius of a metropolitan city in a rural state).

However, clinicians need to keep in mind that bias could be introduced at each point where a subgroup is selected. For example, the study population will include some people willing to participate and others who refuse to participate in the study. If participants volunteer to be involved in the study (i.e., a convenience sample), the volunteers may differ from those who do not volunteer in some characteristic that influences the outcomes in some way. For example, in a study of the impact of exercise on the health of adults older than 80 years, those who volunteer for a study may start with a more positive attitude toward exercise and adhere to the study protocol better. If the study involved only such people, this could affect the study outcomes and make them inapplicable to the reference population. This type of effect is particularly relevant in studies where people's attitudes or beliefs are being explored because these may be the very characteristics that influence their decision to participate or not (Polit & Beck, 2007). Evidence users must be aware that despite the best efforts of the investigators to select a sample that is representative of the reference population, there may be significant differences between the study sample and the general population.

Knowing Who Receives Which Intervention. Another type of bias in RCTs is introduced by participants or researchers knowing who is receiving which intervention. To minimize this bias, participants and those evaluating outcomes of the study are kept blind or "in the dark" about who receives which intervention (i.e., the experimental and the comparison groups). These studies are called double-blind studies.

Gatekeepers. Another element known to introduce bias is a well-intentioned person acting as a gatekeeper, particularly in studies involving vulnerable populations. For example, researchers conducting a study with patients receiving palliative care may have difficulty recruiting sufficient number of people into the study because the patients' caregivers may consider it too burdensome to ask the patients to participate in research at a difficult time in their lives. This introduces bias as healthier patients may respond differently to the intervention and thus lead to different outcomes than if a more representative sample was enrolled in the study.

Measurement Bias. Another concern that may influence study results is measurement bias (i.e., how the data are measured). For example, *systematic error* can occur through using an incorrectly calibrated device that consistently gives higher or lower measurements than the true measurement. Data collectors may deviate from established data collection protocols or their individual personality traits may affect the eliciting of information from patients in studies involving interviews or surveys. Longitudinal studies, in general, have challenges with measurement bias.

Recall Bias. One type of longitudinal, retrospective study that compares two groups is a **case–control** study, in which researchers select a group of people with an outcome of interest, the cases (e.g., cases of infection), and another group of people without that outcome, the control cases (e.g., no infection). Both groups are surveyed in an attempt to find the key differences between the groups that may suggest why one group had the outcome (i.e., infection) and the other did not. Participants respond to surveys about what they did in the past. This is referred to as *recall*. Studies that rely on patients remembering data are subject to "recall bias" (Callas & Delwiche, 2008). Recall may be affected by a number of factors. For example, asking patients with brain tumors about their past use of cellular phones might generate highly accurate or falsely inflated responses because those patients seek an explanation for their disease, compared with people who do not have tumors and whose recall of phone use may be less accurate in the absence of disease (Muscat et al., 2000). Bias can be a challenge with case–control studies in that people may not remember things correctly.

Information Bias. Another related form of bias occurs when researchers record different information from interviews or patient records. The risk of such information bias is higher when researchers know which participants are in the case group and which are controls (Callas & Delwiche, 2008). One form of longitudinal study that has to battle information bias is a **cohort study**. This type of study focuses prospectively on one group of people who have been exposed to a condition and another group that has not. For example, people living in one town might be put into one cohort and those in another town into a second cohort—the town they lived in would be the selection criterion. All of the participants would be followed over a number of years to identify differences between the two cohorts that might be associated with differences between the towns and specific outcomes (e.g., environmental factors and breast cancer).

Loss to Follow-Up. In longitudinal studies like cohort studies, loss of participants to follow-up may contribute to measurement bias. For example, if people stop the intervention because of an adverse event, and this is not followed up on or reported, the reported outcomes may mask important reasons for observed differences between the experimental intervention and control groups. Possible reasons for loss of participants (i.e., study attrition) could include unforeseen side effects of the intervention or burdensome data collection procedures. While such factors are often out of the control of researchers, they can lead to noncomparable groups and biased results. Therefore, they should be noted and addressed in reports of studies.

Contamination. Contamination is another form of measurement bias. This occurs when participants originally allocated to a particular group or arm of a study are exposed to the alternative group's intervention (i.e., the comparison intervention). For example, in a study of asthmatic school children that compares retention of asthma management information given to the children in written form and by video, results may be compromised if those in the video group lend their videos to those in the written information group. Another example would be if patients in a placebo-controlled trial somehow become aware that they have been assigned to the placebo group and, believing they should be in the intervention arm of the study, find some way to access the intervention.

In critical appraisal of a research study, specific questions should be asked about the report to identify whether the study was well designed and conducted or whether risks of bias were introduced at different points. Chapter 17 contains more information on these quantitative designs and ways of reducing bias. Appendix B contains rapid critical appraisal checklists for quantitative study designs as well as qualitative studies that provide standardized criteria to be applied to each study methodology to determine if it is a valid study.

Confounded Study Results

When interpreting results presented in quantitative research papers, clinicians should always consider that there may be multiple explanations for any effect reported in a study. A study's results may be confounded when a relationship between two variables is actually due to a third, either known or unknown variable (i.e., a confounding variable). The confounding variable relates to both the intervention (i.e., the exposure) and the outcome, but is not directly a part of the causal pathway (i.e., the relationship) between the two. Confounding variables are often encountered in studies about lifestyle and health. For example, clinicians confounding variables should be considered in a report linking caffeine intake with the incidence of headaches among hospital workers fasting for Ramadan (Awada & Al Jumah, 1999). Headache sufferers consumed significantly more caffeine in beverages such as tea and coffee compared to those who did not get headaches. The reduction in caffeine consumption during fasting for Ramadan led to caffeine withdrawal, which the researchers stated was the most likely cause of the headaches. Intuitively, this may sound likely; however, if the study population includes people engaged in shift work, which is very likely since the participants were hospital staff, the irregular working hours or a combination of variables may have contributed to the headaches, not solely caffeine withdrawal. Figure 5.4 demonstrates how confounding variables can lead to confusing results. The shift work is related to both the exposure (i.e., reduced high caffeine intake and subsequent withdrawal) and the outcomes (i.e., headaches). However, it is not directly causal (i.e., irregular working hours do not cause headaches).

When critically appraising a study, clinicians must evaluate whether investigators considered the possibility of confounding variables in the original study design, as well as in the analysis and interpretation of their results. Minimizing the possible impact of confounding variables on a study's results is best addressed by a research design that utilizes a randomization process to assign participants to each study group. In this way, confounding variables, either known or unknown, are expected to equally influence the outcomes of the different groups in the study.

Confounding variables may still influence a study's results despite investigators' best efforts. Unplanned events occurring at the same time as the study may have an impact on the observed outcomes. This is often referred to as *history*. For example, a study is launched to determine the effects of an educational program regarding infant nutrition (i.e., the experimental intervention group). The control group receives the usual information on infant growth and development provided at maternal and child health visits. Unknown to the researchers, the regional health department simultaneously begins a widespread media campaign to promote child health. This confounding historical event could impact the results and thereby make it difficult to directly attribute any observed outcomes solely to the experimental intervention (i.e., information on infant nutrition). Finally, inclusion and exclusion criteria should be used to select participants and should be prespecified (i.e., a priori). Often these criteria can be controls for possible confounding variables (see Appendix B).

What Are the Results? (Reliability)

Quantitative studies use statistics to report their findings. Having evaluated the validity of a study's findings, the numerical study results need to be examined. Clinicians planning to use the results of quantitative studies need a general understanding of how to interpret the numerical results. The main concerns are the size of the intervention's effect (the effect size) and how precisely that effect was

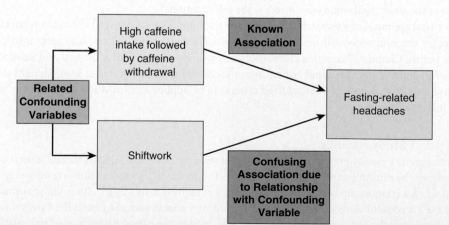

Figure 5.4: Model of possible confounding variables in a study examining the association between caffeine intake and symptoms.

estimated. Together, these determine the reliability of the study findings. This goes beyond understanding the study's results to evaluating how likely it is that the intervention will have the same effect when clinicians use it in their practices. This part of critical appraisal examines the numerical data reported in the results section of a study.

....

Nothing in the world can take the place of Persistence ... Persistence and determination alone are omnipotent. The slogan 'Press On' has solved and always will solve the problems of the human race.
—Calvin Coolidge

....

Reporting the Study Results: Do the Numbers Add Up?

In all studies, the total number of participants approached and the number consenting to participate in the study should be reported. The total number of those participating is abbreviated as N (i.e., the total sample). In addition, in RCTs, the *total number* in each group or arm of a study (e.g., intervention or comparison group) should be reported, as these values will usually be included in the statistical calculations involving the study findings (Table 5.2).

In the results section and subsequent analyses, the numbers of participants with various outcomes of interest are reported as n. When appraising a study, clinicians should check whether the sum of all n values equals the original N reported (see Table 5.2). This is particularly important, as a discrepancy represents loss of subjects to follow-up (i.e., attrition). Participants may withdraw from a study for various reasons, some of which are very relevant to the validity of the study results. Regardless of the reasons, researchers should account for any difference in the final number of participants in each group compared to the number of people who commenced the study. For example, a study reporting the effectiveness of depression management that uses frequent individual appointments with a professional may report fewer participants at the end of the study than were originally enrolled. A high attrition rate may have occurred because participants found it difficult to attend the frequent appointments. A well-conducted study would attempt to discover participants' reasons for withdrawing. These factors are important to consider because sometimes even if interventions were found to be effective in a study, they may be difficult to implement in the real world.

Table 5.2   Measures of Effect

Exposure to Intervention	Expected Outcome Occurred		
	Yes	No	Total
Yes	a	b	$a + b$
No	c	d	$c + d$
Total	$a + c$	$b + d$	$a + b + c + d$

Notes: $a + b + c + d$ is the total number of study participants, N.
$a + b$ is the total number of study participants in the intervention arm of the study.
a is the number of participants exposed to the intervention who had the expected outcome.
b is the number of participants exposed to the intervention who did not have the expected outcome.
$c + d$ is the total number of study participants in the unexposed or comparison arm of the study.
c is the number of participants not exposed to the intervention who nevertheless had the expected outcome.
d is the number of participants not exposed to the intervention and who did not have the expected outcome.
$a + c$ is the total number of study participants, both exposed and not exposed to the intervention, who had the expected outcome occur.
$b + d$ is the total number of study participants in the control and intervention groups who did not have the expected outcome occur.

Magnitude of the Effect

Quantitative studies are frequently conducted to find out if there is an important and identifiable difference between two groups. Some examples could be: (a) why one group is diagnosed with breast cancer and not the other group, (b) the quality of life for older people living at home compared to those living in nursing homes, or (c) outcomes of taking drug A compared to taking drug B. A study will pick one or more outcomes to determine whether there are important differences between the groups. The **magnitude of effect** refers to the degree of the difference or lack of difference between the various groups (i.e., experimental and control) in the study. The effect is the **rate of occurrence** in each of the groups for the outcome of interest. It is helpful when trying to determine the magnitude of effect to use what is called a two-by-two table—two columns and two rows. Table 5.3 is a two-by-two table in which one column lists those who had the outcome and the other column lists those without the outcome. Each row provides the outcomes for those exposed to the different interventions or those with or without the different conditions.

Statistical tests that researchers may conduct to determine if the effects differ significantly between groups may be included in such tables. While it is important for clinicians to understand what these statistics mean, they do not need to carry statistical formulas around in their heads to critically appraise the literature. Some knowledge of how to interpret commonly used statistical tests and when they should be used is adequate for the appraisal process. However, keeping a health sciences statistics book nearby or using the Internet to refresh one's memory can be helpful when evaluating a study.

Table 5.3 presents data to assist in understanding how to use this kind of table. The outcome chosen here is dichotomous, meaning that the outcome is either present or absent (e.g., Do you smoke? Either a "yes" or "no" answer is required). Data can also be continuous across a range of values (e.g., 1 to 10). Examples of continuous data include age, blood pressure, or pain levels. Dichotomous and continuous data are analyzed using different statistical tests. For example, the effect measured in the hypothetical study was whether smokers or nonsmokers developed a hypothetical disease, *ukillmeousus*, or not (i.e., dichotomous data, with an outcome of either "yes" or "no").

Another approach to evaluating the response of a population to a particular disease is reporting the risk of developing a disease (e.g., how likely it is that a smoker will develop the disease at some point). Other terms used to describe outcomes are *incidence* (i.e., how often the outcome occurs or the number of newly diagnosed cases during a specific time period) or *prevalence* (i.e., the total number of people at risk for the outcome or total number of cases of a disease in a given population in a given time frame). For the purposes of this discussion about understanding the magnitude of a treatment effect, the focus will be on risk. People are often concerned about reducing the risk of a perceived bad outcome (e.g., developing colon cancer), usually through choosing the treatment, screening, or lifestyle change that best minimizes the risk of the outcome occurrence.

Strength of Association

In the context of the example in Table 5.3, the risk is the probability that a smoker who is currently free from *ukillmeousus* will develop the disease at some point. This risk can be expressed in a few different

Table 5.3   Two-by-Two Table of Smokers and Nonsmokers Incidence of Ukillmeousus*

Condition	Outcome: Incidence of Ukillmeousus		
	Yes	No	Total
Smokers	3	97	100
Nonsmokers	2	98	100

Ukillmeousus is a hypothetical disease.

ways. The absolute risk of smokers developing *ukillmeousus*, often referred to as the probability (i.e., risk) of the outcome in the exposed group (Re), is 3 out of 100, (i.e., 0.03, 1 in 33, or 3%). This is derived by dividing the number of those who had the outcome by the total number of those who could have had the outcome (i.e., 3/100). The risk for nonsmokers developing *ukillmeousus* (i.e., the probability of the outcome occurring in the unexposed group [Ru]) is 2 out of 100. This risk can also be expressed as a proportion, 1 in 50 (0.02), or percentage, 2%. Table 5.4 contains the general formulas for these and other statistics. The following paragraphs will use the data and formulas in Tables 5.2, 5.3, and 5.4 to show how the results of studies can be used to make clinical decisions.

When comparing groups, whether testing an intervention or examining the impact of a lifestyle factor or policy, people are often concerned about risk. Some examples of common concerns about risk include (a) colon screening to reduce the risk of colon cancer deaths; (b) high-fiber, low-fat diets to reduce the risk of cardiovascular disease; (c) high-school coping intervention programs to reduce the risk of suicide in adolescents; and (d) lipid medications reducing the risk of cardiovascular disease. Often, we are interested in the difference in risks of an outcome between a group that has a particular intervention and one that does not. When groups differ in their risks for an outcome, this can be expressed in a number of different ways. One way to report this is the absolute difference in risks between the groups. The **absolute risk reduction** (ARR) for an undesirable outcome is when the risk is less for the experimental/condition group than for the control/comparison group. The **absolute risk increase** (ARI) for an undesirable outcome is when the risk is more for the experimental/condition group than the control/comparison group. These values can also be referred to as the risk difference (RD).

In the previous example, the risk for the undesirable outcome of *ukillmeousus* is higher in the smoker (i.e., condition) group than in the comparison group (i.e., nonsmokers). Therefore, the ARI is calculated as 3% (risk [or probability] of *ukillmeousus* for smokers) – 2% (risk of *ukillmeousus* for nonsmokers) = 1% (or, in proportions, 0.03 – 0.02 = 0.01). To put it in a sentence, the absolute risk for developing *ukillmeousus* is 1% higher for smokers than the risk for nonsmokers.

Risks between two groups can also be compared using what is called **relative risk** or risk ratio (RR). This indicates the likelihood (i.e., risk) that the outcome would occur in one group compared to the other. The group with the particular condition or intervention of interest is usually the focus of the

Table 5.4   Statistics to Assist in Interpreting Findings in Healthcare Research

Statistic	Formula	*Ukillmeousus* Example
Absolute risk (AR)	Risk in exposed (Re) = $a/(a + b)$ Risk in unexposed (Ru) = $c/(c + d)$	3/(3 + 97) = 3/100 = 0.03 2/(2 + 98) = 2/100 = 0.02
Absolute risk reduction (ARR)	Ru – Re = ARR	Not appropriate
Absolute risk increase (ARI)	Re – Ru = ARI	0.03 – 0.02 = 0.01 0.01 × 100 = 1%
Relative risk (RR)	RR = Re/Ru	0.03/0.02 = 1.5
Relative risk reduction (RRR)	RRR = {|Re – Ru|/Ru} × 100%	{|0.03–0.02|/0.02} = 0.01/0.02 = 0.5 × 100 = 50%
Odds ratio (OR)	Odds of exposed = a/b Odds of unexposed = c/d OR = $(a/b)/(c/d)$	Odds of smokers 3/97 = 0.03 Odds of nonsmokers 2/98 = 0.02 OR 0.03/0.02 = 1.5

study. In the example, the condition is smoking. Relative risk is calculated by dividing the two absolute risk values (condition of interest/intervention group divided by control group). In the example, the RR is AR for smokers/AR for nonsmokers: 0.03/0.02 = 1.5. To use it in a sentence, smokers are 1.5 times more likely to develop *ukillmeousus* compared to nonsmokers. Relative risk is frequently used in prospective studies, such as RCTs and cohort studies. If the outcome is something we want, an RR greater than 1 means the treatment (or condition) is better than control. If the outcome is something we do not want (*ukillmeousus*), an RR greater than 1 means the treatment (or condition) is worse than control. In the example, the outcome of *ukillmeousus* is not desirable and the RR is greater than 1; therefore, the condition of a smoker is worse than the condition of a nonsmoker.

A related way to express this term is the **relative risk reduction** (RRR). This expresses the proportion of the risk in the intervention/condition group compared to the proportion of risk in the control group. It can be calculated by taking the risk of the condition (Re = 0.03) minus the risk of the control (Ru = 0.02), dividing the result by the risk for the control (Ru), and then multiplying by 100 (to make it a percentage) ([0.03 – 0.02]/0.02) × 100 = 50%. To state this in a sentence, being a nonsmoker reduces the risk of developing *ukillmeousus* by 50% relative to being a smoker.

Notice here the importance of understanding what these terms mean. An RRR of 50% *sounds* more impressive than a 1% RD (i.e., ARI). Yet both of these terms have been derived from the same data. Other factors must be taken into account. For example, a 1% RD may not be very significant if the disease is relatively mild and short-lived. However, it may be very significant if the disease is frequently fatal. If the differences between the groups are due to treatment options, the nature and incidence of adverse effects will also need to be taken into account (see Example One later in this chapter).

When trying to predict outcomes, "odds" terminology arises frequently. In quantitative studies, calculating the odds of an outcome provides another way of estimating the strength of association between an intervention and an outcome. The odds of the outcome occurring in a particular group are calculated by dividing the number of those exposed to the condition or treatment who had the outcome by the number of people without the outcome, not the total number of people in the study (see Table 5.4). In the example comparing smokers and nonsmokers, the odds of a smoker getting the disease are 3/97 = 0.031. The odds of a nonsmoker getting *ukillmeousus* are 2/98 = 0.020. The **odds ratio** (OR) is the odds of the smokers (0.031) divided by the odds of the nonsmokers (0.020) = 1.5. To use it in a sentence, smokers have 1.5 greater odds of developing *ukillmeousus* than nonsmokers. As seen in this example, the OR and RR can be very similar in value. This happens when the number of events of interest (i.e., how many developed the observed outcome) is low; as the event rate increases, the values can diverge.

Interpreting results that are presented as an ARR, ARI, RR, or OR sometimes can be difficult not only for the clinician but also for the patient—an essential contributor to the healthcare decision-making process. A more meaningful way to present the study results is through the calculation of the **number needed to treat** (NNT). NNT is a value that can permit all stakeholders in the clinical decision to better understand the likelihood of developing the outcome if a patient has a given intervention or condition. The NNT represents the number of people who would need to receive the therapy or intervention to prevent one bad outcome or cause one additional good outcome. If the NNT for a therapy was 15, this would mean 15 patients would need to receive this therapy before you could expect one additional person to benefit. Another way of putting this is that a person's chance of benefiting from the therapy is 1 in 15. The NNT is calculated by taking the inverse of the ARR (i.e., 1/ARR). For example, if smoking cessation counseling is the treatment, the outcome is smoking cessation, and the ARR for smoking cessation is 0.1, the NNT to see one additional person quit smoking using this treatment is 1/0.1 or 10. Ten people would need to receive the counseling to result in one additional person stopping smoking.

A related parameter to NNT is the **number needed to harm** (NNH). This is the number of people who would need to receive an intervention before one additional person would be harmed (i.e., have a bad outcome). It is calculated as the inverse of the ARI (i.e., 1/ARI). In the *ukillmeousus* example, the ARI for the condition of smoking versus nonsmoking was 0.01; the NNH is 1/0.01 = 100. For every 100 persons who continue to smoke, there will be one case of *ukillmeousus*. While one case of *ukillmeousus* in 100 smokers may seem small, if we assume that this disease is fatal, clinicians may choose to put more effort and resources toward helping people stop smoking. The interpretation of a statistic must be made in the context of the severity of the outcome (e.g., *ukillmeousus*) and the cost and feasibility of the removal of the condition (e.g., smoking) or the delivery of the intervention (e.g., smoking cessation counseling).

Interpreting the Results of a Study: Example One. You are a clinician who is working with patients who want to quit smoking. They have friends who have managed to quit by using nicotine chewing gum and wonder whether this also might work for them. You find a clinical trial that measured the effectiveness of nicotine chewing gum versus a placebo (Table 5.5). Among those using nicotine chewing gum, 18.2% quit smoking (i.e., risk of the outcome in the exposed group [Re]). At the same time, some participants in the control group also gave up smoking (10.7%; i.e., risk of the outcome in the unexposed group [Ru]). The RD for the outcome between these groups (i.e., these two percentages subtracted from one another) is 7.5% (i.e., the ARR is 0.075). The NNT is the inverse of the ARR, or 13.3. In other words, 13 smokers need to use the gum for one additional person to give up smoking. Nicotine gum is a relatively inexpensive and easy-to-use treatment, with few side effects. Given the costs of smoking, treating 13 smokers to help 1 stop smoking is reasonable.

The size of the NNT influences decision making about whether or not the treatment should be used; however, it is not the sole decision-making factor. Other factors will influence the decision-making process and should be taken into account, including patient preferences. For example, some smokers who are determined to quit may not view a treatment with a 1 in 13 chance of success as good enough. They may want an intervention with a lower NNT, even if it is more expensive. In other situations, a treatment with a low NNT may also have a high risk of adverse effects (i.e., a low NNH). Clinicians may use NNT and NNH in their evaluation of the risks and benefits of an intervention; however, simply determining that an NNT is low is insufficient to justify a particular intervention (Barratt et al., 2004). Evidence-based clinical decision making requires not only ongoing consideration but also an active blending of the numerical study findings, clinicians' expertise, and patients' preferences.

....

Energy and persistence conquer all things.
—Benjamin Franklin

....

Measures of Clinical Significance

Clinicians involved in critical appraisal of a study should be asking themselves: Are the reported results of actual clinical significance? In everyday language, "significant" means "important," but when statistics is used to determine that a study's results use significant, this has a very specific meaning (to be discussed later). When appraising a study, clinicians (and patients) want to know the importance of these results for the clinical decision at hand. This is referred to as *clinical* significance, which may be very different from *statistical* significance (Fethney, 2010). Without understanding this, the reported significance of study findings may be misleading. For example, the ARR reported in study results is

Table 5.5 **The Effectiveness of Nicotine Chewing Gum**

	Outcome		
Exposure	**Quit, *n* (%)**	**Did Not Quit, *n* (%)**	**Total**
Nicotine gum	1,149 (18.2)	5,179 (81.8)	6,328
Placebo	893 (10.7)	7,487 (89.3)	8,380
Total	2,042	12,666	

calculated in a way that considers the underlying susceptibility of a patient to an outcome and thereby can distinguish between very large and very small treatment effects. In contrast, RRR does not take into account existing baseline risk and therefore fails to discriminate between large and small treatment effects.

Interpreting the Results of a Study: Example Two. In a hypothetical example, assume that researchers conducted several RCTs evaluating the same antihypertensive drug and found that it had an RRR of 33% over 3 years (Barratt et al., 2004). A clinician is caring for two 70-year-old women: (a) Pat, who has stable, normal blood pressure, and her risk of stroke is estimated at 1% per year; and (b) Dorothy, who has had one stroke, and although her blood pressure is normal, her risk of another stroke is 10% per year. With an RRR of stroke of 33%, the antihypertensive medication seems like a good option. However, the underlying risk is not incorporated into RRR, and therefore ARR must be examined in making clinically relevant decisions.

In the first study conducted on a sample of people with low risk for stroke, the ARR for this medication was 0.01 or 1%. In the second study, conducted on a sample of individuals at high risk for stroke, the ARR was 0.20 or 20%.

Without treatment, Pat has a 1% risk per year of stroke, or 3% risk over 3 years. An ARR of 1% means that treatment with this drug will reduce her risk to 2% over 3 years. From the low-risk study (i.e., the participants looked most like Pat), 100 patients would need to be treated before one stroke would be avoided (i.e., NNT). Without treatment, Dorothy has a 10% risk of stroke each year, or 30% over 3 years. From the second study (i.e., the participants looked most like Dorothy), with an ARR of 20%, the drug would reduce her risk to 10% over 3 years, and five patients would need to be treated to reduce the incidence of stroke by one (i.e., NNT). In this case, it appears that this medication can be beneficial for both women; however, Dorothy will receive more benefit than Pat. The clinical significance of this treatment is much higher when used in people with a higher baseline risk. The ARR and NNT reveal this, but the RRR does not.

For both of these patients, the risk of adverse effects must be taken into account. In these hypothetical RCTs, researchers found that the drug increased the RR of severe gastric bleeding by 3%. Epidemiologic studies have established that women in this age group inherently have a 0.1% per year risk of severe gastric bleeding. Over 3 years, the risk of bleeding would be 0.3% without treatment (i.e., Ru) and 0.9% with the medication (i.e., Re), giving an ARI of 0.6%. If Pat takes this drug for 3 years, she will have a relatively small benefit (ARR of 1%) and an increased risk of gastric bleeding (ARI of 0.6%). If Dorothy takes the drug for 3 years, she will have a larger benefit (ARR of 20%) and the same increased risk of gastric bleeding (ARI of 0.6%). The evidence suggests that Dorothy is more likely to benefit from treatment than Pat; however, the final decision will depend on their preferences (i.e., how they weigh these benefits and harms).

Precision in the Measurement of Effect

Random Error. Critical appraisal evaluates systematic error when checking for bias and confounding variables. This addresses validity and accuracy in the results. However, error can also be introduced by chance (i.e., random error). Variations due to chance occur in almost all situations. For example, a study might enroll more women than men for no particular reason other than pure chance. If a study was to draw some conclusion about the outcome in relationship to it occurring in men or women, the interpretation would have to consider that the variations in the outcome could have occurred due to the random error of the unplanned disproportionate number of men to women in the sample. If participants were not randomly assigned to groups, very sick people could enroll in one group purely by chance and that could have an impact on the results. A hospital could be particularly busy during the time a research study is being conducted there, and that could distort the results. Random error can lead to reported effects that are smaller or greater than the true effect (i.e., the actual impact of an intervention which researchers do their best to determine, without being 100% certain they have found it). Random error influences the precision of a study finding.

The chances of random error having an impact on the results can be reduced up to a point by study design factors such as increasing the sample size or increasing the number of times measurements are made (i.e., avoiding measurements that are a snapshot in time). When repeated measures of the same outcome are similar in a study, it is presumed that there is low random error. The extent to which random error may influence a measurement can be reported using statistical significance (p values) or by CIs.

Statistical Significance. The aim of statistical analysis is to determine whether an observed effect arises from the study intervention or has occurred by chance. In comparing two groups, the research question can be phrased as a hypothesis (i.e., what we think will happen) and data collected to determine if the hypothesis is confirmed. For example, the hypothesis might be that an experimental drug relieves pain better than a placebo (i.e., the drug has effects beyond those of suggestion or the personal interactions between those involved in the study). Usually, researchers describe what they expect to happen as their study hypothesis. The **null hypothesis** is that there will be *no difference* in effect between the drug and placebo (i.e., the opposite position to the primary hypothesis). When an intervention study is conducted and statistical analysis is performed on study data (i.e., hypothesis testing), a p value is calculated that indicates the probability that the null hypothesis is true. The smaller the p value, the less likely that the null hypothesis is true (i.e., the decreased likelihood that the study findings occurred by chance); therefore, the more likely that the observed effect is due to the intervention. By convention, a p value of 0.05 or less is considered a statistically significant result in healthcare research. This means that it has become acceptable for the study findings to occur by chance 1 in 20 times.

While p values have been commonly reported in healthcare literature, they have been debated for many years (Rothman, 1978). Very small p values can arise when small differences are found in studies with large samples. These findings can be interpreted as statistically significant, but may have little clinical meaningfulness. Conversely, studies with small sample sizes can have strongly associated outcomes with large p values, which may be dismissed as statistically insignificant, but could be clinically meaningful. Part of the problem is that p values lead to an "either-or" conclusion (i.e., statistically significant or not significant) and do not assist in evaluating the strength of an association. In spite of its reputation, "significance testing is not an objective procedure and does not alleviate the need for careful thought and judgment relevant to the subject matter being studied" (Hayat, 2010, p. 219). For example, the "cutoff" of $p \leq 0.05$ is set arbitrarily, and it contributes to dichotomous decision making. Hence, studies reporting only p values tend to be classified as statistically significant (i.e., a positive finding) or statistically not significant (i.e., a negative study finding). The impression given is that the intervention is either useful or useless, respectively. In clinical settings, the study finding is more or less likely to be useful depending on several other factors that clinicians have to take into account when hoping to obtain similar results with their patients.

For example, patients can require mechanical ventilation because of different injuries and diseases. However, mechanical ventilation itself can cause further lung damage, especially if high tidal volumes are used. In an RCT, patients were randomly assigned to receive either low or high levels of a therapy called positive end-expiratory pressure (PEEP). The number of deaths in each group in this study are given in Table 5.6 (Brower et al., 2004). The ARI for death in the high-PEEP group was 13%. When researchers investigated whether or not there was a difference between the two groups, they found that the probability of the null hypothesis (i.e., no differences in the groups) being true was $p = 0.48$. Therefore, the researchers concluded that there were no significant differences in mortality between the two levels of PEEP. However, if the study was simply classified as "statistically not significant," other important information would have been missed, as will be shown later.

Interpreting the Results of a Study: Example Three. Another potential problem with p values occurs if researchers collect a lot of data without clear objectives (i.e., hypotheses) and then analyze everything looking for some significant correlation. In these situations, it is more likely that chance alone will lead to significant results. When the level of statistical significance for the p value is set at 0.05, the probability of saying that the intervention worked when it did not (i.e., getting a false-positive result) can be calculated as $(1 - 0.95)$ or 0.05 (i.e., 1 in 20 positive results will be found by chance). Multiple hypothesis testing is a

Table 5.6   **Two-by-Two Table of the Incidence of Death in Comparing High PEEP to Low PEEP**

Exposure	Outcome (Death)		
	Yes	No	Total
High PEEP	76	200	276
Low PEEP	68	205	273
Calculations			
Absolute Risk (AR)	$Re = a/(a + b)$ $Ru = c/(c + d)$	$Re = 76/(76 + 200) = 0.28$ $Ru = 68/(68 + 205) = 0.25$	
Absolute Risk Increase (ARI)	$ARI = Re - Ru$	$= 0.28 - 0.25 = 0.03$ $0.03 \times 100 = 3\%$ increase in risk of death with high PEEP	
CI for ARI	$CI = ARI \pm 1.96 \sqrt{[Re(100-Re)/a+b]+[Ru(100-Ru)/c+d]}$ $= 0.03 \pm 0.44$ 95% CI : -0.44 to 0.47		

commonly found example of poor research design (Goodacre, 2008b). When two hypotheses are tested, the probability of a chance finding is increased to $[1 - (0.95 \times 0.95)]$ or 0.0975 (i.e., about 1 in 10 positive results will be found by chance). With five tests, the probability moves to 0.23 (i.e., almost a one in four chance that a positive result will be found by random chance).

There are circumstances in which testing several hypotheses may be legitimate (e.g., when several factors are known to impact an outcome). In such cases, there are statistical analyses that can avoid the problems of multiple hypothesis testing (e.g., the Bonferonni Correction; Bono & Tornetta, 2006). Researchers generally select one primary outcome; however, secondary outcomes may also be appropriate when they arise from the study's conceptual background and objectives. In contrast, "fishing expeditions" or "data dredging" occurs when the sole purpose of data collection is to find statistically significant results. Often a clue to data dredging is when subgroups are created without any conceptual basis and these groups differ significantly on an outcome. Subgroups should be planned prior to starting the study (i.e., a priori) and should be formed based on the conceptual framework that underpins the study. For example, a large RCT of high-dose steroids to treat spinal cord injuries has been criticized for its multiple statistical tests (Bracken et al., 1997). More than 100 p values were presented in the report without specifying which one was planned as the primary analysis (Bono & Tornetta). The main results table gave 24 p values for various outcomes at different time intervals, of which one was statistically significant. With the convention for probability set at $p < 0.05$, 1 positive test in every 20 tests is likely to be found by chance; therefore, 1 positive test out of the 24 tests in the study example would very likely be due to chance. One positive finding was that patients had statistically significant better neurologic outcome scores when treated with intravenous steroids within 8 hours of a spinal cord injury. However, no significant differences in neurologic outcomes were found for the entire study population. One problem was that the 8-hour cutoff was not identified prior to the study being conducted, nor was there evidence from basic research as to why treatment prior to 8 hours would make a significant difference (Coleman et al., 2000). Researchers, including one involved in the original study, have expressed concerns that multiple statistical tests were run until a statistically significant difference was discovered, resulting in an artificially created subgroup (Lenzer, 2006). This has important clinical implications as this study continues to determine the standard of care even though many clinicians and researchers have questioned the reliability of its conclusion (Lenzer & Brownlee, 2008). Statistical significance cannot be the sole marker for whether or not a study finding is valuable to practice. Clinical meaningfulness (i.e., the clinician can achieve similar outcomes to the study) is another mechanism that can assist the practitioner in evaluating the value of a study's results to patient care.

Confidence Intervals (CIs). A CI describes the range in which the true effect lies with a given degree of certainty. In other words, the CI provides clinicians a range of values in which they can be reasonably confident (e.g., 95%) that they will find a result when implementing the study findings. The two most important values for clinicians are the study point estimate and the CI. The point estimate, given the study sample and potentially confounding variables, is the best estimate of the magnitude and direction of the experimental intervention's effect compared with the control (Higgins & Green, 2008). Clinicians need to know the degree to which the intervention brought about the study outcome, and they need to know how confident they can be that they can achieve similar outcomes to the study. In general, researchers present a 95% CI, which means that clinicians can have 95% confidence that the value they can achieve (i.e., the true value) falls within this range of values. Studies can report 90% or 99% CI if this level of confidence is more appropriate, although 95% CI remains the most common in healthcare research (Fethney, 2010).

Although a CI can be calculated easily, it is not the calculation that clinicians need to remember; rather, they need to understand what information the CI provides. A CI is appropriate to provide clinical meaningfulness for the measured effect of (a) an intervention in one group, (b) the difference the intervention made between two groups, or (c) the intervention's effect with multiple samples pooled together in a **meta-analysis**. A CI's range can be expressed numerically and graphically (Figure 5.5).

The width of the CI is the key to its interpretation. In general, narrower CIs are more favorable than wider CIs. The narrower the CI around the study point estimate, the less the margin of error for the clinician who is choosing to implement the study findings. In Figure 5.5, the CI is wider, leading to lesser confidence in the study findings. When the CI contains the line of no difference (also called the line of no effect), the difference between the groups (i.e., the study point estimate) is not statistically significant. The actual numerical value for this line can vary depending on the statistic used (e.g., for OR or RR, no effect = 1; for effect size, no effect = 0). The CI in Figure 5.5 crosses the center line of no effect, and therefore the results are not statistically significant.

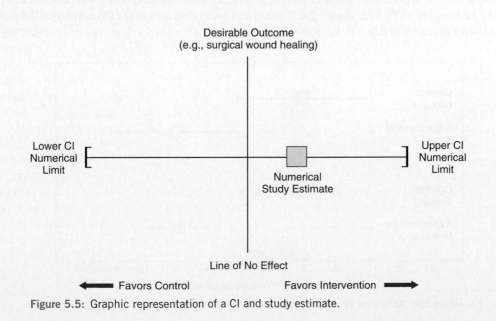

Figure 5.5: Graphic representation of a CI and study estimate.

CI width can be influenced by sample size. Larger samples tend to give more precise estimates of effects (i.e., a narrower CI) and tend to more likely yield statistically significant effects. In Figure 5.6, outcome estimates for the intervention and control groups and the accompanying CIs are shown for two studies. In the second study, the sample size is doubled and the same values are found. Though the mean values remain the same, the 95% CI is more narrowly defined. Clinicians can have more confidence in the findings of the second study. For continuous outcomes (e.g., blood pressure), in addition to sample size, the CI width also depends on the natural variability in the outcome measurements. Because of the limitations of p values, healthcare journals, more commonly, ask for the statistical analyses to report CIs (Goodacre, 2008b).

The information provided by a CI accommodates the uncertainty that is inherent in real-world clinical practice. This uncertainty is not reflected when interventions are described solely as either statistically significant or not. While we can never be absolutely certain whether or not an intervention will help our patients, we can be reasonably confident in the outcome when we have a narrow CI and an effective intervention.

Interpreting the Results of a Study: Example Four. Look over the data in Table 5.6 from the study comparing the incidence of death with high PEEP and low PEEP in mechanical ventilation (Brower et al., 2004). The study point estimate indicates that those participants with low PEEP had lower mortality rates. While the difference in death rate between the two groups was not statistically significant (CI crosses the line of no effect with ARI = 0; $p = 0.48$), the 95% CI provides additional information that is clinically meaningful for patient care. The 95% CI for ARI is narrow (−0.41 to 0.47), indicating that clinicians can have confidence that they too can get a very small increase in mortality rates using high PEEP (Figure 5.7). Although the small increase in death rate is not statistically significant, it is clinically meaningful. However, it would be unwise to decide whether or not to use high PEEP based solely on results of this single study. A more definitive conclusion would require further trials with more subjects. In addition, since the outcome is death, it would be advisable to decrease the acceptable error to 1 in 100 or a 99% CI.

Interpreting the Results of a Study: Example Five. CIs can also be useful in examining the clinical significance of trials with statistically significant results. A blinded, multicenter trial enrolled almost 20,000 patients with vascular disease and randomized them to either aspirin or clopidogrel (CAPRIE Steering Committee, 1996). Both drugs have been recommended to reduce the risk of serious adverse events, especially ischemic stroke, myocardial infarction, or vascular death. Researchers found an annual risk of these outcomes of 5.32% with clopidogrel (i.e., Re) and 5.83% with aspirin (i.e., Ru), giving an RRR of 8.7% in favor of clopidogrel ($p = 0.043$; 95% CI, 0.3 to 16.5).

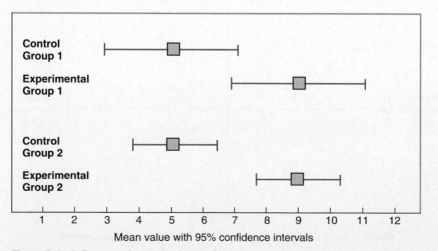

Figure 5.6: Influence of sample size on CIs.

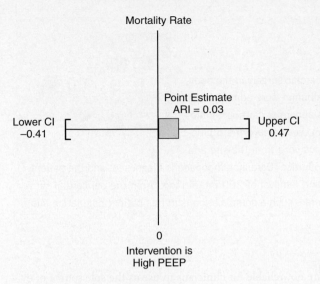

Figure 5.7: Interpretation of study findings.

As discussed earlier, for clinical decision making, the NNT expresses study results more meaningfully. This is calculated as the inverse of the ARR. In this case, the ARR = 0.51% (95% CI, 0.02 to 0.9) and the NNT = 1/(0.51%) = 100/0.51 = 196. Put into a sentence, 196 patients would need to be treated with clopidogrel instead of aspirin for one serious adverse event to be avoided each year. Sometimes, clinicians consider comparing NNT per 1,000 patients; for this example, for every 1,000 patients treated with clopidogrel instead of aspirin, about five serious adverse events would be avoided each year (i.e., adverse events avoided per 1,000 patients = 1,000/196 = 5.1).

Expressing data in terms of NNT may help clinicians discuss these results with patients. They may get a better sense of the risks involved when expressed this way. On the other hand, patients and clinicians may realize that the evidence is not available to provide clear recommendations. They may need to await the results of larger clinical trials to provide the needed evidence for more confident decision making.

Will the Results Help Me in Caring for My Patients? (Applicability)

The last couple of examples have moved into the area of applying results to an individual patient or local situation. Clinicians who are appraising evidence should always keep application to patients in mind as the ultimate goal. Each study design has specific questions that, when answered, assist clinicians in critically appraising those studies to determine their worth to practice (i.e., validity, reliability, and usefulness for clinical decision making). Several study designs will be discussed later in the chapter regarding their distinctive appraisals and how to interpret the results for application to patient care.

CRITICAL APPRAISAL OF CASE STUDIES

Case studies, also called case reports, are historically ranked lower in the hierarchy of evidence for intervention questions because of their lack of objectivity (Chapter 1, Box 1.2). In addition, publication bias could be a factor, since most case studies found in the literature have positive outcomes. Evidence for this was found in a review of case reports published in one typical clinical dermatology journal (Albrecht, Meves, & Bigby, 2009). Of the 100 case reports or short case series reviewed, 96 reported treatment successes (and the reviewers considered one case reported as a success to be a failure when viewed from the patient's perspective).

Case reports describe the history of a single patient (or a small group of patients), usually in the form of a story. These publications are often of great interest to clinicians because of the appealing way in which they are written and because of their strong clinical focus. However, since case reports describe

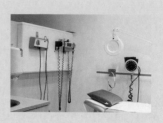

Clinical Scenario 5.1

You are caring for an infant 4 days after cardiac surgery in the pediatric intensive care unit. Platelets and albumin were administered the night before because of the infant's abnormal clotting profile. In consultation with the healthcare team, you remove the pulmonary artery catheter. You notice continuous ooze from the site and a marked deterioration in the patient's condition. Cardiac tamponade is diagnosed, and the patient requires a reopening of the sternotomy and removal of 200 mL of blood from the pericardial sac. At the end of your shift, you wonder how rare such a complication is in this patient population and decide to look at the literature.

one person's situation (or very few), they are not reliable for clinicians to use as the sole source of evidence. They must be used with caution to inform practice, and any application requires careful evaluation of the outcomes. Case studies play important roles in alerting clinicians to new issues and rare and/ or adverse events in practice and to assist in hypothesis generation. Any such hypotheses must be tested in other, less bias-prone research.

Case studies are also beneficial in providing information that would not necessarily be reported in the results of clinical trials or survey research. Publications reporting a clinician's experience and a discussion of early indicators and possible preventive measures can be an extremely useful addition to the clinician's knowledge base. Given that a case series would present a small number of patients with similar experiences or complications and their outcomes, statistical analyses are rarely, if ever, appropriate. A major caution that impacts critical appraisal of case studies is that the purpose of such studies is to provide a patient's story about little-known health issues and not to make generalizations applicable to the general population.

What the Literature Says: Answering a Clinical Question

In Clinical Scenario 5.1, the clinical question you may want to ask is: In infants who have had cardiac surgery (*P*), how often does removing pulmonary artery catheters (*I*) influence cardiac tamponade (*O*) within the first week after surgery (*T*)? In your search, you find a case study that describes a similar complication to one you have just experienced: Johnston and McKinley (2000).

The article is a case report of one patient who experienced cardiac tamponade after removal of a pulmonary artery catheter. The article focuses on describing the pathophysiology of tamponade. The report states that this complication occurs with a frequency rate of 0.22%. The authors give details of their experience with a single patient and provide some recommendations for limiting the potential for bleeding complications in this patient population. You take a copy of the paper to your unit for discussion. You realize that this one case study is not enough to make practice change, so you search for stronger studies (e.g., controlled trials) to assist in developing an addition to your unit protocol manual to create awareness of possible complications arising from removal of monitoring catheters and how to prevent such complications.

CRITICAL APPRAISAL OF CASE–CONTROL STUDIES

A **case–control** study investigates why certain people develop a specific illness, have an adverse event with a particular treatment, or behave in a particular way. An example of a clinical question (written in the PICO format discussed in Chapter 2) for which a case–control study could be the appropriate design to provide an answer would be, In patients who have a family history of obesity (BMI > 30) (**P**), how does dietary carbohydrate intake (**I**) influence healthy weight maintenance (BMI < 25) (**O**) over 6 months (**T**)? Another clinical question that could be answered by a case–control study could be, In patients who have cystic fibrosis (**P**), how does socioeconomic status (**I**) influence their engagement with and adherence to their healthcare regimen (**O**)?

Investigators conducting a case–control study try to identify factors that explain the proposed relationship between a condition and a disease or behavior. The case–control method selects individuals who have an outcome (disease, adverse event, behavior) and retrospectively looks back to identify possible conditions that may be associated with the outcome. The characteristics of these individuals (the cases) are compared with those of other individuals who do not have the outcome (the controls). The assumption underpinning this methodological approach is that differences found between the groups may be likely indicators of why the "cases" became "cases."

For example, case–control methodology was used to address a clinical issue in identifying the connection between a rare cancer in women and diethylstilbestrol (DES) use by their mothers when they were pregnant (Herbst, Ulfelder, & Poskanzer, 1971). A prospective design would have been challenging because the adverse event took 20 years to develop and an RCT could not be used for ethical reasons (i.e., it would be unethical to ask pregnant women to take a drug to determine whether or not it increased the risk of birth defects). Eight women with cancer (vaginal adenocarcinoma) were enrolled in the study as cases, and 32 women without cancer were enrolled as controls in the study. Various risk factors were proposed, but found to be present in cases and controls. In contrast, mothers of seven of the women with cancer (i.e., cases) received DES when pregnant, while none of the controls' mothers did. The association between having the cancer and having a mother who took DES was highly significant ($p < 0.00001$) and was subsequently demonstrated in cohort studies (Troisi et al., 2007). The combination of (a) the huge impact vaginal adenocarcinoma had on women's lives, (b) the final outcome of death, and (c) the strong association established between the occurrence of the cancer and mothers taking DES while pregnant led to a common acceptance that DES causes this cancer (Reed & Fenton, 2013). However, causation cannot be established by a case–control study. Instead, a strong association was found between taking DES while pregnant and vaginal adenocarcinoma in the adult child. In addition, this case–control study played an important role is alerting people to the potential adverse effects of using any medications during pregnancy.

Rapid Appraisal Questions for Case–Control Studies

There are three rapid appraisal questions for all studies: Are the results of the study valid? What are the results? Do the results apply to my patients? Each of these questions has design-specific issues that must be answered before case–control studies can assist the clinician in decision making. Rapid critical appraisal is intended to quickly determine if a study is worthy of consideration (Box 5.2).

Are the Results of the Study Valid? (Validity)

How Were the Cases Obtained?   When appraising a case–control study, the clinician first determines how the cases were identified. The investigators should provide an adequate description or definition of what constitutes a case, including the diagnostic criteria, any exclusion criteria, and an explanation of how the cases were obtained (e.g., from a specialist center, such as an oncology unit, or from the general population). In the DES study, all the cases were identified in the same hospital in Boston over a period of a few years (Herbst et al., 1971). Cases coming from one geographical area could represent another explanation for the findings. Controls would need to be from the same geographical area to control for that possible confounding variable.

The source of the cases has important implications for the appraisal of the study. For example, recruitment of patients from an outpatient chemotherapy unit could include patients with well-established and managed disease and exclude those who are newly diagnosed. Bias could be introduced when cases are recruited from a general population because the potential participants could be at various stages in

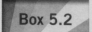

Box 5.2 — Rapid Critical Appraisal Questions for Case–Control Studies

1. Are the Results of the Study Valid?
   a. How were the cases obtained?
   b. Were appropriate controls selected?
   c. Were data collection methods the same for the cases and controls?
2. What Are the Results?
   a. Is an estimate of effect given (do the numbers add up)?
   b. Are there multiple comparisons of data?
   c. Is there any possibility of bias or confounding?
3. Will the Results Help Me in Caring for My Patients?
   a. Were the study patients similar to my own?
   b. How do the results compare with previous studies?
   c. What are my patient's/family's values and expectations for the outcome?

their disease or have a degree of the behavior of interest. Similarly, bias may arise if some of those cases sought are not included in the study for whatever reason. Patients who choose to become involved in research studies can have characteristics that distinguish them from those who avoid research studies. Care must be taken to ensure that these characteristics are not confounding variables that may influence the relationship between the condition being investigated and the outcome.

Were Appropriate Controls Selected? Selection of controls should be done so that the controls are as similar as possible to the cases in all respects except that they do not have the disease or observed behavior under investigation. In the DES study, the control women were born within 5 days of a case in the same hospital and with the same type of delivery and were from the same geographical area (Herbst et al., 1971). In general, controls may be selected from a specialist source or from the general population. The controls in case–control studies may be recruited into the study at the same time as the cases (concurrent controls). Alternatively, they may be what are referred to as historical controls (i.e., the person's past history is examined, often through medical records). Case–control studies with historical controls are generally viewed as lower on the hierarchy of evidence than those studies with concurrent controls, because the likelihood of bias is higher.

Were Data Collection Methods the Same for the Cases and Controls? Data collection is another potential source of bias in a case–control study. Recall bias, which is inaccurately remembering what occurred, needs to be considered because of the retrospective approach to determining the possible predictive factors. For example, people who have developed a fatal disease may have already spent a considerable amount of time thinking about why they might have developed the disease and therefore be able to recall in great detail their past behaviors. They may have preconceived ideas about what they think caused their illness and report these rather than other factors they have not considered.

In contrast, the disease-free controls may not have considered their past activities in great detail and may have difficulty recalling events accurately. The time since the event can influence how accurately details are recalled. Therefore, the data should ideally be collected in the same way for both the case and control groups. Blinding of the data collector to either the case or the control status or the risk factors of interest assists in reducing the inherent bias in a case–control approach and thus provides more accurate information.

Additional Considerations. The possibility of confounding variables needs to be considered when interpreting a case–control study. Confounding variables are other extrinsic factors that unexpectedly (or unknowingly) influence the variables expected to be associated with the outcome. A case–control study reported a strong association ($p = 0.001$) between coffee consumption and pancreatic cancer (MacMahon, Yen, Trichopoulos, Warren, & Nardi, 1981). The researchers stated that if the association was borne out by other research, it would account for a substantial proportion of the cases of pancreatic cancer in the United States. However, other research failed to replicate these findings, which are now regarded as false-positive results (Type I error—accepting that there was an effect when in fact there was none). Individuals with a history of diseases related to cigarette smoking or alcohol consumption were excluded from the control group, but not the cases (Boffetta et al., 2008). These activities are highly correlated with coffee consumption, suggesting that coffee consumption may have been lower among the controls than among the cases because of how the cases were selected. This methodological error generated an uncontrolled confounding variable that may have been the reason for the apparent association between coffee and pancreatic cancer and gives an alert appraiser reason to question the validity of the study findings. Subsequent case–control and cohort studies have failed to support an association between coffee and pancreatic cancer (Turati et al., 2012). All findings must be carefully evaluated to determine the validity of a study's conclusions and how applicable they are to practice.

Clinical Scenario 5.2

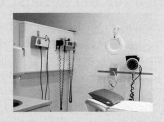

A concerned relative follows you into the hall from the room of a family member who has just been diagnosed with a rare brain tumor. He tells you he recently saw a program on television that described research linking cellular phone use to the development of some forms of cancer. His relative has used a cellular phone for many years, and he wonders whether that may have caused the tumor. You would like to know what the research literature has to say about this issue.

What the Literature Says: Answering a Clinical Question

The clinical question for Clinical Scenario 5.2 could be: In patients admitted with brain tumors (**P**), how does cell phone usage (**I**) influence brain tumor incidence (**O**)? When conducting a quick search of the literature, you find the following study and believe it may help answer the question from the family member in your practice: Inskip et al. (2001).

Enrolled in the study were 782 case participants with histologically confirmed glioma, meningioma, or acoustic neuroma. Participants came from a number of hospitals. The control participants were 799 patients admitted to the same hospitals as the cases but with nonmalignant conditions. The predictor measured was cellular phone usage, which was quantified using a personal interview to collect information on duration and frequency of use. Once the details of the study are evaluated, the general critical appraisal questions should be answered. The rapid critical appraisal questions for case–control studies found in Box 5.2 can assist in critically appraising this study to determine its value in answering this relative's question.

Are the Results of the Study Valid? (Validity)

This case–control study describes in detail how cases were selected from eligible patients who had been diagnosed with the various types of tumors. Tumor diagnosis was confirmed by objective tests. Validity can be compromised in case–control studies if cases are misdiagnosed. Control patients were concurrently recruited from the same healthcare centers and were matched for age, sex, and ethnicity.

A research nurse administered a computer-assisted personal interview with the patient or a proxy if the patient could not participate. Participants were asked about the frequency of cellular phone usage. Reliance on recall rather than a more objective way to measure cell phone usage is a weakness in this study. Other studies have used computer databases of actual cell phone usage to overcome this limitation (Guyatt et al., 2008). While case patients were matched on certain demographic variables, other variables that influenced the outcome may not have been considered. In addition, recall bias would be a serious threat to the validity of this study. Although the data analysis did not support the hypothesis that cellular phone usage causes brain tumors, possible inaccuracies in patient recall or use of different types of cellular phones raise questions about the validity of the results. Overall, the study suggested that cellular phone usage does not increase or decrease the risk of brain tumors. However, subsequent research has raised conflicting results, leading to the World Health Organization declaring wireless devices a "possible human carcinogen" in 2011 (Hardell, Carlberg, & Hansson Mild, 2013). Given the widespread use of cellular phones, and the controversy surrounding their risks, further research is needed and being conducted on this issue. Clinicians will need to keep abreast of this field if they are to have confidence in the validity of any individual study's findings.

What Are the Results? (Reliability)

Returning to the Inskip et al. study, comparisons were made between those who never or very rarely used a cellular phone and those who used one for more than 100 hours. The RR for cellular phone usage were RR = 0.9 for glioma (95% CI, 0.5 to 1.6); RR = 0.7 for meningioma (95% CI, 0.3 to 1.7); RR = 1.4 for acoustic neuroma (95% CI, 0.6 to 3.5); and the overall RR = 1.0 (95% CI, 0.6 to 1.5) for all tumor types combined. While some studies indicated that the RR of certain types of brain tumors increased with cell phone use, the overall result from this group of studies indicated an RR of 1. This indicates that a person who has used a cell phone for more than 100 hours is just as likely (RR = 1.0) to have a tumor as someone who has not used a cell phone. The CIs reportedly give us an estimate of the precision of the measurement of effect of cell phone use in this study. Note that all the CIs in this example include the value of 1. Remember that when the CI contains what is called the line of no effect, which for RR is 1, the results are not statistically significant.

For example, from this study's findings, the RR for meningioma was 0.7 with a CI of 0.3 to 1.7, which includes 1 and therefore is not statistically significant. Since in this study the sample size is moderate to large, we would expect the CIs to be narrow. The narrower the CI, the more precise the finding is for the clinician (i.e., the more likely clinicians can get close to the study finding). A 95% CI enables clinicians to be 95% confident that their findings, if they do the same thing (e.g., use the cell phone for so many hours), will be within the range of the CI. In studies with a high-risk outcome (e.g., death), having 95% confidence in knowing the outcome they will achieve may not be sufficient. In studies of these types, clinicians will want to know more specifically what they can expect and would be likely to choose a 99% CI.

Will the Results Help Me in Caring for My Patients? (Applicability)

When evaluating the results of this study and the associated limitations, it is difficult to find helpful information for clinical decision making. When critically appraising all studies, a basic aspect of applicability is to evaluate the study patients in comparison with the patients to whom the evidence would be applied (i.e., the clinician's own patients). Since this study has known limitations, it is more challenging to determine if the results would lead directly to selecting or avoiding cell phone use. However, the results of the study assist researchers in understanding the need for more research about cell phone usage and the possible sequelae of brain tumors. For the patient's family members, the information from this one study would not be definitive. To provide appropriate counsel to healthcare consumers, it would be important to find other studies that could help answer the clinical question (e.g., Hardell et al., 2013).

CRITICAL APPRAISAL OF COHORT STUDIES

The **cohort study** design is especially suitable for investigating the course of a disease or the unintended consequences of a treatment (Fineout-Overholt & Melnyk, 2007; Guyatt et al., 2008). A *cohort* refers to a study population sharing a characteristic or group of characteristics. Cohort studies can be conducted with and without a control group. Without a control group, researchers identify a cohort exposed to the characteristic of interest and monitor them over time to describe various outcomes. For example, a cohort could be adolescents experiencing their first episode of psychosis. The study could follow the cohort over time and report on what was observed and measured. Alternatively, a control group could be included by selecting another cohort of adolescents that is similar in every way, yet who have not experienced psychosis. As with case–control studies, exposed and unexposed cohorts should have a similar risk of the target outcome.

The largest long-term cohort study of women's health is the Nurses' Health Study. More than 121,000 nurses were enrolled in the study in 1976 and were mailed questionnaires every 2 years. A new cohort was enrolled in 1989 and, as of 2013, Nurses' Health Study 3 is enrolling a third cohort. Several correlations have been identified through these cohorts. For example, women under 60 years (but not older) who sleep 5 or fewer hours per night are more likely to have high blood pressure compared to those sleeping 7 hours per night (Gangwisch, Feskanich, Malaspina, Shen, & Forman, 2013). The results were statistically significant (OR = 1.19 and 95% CI = 1.14 to 1.25). The cohorts were selected from within Nurses' Health Study I and II based on answers to a question about sleep duration.

Since cohort studies generally follow people over a period of time to determine their outcomes, they are longitudinal. In prospective studies, a cohort exposed to a drug, surgery, or particular diagnosis may be followed for years while collecting data on outcomes. For example, in studying DES and cancer, cohort studies have been running since the initial case studies reported in the 1970s and now involve three generations of people who have been impacted by this association (Troisi et al., 2007). Since such prospective studies can take many years to complete, cohort studies are often retrospective. In retrospective studies, the outcome under investigation (e.g., occurrence of a disease or condition) has already occurred and researchers go even further into the past to select those characteristics they believe might be associated with the given outcome. The cohort is followed from that point forward to determine what influenced the development of the outcome and when those influences occurred. Since participants are not randomly assigned to a cohort, cohort studies do not have an experimental research design. These studies therefore have the limitations of all observational studies.

An example of the limitations that may accompany a cohort study can be seen in the data supporting or refuting the benefits of hormone replacement therapy for heart health. A meta-analysis of 16 cohort studies of women taking postmenopausal estrogen therapy concluded that the medication gave women a lower risk of coronary heart disease (CHD) with an RR of 0.5 and 95% CI of 0.44 to 0.57 (Stampfer & Colditz, 1991). Practice was based on these studies for quite a long time; however, standards of care were challenged when the highly publicized Women's Health Initiative RCT showed that hormone replacement therapy actually increased the risk of CHD in postmenopausal women (Rossouw et al., 2002). The quandary for clinicians is which studies provide the most valid and reliable evidence for making decisions with their patients. RCTs are the strongest evidence for making decisions about interventions; however, without the existence of this type of evidence, cohort studies may be the only evidence to guide practice.

Rapid Appraisal Questions for a Cohort Study

The design-specific rapid critical appraisal questions for cohort studies that can assist the clinician in quickly determining the value of a cohort study can be found in Box 5.3.

Box 5.3 Rapid Critical Appraisal Questions for Cohort Studies

1. Are the Results of the Study Valid?
   a. Was there a representative and well-defined sample of patients at a similar point in the course of the disease?
   b. Was follow-up sufficiently long and complete?
   c. Were objective and unbiased outcome criteria used?
   d. Did the analysis adjust for important prognostic risk factors and confounding variables?
2. What Are the Results?
   a. What is the magnitude of the relationship between predictors (i.e., prognostic indicators) and targeted outcome?
   b. How likely is the outcome event(s) in a specified period of time?
   c. How precise are the study estimates?
3. Will the Results Help Me in Caring for My Patients?
   a. Were the study patients similar to my own?
   b. Will the results lead directly to selecting or avoiding therapy?
   c. Would the results be used to counsel patients?

Are the Results of the Study Valid? (Validity)

Was There a Representative and Well-Defined Sample of Patients at a Similar Point in the Course of the Disease? When appraising a cohort study, establishing the characteristics of the patients or clients under study is important. These characteristics, such as the severity of symptoms or stage in the illness trajectory, will strongly influence the impact an intervention may have on the patient's condition or the resulting outcomes. A suitably detailed description of the population and how the cohorts were defined (i.e., how the exposure [and nonexposure, if appropriate] cohorts were established) is necessary for the clinician to draw any conclusions about the validity of the results and whether they are generalizable to other populations.

Was Follow-Up Sufficiently Long and Complete? The length of follow-up for a cohort study will depend on the outcomes of interest. For example, wound breakdown as a consequence of an early discharge program after surgery would require a shorter follow-up period than a study examining hospital admissions for management of acute asthma subsequent to an in-school education strategy. Insufficient time for outcomes to be demonstrated will bias the study findings.

Clinicians appraising a cohort study would need to evaluate if people withdrew from the study, and if so, why (i.e., to determine if there was something unique about those participants). Patients enrolled in a cohort study, particularly over a long time, may be lost to follow-up. Furthermore, the condition of interest in a cohort study may predispose patients to incomplete or nonadherent participation in a study. Cohort studies involving patients with a terminal or end-stage illness commonly must deal with patients dying during the study before follow-up data are completely collected. While unavoidable, the extent of loss to follow-up may bias the study results.

Were Objective and Unbiased Outcome Criteria Used? When evaluating outcomes in the cohort, researchers can use both subjective and objective measurements. Subjective measures introduce bias (e.g., recall) into the study; whereas, ideally, objective measures have less bias and provide more reliable data. Patient self-reporting and clinician diagnosis are outcome measures that are subject to some bias. Objective measures will be based on a reference standard, such as a biochemical test or clinical interview conducted by a psychologist. Research reports should contain the validity and reliability of the measures that were used. The clinician should also integrate clinical expertise with appraisal skills when thinking about the measurement of the outcomes of interest.

Did the Analysis Adjust for Important Prognostic Risk Factors and Confounding Variables? Clinicians need to consider what, if any, other prognostic (i.e., predictive) factors could have been included in the study, but were not. If there are other factors identified, clinicians must determine how those would affect the validity of the current findings. In addition, other factors must be considered that could muddy the relationships among the existing identified factors and the outcomes. For example, a cohort study may be designed to study the risk of gastric bleeding in nonsteroidal anti-inflammatory drug (NSAID) users compared to nonusers. Incidence of gastric bleeding (i.e., the event rate) is so low that an enormous number of participants would be needed for an RCT, making a cohort study more feasible. However, a cohort of NSAID users may inherently be older than a cohort of NSAID nonusers and bring with them increased risk for gastric bleeding. In this case, age could be a confounding variable if it is not controlled for when selecting the cohorts.

What Are the Results? (Reliability)

What Is the Magnitude of the Relationship Between Predictors (i.e., Prognostic Indicators) and Targeted Outcome? For cohort studies, clinicians must evaluate the final results. Often studies may report an incident rate or a proportion for the outcome occurring within the exposed and unexposed cohorts as well as the differences in those rates or proportions. Evaluating the strength of association between exposure and outcome is imperative (e.g., RR, ARR, or NNT).

How Likely Is the Outcome Event(s) in a Specified Period of Time? Often the strength of association is provided for a given time period. For example, researchers may state that the NNT is 15 with an antihypertensive medication to prevent one more stroke within 3 years.

How Precise Are the Study Estimates? CIs must be provided, along with *p* values, to determine precision of the findings (i.e., whether a clinician can replicate the results).

Will the Results Help Me in Caring for My Patients? (Applicability)

Were the Study Patients Similar to My Own? As with all studies, it is important to note how similar or dissimilar the sample is to the clinicians' patients.

Will the Results Lead Directly to Selecting or Avoiding Therapy? and Would the Results Be Used to Counsel Patients? After clinicians evaluate the findings to see if they are reliable and applicable to their patients, they must determine how they can be used to assist those patients in their healthcare management. Caution must be used here, as cohort studies are not RCTs and inherently have bias in their design; therefore, confidence in replicating their findings should always be lower. Nevertheless, providing information to patients regarding the study findings is important to having evidence-based consumers who use the best evidence to make their healthcare decisions.

Clinical Scenario 5.3

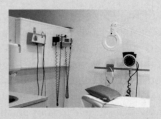

You have been working in a community mental health program for a number of years. Young people who have experienced their first episode of schizophrenia make up a large proportion of your client base. Your colleagues have suggested that differences in the disease and social course of schizophrenia may arise depending on clients' age at onset. You volunteer to find a paper for the next journal club that investigates the influence of age at onset on the symptom-related course of the disease.

What the Literature Says: Answering a Clinical Question

The clinical question for Clinical Scenario 5.3 could be: In adolescent patients who have schizophrenia (*P*), how does age of onset (*I*) influence the social course of the disease (*O*)? The following study may help answer the question about adolescents and schizophrenia: Häfner, Hambrecht, Löffler, Munk-Jøgensen, and Riecher-Rössler (1998). Using the rapid critical appraisal questions, this study will be evaluated to determine whether it provides valid, relevant evidence to address this clinical question.

The participants in the study were 1,109 patients first admitted to a mental health institution with a broad diagnosis of schizophrenia at age 12 to 20, 21 to 35, or 36 to 59 years. Symptoms were assessed at 6 months and at 1, 2, 3, and 5 years after first admission. The outcome measured was symptom severity as determined by scores on the symptom-based Present State Examination (PSE), using a computer program to arrive at diagnostic classifications (PSE-CATEGO). The higher the score on the PSE-CATEGO, the more severe the illness.

Are the Results of the Study Valid? (Validity)

There are several questions that help determine if a cohort study is valid. The first is: Was there a representative and well-defined sample of patients at a similar point in the course of the disease? Since the participants in this study were admitted into the study at their first admission and their onset and course before the first admission were assessed retrospectively with a standardized instrument, the study sample seems representative for patients at similar points for schizophrenia. The second question is: Was follow-up sufficiently long and complete? In this study, ensuing symptoms and social consequences were prospectively followed over 5 years. Although there was no explanation for why a 5-year follow-up period was chosen, nor was any information given on losses to follow-up, 5 years is probably sufficiently long enough for follow-up. The third question is: Were objective and unbiased outcome criteria used? Symptomatology, functional impairment, and social disability were assessed by clinically experienced, trained psychiatrists and psychologists using previously validated instruments. The fourth and final question to assess study validity is: Did the analysis adjust for important prognostic risk factors? In the study, symptoms of schizophrenia as well as onset of formal treatment were considered for their impact on functional impairment and social disability. Given these methods, the study findings are valid and can help in determining practice.

What Are the Results? (Reliability)

In this study, participants with early-onset schizophrenia, especially men, presented with higher PSE-CATEGO scores than did study participants with late-onset disease. In men, symptom severity decreased with increasing age of onset. In women, symptom severity remained stable, although there was an increase in negative symptoms with late onset. Disorganization decreased with age, but delusions increased markedly across the whole age of onset range. The main determinant of social course was level of social development at onset. Inferential statistics were used to determine any differences between groups, and *p* values were reported; however, there were no CIs provided, and precision of the effect is difficult to determine.

Will the Results Help Me in Caring for My Patients? (Applicability)

Some of the study participants are similar in age and social development to those in your clinic population. Although much of the data show trends rather than statistically significant differences, the authors of the study developed some suggestions about why any differences exist that are clinically meaningful. You and your colleagues could use this information, along with other studies, to plan early intervention programs with the goal of limiting the negative consequences of schizophrenia in young people. This study is applicable to your practice and should assist in making decisions. Always keep in mind, however, that any time you use evidence to make clinical decisions, subsequent evaluation of the difference the evidence makes in your own practice is essential.

....
**Persistence is the twin sister of excellence. One is a matter of quality;
the other, a matter of time.**
—Marabel Morgan
....

CRITICAL APPRAISAL OF RCTS

RCTs are the most appropriate research design to answer questions of efficacy and effectiveness of interventions because their methodology provides confidence in establishing cause and effect (i.e., increased confidence that a given intervention leads to a particular outcome). As individual studies, RCTs rank as Level II evidence in this hierarchy of evidence because a well-conducted study should have a low risk of bias. A synthesis of RCTs is considered Level I evidence for answering questions about interventions for the same reason (see Chapter 1, Box 1.3). An RCT compares the effectiveness of different interventions. This can involve one treatment group getting the intervention under investigation and a comparison treatment group receiving another intervention (e.g., current standard of care for the same outcome) to determine which is better at producing the outcome. The interventions studied could be the experimental treatment compared to a comparison group, with the comparison group receiving no intervention (i.e., true control group), a placebo, or the usual standard of care. RCTs are experimental studies in which participants are *randomly* assigned to each intervention in what are often referred to as the "arms" of a study. An RCT often has two arms, but may have more than two, such as when an intervention is being compared with no intervention and a placebo. RCTs are also prospective and longitudinal in that participants are studied over a period of time to assess the effects of an intervention or treatment on selected outcomes.

In crossover trials, participants are given the experimental intervention and then the comparison or placebo-controlled intervention in consecutive periods and thus serve as their own controls. For example, a crossover design was used to study the effectiveness of two combinations of dental hygiene products on bad mouth odor (Farrell, Barker, Walanski, & Gerlach, 2008). The study used four periods in which participants were randomly assigned to either combination A (antibacterial toothpaste, antibacterial mouth rinse, and an oscillating-rotating toothbrush) or combination B (regular toothpaste and manual toothbrush). The participants were allowed 2 days between each intervention to permit the effects of the previous intervention to subside or washout, hence the name "washout period." Combination A led to a 35% reduction in bad breath as determined by an instrument widely used to measure breath volatiles ($p < 0.001$). Crossover trials allow comparisons of the same participants' responses to the two interventions, thus minimizing variability caused by having different people in each intervention group. The crossover design works well for short-lasting interventions, such as the dental hygiene products used in this study. The major concern with crossover trials is carryover, in which the effects of the first intervention linger into the period of testing of the second intervention (Higgins & Green, 2008). It is important to consider this introduction of bias when critically appraising a crossover trial.

RCTs, in general, are sometimes considered to be overly artificial because of the control investigators exert over most aspects of the study. Predetermined inclusion and exclusion criteria are used to select participants and provide a homogeneous study population (i.e., all the participants in the sample are alike). The investigators must carefully consider how to recruit participants for the intervention, the control, and the comparison groups before starting the study. The outcomes of interest are also predetermined. Since some suggest that the results of an RCT are really only generalizable to the particular population studied in the trial because of this artificiality, two approaches to conducting RCTs have been developed.

The two approaches to conducting RCTs are called the efficacy study and the effectiveness study (Kim, 2013). The efficacy has to be established first (i.e., how well does the intervention actually work) before an effectiveness trial is done (i.e., how well does the intervention work in the real world).

The distinction rests with the sort of research question that each study attempts to answer. In an efficacy study (sometimes also called an explanatory study), everything is controlled as tightly as possible to ensure the two groups differ only in regard to how they respond to the intervention. Such studies give the best information on whether and how well the intervention works, but may not be as readily applicable to clinical practice. Effectiveness studies are about the pragmatic value of an intervention in clinical practice. In an effectiveness study, controls are kept to a minimum to ensure the research setting is as similar to routine practice as possible. In contrast, efficacy studies are designed to explain how or why an intervention works, usually in ideal circumstances. While the degree to which RCT findings are generalizable must be kept in mind when applying the results to individual patients, RCTs remain the most valid and rigorous study design for assessing the benefits or harms of an intervention and supporting cause and effect relationships.

Rapid Appraisal Questions for Randomized Controlled Trials

Are the Results of the Study Valid? (Validity)

Although all the issues and standard appraisal questions discussed earlier in this chapter apply to RCTs, there are additional questions that are specific to this methodology. Rapid appraisal questions for RCTs can assist the clinician in quickly determining a particular study's value for practice (Box 5.4).

Were the Subjects Randomly Assigned to the Experimental and Control Groups? Because the purpose of an RCT is to determine the efficacy or effectiveness of an intervention in producing an outcome, with-

Box 5.4 — Rapid Critical Appraisal Questions for Randomized Controlled Trials

1. Are the Results of the Study Valid?
   a. Were the subjects randomly assigned to the experimental and control groups?
   b. Was random assignment concealed from the individuals who were first enrolling subjects into the study?
   c. Were the subjects and providers kept blind to study group?
   d. Were reasons given to explain why subjects did not complete the study?
   e. Were the follow-up assessments conducted long enough to fully study the effects of the intervention?
   f. Were the subjects analyzed in the group to which they were randomly assigned?
   g. Was the control group appropriate?
   h. Were the instruments used to measure the outcomes valid and reliable?
   i. Were the subjects in each of the groups similar on demographic and baseline clinical variables?

2. What Are the Results?
   a. How large is the intervention or treatment effect (NNT, NNH, effect size, level of significance)?
   b. How precise is the intervention or treatment effect (CI)?

3. Will the Results Help Me in Caring for My Patients?
   a. Were all clinically important outcomes measured?
   b. What are the risks and benefits of the treatment?
   c. Is the treatment feasible in my clinical setting?
   d. What are my patient's/family's values and expectations for the outcome being pursued and the treatment itself?

out it being by chance, the groups assigned to either the experimental treatment or the comparison need to be equivalent in all relevant characteristics (e.g., age, disease severity, socioeconomic status, gender) at the beginning of the study, before the intervention is delivered. The best method to ensure baseline equivalency between study groups is to randomly assign participants to the experimental treatment or intervention and to the comparison or placebo-controlled group. This became more obvious when awareness of bias in observational studies arose in the 1980s. Several studies were published that showed how observational studies tended to have more favorable outcomes than an RCT on the same research question (Kunz & Oxman, 1998). In one early review, the researchers found significant differences between the outcomes of 145 trials investigating different treatments for acute myocardial infarction (Chalmers, Celano, Sacks, & Smith, 1983). Within this body of evidence, the frequency of significant outcomes for observational trials for a given treatment was 25%, for nonconcealed RCTs was 11%, and for concealed RCTs was 5%. The average RRR for a myocardial infarction per study type was 34%, 7%, and 3%, respectively. More recent comparisons of study designs have found that observational studies can produce similar results to RCTs with certain types of interventions, which suggests that the general quality of observational studies has improved (Benson & Hartz, 2000; Concato, Shah, & Horwitz, 2000). However, this is not always the case. A review of studies comparing oral and depot antipsychotics for schizophrenia found no significant difference between the two formulations in RCTs, while observational trials showed a significant benefit for depot injections (Kirson et al., 2013). This shows the importance of examining the impact of research design on study outcomes.

In a large review of treatments for 45 conditions, researchers found that while randomized and nonrandomized trials of the same treatment tend to agree on whether the treatment works, they often disagree on the size of the effect (Ioannidis et al., 2001). Observational studies may often be preferred in evaluating the harms of medical treatments; however, RCTs of the same treatments usually found larger risks of harm than observational trials, though not always (Papanikolaou, Christidi, & Ioannidis, 2006). In general, it appears that if the clinician chooses which patients receive which treatment or if patients self-select the treatment they will receive, important demographic and clinical variables are introduced that impact the outcomes. Where possible, random assignment should be used to minimize such bias.

The method of randomization should be reported in the methods section of the published research report. To avoid selection bias, the random sequence for assigning patients should be unpredictable (e.g., a random number table, a computer random number generator, or tossing a coin). Researchers sometimes assign participants to groups on an alternate basis or by such criteria as the participant's date of birth or the day of the week, but these methods are not adequate because the sequence can introduce bias. For example, significantly higher death rates after elective surgery have been demonstrated if the surgery is carried out on Friday or at the weekend compared to other days of the week (Aylin, Alexandrescu, Jen, Mayer, & Bottle, 2013). If participants in a study were assigned to a surgical intervention according to the day of the week, the day would be a confounding variable. Such kinds of assignment methods are called *pseudo-* or *quasi-randomization*, and have been shown to introduce assignment bias (Schulz & Grimes, 2002b). Often such approaches are used because they are more convenient; however, the higher risk of bias makes them less desirable.

Variations on the simple randomization method described previously do exist. *Cluster randomization* is a method whereby groups of participants are randomized to the same treatment together (Torgerson, 2001). The unit of measurement (e.g., individual clinician, patient unit, hospital, clinic, or school) in such a study is the experimental unit rather than individual participants. When critically appraising a cluster randomized trial, attention must be paid to whether the results were analyzed properly. A review of such trials in primary care found that 41% did not take account of the clustering in their analyses (Eldridge, Ashby, Feder, Rudnicka, & Ukoumunne, 2004). *Block randomization* is where participants from groups with characteristics that cannot be manipulated (e.g., age, gender) are randomly assigned to the intervention and control groups in equal numbers (i.e., 40 men out of a group of 100 men and 40 women out of a group of 100 women). *Stratified randomization* ensures an equal distribution of certain patient characteristics (e.g., gestational age or severity of illness) across the groups.

Was Random Assignment Concealed From the Individuals Who Were First Enrolling Subjects Into the Study? Bias can be introduced when recruiting participants into a study. If those recruiting know to which group the participants will be assigned, they may recruit those going into the intervention group differently than those going into the comparison or control group. Therefore, random assignment should be concealed until after the participants are recruited into the study. This can be accomplished with a method as simple as having designated recruiters who are not investigators or by placing the assignment in an envelope and revealing the assignment once recruitment is complete, to something as elaborate as using an assignment service independent of the study investigators. Using a sealed, opaque envelope to conceal the randomly generated treatment allocation can be susceptible to bias if recruiters are determined to ensure a specific allocation for a particular participant (Schulz & Grimes, 2002a). This susceptibility was illustrated in a study in which researchers anonymously admitted they had held semiopaque envelopes up to a bright light to reveal the allocation sequence or searched a principal investigator's files to discover the allocation list (Schulz, 1995). While such investigators may have rationalized that their actions were well intended, they probably introduced bias into their studies, which could have undermined the conclusions. To avoid such issues, a central research facility could be used where someone other than the study researchers phone or fax the enrollment of a new participant. The central facility determines the treatment allocation and informs the researcher. Such *distance randomization* removes the possibility of researchers introducing bias by attempting to ensure that a patient receives the treatment they believe would be most beneficial; however, the increased cost of this option may prohibit using it.

Were the Subjects and Providers Kept Blind to Study Group? Blinding, sometimes referred to as "masking," is undertaken to reduce the bias that could arise when those observing the outcome know what intervention was received by the study participants. Clinicians may be familiar with the term *double blind*, in which neither the person delivering the intervention nor the participant receiving it knows whether it is the treatment or comparison intervention; however, they may not be as familiar with other degrees of blinding, such as *single blind* and *triple blind* (Devereaux et al., 2001). All research reports need to describe precisely how groups were blinded to treatment allocation. Double-blinding is very important because it mitigates the placebo effect (i.e., participants respond to an intervention simply because they received something rather than the intervention itself being effective). Studies have demonstrated that the size of a treatment effect can be inflated when patients, clinicians, data collectors, data analyzers, or report authors know which patients received which interventions (Devereaux et al., 2001). When everyone involved is blinded, the expectations of those involved in the study are less likely to influence the results observed.

The degree of blinding utilized in a study partly depends on the intervention being studied and the outcome of interest. For example, death as an outcome is objective and unlikely to be influenced by knowledge of the intervention. However, quality of life or pain scores are relatively subjective measures and may be influenced by the participant's knowledge, if outcomes are self-reporting, or by the health professionals' knowledge, if they are collecting the data.

The **placebo** intervention is another method used for blinding. When investigators report on using a placebo, it should appear like the treatment in all aspects. For example, a placebo medication should look, smell, and taste just like the experimental drug and should be given via the same mode of delivery. A placebo can be developed for many types of interventions. Surgical procedures have been tested in patient-blinded trials using "sham surgery" in which patients receive only an incision. Although ethically controversial, they are viewed by some as necessary to adequately evaluate surgical procedures (Swift, 2012).

When the intervention cannot be blinded, usually due to ethical considerations, researchers can ensure that outcome assessment is blinded to reduce bias. For example, patients with burns could be allocated to either the currently used dressing type or an experimental bioengineered dressing. The patients and their caregivers would be aware of the dressing that they were receiving; however, through taking photographs of the wounds and having assessors score the degree of healing without knowing which patients received which dressing, healing could be measured in a blinded fashion.

Were Reasons Given to Explain Why Subjects Did Not Complete the Study? Researchers conducting RCTs prospectively follow people over a period of time, sometimes for years. When critically appraising such studies, the research consumer should examine the number of participants originally enrolled in the study and compare that number with the final numbers in the analyzed outcome data. Ideally, the status of every patient enrolled in the study will be known at the study's completion and reported. When large numbers of participants leave a study and therefore have unknown outcomes, the validity of the study is potentially compromised or bias may be introduced. Participants may leave a study for many reasons, including adverse outcomes, death, a burdensome protocol, or because their symptoms resolved and they did not return for assessment. When critically appraising a study, consider whether those who were lost to follow-up differed from those who finished the trial. Although a commonly accepted dropout rate is 20% or less (i.e., 80% retention), this arbitrary rate is inadvisable as a sole marker of study validity.

Consider an example where researchers conducting a well-done study with severely ill participants plan to enroll more participants than they know is necessary according to a **power analysis**. These are done to reduce making a Type II error (i.e., accepting that the intervention really did not work, when it did). They enroll additional participants because they anticipate a high dropout rate. For example, if the power calculation determines they need 100 participants to avoid a Type II error, and they anticipate a 50% dropout rate, they may enroll 200 participants to ensure that at least 100 participants complete the study. This is why it is important to note not only the number of participants who completed the study but also other factors that influence such studies (e.g., conducted over very long periods or involving severely ill participants) that may lead to unavoidable higher dropout rates. Often researchers will compare the demographic variables of those who dropped out of the study to those who remained in the study. They may also assess the impact of loss to follow-up by assuming the worst outcome for those who withdrew and by repeating the analysis. If researchers find that this worst case scenario has the same treatment effect, clinicians can consider that the validity of the study has not been compromised.

Were the Follow-Up Assessments Conducted Long Enough to Fully Study the Effects of the Intervention? In critically appraising an intervention study, clinicians consider how long it takes for the intervention to produce the outcome. For example, if an intervention was given in hospital, and a study measured the outcome at discharge, insufficient time may have passed to adequately evaluate the outcome. Follow-up assessment might need to be weeks or months later. In critically appraising a study, clinicians should use their experience with patient populations to guide them in determining the appropriate timeframe for a study.

Were the Subjects Analyzed in the Group to Which They Were Randomly Assigned? Another way to ask this question is: Was an intention to treat analysis conducted? Despite the best efforts of investigators, some patients assigned to a particular group may not receive the allocated treatment throughout the entire study period. For example, some people allocated an experimental drug might not take it. In the Chocolate Happiness Undergoing More Pleasantness (CHUMP) study (Chan, 2007), participants in one treatment group traded treatments with another treatment arm of the study, muddying the analysis for both arms of the study.

One approach to addressing these cross-contamination issues could be to exclude from the analysis the data of everyone who did not adhere to their assigned intervention. However, this approach could potentially introduce bias as patients who change treatment or drop out of a study may be systematically different from those who do not. The intention to treat principle states that data should be analyzed according to the group to which the patient was originally allocated. Researchers follow this principle to preserve the value of random assignment (Busse & Heetveld, 2006). If the comparability of groups is to be maintained through the study, patients should not be excluded from the analysis or switched.

The intention to treat principle tends to minimize Type I errors but is more susceptible to Type II errors (Table 5.1). The alternative approach would be to analyze patient data according to the intervention they actually obtained in the study (i.e., per protocol analysis), but this method is vulnerable to bias. Any study that deviates substantially from its protocol may have methodological problems or a higher risk of bias and should be evaluated carefully before being applied to practice (Ruiz-Canela, Martínez-González, & de Irala-Estévez, 2000).

Another alternative would be for researchers to exclude patients from final data analysis. It is commonly accepted that patients who were actually ineligible to be enrolled in the trial and who were mistakenly randomized may be excluded, as well as patients who were prematurely enrolled in a trial but who never received the intervention. Excluding such patients from analysis may not introduce bias; however, clinicians should consider the implications these reductions would have on sample size and the study's ability to detect important differences (Fergusson, Horwood, & Ridder, 2005).

Was the Control Group Appropriate? The only difference between the experimental and control groups should be the study intervention. What the researchers choose for the comparison or control intervention can assist in understanding whether or not the study results are valid. If an intervention involves personal attention, time spent with participants, or other activities, the participants in the treatment group must be provided the same attention, time, or activities as the comparison group. This is because the attention, time, or other activity could impact the outcomes. For example, an RCT was conducted to evaluate the effect of a complementary therapy, Therapeutic Touch (TT), on women's mood (Lafreniere et al., 1999). Participants in the experimental group removed their shoes, laid on a hospital bed, and listened to soft music while receiving TT. They rested for 5 to 10 minutes and were taken to a testing room where they completed study questionnaires. Those in the control group went directly to the testing room to complete the questionnaires, without any of the attention or time that the experimental group received. The indicators of mood differed significantly between the groups, but the choice of control made it inappropriate to attribute the differences to TT alone. The soft music, relaxing environment, 10 minutes of rest, or any combination of those confounding variables could have contributed to the observed outcomes, making the study findings unreliable for clinicians to use in practice. Another study found that when irritable bowel syndrome patients were informed that they would be given a placebo, their outcomes were significantly better than those assigned to a no treatment control (Kaptchuk et al., 2010). In this case, the professional interaction between patients and researchers impacted the outcomes, even though the patients knew their treatment was an inert placebo.

If treatments used in a research study are to be used in clinical practice, a clear description of the intervention and control is essential. If the detail is unclear, clinicians' delivery of the interventions may differ, thereby resulting in a different outcome. For example, drug dosages, details of written information given to participants, or number of clinic visits, if relevant, should be described adequately. The description of the interventions in the methods section also should report any other interventions that differed between the two groups, such as additional visits from practitioners or telephone calls, because these may affect the reported outcomes.

Were the Instruments Used to Measure the Outcomes Valid and Reliable? The instruments researchers use to measure study outcomes are important in determining how useful the results are to clinicians. If the measures are valid (i.e., they measure what they are intended to) and they are reliable (i.e., the items within the instrument are consistent in their measurement, time after time), then clinicians can have more confidence in the study findings. Chapter 17 has more information on validity and reliability of outcome measurement.

Were the Subjects in Each of the Groups Similar on Demographic and Baseline Clinical Variables? Sufficient information about how the participants were selected should be provided in the research paper, usually in the methods section. The study population should be appropriate for the question the study is addressing. Clinicians can decide whether the results reported are relevant to the patients in their care. The choice of participants may affect the size of the observed treatment effect. For example, an intervention delivered to people with advanced disease and cared for in a specialist center may not be as effective for or relevant to those with early-stage disease managed in the community.

The characteristics of all intervention groups should be similar at baseline if randomization did what it is expected to do. These data are often the first data reported in the results section of a research paper. This can include demographic variables of the groups, such as age and gender, stage of disease, or illness severity scores. Investigators generally indicate if the groups differed significantly on any variables. If the groups are different at baseline, clinicians must decide whether these reported differences invalidate the findings, rendering them clinically unusable.

As an example, let's say that researchers attempted to determine the effectiveness of oral sucrose in alleviating procedural pain in infants. The participating infants were randomized to treatment (sucrose) or control (water) groups. Statistical tests found that the two groups did not differ significantly in gestational age, birth weight, and the like. However, by chance and despite the appropriate randomization, a statistically significant difference in the severity of illness scores existed between the two groups and in the number of infants in each group who used a pacifier as a comfort measure. As clinicians evaluate these results, they must decide about the usefulness of the study findings. If the outcome of interest was incidence of infection, these differences may be irrelevant. However, in the hypothetical study described here, the outcome (i.e., pain scores associated with a procedure) could very well be influenced by the infants' use of a pacifier for comfort. In this case, the baseline differences should be taken into account when reporting the observed effects. If the groups are reported as being significantly different on certain baseline variables, clinicians should look for how investigators controlled for those baseline differences in their statistical analyses (e.g., analysis of covariance tests).

What Are the Results? (Reliability)

How Large Is the Intervention or Treatment Effect and How Precise Is the Intervention or Treatment Effect? How the size and precision of the effect are reported is extremely important. As discussed earlier in this chapter, trials should report the total number of study participants assigned to the groups, the numbers available for measurement of outcomes, and the occurrence or event rates in the groups. If these data are not reported, the measures of effect, such as RR and OR, cannot be calculated. CI and/or p values (or the information required to calculate these) should also be included in the results presented to identify the precision of the effect estimates.

Clinicians have to decide on the usefulness or clinical significance of any statistical differences observed. As discussed earlier, statistically significant differences and clinically meaningful differences are not always equivalent. If the CI is wide and includes the point estimate of no effect, such as an RR of 1 or a reported p value of greater than 0.05, the precision of the measurement is likely to be inadequate and the results unreliable. Clinicians cannot have confidence that they can implement the treatment and get similar results. Clinicians must also ask, since the results are not significant and the CI is wide, if it is possible that the sample size was not large enough. A larger sample would likely produce a shorter CI. In addition, trials are increasingly conducted across a large number of healthcare sites. If the findings are consistent across different settings, clinicians could be more confident that the findings were reliable.

Will the Results Assist Me in Caring for My Patients? (Applicability)

Are the Outcomes Measured Clinically Relevant? EBP requires integration of clinical expertise with the best available research evidence and patient values, concerns, and choices. Clinicians need to utilize their own expertise at this point in the critical appraisal process to decide whether the outcomes measured in a study were clinically important. They also need to assess whether the timing of outcome measurement in relation to the delivery of the intervention was appropriate. For example, it may be important to measure the effectiveness of an intervention, such as corticosteroid administration in the management of traumatic brain injury, by measuring survival to discharge from the intensive care unit. However, in determining the effectiveness of a cancer therapy, survival up to 5 years may be more relevant. Outcome measures such as mortality would appear appropriate in these examples but would not likely be relevant in trials with patients with dementia or chronic back pain. Quality of life scores or days lost from work would be more useful measures in the studies of these types of conditions.

Investigators may be interested in more than one outcome when designing a study, such as less pain and an improved quality of life. Researchers should designate the primary outcome of interest in their research report, and should clarify what outcome formed the basis of their a priori power calculation (assuming one was carried out). This should minimize problems with multiple measures or data dredging in attempts to ensure that a significant result is found.

Clinical Scenario 5.4

At a recent meeting of the surgical division managers of your hospital, the budget was discussed. An idea was proposed that a legitimate cost-cutting measure may be found by discharging women earlier after surgery for breast cancer. Debate about the advantages and disadvantages of such a change to health service provision continued until it was decided to investigate the available evidence.

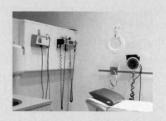

What the Literature Says: Answering a Clinical Question

The following study may begin to help answer the question that arises from Clinical Scenario 5.4. In women who have had surgery for breast cancer (**P**), how does early discharge (**I**) compared to current length of stay (**C**) affect coping with the challenges of recovery (**O**) (physical and psychosocial)? Bundred et al. (1998). Using the general critical appraisal questions, clinicians can critically appraise this study to determine whether it provides valid, reliable, and relevant evidence.

The participants in the study were 100 women who had early breast cancer and who were undergoing (a) mastectomy with axillary node clearance ($n = 20$) or (b) breast conservation surgery ($n = 80$). The intervention and comparison were early discharge program versus routine length of stay. The outcomes measured were physical illness (i.e., infection, seroma formation, shoulder movement) and psychological illness (i.e., depression and anxiety scores). The timing of follow-up was first preoperatively, then 1 and 3 months postoperatively.

Are the Results of the Study Valid? (Validity)

After patients were recruited into the study, they were randomized in clusters for each week of admissions by a research nurse who opened a sealed envelope containing the randomization code. A flowchart was provided in the report to identify the recruitment, participation, and follow-up of participants. Before the study began (i.e., a priori), a power calculation was undertaken to determine how large the sample needed to be to lessen the chance of accepting that there was no effect when there was one (i.e., Type II error). Participants were analyzed using an intention to treat analysis. Participants were not blinded to the intervention and no mention was made of whether the investigators assessing the outcomes were blinded. A detailed description of the intervention and the control management was given. The groups were reported as similar at baseline. Based on these methods, the study results should be considered valid.

What Are the Results? (Reliability)

Results are expressed as OR with 95% CI, and p values are provided where there was statistical significance. Women discharged early had greater shoulder movement (OR 0.28; 95% CI, 0.08 to 0.95) and less wound pain (OR 0.28; 95% CI, 0.10 to 0.79) at 3 months compared with the standard length of stay group. Symptom questionnaire scores were significantly lower in the early discharge group at 1 month. It is difficult to determine whether there were clinically meaningful differences in the psychological measures because a total of six tools were used to measure psychological illness. Multiple measurements in themselves are more likely to lead to significant results.

Will the Results Help Me in Caring for My Patients? (Applicability)

The results presented in this research report are those of a planned interim analysis (i.e., the analysis was done to confirm that there were no adverse consequences of early discharge). This approach is reasonable to protect the participants. The results of the full study, when and if completed, would be important to evaluate. From this interim analysis, it would appear that early discharge might be appropriate if women are given sufficient support and resources. However, an outcome that may affect the usefulness of the findings is cost. A cost analysis was not undertaken, so further research that addresses this point may need to be found and appraised before making any final decisions about changing an entire health service model. Based on these issues, this evidence will assist clinicians to consider early discharge but will not answer the clinical question of whether it is the best option for most women who have had surgery for breast cancer.

CRITICAL APPRAISAL OF SYSTEMATIC REVIEWS

A systematic review is a compilation of similar studies that address a specific clinical question (Table 5.7). To conduct a systematic review, a detailed search strategy is employed to find the relevant evidence to answer a clinical question. The researchers determine beforehand what inclusion and exclusion criteria will be used to select identified studies. Systematic reviews of RCTs, considered Level I evidence, are found at the top of the hierarchy of evidence for intervention studies (see Chapter 1, Box 1.2). Systematic review methodology is the most rigorous approach to minimization of bias in reviewing studies.

A systematic review is not the same as a literature review or narrative review (O'Mathúna, 2010a). The methods used in a systematic review are specific and rigorous, whereas a narrative review usually compiles published papers that support an author's particular point of view or serve as general background

Table 5.7   Definitions of Different Types of Research Evidence Reviews

Review	Definition
Systematic review	A compilation of like studies to address a specific clinical question using a detailed, comprehensive search strategy and rigorous appraisal methods for the purpose of summarizing, appraising, and communicating the results and implications of all the research available on a clinical question. A systematic review is the most rigorous approach to minimization of bias in summarizing research
Meta-analysis	A statistical approach to synthesizing the results of a number of studies that produces a larger sample size and thus greater power to determine the true magnitude of an effect. Used to obtain a single-effect measure (i.e., a summary statistic) of the results of all studies included in a systematic review
Integrative review	A systematic review that does not have a summary statistic because of limitations in the studies found (usually due to heterogeneous studies or samples)
Narrative review	A research review that includes published papers that support an author's particular point of view and usually serves as a general background discussion of a particular issue. An explicit and systematic approach to searching for and evaluating papers is usually not used

discussion for a particular issue. A systematic review is a scientific approach to summarize, appraise, and communicate the results and implications of several studies that may have contradictory results.

Research trials rarely, if ever, have flawless methodology and a large enough sample size to provide a conclusive answer to questions about clinical effectiveness. Archie Cochrane, an epidemiologist after whom the Cochrane Collaboration is named, recognized that the increasingly large number of RCTs of variable quality and differing results were seldom made available to clinicians in useful formats to improve practice. "It is surely a great criticism of our profession that we have not organised a critical summary, by specialty or subspecialty, adapted periodically, of all relevant randomised controlled trials" (Cochrane, 1979, p. 9). For this reason, the systematic review methodology has been gradually adopted and adapted to assist healthcare professionals take advantage of the overwhelming amount of information available in an effort to improve patient care and outcomes. According to the Cochrane Collaboration, which facilitates the production of healthcare systematic reviews and provides much helpful information on the Internet, the key characteristics of a systematic review are (Higgins & Green, 2008):

- ◆ A clearly stated set of objectives with predefined eligibility criteria for studies
- ◆ An explicit, reproducible methodology
- ◆ A systematic search that attempts to identify all studies that would meet the eligibility criteria
- ◆ A standardized assessment of the validity of the findings of the included studies, for example, through the assessment of risk of bias
- ◆ A systematic presentation of the synthesis of studies, including the characteristics and findings of the studies included in the review

A systematic review is a form of *secondary research* because it uses previously conducted studies. The study types discussed previously in this chapter would be *primary research* studies. Because it is such an obviously different research approach, it requires unique critical appraisal questions to address the quality of a review.

....

Life is either a daring adventure or nothing.
—Helen Keller

....

Specific Critical Appraisal Questions for Systematic Reviews

Systematic reviews have multiple phases of development, with each one designed to reduce bias. This entire process requires attention to detail that can make it time consuming and costly (O'Mathúna, Fineout-Overholt, & Kent, 2008). Clinicians have specific questions that they must ask in appraising a systematic review (Box 5.5), just as they should do with other study designs to determine their value for practice (O'Mathúna, 2010b). (Please note that the discussion below of critical appraisal of systematic reviews follows a slightly different format than prior research design sections.)

Are the Results of the Study Valid? (Validity)

Phase 1 of a systematic review identifies the clinical practice question to be addressed and the most suitable type of research design to answer it. The next step, Phase 2, develops inclusion criteria for the studies to be included and exclusion criteria for those studies that will not be included in the analysis. These steps are completed prior to gathering any evidence.

Once Phase 2 of planning is completed, Phase 3 begins the process of searching for and retrieving published and unpublished literature related to the study question. Rigorous search strategies are developed to ensure that research findings from all relevant disciplines and in all languages are found. Multiple computer databases (e.g., MEDLINE, CINAHL, EMBASE) are searched, as well as conference proceedings, dissertations, and other "grey literature." Grey literature is unpublished studies or studies published by governmental agencies or other organizations that are not peer-reviewed (Hopewell, McDonald, Clarke, & Egger, 2007). The section of the research report that discusses Phase 3 includes

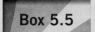

Rapid Critical Appraisal Questions for Systematic Reviews

Box 5.5

1. Are the Results of the Review Valid?
   a. Are the studies contained in the review RCTs?
   b. Does the review include a detailed description of the search strategy to find all relevant studies?
   c. Does the review describe how validity of the individual studies was assessed (e.g., methodological quality, including the use of random assignment to study groups and complete follow-up of the subjects)?
   d. Were the results consistent across studies?
   e. Were individual patient data or aggregate data used in the analysis?
2. What Were the Results?
   a. How large is the intervention or treatment effect (OR, RR, effect size, level of significance)?
   b. How precise is the intervention or treatment effect (CI)?
3. Will the Results Assist Me in Caring for My Patients?
   a. Are my patients similar to the ones included in the review?
   b. Is it feasible to implement the findings in my practice setting?
   c. Were all clinically important outcomes considered, including risks and benefits of the treatment?
   d. What is my clinical assessment of the patient and are there any contraindications or circumstances that would inhibit me from implementing the treatment?
   e. What are my patient's and his or her family's preferences and values about the treatment under consideration?

answers to the critical appraisal questions: Are the studies contained in the review RCTs? Does the review include a detailed description of the search strategy to find all relevant studies?

Systematic reviews minimize bias by the way in which the literature pertaining to the research question is identified and obtained. The research literature comprises the raw data for a review. When appraising a systematic review, the clinician looks for a detailed description of the databases accessed, the search strategies used, and the search terms. The databases should be specified, as should the years searched. The authors should indicate whether the retrieved information was limited to English language studies only. MEDLINE and CINAHL are probably the best-known healthcare publication databases for such studies. Although these databases index thousands of journals, not all journals are indexed by any one database. If reviewers limit their search to English language sources, they risk biasing the research they may find that addresses that particular research question. EMBASE is a European database of healthcare research, and many other databases exist in non-English languages. However, the cost of accessing these databases and translating non-English language papers may create challenges.

Search terms used should be clearly described so the reader can make an informed decision about whether all relevant publications were likely to be found. For example, a review of antibiotic therapy for otitis media might use the search terms *otitis media* and *glue ear*. However, *red ear* is also used commonly for this disorder, and omission of the term from the search strategy may lead to the review missing some studies. Most electronic databases provide an index or thesaurus of the best terms to use in searching, such as MeSH terms in MEDLINE (O'Mathúna et al., 2008).

Clinicians should be able to clearly see from the systematic review which studies were included and which were excluded. The studies are usually presented in a table format and provide clinicians with information about the study populations, settings, and outcomes measured. Ideally, included studies should be relatively homogenous (i.e., the same) with respect to these aspects. Reasons for exclusion, such as study design or quality issues, also should be included in a table. The information presented in these tables assists clinicians to decide whether it was appropriate to combine the results of the studies.

Both published and unpublished research should be identified and retrieved where possible because of publication bias. This term applies to the finding that studies reporting positive or highly significant results have a greater chance of being published compared to those with nonsignificant results (*PLoS Medicine*, 2011). Publication bias arises for several reasons and means that the results of systematic reviews or meta-analyses that include only published results could be misleading. Including grey literature in the search strategy is one way to overcome publication bias. Reviewers will commonly search relevant journals by hand, called hand searching, and examine the reference lists of previously retrieved papers for possible studies. In addition, a review will usually specify whether researchers in the field of interest were contacted to identify other studies. Additionally, authors of retrieved studies may be contacted if information in the publication is missing or insufficient to make a decision regarding inclusion. This process of literature retrieval can be costly, and clinicians need to consider whether the absence of such an exhaustive search affects the conclusions drawn in the review.

Clinicians need to be reassured that all reasonable attempts were made to retrieve both published and unpublished studies. When unpublished studies are not included, the size of any effect is likely to be exaggerated. One way researchers may indicate that they evaluated the presence of selection bias is through the use of a statistical test called the "funnel plot." This method is a scatterplot in which each study's sample size is plotted on the horizontal axis and each study's effect size is plotted on the vertical axis of the graph. When the risk of publication bias is low, a symmetrical inverted funnel is expected. An asymmetrical plot may indicate selection bias through the absence of some studies.

The next critical appraisal question is, Does the review describe how validity of the individual studies was assessed (e.g., methodological quality, including the use of random assignment to study groups and complete follow-up of the subjects)? This can be answered in the section addressing Phases 4 and 5 of a systematic review. These phases involve assessing the quality and validity of the included studies. The systematic review should report precisely how this was conducted and against what criteria evaluations were made. A clear report of how the review was conducted can assist the clinician in determining the worth of the gathered studies for practice.

The critical appraisal process itself shows that primary research is of varying quality. A rigorous, high-quality systematic review should base its primary conclusions only on high-quality studies. A clear description of the basis for quality assessment should be included in the review. Although a review with a rigorous methodology that includes only RCTs is considered the highest level of evidence for intervention questions, other clinical questions (e.g., questions of prognosis) that are not appropriate for an RCT design should also include the types of study designs that are most appropriate to answer those questions (e.g., cohort studies).

The systematic review report should inform clinicians about how data were extracted from the individual studies (Phase 6) and provide an overview of the evaluation of the included studies (Phase 7). Data should be extracted and the quality of included studies assessed independently by at least two members of the review team. The independent assessment further reduces the possibility of bias regarding evaluation of the studies. This process should be discussed in a systematic review as well as how the researchers resolved any disagreement they may have had regarding study findings.

The studies included in a systematic review often have varying designs and inconsistent results, which may allow for only a descriptive evaluation of the studies. When studies are similar enough to be combined in a quantitative synthesis (e.g., comparing effect size, ORs), this can be very helpful to clinicians. The statistical approach to synthesizing the results of two or more studies is called a meta-analysis. A meta-analysis is a quantitative systematic review, but not all systematic reviews are meta-analyses (Fineout-Overholt et al., 2008). When critically appraising these studies, clinicians must keep in mind that overviews or integrative reviews do not apply statistical analyses to the results across studies, generally because the studies are not amenable to that kind of analysis. Instead, these reviews or evidence syntheses often culminate in recommendations based on descriptive evaluations of the findings, or they indicate to clinicians that the included studies on a given topic cannot be synthesized, for a myriad of reasons.

This section of the study report is helpful in answering the following critical appraisal questions: Were the results consistent across studies? Were individual patient data or aggregate data used in the analysis? The latter question reflects whether pooling the data was suitable or not from across the included studies. If it is possible (i.e., the researchers studied the same variables, defined them the same way, measured them the same way), given what you know about the sample size from your prior reading, consider how researchers could have more reliable findings with a larger pooled sample (e.g., 1,000), than 10 smaller samples (e.g., 100).

Chance alone would suggest that some variation will arise in the results of individual studies examining the same question. The differences in studies and the reported findings (i.e., heterogeneity) can be due to study design. Formal statistical methods can be used to test whether there is significant heterogeneity among the studies that precludes them being combined. Generally, reviewers will report using such a test. However, as with all statistical tests, statistical significance is not the same as clinical meaningfulness.

What Are the Results? (Reliability)

The results section of the systematic review can address the following critical appraisal questions: How large is the intervention or treatment effect (e.g., NNT, NNH, effect size, level of significance)? How precise is the intervention or treatment? Common statistics seen in systematic reviews are ORs and effect sizes. If the study is a meta-analysis, these values will assist the clinician in determining the magnitude of effect. The CI is the indicator of the preciseness of the study findings (i.e., can clinicians get what the researcher got, if they repeat the intervention?). A major advantage of a systematic review is the combining of results from many studies. In meta-analyses, combining the results of several studies produces a larger sample size and thus greater power to accurately determine the magnitude of the effect. Because of the strength of this type of evidence, this relatively new methodology has become a hallmark of EBP (Stevens, 2001).

Meta-analysis is the statistical method used to obtain a single-effect measure of the summarized results of all studies included in a review. While the technique may sound complicated, clinicians do not require even moderate understanding of the mathematics involved in such methods. A solid understanding of how to interpret the results is what is needed. The meta-analysis of a number of trials recognizes how sample size of the studies may influence findings and, thereby, provides a more precise estimate of treatment effect than individual studies. A "forest plot" (Figure 5.8) is a diagrammatic representation of the results of trials included in a meta-analysis, along with their CIs. You can now apply what you learned from the explanation of OR and CI given earlier in this chapter. In the forest plot, each square is the measure of effect of an individual study, and the horizontal line shows its CI. The larger the square, the more important the contribution of that particular study is to the meta-analysis

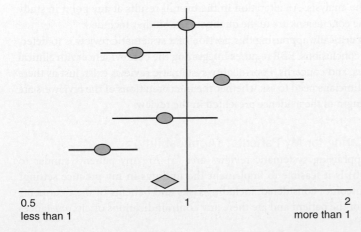

0.5
less than 1

1

2
more than 1

Figure 5.8: Example of a forest plot.

(Lewis & Clarke, 2001). The diamond at the bottom of the forest plot is the summary treatment effect of all studies, with the vertical points of the diamond being the result and the horizontal points of the diamond being the CI for that overall result.

To interpret these data, clinicians must consider the outcome first. If there is no difference in outcomes between the treatment and control groups, the resulting OR is 1.0. If the CI crosses the line of no treatment effect (OR = 1.0), the study is not statistically significant. If the outcome is something you do not want (e.g., death, pain, or infection), a square to the right of the line means that the treatment was worse than the control in the trial (i.e., there were more deaths in the treated group compared to the comparison or control group). Usually, this is not the desired result. For a negative outcome, the desired result is to see the treatment decrease the outcome, and this would be reflected in a square to the left of the line of no effect. A square to the left of the line means that the treatment was better, which is what would be desired for outcomes you want (e.g., stopping smoking or continuation of breast-feeding).

The forest plot gives a way to make an informed estimate of study homogeneity. A forest plot with study estimates that are scattered all over and have wide CIs suggests excessive heterogeneity in the measurement and precision of effect. Bringing together all of the studies to answer a particular clinical question provides important information; however, studies are often too dissimilar to combine their results. If possible, reviewers can quantify the effectiveness of the intervention in a summary statistic that can be compared across these studies. Alternatively, the studies may not be of sufficient quality to combine or compare, which provides information to researchers regarding the need for additional high-quality research.

Clinicians must also watch for reports in which reviewers have analyzed by subgroups when no overall effect was found. Study subsets may be analyzed on the basis of particular patient demographics or methodological quality of the included studies. However, in such an analysis, the purpose of the initial randomization to treatment and control groups in the underlying studies is essentially lost because the balance afforded by randomization does not extend to subgroupings after the fact. However, some subgroup analyses may be legitimate. For example, if an overall effect is found, but individual studies varied widely in quality, subgroup analysis based on study quality may be warranted and important. For example, researchers conducting a meta-analysis of chromium supplements for diabetes found some beneficial outcomes, but when subgroup analyses were conducted based on study quality, those studies with the lowest quality had significantly more favorable outcomes than the high-quality studies (Balk, Tatsioni, Lichtenstein, Lau, & Pittas, 2007). This suggests that the overall beneficial results of the meta-analysis were unduly influenced by low-quality studies, and therefore the overall results of the meta-analysis should be applied with caution in clinical practice.

Another tool for clinicians is a sensitivity analysis, which is done to help determine how the main findings may change as a result of pooling the data. It involves first combining the results of all the included studies. The studies considered of lowest quality or unpublished studies are then excluded, and the data are reanalyzed. This process is repeated sequentially, excluding studies until only the studies of highest quality are included in the analysis. An alteration in the overall results at any point in study exclusion indicates how sensitive the conclusions are to the quality of the studies included.

The final issue for clinicians in critically appraising this portion of a systematic review is to determine if the reviewers justified their conclusions. EBP requires integrating the best evidence with clinical expertise and patient values, choices, and concerns. Poor-quality systematic reviews exist, just as there are poor-quality primary studies. Clinicians need to ask whether the interpretations of the reviewers are justified and valid based on the strength of the evidence presented in the review.

Will the Results Help Me in Caring for My Patients? (Applicability)

The final questions in critically appraising systematic reviews are: (a) Are my patients similar to the ones included in the review? (b) Is it feasible to implement the findings in my practice setting? (c) Were all clinically important outcomes considered, including risks and benefits of the treatment? (d) What is my clinical assessment of the patient and are there any contraindications or circumstances that would inhibit me from implementing the treatment? and (e) What are my patient's and his or her family's preferences and values about the treatment under consideration? Common sense may appear to answer some of the questions, but without careful attention to them, important application issues can be missed.

Interpreting the Results of a Study: Example Six. You are thinking of establishing an early discharge program for first-time mothers, but are concerned that such a program may be associated with unplanned readmissions for breast-feeding-related problems. You find three RCTs with different sample sizes. The smallest study ($n = 50$) reports that there is no difference in readmissions between the early discharge and routine length of stay groups. A study with a larger sample size ($n = 100$) reports an increase in readmissions in the experimental group. The study with the largest sample size ($n = 1,000$) reports an increase in readmissions in the control group. All three studies are rigorously conducted trials with very similar patient demographics. How can these three studies be synthesized for clinical decision making?

While the study with the larger sample size is more likely to capture the variation in the reference population and thus represent a more accurate estimation of the effect of such a program, the other studies need to be considered as well, as they may have small samples, but clinically meaningful results. Ideally, you would like to have a meta-analysis that combines the results of all three studies and pools the study samples. This would provide a sample size of 1,150 and important evidence to guide decision making.

Clinical Scenario 5.5

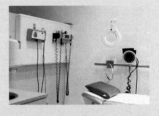

Nursing staff on your unit in a residential elder care facility have just completed an audit of falls in the previous 12 months. A total of 45 falls were documented during the period, but the actual number could have been higher. Interested and concerned clinicians meet to discuss the results and consider options for reducing this incidence. A few people bring copies of trials with them that discuss the efficacy of fall prevention programs that incorporated various interventions. All the trials look like high-quality studies, but they all show different results. Which one to believe? It would be nice to have one study that summarizes all the available evidence for you and presents the implications for clinical practice.

What the Literature Says: Answering a Clinical Question

The following study may help answer the clinical question for Clinical Scenario 5.5. In older adults living in residential care facilities (**P**), how do fall prevention programs (**I**) compared to no fall prevention (**C**) affect fall rates (**O**)? Cameron et al. (2012) conducted a systematic review in which the objective was to assess the effects of interventions designed to reduce the incidence of falls in older people in care facilities and hospitals. The literature search was conducted on the Cochrane Bone, Joint and Muscle Trauma Group Specialised Register (March 2012), the Cochrane Library (2012, Issue 3), MEDLINE (1966 to March 2012), EMBASE (1988 to March 2012), CINAHL (1982 to March 2012), and ongoing trial registers (to August 2012). A hand search of reference lists of articles was conducted, and field researchers were contacted. The selection criterion was that studies had to be randomized trials of interventions designed to reduce falls in older people in residential or nursing care facilities or in hospitals. The primary outcomes of interest were the rates or numbers of falls or numbers of fallers. Trials reporting only intermediate outcomes (like improved balance) were excluded. The data collection and analysis methods involved two reviewers independently assessing the trial quality and extracting data. Data were pooled using the **fixed effect model** where appropriate. In the fixed effect model, it is assumed that the event rates are fixed in both control and treatment groups. Therefore, if the event rates have any variation, this can be attributed to chance.

> *If the trials being combined are truly clinically homogeneous and have been designed properly (for example, with balanced arms), which is the situation that will commonly pertain, then in this (and only in this) case it is appropriate to pool raw data.* (Moore, Gavaghan, Edwards, Wiffen, & McQuay, 2002, p. 3)

The systematic review included 60 trials, 43 in care facilities and 17 in hospitals. Thirteen trials tested exercise interventions, but the results were inconsistent, and overall meta-analysis showed no significant differences between intervention and control groups in either rate of falls or risk of falls. However, post hoc subgroup analysis by level of care showed reduced falls in intermediate-level facilities and increased falls in high-level facilities. Vitamin D supplementation reduced the rate of falls but not the risk of falling. Multifactorial interventions showed some benefit in reducing falls in hospitals, but their impact on risk of falling was inconclusive. Many different interventions were tested in different trials, making it difficult to determine the effectiveness of any individual component.

The reviewers' conclusions were that interventions to prevent falls that are likely to be effective are now available. Costs per fall prevented have been established for four of the interventions. Some potential interventions are of unknown effectiveness, and further research is indicated.

Are the Results of the Study Valid? (Validity)

Only RCTs that met quality inclusion criteria were included in the review. A large number of databases were searched, and both English and non-English language sources were searched. Two reviewers independently assessed the quality of trials and extracted the data. Tables of included and excluded studies were provided. These methods produced valid results.

What Are the Results? (Reliability)

A rate ratio (RaR) with 95% CI was used to compare rates of falls and an RR with 95% CI for the risk of falling. For the trials testing exercise interventions, no significant differences were found for the rate of falls (RaR 1.03, 95% CI 0.81 to 1.31) or risk of falling (RR 1.07, 95% CI 0.94 to 1.23). In both cases, the 95% CI crosses the line of no effect at 1. Similar statistics were reported for the other intervention groupings and subgroup analyses. However, since the subgroup analysis by level of care was conducted post hoc (and not a priori), the results should be interpreted somewhat cautiously. The overall protocol was published prior to completion of the review (standard practice for Cochrane reviews), and the pooled study results were tested for heterogeneity. The results of the review can be viewed as reliable.

Will the Results Help Me in Caring for My Patients? (Applicability)

Although there was variation in the study settings, types of patients, and interventions included in this review, the authors provided a description of the circumstances in which a particular intervention may be beneficial. Economic outcomes were not reported, and there were no trials of reducing the serious consequences of falls. Given the clinical question of reducing falls in an elder care facility, the evidence is applicable.

....

When a resolute young fellow steps up to the great bully, the world, and takes him boldly by the beard, he is often surprised to find it comes off in his hand, and that it was only tied on to scare away the timid adventurers.
—Ralph Waldo Emerson

....

EVALUATION AND SYNTHESIS: FINAL STEPS IN CRITICAL APPRAISAL

Critical appraisal includes rapid critical appraisal, as described throughout the chapter, as well as digging deeper. Once studies have been defined as keepers, they should be melded together into a synthesis upon which to base practice and standards of care. Clinical decisions at the point of care may use already synthesized or synopsized resources, as described in Chapter 3; however, when sustainable practice changes are required, careful evaluation and synthesis of evidence are necessary. To provide best care, we must act on what we currently know and understand from what we synthesize as the best available evidence (Fineout-Overholt, 2008).

Each study should be evaluated using an evaluation table like the one found in Table 5.8. The essential elements are listed as headings for the table. There may be other headings that clinicians feel are important to their studies, which can be added. The PICOT question is the driver for the evaluation table and synthesis tables. For example, with data analysis, while many statistics may be reported in a study, only those statistics that assist you in answering your clinical question should be placed in the table. As well, only the findings that are relevant to the clinical question should be placed in the table. Keeping the order of information placed in the table clear and simple is imperative for comparisons across studies for synthesis. Some suggestions to make the table user-friendly are to (a) use abbreviations (e.g., RCT) with a legend for interpretation, (b) keep the order of the information the same in each study (e.g., MS would appear at the top of the variables section for each study), and (c) place similar statistics in the same order in each study for easy comparison (Fineout-Overholt, 2008). Appendix C contains templates for evaluation and synthesis tables for conducting an evidence review.

Synthesis occurs as clinicians enter the study data into the evaluation table (Fineout-Overholt, 2008). Each study is compared to the others for how it agrees or disagrees with the others in the table. Some examples of the columns that would be included in the table are study design, sample characteristics, and major variables studied. Using the last column to document the level of evidence as well as the quality assists the clinician to quickly peruse the strength of the evidence that leads to the confidence to act on that evidence to impact outcomes (Fineout-Overholt).

Table 5.8   Example of Headings for an Evaluation Table*

Citation of a Single Study	Theoretical or Conceptual Framework	Study Design and Method	Sample Characteristics and Setting	Names and Definitions of Major Variables	Outcomes Measures	Data Analysis	Findings	Level and Quality of Evidence
Jones and Smith (2009)	ARCC	RCT	EBPM ACC	IV = MS	WSI	t-Test	NSD	Level II
			EBPM M/S	DV = NrsS				
Smith and Jones (2007)	ARCC	RCT	EBPM Peds NM	MS NrsS	WSI JS	t-Test	EBPM SD NM, $p < 0.001$	Level II

*Example is hypothetical.
Notes: ACC, acute and critical care; ARCC, Advancing Research & Clinical practice through close collaboration; DV, dependent variable; EBPM, EBP mentors; IV, independent variable; JS, job satisfaction; M/S, Medical/Surgical; MS, managerial style; NM, nurse managers; NrsS, nurse satisfaction; NSD, no significant difference; Peds, Pediatrics; RCT, randomized controlled trial; SD, significantly different; WSI, Work Satisfaction Index.

Fineout-Overholt (2008) outlines some principles of synthesis that can assist clinicians in making determinations about how to use the data extracted from across the studies. These principles of synthesis include making decisions about which study details and findings need to be synthesized. The clinical question drives this decision making. Often, clinicians can cluster studies around different aspects of methods or findings (e.g., study design, interventions, outcome measurement, or findings). Synthesis requires a thoughtful consideration of inconsistencies as well as consistencies across studies. These can give great insights into what is not known, what is known, and what researchers need to focus on to improve the body of evidence to address a particular clinical question. Pulling together the conclusions or major findings from a study can be of great help in clinical decision making. In addition, carefully discussing how studies' strengths, limitations, and level of evidence match or do not match can assist in the final conclusion of what should be done in practice. Synthesis tables are the best way to formulate and communicate the information that is essential for comparison across studies (Table 5.9). A caveat about synthesis is in order here: Synthesis is not reporting the findings of consecutive studies; rather, it is combining, contrasting, and interpreting a body of evidence to reach a conclusion about what is known and what should be done with that knowledge to improve healthcare outcomes, which adds confidence to the final step of critical appraisal, making recommendations for practice.

Evaluation and synthesis tables differ in that evaluation tables contain information about each individual study, while synthesis tables contain only those aspects of the individual studies that are common or unique across studies (e.g., study design, outcomes, findings). Such tables should have the advantages of clarity and simplicity. Synthesis tables enable clinicians to confidently make clinical decisions about the care that is provided to their patients by making evidence from studies readily useable for clinical decision making (Fineout-Overholt, 2008). Chapter 9 speaks to implementation of evidence, which is the next step after critical appraisal (i.e., rapid critical appraisal, evaluation, synthesis and recommendations).

Table 5.9   Example of Headings for a Synthesis Table*

Sample Clinical Question: In adolescents at risk for depression (P), how does relaxation and visual imagery (I_1) and/or music (I_2) compared to yoga (C) affect depression (O) over 5 months (T)?

Study Author	Year	Number of Participants	Mean Age (or Other Sample Characteristic That Is Pertinent to Your Question)	Study Design	Intervention	Major Finding That Addresses Your Question
Carrigan	2001	15	15	R	Yoga	↓ D
Johnson	2005	280	17	Q	Relaxation/visual imagery	— D
Meade	1999	51	19	Q	Music	↓ D
Smith	2008	1,400	14	R	Relaxation/visual imagery + music	↑ D

*Example is hypothetical.
Notes: D, depression; Q, quasi-experimental study; R, randomized controlled trial (all studies measured depression using the Beck Depression Scale); ↓, decreased; ↑, increased; —,

CONCLUSIONS

Evidence-based healthcare decision making requires the integration of clinical expertise with the best available research evidence and the patients' values, concerns, and choices. To do this, clinicians must develop skills in critically appraising available research studies and applying the findings. The validity of study findings depends on how well researchers use study design principles and how different designs best match the clinical question under investigation. Clinicians must understand these aspects of studies to utilize research appropriately to improve practice. Accessing and regularly using one of the many critical appraisal skills guides available will help the clinician learn more about the scientific basis for health management and lead to more informed decision making and better patient outcomes (see Appendix B). Completing the critical appraisal process with evaluation and synthesis of studies will boost clinicians' confidence to act on strong evidence to change outcomes.

EBP FAST FACTS

◆ EBP requires critical appraisal of the results of all studies before they influence practice, even if they are published in high-impact, peer-reviewed journals.
◆ The three key questions to ask of all studies are (1) whether the results are valid, (2) what the results are, and (3) whether the results will help in caring for my patients.
◆ Additional questions should be asked of each study, which depend on the specific research methodology used in the study.
◆ Some knowledge of statistics is required to appraise research studies, especially to be able to distinguish between statistical significance and clinical significance.
◆ Having critically appraised relevant studies, the final step is to synthesize the results before using them to influence practice and standards of care.

References

Albrecht, J., Meves, A., & Bigby, M. (2009). A survey of case reports and case series of therapeutic interventions in the *Archives of Dermatology. International Journal of Dermatology, 48*(6), 592–597.

Awada, A., & Al Jumah, M. (1999). The first-of-Ramadan headache. *Headache, 39*(7), 490–493.

Aylin, P., Alexandrescu, R., Jen, M. H., Mayer, E. K., & Bottle, A. (2013). Day of week of procedure and 30 day mortality for elective surgery: Retrospective analysis of hospital episode statistics. *BMJ, 346*, f2424.

Balk, E. M., Tatsioni, A., Lichtenstein, A. H., Lau, J., & Pittas, A. G. (2007). Effect of chromium supplementation on glucose metabolism and lipids: A systematic review of randomized controlled trials. *Diabetes Care, 30*(8), 2154–2163.

Barratt, A., Wyer, P. C., Hatala, R., McGinn, T., Dans, A. L., Keitz, S., ... The Evidence-Based Medicine Teaching Tips Working Group. (2004). Tips for learners of evidence-based medicine: 1. Relative risk reduction, absolute risk reduction and number needed to treat. *Canadian Medical Association Journal, 171*(4), 353–358.

Benson, K., & Hartz, A. J. (2000). A comparison of observational studies and randomized, controlled trials. *New England Journal of Medicine, 342*(25), 1878–1886.

Boffetta, P., McLaughlin, J. K., La Vecchia, C., Tarone, R. E., Lipworth, L., & Blot, W. J. (2008). False-positive results in cancer epidemiology: A plea for epistemological modesty. *Journal of the National Cancer Institute, 100*(14), 988–995.

Bono, C. M., & Tornetta III, P. (2006). Common errors in the design of orthopaedic studies. *Injury, 37*(4), 355–360.

Bracken, M. B., Shepard, M. J., Holford, T. R., Leo-Summers, L., Aldrich, E. F., Fazl, M., ... Young, W. (1997). Administration of methylprednisolone for 24 or 48 h or tirilazad mesylate for 48 h in the treatment of acute spinal cord injury: Results of the Third National Acute Spinal Cord Injury Randomized Controlled Trial. National Acute Spinal Cord Injury Study. *Journal of the American Medical Association, 277*(20), 1597–1604.

Brower, R. G., Lanken, P. N., MacIntyre, N., Matthay, M. A., Morris, A., Ancukiewicz, M., ... National Heart, Lung, and Blood Institute ARDS Clinical Trials Network. (2004). Higher versus lower positive end-expiratory pressures in patients with the acute respiratory distress syndrome. *New England Journal of Medicine, 351*(4), 327–336.

Bundred, N., Maguire, P., Reynolds, J., Grimshaw, J., Morris, J., Thomson, L., … Baildam, A. (1998). Randomised controlled trial of effects of early discharge after surgery for breast cancer. *British Medical Journal, 317*(7168), 1275–1279.

Busse, J. W., & Heetveld, M. J. (2006). Critical appraisal of the orthopaedic literature: Therapeutic and economic analysis. *Injury, 37*(4), 312–320.

Callas, P. W., & Delwiche, F. A. (2008). Searching the biomedical literature: Research study designs and critical appraisal. *Clinical Laboratory Science, 21*(1), 42–48.

Cameron, I. D., Murray, G. R., Gillespie, L. D., Robertson, M. C., Hill, K. D., Cumming, R. G., & Kerse, N. (2012). Interventions for preventing falls in older people in nursing care facilities and hospitals. *Cochrane Database of Systematic Reviews, 12*, CD005465.

CAPRIE Steering Committee. (1996). A randomised, blinded, trial of clopidogrel versus aspirin in patients at risk of ischaemic events (CAPRIE). *Lancet, 348*(9038), 1329–1339.

Chalmers, T. C., Celano, P., Sacks, H. S., & Smith Jr., H. (1983). Bias in treatment assignment in controlled clinical trials. *New England Journal of Medicine, 309*(22), 1358–1361.

Chan, K. (2007). A clinical trial gone awry: The Chocolate Happiness Undergoing More Pleasantness (CHUMP) study. *Canadian Medical Association Journal, 177*(12), 1539–1541.

Cochrane, A. L. (1979). 1931–1971: A critical review, with particular reference to the medical profession. In *Medicines for the Year 2000* (pp. 1–11). London: Office of Health Economics.

Coleman, W. P., Benzel, E., Cahill, D., Ducker, T., Geisler, F., Green, B., … Zeidman, S. (2000). A critical appraisal of the reporting of the National Acute Spinal Cord Injury Studies (II and III) of methylprednisolone in acute spinal cord injury. *Journal of Spinal Disorders, 13*(3), 185–199.

Concato, J., Shah, N., & Horwitz, R. I. (2000). Randomized, controlled trials, observational studies, and the hierarchy of research designs. *New England Journal of Medicine, 342*(25), 1887–1892.

Crombie, I. (1996). *The pocket guide to critical appraisal.* London: BMJ Publishing Group.

Devereaux, P. J., Manns, B. J. H., Ghali, W. A., Quan, H., Lacchetti, C., Montori, V. M., … Guyatt, G. H. (2001). Physician interpretations and textbook definitions of blinding terminology in randomized controlled trials. *Journal of the American Medical Association, 285*(15), 2000–2003.

Eldridge, S. M., Ashby, D., Feder, G. S., Rudnicka, A. R., & Ukoumunne, O. C. (2004). Lessons for cluster randomized trials in the twenty-first century: A systematic review of trials in primary care. *Clinical Trials, 1*(1), 80–90.

Farrell, S., Barker, M. L., Walanski, A., & Gerlach, R. W. (2008). Short-term effects of a combination product night-time therapeutic regimen on breath malodor. *Journal of Contemporary Dental Practice, 9*(6), 1–8.

Fergusson, D. M., Horwood, L. J., & Ridder, E. M. (2005). Tests of causal linkages between cannabis use and psychotic symptoms. *Addiction, 100*(3), 354–366.

Fethney, J. (2010). Statistical and clinical significance, and how to use confidence intervals to help interpret both. *Australian Critical Care, 23*(2), 93–97.

Fineout-Overholt, E. (2008). Synthesizing the evidence: How far can your confidence meter take you? *AACN Advanced Critical Care, 19*(3), 335–339.

Fineout-Overholt, E., & Melnyk, B. (2007). Evaluating studies on prognosis. In N. Cullum, D. Ciliska, & B. Hayne (Eds.), *Evidence-based nursing: An introduction.* London: Blackwell, 168–178.

Fineout-Overholt, E., O'Mathúna, D. P., & Kent, B. (2008). Teaching EBP: How systematic reviews can foster evidence-based clinical decisions: Part I. *Worldviews on Evidence-Based Nursing, 5*(1), 45–48.

Gangwisch, J. E., Feskanich, D., Malaspina, D., Shen, S., & Forman, J. P. (2013). Sleep duration and risk for hypertension in women: Results from the Nurses' Health Study. *American Journal of Hypertension, 26*(7), 903–911.

Goodacre, S. (2008a). Critical appraisal for emergency medicine: 1. Concepts and definitions. *Emergency Medicine Journal, 25*(4), 219–221.

Goodacre, S. (2008b). Critical appraisal for emergency medicine 2: Statistics. *Emergency Medicine Journal, 25*(6), 362–364.

Guyatt, G., Rennie, D., Meade, M. O., & Cook, D. J. (2008). *Users' guide to the medical literature: A manual for evidence-based clinical practice* (2nd ed.). New York: McGraw Hill.

Häfner, H., Hambrecht, M., Löffler, W., Munk-Jørgensen, P., & Riecher-Rössler, A. (1998). Is schizophrenia a disorder of all ages? A comparison of first episodes and early course across the life-cycle. *Psychological Medicine, 28*(2), 351–365.

Hardell, L., Carlberg, M., & Hansson Mild, K. (2013). Use of mobile phones and cordless phones is associated with increased risk for glioma and acoustic neuroma. *Pathophysiology, 20*(2), 85–110.

Hayat, M. J. (2010). Understanding statistical significance. *Nursing Research, 59*(3), 219–223.

Hellems, M. A., Gurka, M. J., & Hayden, G. F. (2007). Statistical literacy for readers of *Pediatrics*: A moving target. *Pediatrics, 119*(6), 1083–1088.

Herbst, A. L., Ulfelder, H., & Poskanzer, D. C. (1971). Adenocarcinoma of the vagina: Association of maternal stilbestrol therapy with tumor appearance in young women. *New England Journal of Medicine, 284*(15), 878–881.

Higgins, J. P. T., & Green, S. (Eds.). (2008). *Cochrane handbook for systematic reviews of interventions, Version 5.0.1.* Retrieved January 8, 2009, from http://www.cochrane-handbook.org

Hopewell, S., McDonald, S., Clarke, M., & Egger, M. (2007). Grey literature in meta-analyses of randomized trials of health care interventions. *Cochrane Database of Systematic Reviews, 2.*

Howland, R. H. (2011). Publication bias and outcome reporting bias: Agomelatine as a case example. *Journal of Psychosocial Nursing and Mental Health Services, 49*(9), 11–14.

Inskip, P., Tarone, R., Hatch, E., Wilcosky, T., Shapiro, W., Selker, R., … Linet, M. S. (2001). Cellular-telephone use and brain tumors. *New England Journal of Medicine, 344*(2), 79–86.

Ioannidis, J. P. A., Haidich, A. B., Pappa, M., Pantazis, N., Kokori, S. I., Tektonidou, M. G., … Lau, J. (2001). Comparison of evidence of treatment effects in randomized and nonrandomized studies. *Journal of the American Medical Association, 286*(7), 821–830.

Johnston, L. J., & McKinley, D. F. (2000). Cardiac tamponade after removal of atrial intracardiac monitoring catheters in a pediatric patient: Case report. *Heart and Lung, 29*(4), 256–261.

Kaptchuk, T. J., Friedlander, E., Kelley, J. M., Sanchez, M. N., Kokkotou, E., Singer, J. P., … Lembo, A. J. (2010) Placebos without deception: A randomized controlled trial in irritable bowel syndrome. *PLoS ONE, 5*(12), e15591.

Kim, S. Y. (2013). Efficacy versus effectiveness. *Korean Journal of Family Medicine, 34*(4), 227.

Kirson, N. Y., Weiden, P. J., Yermakov, S., Huang, W., Samuelson, T., Offord, S. J., … Wong, B. J. (2013). Efficacy and effectiveness of depot versus oral antipsychotics in schizophrenia: Synthesizing results across different research designs. *Journal of Clinical Psychiatry, 74*(6), 568–575.

Kunz, R., & Oxman, A. D. (1998). The unpredictability paradox: Review of empirical comparisons of randomised and nonrandomised clinical trials. *British Medical Journal, 317*(7167), 1185–1190.

Lafreniere, K. D., Mutus, B., Cameron, S., Tannous, M., Giannotti, M., Abu-Zahra, H., & Laukkanen, E. (1999). Effects of therapeutic touch on biochemical and mood indicators in women. *Journal of Alternative and Complementary Medicine, 5*(4), 367–370.

Lenzer, J. (2006). NIH secrets government funded data concealment. *New Republic.* Retrieved January 8, 2009, from http://www.ahrp.org/cms/index2.php?option=com_content&do_pdf = 1&id = 398

Lenzer, J., & Brownlee, S. (2008). An untold story? *British Medical Journal, 336*(7643), 532–534.

Lewis, S., & Clarke, M. (2001). Forest plots: Trying to see the wood and the trees. *British Medical Journal, 322*(7300), 1479–1480.

Loher-Niederer, A., Maccora, J., & Ritz, N. (2013). Positive linking: A survival guide on how to keep up-to-date with pediatric infectious diseases literature using internet technology. *Pediatric Infectious Disease Journal, 32*(7), 786–787.

MacMahon, B., Yen, S., Trichopoulos, D., Warren, K., & Nardi, G. (1981). Coffee and cancer of the pancreas. *New England Journal of Medicine, 304*(11), 630–633.

Moore, R., Gavaghan, D., Edwards, J., Wiffen, P., & McQuay, H. (2002). Pooling data for number needed to treat: No problems for apples. *BMC Medical Research Methodology, 2,* 2.

Muscat, J., Malkin, M., Thompson, S., Shore, R., Stellman, S., McRee, D., … Wynder, E. L. (2000). Handheld cellular telephone use and risk of brain cancer. *Journal of the American Medical Association, 284*(23), 3001–3007.

O'Mathúna, D. P. (2010a). The role of systematic reviews. *International Journal of Nursing Practice, 16*(2), 205–207.

O'Mathúna, D. P. (2010b). Critical appraisal of systematic reviews. *International Journal of Nursing Practice, 16*(4), 414–418.

O'Mathúna, D. P., Fineout-Overholt, E., & Kent, B. (2008). Teaching EBP: How systematic reviews can foster evidence-based clinical decisions: Part II. *Worldviews on Evidence-Based Nursing, 5*(2), 102–107.

Papanikolaou, P. N., Christidi, G. D., & Ioannidis, J. P. A. (2006). Comparison of evidence on harms of medical interventions in randomized and nonrandomized studies. *Canadian Medical Association Journal, 174*(5), 635–641.

PLoS Medicine (Ed.). (2011). Best practice in systematic reviews: The importance of protocols and registration. *PLoS Medicine, 8*(2), e1001009.

Polit, D., & Beck, C. (2007). *Nursing research: Generating and assessing evidence for nursing practice* (8th ed.). Philadelphia, PA: Lippincott Williams & Wilkins.

Reed, C. E., & Fenton, S. E. (2013). Exposure to diethylstilbestrol during sensitive life stages: A legacy of heritable health effects. *Birth Defects Research. Part C, Embryo Today, 99*(2), 134–146.

Rossouw, J. E., Anderson, G. L., Prentice, R. L., LaCroix, A. Z., Kooperberg, C., Stefanick, M. L., … Writing Group for the Women's Health Initiative Investigators. (2002). Risks and benefits of estrogen plus progestin in healthy postmenopausal women: Principal results from the women's health initiative randomized controlled trial. *Journal of the American Medical Association, 288*(3), 321–333.

Rothman, K. J. (1978). A show of confidence. *New England Journal of Medicine, 299*(24), 1362–1363.

Ruiz-Canela, M., Martínez-González, M. A., & de Irala-Estévez, J. (2000). Intention to treat analysis is related to methodological quality [letter]. *British Medical Journal, 320*(7240), 1007–1008.

Schulz, K. F. (1995). Subverting randomization in controlled trials. *Journal of the American Medical Association, 274*(18), 1456–1458.

Schulz, K. F., & Grimes, D. A. (2002a). Allocation concealment in randomised trials: Defending against deciphering. *Lancet, 359*(9306), 614–618.

Schulz, K. F., & Grimes, D. A. (2002b). Generation of allocation sequences in randomised trials: Chance, not choice. *Lancet, 359*(9305), 515–519.

Sirriyeh, R., Lawton, R., Gardner, P., & Armitage, G. (2012). Reviewing studies with diverse designs: The development and evaluation of a new tool. *Journal of Evaluation in Clinical Practice, 18*(4): 746–752.

Stampfer, M. J., & Colditz, G. A. (1991). Estrogen replacement therapy and coronary heart disease: A quantitative assessment of the epidemiologic evidence. *Preventive Medicine, 20*(1), 47–63.

Stevens, K. R. (2001). Systematic reviews: The heart of evidence-based practice. *AACN Clinical Issues, 12*(4), 529–538.

Strasak, A. M., Zaman, Q., Pfeiffer, K. P., Göbel, G., & Ulmer, H. (2007). Statistical errors in medical research—A review of common pitfalls. *Swiss Medical Weekly, 137*(3–4), 44–49.

Swift, T. L. (2012). Sham surgery trial controls: perspectives of patients and their relatives. *Journal of Empirical Research on Human Research Ethics, 7*(3), 15–28.

Torgerson, D. J. (2001). Contamination in trials: Is cluster randomisation the answer? *British Medical Journal, 322*(7282), 355–357.

Troisi, R., Hatch, E. E., Titus-Ernstoff, L., Hyer, M., Palmer, J. R., Robboy, S. J., … Hoover, R. N. (2007). Cancer risk in women prenatally exposed to diethylstilbestrol. *International Journal of Cancer, 121*(2), 356–360.

Turati, F., Galeone, C., Edefonti, V., Ferraroni, M., Lagiou, P., La Vecchia, C., & Tavani, A. (2012). A meta-analysis of coffee consumption and pancreatic cancer. *Annals of Oncology, 23*(2), 311–318.

Turner, T. L., Balmer, D. F., & Coverdale, J. H. (2013). Methodologies and study designs relevant to medical education research. *International Review of Psychiatry, 25*(3), 301–310.

University College London. (2011). *Critical appraisal of a journal article.* Retrieved July 22, 2013, from http://www.ucl.ac.uk/ich/services/library/training_material/critical-appraisal

Verhagen, A. P., de Vet, H. C., de Bie, R. A., Boers, M., & van den Brandt, P. A. (2001). The art of quality assessment of RCTs included in systematic reviews. *Journal of Clinical Epidemiology, 54*(7), 651–654.

Chapter 6

Critically Appraising Qualitative Evidence for Clinical Decision Making

Bethel Ann Powers

What is important is to keep learning, to enjoy challenge, and to tolerate ambiguity. In the end there are no certain answers

—Martina Horner

All scientific evidence is important to clinical decision making, and all evidence must be critically appraised to determine its contribution to that decision making. Part of critical appraisal is applying the clinician's understanding of a field of science to the content of a research report, that is, how well does the research answer my clinical question (for more on clinical questions, see Chapter 2). Qualitative evidence may not be as familiar to practitioners as quantitative evidence—methods, language, and especially how it can be useful in guiding practice. Qualitative evidence is defined as information that is narrative, reflective, or anecdotal and requires judgment to interpret the data. Qualitative evidence answers clinical questions about the human experience, such as How do parents with a child newly diagnosed with cancer perceive their parenting? Answering these questions can be considered as providing clinicians with the *why* for practice, whereas answering questions that require quantitative evidence tends to provide the *how*. Therefore, this chapter offers information to help clinicians with principles and queries for appraising of qualitative evidence for clinical decision making, including:

◆ Language and concepts that will be encountered in the qualitative literature
◆ Aspects of qualitative research that are known to have raised concerns for readers less familiar with different qualitative methods
◆ Issues surrounding the use of evaluative criteria that, if not understood, could lead to their misuse in the appraisal of studies and subsequent erroneous conclusions

With adequate knowledge, practitioners can extract what is good and useful to clinical decision making by applying appropriate method-specific and general appraisal criteria to qualitative research reports. Glossary boxes are provided throughout the chapter to assist the reader in understanding common terms and concepts that support and structure the chapter discussion.

It is important for clinicians to gain the knowledge and ability required to appreciate qualitative studies as sources of evidence for clinical decision making. As with all knowledge, application is the best way to gain proficiency. Readers are invited to review a demonstration of how to use the rapid critical appraisal checklist in Box 6.1 with a variety of sample articles found in Appendix D. Reading these articles is the best way to fully appreciate how to apply the checklist. First-hand appraisal of qualitative studies requires active engagement with the evidence. This chapter prepares clinicians to engage with and move beyond the material presented to apply it when appraising the research in their particular fields of practice.

....

Learning is not attained by chance; it must be sought for with ardor and attended to with diligence.
—Abigail Adams

....

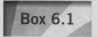

Rapid Critical Appraisal of Qualitative Evidence

Box 6.1

Are the Results Valid/Trustworthy and Credible?

1. How were study participants chosen?
2. How were accuracy and completeness of data assured?
3. How plausible/believable are the results?

Are Implications of the Research Stated?

1. May new insights increase sensitivity to others' needs?
2. May understandings enhance situational competence?

What Is the Effect on the Reader?

1. Are results plausible and believable?
2. Is the reader imaginatively drawn into the experience?

What Were the Results of the Study?

1. Does the research approach fit the purpose of the study?

How Does the Researcher Identify the Study Approach?

1. Are language and concepts consistent with the approach?
2. Are data collection and analysis techniques appropriate?

Is the Significance/Importance of the Study Explicit?

1. Does review of the literature support a need for the study?
2. What is the study's potential contribution?

Is the Sampling Strategy Clear and Guided by Study Needs?

1. Does the researcher control selection of the sample?
2. Do sample composition and size reflect study needs?
3. Is the phenomenon (human experience) clearly identified?

Are Data Collection Procedures Clear?

1. Are sources and means of verifying data explicit?
2. Are researcher roles and activities explained?

Are Data Analysis Procedures Described?

1. Does analysis guide direction of sampling and when it ends?
2. Are data management processes described?
3. What are the reported results (description or interpretation)?

How Are Specific Findings Presented?

1. Is presentation logical, consistent, and easy to follow?
2. Do quotes fit the findings they are intended to illustrate?

How Are Overall Results Presented?

1. Are meanings derived from data described in context?
2. Does the writing effectively promote understanding?

Will the Results Help Me in Caring for My Patients?

1. Are the results relevant to persons in similar situations?
2. Are the results relevant to patient values and/or circumstances?
3. How may the results be applied in clinical practice?

THE CONTRIBUTION OF QUALITATIVE RESEARCH TO DECISION MAKING

In the past, critical appraisal seems to have been the portion of the EBP paradigm that has received the most attention, with literature focusing on helping practitioners develop their skills in retrieving, critically appraising, and synthesizing largely quantitative studies. There is growing awareness, however, that "qualitative research may provide us with some guidance in deciding whether we can apply the findings from quantitative studies to our patients [and] can help us to understand clinical phenomena with emphasis on understanding the experiences and values of our patients" (Straus, Richardson, Glasziou, & Haynes, 2005, p. 143). Clinical practice questions that focus on interventions, risk, and etiology require different hierarchies of evidence that do not designate qualitative evidence as "best evidence" (for more on hierarchies (Levels) of evidence and associated clinical questions, see Chapter 2). Multiple types of qualitative research are present in cross-disciplinary literature. When addressing a meaning question (i.e., about the human experience), synthesis of qualitative research is considered Level 1 evidence—the top of the hierarchy. Knowledge derived from syntheses of qualitative and quantitative research evidence to answer respective clinical questions enables the integration of all elements of EBP in a manner that optimizes clinical outcomes. Therefore, both a challenge and an opportunity are present for clinicians—to utilize the appropriate evidence to answer their questions about quality patient care.

Expanding the Concept of Evidence

From its inception as a clinical learning strategy used at Canada's McMaster Medical School in the 1980s, clinical trials and other types of intervention research have been a primary focus of evidence-based practice (EBP). As well, the international availability of systematic reviews (for more information on systematic reviews, see Chapter 5) provided by the Cochrane Collaboration and the incorporation of intervention studies as evidence in clinical decision support systems have made this type of evidence readily available to point-of-care clinicians. Previously, when compared with quasi-experimental and nonexperimental (i.e., comparative, correlational, and descriptive) designs, RCTs easily emerged as the designated gold standard for determining the effectiveness of a treatment. The one-size-fits-all "rules of evidence" (determination of weakest to strongest evidence with a focus on the effectiveness of interventions) often used to dominate discussions within the EBP movement. That has been minimized with new hierarchies of evidence that assist in identifying the best evidence for different kinds of questions. Now, evidence hierarchies that focus on quantitative research provide the guidance for selection of studies evaluated in EBP reviews to answer **intervention** questions. In turn, evidence hierarchies focused on qualitative research guide selection of studies to answer meaning questions.

Nevertheless, the use of qualitative studies still remains less clear than is desirable for clinical decision making (Milton, 2007; Powers & Knapp, 2011b). In strength-of-evidence pyramids (i.e., a rating system for the hierarchy of evidence) that are proposed as universal for all types of clinical questions, qualitative studies continue to be ranked as weaker forms of evidence at or near the base of the pyramids, along with descriptive, evaluative, and case studies and the strongest research design being RCTs at or near the apex. This misrepresents qualitative research genres, because applying the linear approach used to evaluate intervention studies does not fit the divergent purposes and nonlinear nature of these research traditions and designs.

Now we know that systematic reviews of RCTs provide best evidence for intervention questions. Best evidence for diagnosis and prognosis questions are systematic reviews of descriptive prospective cohort studies. Grace and Powers (2009) have proposed recognition of two additional question domains: human response and meaning, of particular importance for patient-centered care. They argue that the strongest evidence for these question types arise from qualitative research traditions. This supports the use of different evidence hierarchies for different types of questions (see Chapter 2 for more information on levels of evidence that are appropriate for different types of questions).

Furthermore, a need to balance scientific knowledge gained through empirical research with practice-generated evidence and theories in clinical decision making is part of the work of expanding the concept of evidence (Fineout-Overholt, Melnyk, & Schultz, 2005; Powers & Knapp, 2011a). That is, there is a need to extend the concept of evidence beyond empirical research and randomized clinical trials. Evidence should also include theoretical sources, such as ethical standards and philosophies, personal experiences and creative, aesthetic arts (Fawcett, Watson, Neuman, Hinton-Walker, & Fitzpatrick, 2001).

Efforts to expand the concept of evidence are consistent with fundamental tenets of the EBP movement. A clear example is the conceptual framework put forward in this chapter in which the goal of EBP is the successful integration of the following elements of clinical care (see Figure 1.2):

- Best research (e.g., valid, reliable and clinically relevant) evidence
- Clinical expertise (e.g., clinical skills, past experience, interpretation of practice-based evidence)
- Patient values (e.g., unique preferences, concerns, and expectations)
- Patient circumstances (e.g., individual clinical state, practice setting, and organizational culture)

Recognizing Research Relevant to Practice

Science and art come together in the design and execution of qualitative studies. Before clinicians can critically appraise qualitative research, they must have an appreciation for and basic knowledge of its many methodologies and practices, which are rooted in the social and human sciences. Questions asked by qualitative researchers are influenced by focus of these traditions on in-depth understanding of human experiences and the contexts in which the experiences occur.

In the health sciences, knowledge generated by qualitative studies may contain the theoretical bases for explicit (specific) interventions. However, studies that promote better understanding of what health and illness situations are like for people, how they manage, what they wish for and expect, and how they are affected by what goes on around them may also influence practice in other ways. For example, heightened sensitivity or awareness of life from others' vantage points may lead to changes in how persons feel about and behave toward one another, as well as prompt reflection on and discussions about what practical actions might be taken on an individual basis or a larger scale.

Significant growth in qualitative health science literature over recent decades has occurred at least in part because these approaches were capable of addressing many kinds of questions that could not be answered by quantitative, including quantitative descriptive, research methods. Because of the expansion and evolution of qualitative methods, clinicians across disciplines will encounter a more varied mix of articles on different clinical topics. Therefore, to keep up to date on the latest developments in their fields, practitioners need to be able to recognize and judge the validity of relevant qualitative as well as quantitative research studies.

....

The heights by great men reached and kept were not obtained by sudden flight. But they, while their companions slept, were toiling upward in the night.
—Thomas S. Monson

....

SEPARATING WHEAT FROM CHAFF

When we critically appraise a study, we're separating the wheat from the chaff (imperfections) so only the good and useful remains. There are no perfect studies, so the task becomes one of sifting through and deciding whether good and useful elements outweigh a study's shortcomings. To critically appraise qualitative research reports, the reader needs a sense of the diversity that exists within this field (i.e., a flavor of the language and mindset of qualitative research) to appreciate what is involved in using any set of criteria to evaluate a study's validity (or trustworthiness) and usefulness. This decreases the possibility of misconstruing such criteria because of preconceived notions about what they signify and how they should be used. The following sections provide brief overviews of how qualitative approaches differ and a synthesis of basic principles for evaluating qualitative studies.

Managing Diversity

Qualitative research designs and reporting styles are very diverse. In addition, there are many ways to classify qualitative approaches. Therefore, it is necessary to be able to manage this diversity through an awareness of different scientific traditions and associated research methods and techniques used in qualitative studies.

External Diversity Across Qualitative Research Traditions

Qualitative research traditions have origins within academic disciplines (e.g., the social sciences, arts, and humanities) that influence the language, theoretical assumptions, methods, and styles of reporting used to obtain and convey understanding about human experiences. Therefore, despite similarities in techniques for data gathering and management, experiences are viewed through different lenses, studied for different purposes, and reported in language and writing styles consistent with the research tradition's origins. Among qualitative traditions commonly used in health sciences research (i.e., research about health care) are ethnography, grounded theory, phenomenology, and hermeneutics.

Ethnography. Ethnography involves the study of a social group's **culture** through time spent combining **participant observation** (Box 6.2), in-depth interviews, and the collection of artifacts (i.e., material evidence of culture) in the informants' natural setting. This appreciation of culture—drawing on anthropologic (i.e., human development) theory and practice—provides the context for a better understanding of answers to specific research questions. For example, cultural understanding may help answer questions about:

◆ People's experiences of health/illness in their everyday lives (e.g., methods-focused article on use of ethnography in breast-feeding disparities [Cricco-Lizza, 2007]; study about everyday life of children living with juvenile arthritis [Guell, 2007]).

◆ Issues of concern to caregivers (e.g., study of the role of pediatric critical care nursing unit culture in shaping research utilization behaviors [Scott & Pollock, 2008]; study of nursing assessment of pain on two postoperative units [Clabo, 2007]).

◆ Individuals' experiences in certain types of settings (e.g., study of experiences of adult patients and staff in the ward culture of a trauma unit [Tutton, Seers, & Langstaff, 2007]; study of dying in a nursing home [Kayser-Jones, 2002; Kayser-Jones et al., 2003]).

Box 6.2	Ethnography Research Terms

Culture: Shared knowledge and behavior of people who interact within distinct social settings and subsystems.

Participant observation: The active engagement (i.e., observation and participation) of the researcher in settings and activities of people being studied (i.e., everyday activities in study informants' natural settings).

Fieldwork: All research activities carried out in and in relation to the field (informants' natural settings).

Key informant: A select informant/assistant with extensive or specialized knowledge of his/her own culture.

Emic and etic: Contrasting "insider" (emic) views of informants and the researcher's "outsider" (etic) views.

Fieldwork is the term that describes all research activities taking place in or in connection with work in the study setting (i.e., field). These activities include the many social and personal skills required when gaining entry to the field, maintaining field relationships, collecting and analyzing data, resolving political and ethical issues, and leaving the field. Researchers may have **key informants** (in addition to other informants) who assist them in establishing rapport and learning about cultural norms. Research reports are descriptions and interpretations that attempt to capture study informants' **emic** points of view balanced against the researcher's **etic** analytic perspectives. These efforts to make sense of the data may also provide a basis for generating a theory (Wolf, 2007).

Grounded Theory.   The purpose of grounded theory, developed by sociologists Glaser and Strauss (1967), is to generate a theory about how people deal with life situations that is grounded in empirical data and that describes the processes by which they move through experiences over time. Movement is often expressed in terms of stages or phases (e.g., stages/phases of living with a chronic illness, adjusting to a new situation, or coping with challenging circumstances). For example, Beck (2007) described an emerging theory of postpartum depression using grounded theory. In an additional example, Copeland and Heilemann (2008) used grounded theory to describe the experience of mothers striving to obtain assistance for their adult children who are violent and mentally ill. Philosophical underpinnings of this tradition are **symbolic interaction** and **pragmatism** (Wuest, 2007; Box 6.3). Data collection and analysis procedures are similar to those of ethnographic research, but the focus is on symbolic meanings conveyed by people's actions in certain circumstances, resultant patterns of interaction, and their consequences.

The goal is to discover a core variable through procedures of constant comparison and theoretical sampling. **Constant comparison** is coding, categorizing, and analyzing incoming data while consistently seeking linkages by comparing informational categories with one another and with new data. **Theoretical sampling** directs data gathering toward **saturation** of categories (i.e., completeness).

The *core variable*, or **basic social process** (BSP), is the basis for theory generation. It recurs frequently, links all the data together, and describes the pattern followed, regardless of the various conditions under which the experience occurs and different ways in which persons go through it. In the literature, the reader may encounter terms that are used to further describe the types of BSP (e.g., a basic social psychological process [BSPP] and a basic social structural process [BSSP]). Researchers will typically describe the meaning of these terms within the context of the study. Mordoch and Hall

---

Box 6.3	Grounded Theory Research Terms

Symbolic interaction: Theoretical perspective on how social reality is created by human interaction through ongoing, taken-for-granted processes of symbolic communication.

Pragmatism: Theoretical perspective that problems of truth and meaning need to be arrived at inductively; understood in terms of their utility and consequences; and modified to fit the circumstances of time, place, and the advent of new knowledge.

Constant comparison: A systematic approach to analysis that is a search for patterns in data as they are coded, sorted into categories, and examined in different contexts.

Theoretical sampling: Decision making, while concurrently collecting and analyzing data, about the data and data sources that are needed further to develop the emerging theory.

Saturation: The point at which categories of data are full and data collection ceases to provide new information.

Core variable: A theoretical summarization of a process or pattern that people go through in specified life experiences.

(2008) described two interrelated BSPPs in their study of children's perceptions of living with a parent with a mental illness. One process—"finding the rhythm"—helped children manage day-to-day living and staying connected to parents through stages of "monitoring" and "adjusting." The other process— "maintaining the frame"—was used to create a safe distance in relationships with parents through stages identified as "preserving myself" and "gauging."

Phenomenology. Phenomenology is the study of **essences** (i.e., meaning structures, Box 6.4) intuited or grasped through descriptions of **lived experience**. Husserl's philosophy described lived experience (i.e., the lifeworld) as understandings about life's meanings that lie outside of a person's conscious awareness. Thus, in studying the meaning, or essence, of an experience (phenomenon), researchers need to recognize their own personal feelings (**introspection**) and suspend their beliefs about what the experience is like (**bracketing**), particularly if they are using the Husserlian approach to phenomenology. Interpretive insights are derived by collecting experiential descriptions from interviews and other sources and engaging in intellectual analytic processes of reflection, imagination, and intuition (**phenomenological reduction**). Use of certain philosophers' perspectives to direct the analysis (e.g., Husserl, Heidegger, Merleau-Ponty) can affect methodological processes.

Phenomenology, represented as a school of thought within philosophy, offers perspectives shaped through ongoing intellectual dialogues rather than explicit procedures. Descriptions of research processes have come from outside of the parent discipline of philosophy. Processes often cited are as follows:

◆ The philosophically, language-oriented, descriptive-interpretive phenomenology of educator Max van Manen (the German Dilthey-Nohl and the Dutch Utrecht schools of phenomenological pedagogy). An example of this type of phenomenology would be a study of the experience of parents who have a child with autism (Woodgate, Ateah, & Secco, 2008).
◆ The empirical descriptive approaches of the Duquesne school of phenomenological psychology (i.e., Giorgi, Colaizzi, Fischer, and van Kaam). An example of this type of phenomenology would be a study of the impact of birth trauma on breast-feeding (Beck & Watson, 2008).

Examples of phenomena of interest to clinical researchers include what various illness experiences are like for persons or how a sense of hope, trust, or being understood is realized in their lives. Insights offered through research reports range in style from lists of themes and straightforward descriptions (i.e., empiric descriptions) to philosophical theorizing and poetizing (i.e., interpretations). In writing about the usefulness of phenomenology in pediatric cancer nursing research, Fochtman (2008) asserts the perspective that "only when we truly understand the meaning [e.g. what it means to have cancer as a child or adolescent] can we design interventions to ease suffering and increase quality of life" (p. 191).

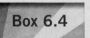

Phenomenology/Hermeneutics Research Terms

Box 6.4

Essences: Internal meaning structures of a phenomenon grasped through the study of human lived experience.
Lived experience: Everyday experience, not as it is conceptualized, but as it is lived (i.e., how it feels or what it is like).
Introspection: A process of recognizing and examining one's own inner state or feelings.
Bracketing: Identifying and suspending previously acquired knowledge, beliefs, and opinions about a phenomenon.
Phenomenological reduction: An intellectual process involving reflection, imagination, and intuition.
Hermeneutics: Philosophy, theories, and practices of interpretation.

Hermeneutics. Hermeneutics has a distinct philosophical history as a theory and method of interpretation (originally associated with the interpretation of Biblical texts). However, various philosophers (e.g., Dilthey, Heidegger, Gadamer, Hirsch, and Ricoeur) have contributed to its development beyond a focus on literal texts to viewing human lived experience as a text that is to be understood through the interpreter's dialogical engagement (i.e., thinking that is like a thoughtful dialog or conversation) with life.

There is not a single way to practice hermeneutics. A variety of theories and debates exist within the field. However, although separated by tradition, it may also be associated with phenomenology and certain schools of phenomenological thought. Thus, *hermeneutic phenomenology* sometimes is the terminology used to denote orientations that are interpretive, in contrast to, or in addition to, being descriptive (van Manen, 1990/1997). For instance, Evans and Hallett (2007) draw on the hermeneutic traditions of Heidegger and Gadamer in their study of the meaning of comfort care for hospice nurses. The complex realities of nurses' work in comfort care settings are presented under the thematic headings of comfort and relief, peace and ease, and spirituality and meaning. Clinicians can obtain a fuller appreciation of how hermeneutic research contributes to understanding clinical practice through firsthand reading of these types of reports, engaging reflectively with the actual words of the written text, and experiencing the total effect of the narrative.

Internal Diversity Within Qualitative Research Traditions

Qualitative research traditions vary internally as well as externally. For example, there are several reasons why ethnographic, grounded theory, or phenomenological accounts may assume a variety of forms, including:

◆ When a tradition acts as a vehicle for different representational styles and theoretical or ideological conceptualizations
◆ When historical evolution of a tradition results in differing procedural approaches
◆ When studies differ individually in terms of their focus on description, interpretation, or theory generation

Representation and Conceptualization. **Representation** of research findings (i.e., writing style, including authorial voice and use of literary forms and rhetorical devices) should not be a matter of dictate or personal whim. Rather, it is part of the analytic process that, in qualitative research, gives rise to a great variety of representational styles. Articles and entire texts have been devoted to the topic of representation (Atkinson, 1992; Denzin, 1997; Mantzoukas, 2004; Morse, 2007; Richardson, 1990; Sandelowski, 1998b, 2004, 2007; van Manen, 1990/1997, 2002; Van Maanen, 1988; Wolcott, 2001, 2002). Qualitative research reports may be conversational dialogs. They may contain researchers' personal reflections and accounts of their experiences; poetry, artistic, and literary references; hypothetical cases; or fictional narratives and stories that are based on actual data, using study informants' own words in efforts to increase sensitivity and enhance understanding of a phenomenon.

Although researchers should not abuse artistic license, readers should also not see a research report as unconventional if that report is enriched by using an alternative literary form as a faithful representation that best serves a legitimate analytic purpose. If the representation is meaningful to the reader, it meets a criterion of analytic significance in keeping with these traditions' scholarly norms. For example, qualitative researchers have used *health theater* (i.e., dramatic performance scripts) to make research findings more accessible and relevant to select audiences (Kontos & Naglie, 2006, 2007; Sandelowski, Trimble, Woodard, & Barroso, 2006; Smith & Gallo, 2007). Further examples of different representational strategies in qualitative health research are the uses of poetic forms (Furman, 2006) and *autoethnography* (i.e., personal/autobiographical experience; Foster, McAllister, & O'Brien, 2005).

Some standard forms of representation are also used with ethnographic, phenomenological, and grounded theory designs to bring out important dimensions of the data. For example, Creswell (2007) discussed how case studies and biography can serve as adjuncts to these types of studies as well as traditions in their own right.

Major qualitative traditions may also be vehicles for distinctive theoretical or ideological concepts. For example, a critical ethnography combines ethnographic methods with methods of **critical inquiry** or cultural critique. The result has been described as "conventional ethnography with a political purpose" (Thomas, 1993, p. 4). The reader should expect to find an integration of empirical analysis and theory related to a goal of emancipation from oppressive circumstances or false ideas. For example, Varcoe (2001) conducted a critical ethnography of how the social context of the emergency room influenced the nursing care of women who had been abused.

Similarly, feminist research, traditionally, has focused critique on "issues of gender, gender relations, inequality, and neglect of diversity" (Flick, 2006, p. 77). However, a feminist perspective may be brought to bear on research interest in any area of social life that would benefit from the establishment of collaborative and nonexploitative relationships and sensitive, ethical approaches. Examples include how researchers deal with boundary issues that arise in qualitative health research on sensitive topics (Dickson-Swift, James, Kippen, & Liamputtong, 2006) and how the quality of written reports may be enriched by inclusion of researchers' embodied experiences (Ellingson, 2006). "In short, rather than a focus on [feminist] methods, [current] discussions have now turned to how to use the methods [informed by a variety of different **feminist epistemologies**, i.e., ways of knowing and reasoning] in a self-disclosing and respectful way" (Creswell, 2007, p. 27) (Box 6.5).

Historical Evolution. Use over time may refine, extend, or alter and produce variations in the practice of a research tradition. One example of this within anthropology is the developing interest in **interpretive ethnography** (Box 6.6). This occurred as researchers crossed disciplinary boundaries to combine theoretical perspectives from practices outside of the discipline to inform their work (e.g., the humanistic approaches of phenomenology and hermeneutics; **discourse analysis**, evolving from **semiotics** and **sociolinguistics**; and **critical theory**). Of course, said influencing practices may also be qualitative approaches in their own right. Examples include Starks and Trinidad's (2007) inclusion of discourse analysis in a comparison of three qualitative approaches that can be used in health research and Stewart and Usher's (2007) discussion of the use of critical theory in exploring nursing leadership issues.

Another example of historical evolution within a tradition began with controversy between Glaser and Strauss, the originators of grounded theory over Strauss' interpretation of the method (Corbin & Strauss, 2008; Strauss & Corbin, 1990, 1998), which included *axial coding,* a procedure not featured in earlier texts (Chenitz & Swanson, 1986; Glaser, 1978; Glaser & Strauss, 1967). When appraising

---

Box 6.5   General Qualitative Research Terms

Representation: Part of the analytic process that raises the issue of providing a truthful portrayal of what the data represent (e.g., essence of an experience; cultural portrait) that will be meaningful to its intended audience.

Case study: An intensive investigation of a case involving a person or small group of people, an issue, or an event.

Biography: An approach that produces an in-depth report of a person's life. Life histories and oral histories also involve gathering of biographical information and recording of personal recollections of one or more individuals.

Critical inquiry: Cultural critique guided by theories/approaches to the study of power interests between individuals and social groups, often involving hegemony (domination or control over others) associated with ideologies that operate to create oppression and constrain multiple competing interests in order to maintain the status quo.

Feminist epistemologies: A variety of views and practices inviting critical dialog about issues arising in areas of social life that involve such concerns as inequality, neglect of diversity, exploitation, insensitivity, and ethical behavior.

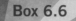

Box 6.6   General Qualitative Research Terms

Interpretive ethnography: Loosely characterized as a movement within anthropology that generates many hybrid forms of ethnographic work as a result of crossing a variety of theoretical boundaries within social science.

Axial coding: A process used to relate categories of information by using a coding paradigm with predetermined subcategories in one approach to grounded theory (Corbin & Strauss, 2008; Strauss & Corbin, 1990).

Emergence: Glaser's (1992) term for conceptually driven ("discovery") vs. procedurally driven ("forcing") theory development in his critique of Strauss and Corbin (1990).

Theoretical sensitivity: A conceptual process to accompany techniques for generating grounded theory (Glaser, 1978).

Discourse analysis: Study of how meaning is created through the use of language (derived from linguistic studies, literary criticism, and semiotics).

Semiotics: The theory and study of signs and symbols applied to the analysis of systems of patterned communication.

Sociolinguistics: The study of the use of speech in social life.

Critical theory: A blend of ideology (based on a critical theory of society) and a form of social analysis and critique that aims to liberate people from unrecognized myths and oppression in order to bring about enlightenment and radical social change.

qualitative evidence, clinicians may see axial coding, which involves the use of a prescribed coding paradigm with predetermined subcategories (e.g., causal conditions, strategies, context, intervening conditions, and consequences) intended to help researchers pose questions about how categories of their data relate to one another. All qualitative researchers did not embrace this new technique. Glaser (1978, 1992) indicated that coding should be driven by conceptualizations about data. These and other concerns (e.g., inattention to earlier developed ideas about BSPs and saturation of categories) led Glaser to assert that Strauss and Corbin's model is a new method no longer oriented to the discovery, or **emergence**, of the grounded theory method as originally conceived by himself and Strauss (Melia, 1996).

These and subsequent developments in grounded theory offer clear choices not only between Straussian and Glaserian methods of analysis but also between both Glaser's and Strauss and Corbin's versions and other approaches that expand its interpretive possibilities, as a growing number of scholars apply grounded theory's basic guidelines to research agendas that involve a wider variety of philosophical perspectives and theoretical assumptions (Bryant & Charmaz, 2007; Charmaz, 2006; Morse et al., 2009). For clinicians, it would be important to note what approach was used in conducting the research to understand the interpretation of the data.

Description, Interpretation, and Theory Generation. Qualitative researchers amass many forms of data: recorded observations (fieldnotes), interview tapes and transcripts, documents, photographs, and collected or received artifacts from the field. There are numerous ways to approach these materials.

All researchers write descriptively about their data (i.e., the empirical evidence). The act of describing necessarily involves interpretation of the facts of an experience through choices made about what to report and how to represent it. Researchers also refer to Geertz's (1973) notion of **thick description** (as opposed to thin description; Box 6.7) as what is needed for interpretations. Thick description not only details reports of what people say and do but also incorporates the textures and feelings of the physical and social worlds in which people move and—always with reference to that context—an interpretation of what their words and actions mean. "Thick description" is a phrase that "ought not to appear in

---

> ### Box 6.7   General Qualitative Research Terms
>
> **Thick description:** Description that does more than describe human experiences by beginning to interpret what they mean.

write-ups of qualitative research at all" (Sandelowski, 2004, p. 215). Rather, it is a quality that needs to be demonstrated in the written presentation.

Describing meaning in context is important because it is a way to try to understand what informants already know about their world. Informants do not talk about what they take for granted (i.e., tacit, personal knowledge) because their attention is not focused on it. And sometimes what they do is different from what they say because everyday actions in familiar settings also draw on tacit understandings of what is usual and expected. Thick descriptions attempt to take this into account. They are the researcher's interpretations of what it means to experience life from certain vantage points through written expression that is "artful and evocative" as well as "factual and truthful" (Van Maanen, 1988, p. 34).

It is the researcher's choice to report research findings in more factual, descriptive terms (allowing the empirical data to speak for itself) or more interpretive terms (drawing out the evidence that illuminates circumstances, meanings, emotions, intentions, strategies, and motivations). But this mostly is a matter of degree for researchers whose work in a designated tradition tends to push them toward more in-depth interpretation. Additionally, the venue and intended audiences influence decisions about how to represent research findings.

Theory generation is also a proper goal in ethnography and an essential outcome in grounded theory. In these traditions, theories are empirical evidence-based explanations of how cultural, social, and personal circumstances account for individuals' actions and interactions with others. Analyzed data supply the evidence in which the theories are grounded. Theory generation is not expected in phenomenological or hermeneutic approaches. The purpose of these studies is to understand and interpret human experience (i.e., to provide a mental picture or image of its meaning and significance), not to explain it (e.g., to describe or theorize about its structure and operation in terms of causes, circumstances, or consequences).

Qualitative Descriptive Studies. Descriptive studies may be used in quantitative research as a prelude to experiments and other types of inquiry. However, qualitative descriptive studies (Box 6.8) serve to summarize factual information about human experiences with more attention to the feel of the data's subjective content than that tends to be found in quantitative description. Sandelowski (2000b) suggests that researchers "name their method as qualitative description [and] if … designed with overtones from other methods, they can describe what these overtones were, instead of inappropriately naming or implementing these other methods" (p. 339).

> ### Box 6.8   General Qualitative Research Terms
>
> **Qualitative description:** Description that "entails a kind of interpretation that is low-inference [close to the 'facts'] or likely to result in easier consensus [about the 'facts'] among researchers" (Sandelowski, 2000b, p. 335).
> **Naturalistic research:** Commitment to the study of phenomena in their naturally occurring settings (contexts).
> **Field studies:** Studies involving direct, firsthand observation and interviews in informants' natural settings.

Generic Qualitative Studies. Researchers may identify their work in accordance with the technique that was used (e.g., observation study or interview study). Other generic terms are **naturalistic research** (Lincoln & Guba, 1985), largely signifying the intellectual commitment to studying phenomena in the natural settings or contexts in which they occur, or **field study**, implying research activities that involve direct, firsthand observations and interviews in the informants' natural settings.

Qualitative Evaluation and Action Research Studies. Some studies that use qualitative research techniques need to retain their unique identities. For example, evaluation of educational and organizational programs, projects, and policies may use qualitative research techniques of interviewing, observation, and document review to generate and analyze data. Also, various forms of **action research**, including **participatory action research** (PAR; see Box 6.9), may use field techniques of observation and interviewing as approaches to data collection and analysis. Examples are the use of PAR to explore the chronic pain experienced in older adults (Baker & Wang, 2006) and as an approach for improving Black women's health in rural and remote communities (Etowa, Bernard, Oyinsan, & Clow, 2007).

Favored Research Techniques

Favored techniques used in qualitative research reflect the needs of particular study designs. It is appropriate for them to appear last in a discussion of methods because techniques do not drive research questions and designs. They are the servants, not the masters, and they are not what make a study qualitative. Nevertheless, a secure knowledge of techniques and their uses has important consequences for successful execution and evaluation of studies.

Observation and Fieldnotes. In fieldwork observation, combined with other activities, takes on different dimensions, sometimes described as complete observer, observer as participant, participant as observer, and complete participant (Flick, 2006). **Participant observation** (i.e., active engagement of the researcher in settings and activities of people being studied; Box 6.10) encompasses all of these social roles with less time spent at the extremes. Most time is spent in the middle where distinctions between observer as participant and participant as observer are blurred. This is similar to everyday life in which the emphasis shifts back and forth as people take more or less active roles in interactions (e.g., speaking and listening, acting and watching, taking the initiative and standing by), depending on the situation.

   Fieldnotes are self-designed observational protocols for recording notes about field observation. Most are not actually recorded in the field, where researchers may only be able to do "jottings" (e.g., phrases and key words as memory aids) until it is possible to compose an expanded account. Fieldnotes are highly detailed records of all that can be remembered of observations, as well as researcher actions and interactions. They may include maps and drawings of the environment, as well as conversations and

---

Box 6.9 Qualitative Research Terms

Qualitative evaluation: A general term covering a variety of approaches to evaluating programs, projects, policies, and so forth using qualitative research techniques.
Action research: A general term for a variety of approaches that aim to resolve social problems by improving existing conditions for oppressed groups or communities.
Participatory action research (PAR): A form of action research that is participatory in nature (i.e., researchers and participants collaborate in problem definition, choice of methods, data analysis, and use of findings); democratic in principle; and reformatory in impulse (i.e., has as its objective the empowerment of persons through the process of constructing and using their own knowledge as a form of consciousness raising with the potential for promoting social action).

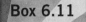

Box 6.10   Qualitative Research Terms

Observation continuum: A range of social roles encompassed by participant observation and ranging from complete observer to complete participant at the extremes.
Fieldnotes: Self-designed observational protocols for recording notes about field observations.
Analytic notes (memos): Notes that researchers write to themselves to record their thoughts, questions, and ideas as a process of simultaneous data collection and data analysis unfolds.

records of events. **Analytic notes** (also called *reflective notes* or *memos*) are notes researchers write to themselves about ideas for analysis, issues to pursue, people to contact, questions, personal emotions, understandings, and confusions brought into focus by writing and thinking about the field experience. This process illustrates how data collection and analysis occur simultaneously throughout the study.

Interviews and Focus Groups. Although a variety of interview forms and question formats are used in qualitative research, their common purpose is to provide ways for informants to express and expand on their own thoughts and remembrances, reflections, and ideas. Informal conversational interviews that occur in the natural course of participant observation are of the **unstructured, open-ended** type (Box 6.11). Formal interviews, however, often involve the use of interview guides that list or outline in advance the topics and questions to be covered. Interviews remain conversational, and the interviewer has the flexibility in deciding sequence and wording of questions on the basis of how the conversation is flowing, but the **semistructured interview** approach makes data collection more comprehensive and systematic from one informant to another.

Some studies also use **structured, open-ended** question formats, where informants answer the same exactly worded question(s) but are free to describe their experiences in their own words and on their own terms. Although this discussion covers several interview methods, it does not exhaust possible interview approaches.

Box 6.11   Qualitative Research Terms

Unstructured, open-ended interviews: Informal conversations that allow informants the fullest range of possibilities to describe their experiences, thoughts, and feelings.
Semistructured interviews: Formal interviews that provide more interviewer control and question format structure but retain a conversational tone and allow informants to answer in their own ways.
Structured, open-ended interviews: Formal interviews with little flexibility in the way the questions are asked but with question formats that allow informants to respond on their own terms (e.g., "What does...mean to you?" "How do you feel/think about...?").
Focus groups: This type of group interview generates data on designated topics through discussion and interaction. Focus group research is a distinct type of study when used as the sole research strategy.

Group interviews may be used in addition to individual interviews in field research. In recent years, **focus groups** have been used in combination with other forms of data collection in both qualitative and quantitative research studies to generate data on designated topics through discussion and interaction. Group moderators direct interaction in structured or semistructured ways, depending on the purpose of the interview. For example, Perkins, Barclay, and Booth (2007) reported a focus group study of palliative care patients' views on priorities for future research that, as the qualitative component of a mixed method study, was used in the development of a questionnaire for a larger quantitative patient survey.

When used as the sole research strategy, the focus group interview represents a distinct type of study with a history in marketing research. Thus, researchers should limit their naming of the method to "focus group" and refer to primary sources for information on specific focus group strategies when planning to use this as the central data collection technique (e.g., Krueger & Casey, 2000).

Narrative and Content Analysis. Analysis in qualitative research involves extracting themes, patterns, processes, essences, and meanings from textual data (i.e., written materials such as fieldnotes, interview transcripts, and various kinds of documents). But there is no single way to go about this. For instance, narrative, discourse, and content analysis are examples of broad areas (paradigms) within which researchers work; each comprises many different approaches.

Narrative analysis is concerned with generating and interpreting stories about life experiences. It is a specific way to understand interview data, representing it in the form of "truthful fictions" (Sandelowski, 1991, p. 165). Kleinman's (1988) *The Illness Narratives* is a well-known example in the medical literature. Other examples include Bingley, Thomas, Brown, Reeve, and Payne's (2008) discussion of narrative analysis approaches that may be of use in palliative care and Edwards and Gabbay's (2007) study of patient experiences with long-term sickness. Although qualitative researchers commonly deal with stories of individuals' experiences, narrative analysis is a particular way of dealing with stories. Therefore, the term should not be used casually to refer to any form of analysis that involves narrative data.

Discourse analysis is a term covering widely diverse approaches to the analysis of recorded talk. The general purpose is to draw attention to how language/communication shapes human interactions. "Discourse analysts argue that language and words, as a system of signs, are in themselves meaningless; it is through the shared, mutually agreed-on use of language that meaning is created" (Starks & Trinidad, 2007, p. 1374).

Current examples from clinical literature of discourse analysis are sparse and varied, primarily due to the existence of multiple discourse analysis techniques but no single method.

> *Discourse analysis uses "conventional" data collection techniques to generate texts... [which] could be interview transcripts, newspaper articles, observations, documents, or visual images... Although the methods of generating texts and the principles of analysis may differ... the premises on which the research being reported has drawn need to be clearly articulated.* (Cheek, 2004, pp. 1145–1146).

An example is Graffigna and Bosio's (2006) analysis of how the setting shapes conversational features of face-to-face versus online discussions about HIV/AIDS.

Qualitative **content analysis** is most commonly mentioned in research reports in connection with procedures that involve breaking down data (e.g., coding, comparing, contrasting, and categorizing bits of information), then reconstituting them in some new form, such as description, interpretation, or theory. Ethnographers refer to this as *working data* to tease out themes and patterns. Grounded theorists describe *procedural sequences* involving different levels of coding and conceptualization of data. Phenomenologists may also use **thematic analysis** as one of many analytic strategies. Hsieh and Shannon (2005) discussed three approaches to qualitative content analysis. To avoid confusion, it should be noted that there are forms of quantitative content analysis that use very different principles to deal with narrative data in predetermined, structured ways.

Sampling Strategies. *Sampling* decisions involve choices about study sites or settings and people who will be able to provide information and insights about the study topic. A single setting may be chosen for in-depth study, or multiple sites may be selected to enlarge and diversify samples or for purposes

Box 6.12	Qualitative Research Terms

Purposeful/purposive sampling: Intentional selection of people or events in accordance with the needs of the study.

Nominated/snowball sampling: Recruitment of participants with the help of informants already enrolled in the study.

Volunteer/convenience sampling: A sample obtained by solicitation or advertising for participants who meet study criteria.

Theoretical sampling: In grounded theory, purposeful sampling used in specific ways to build theory.

of comparison. Some studies of human experiences are not specific to a particular setting. Within and across sites, researchers must choose activities and events that, through observation and interview, will yield the best information. For example, if in a study of older adults' adjustment to congregate living, data gathering is limited to interviews in individuals' private quarters, there will be a loss of other individuals' perspectives (e.g., family members, service providers) and the ability to observe how participants interact with others in different facets of community life.

Choice of participants (i.e., informants or study subjects in qualitative studies) is based on a combination of criteria, including the nature and quality of information they may contribute (i.e., **theoretic interest**), their willingness to participate, their accessibility, and their availability. A prominent qualitative sampling strategy is purposeful.

Purposeful/purposive sampling (Box 6.12) enables researchers to select informants who will be able to provide particular perspectives that relate to the research question(s). In grounded theory, this is called **theoretical sampling** (i.e., sampling is used in specific ways to build theory). **Nominated** or **snowball sampling** may also be used, in which informants assist in recruiting other people they know to participate. This can be helpful when informants are in a position to recommend people who are well informed on a topic and can provide a good interview. **Volunteer/convenience samples** are also used when researchers do not know potential informants and solicit for participants with the desired experience who meet study inclusion criteria. With all types of sampling, researcher judgment and control are essential to be sure that study needs are met.

Researchers' judgments, based on ongoing evaluation of quality and quantity of different types of information in the research database, determine the number and variety of informants needed (Creswell, 2007; Marshall & Rossman, 2011). Minimum numbers of informants needed for a particular kind of study may be estimated, based on historical experience. For example, 30 to 50 interviews typically meet the needs of ethnographic and grounded theory studies, whereas six may be an average sample size for a phenomenological study (Morse, 1994). However, if a study involves multiple interviews of the same people, fewer informants may be needed. And if the quality of information that informants supply is not good or sufficient to answer questions or saturate data categories (the same information keeps coming up), more informants will be needed. Decisions to stop collecting data depend on the nature and scope of the study design; the amount, richness, and quality of useable data; the speed with which types of data move analysis along; and the completeness or saturation (Morse, 2000).

> *An adequate sample size...is one that permits—by virtue of not being too large—the deep, case-oriented analysis that is a hallmark of all qualitative inquiry, and that results in—by virtue of not being too small—a new and richly textured understanding of experience.* (Sandelowski, 1995, p. 183)

Quantitative methods' quality markers should not be applied to qualitative studies. For example, **random sampling**, often used in quantitative studies to achieve statistically representative samples,

---

Box 6.13   Qualitative Research Terms

Qualitative data management: The act of designing systems to organize, catalog, code, store, and retrieve data. (System design influences, in turn, how the researcher approaches the task of analysis.)

Computer-assisted qualitative data analysis: An area of technological innovation that in qualitative research has resulted in uses of word processing and software packages to support data management.

Qualitative data analysis: A variety of techniques that are used to move back and forth between data and ideas throughout the course of the research.

---

does not logically fit with purposes of qualitative designs. Rather purposive sampling in which researchers seek out people who will be the best sources of information about an experience or phenomenon is more appropriate.

Data Management and Analysis. In appraising qualitative studies, it is important to understand how data are managed and analyzed. Qualitative studies generate large amounts of narrative data that need to be managed and manipulated. Personal computers and word processing software facilitate data management (Box 6.13), including:

◆ Data entry (e.g., typing fieldnotes and analytic memos, transcribing recorded interviews)
◆ "Cleaning" or editing
◆ Storage and retrieval (e.g., organizing data into meaningful, easily located units, or files)

Data manipulation involves coding, sorting, and arranging words, phrases, or data segments in ways that advance ongoing analysis. Various types of specialized software have been developed to support management and manipulation of textual data. There is no inherent virtue in using or not using qualitative data analysis software (QDAS). It is wise to consider the advantages and disadvantages (Creswell, 2007). Most important to remember is that QDAS packages, unlike statistical software, may support but do not perform data analyses. Users need to be certain that the analyses they must perform do not suffer as a result of inappropriate fit with the limits and demands of a particular program or the learning curve that may be involved.

Data analysis occurs throughout data collection to ensure that sampling decisions produce an appropriate, accurate, and sufficiently complete and richly detailed data set to meet the needs of the study. Also, to manage the volume of data involved, ongoing analysis is needed to sort and arrange data while developing ideas about how to reassemble and represent them as descriptions, theories, or interpretations.

Sorting may involve making frequency counts, coding, developing categories, formulating working hypotheses, accounting for negative cases (instances that contradict other data or do not fit hypotheses), or identifying concepts that explain patterns and relationships among data. Research design and specific aims determine one of the many analytic techniques that will be used (e.g., phenomenological reduction, constant comparison, narrative analysis, content analysis).

Similarly, the results of data analysis may take many forms. A common example is thematic analysis that systematically describes recurring ideas or topics (i.e., themes) that represent different yet related aspects of a phenomenon. Data may be organized into tables, charts, or graphs or presented as narratives using actual quotes from informants or reconstructed life stories (i.e., data-based hypothetical examples). Data may also be presented as typologies or taxonomies (i.e., classification schemes) that serve explanatory or heuristic (i.e., illustrative and educational) purposes (Porter, Ganong, Drew, & Lanes,

> **Box 6.14**   Qualitative Research Terms
>
> **Paradigm:** A world view or set of beliefs, assumptions, and values that guide all types of research by identifying where the researcher stands on issues related to the nature of reality (ontology), relationship of the researcher to the researched (epistemology), role of values (axiology), use of language (rhetoric), and process (methodology; Creswell, 2007).
>
> **Method:** The theory of how a certain type of research should be carried out (i.e., strategy, approach, process/overall design, and logic of design). Researchers often subsume description of techniques under a discussion of method.
>
> **Techniques:** Tools or procedures used to generate or analyze data (e.g., interviewing, observation, standardized tests and measures, constant comparison, document analysis, content analysis, statistical analysis). Techniques are method-neutral and may be used, as appropriate, in any research design—either qualitative or quantitative.

2004; Powers, 2001, 2005). As noted previously in discussing issues of representation, researchers may also use drama, self-stories, and poetry to immerse the reader in the informants' world, decrease the distance between the author and the reader, and more vividly portray the emotional content of an experience. These kinds of evaluation are important to critical appraisal of qualitative studies.

Mixing Methods. It is unhelpful to view qualitative research as a singular entity that can be divorced from the assumptions of the traditions associated with different methods or reduced to a group of data collection and analysis techniques. Because there are so many choices that necessarily involve multilevel (e.g., paradigm, method, and technique; Box 6.14) commitments (Sandelowski, 2000a), seasoned researchers have cautioned against nonreflective, uncritical mixing of qualitative perspectives, language, and analytic strategies (i.e., hybridized qualitative studies) to produce results that do not meet rigorous scholarly standards, which clinicians should be aware of when appraising qualitative evidence. This is coupled with a concern about researchers who rely on textbooks or survey courses for direction rather than expert mentorship. The concern is that, as more novice researchers, their ability to recognize within-method and across-method subtleties and nuances, identify decision points and anticipate consequences involved in the research choices they make may be compromised as a result of the insufficient depth of understanding afforded by these limited knowledge bases (Morse, 1997a). Clinicians who are novice readers of qualitative research (and beginning researchers) are advised first to learn about pure methods so that they will be able to proceed with greater knowledge and confidence, should they later encounter a hybrid (combined qualitative) or mixed-method (combined qualitative and quantitative) approach.

APPRAISING INDIVIDUAL QUALITATIVE STUDIES

A variety of method-specific and general criteria have been proposed for evaluating qualitative studies. In fact, there is a large variety of rules related to quality standards, but there is no agreed-upon terminology or preset format that bridges the diversity of methods enough to dictate how researchers communicate about the rules they followed. Only part of the judgment involves what researchers say they did. The other part is how well they represent research results, the effect of the presentation on readers, and readers' judgments about whether study findings seem credible and useful.

> ### Box 6.15   Glaser and Strauss' Evaluative Criteria for a Grounded Theory Study
>
> ◆ **Fit:** Categories must be indicated by the data.
> ◆ **Grab:** The theory must be relevant to the social/practical world.
> ◆ **Work:** The theory must be useful in explaining, interpreting, or predicting the study phenomenon.
> ◆ **Modifiability:** The theory must be adaptable over time to changing social conditions.

Method-Specific Criteria for Evaluating Qualitative Studies

Some criteria for evaluating scientific rigor specifically relate to central purposes and characteristics of traditional methods. For example, ethnography's historic emphasis on understanding human experience in cultural context is reflected by six variables proposed by Homans (1955) to evaluate the adequacy of field studies: *time*, *place*, *social circumstance*, *language*, *intimacy*, and *consensus*.

Elaboration on these variables relates to values placed on prolonged close engagement of the researcher with study participants, active participation in daily social events, communication, and confirmation of individual informant reports by consulting multiple informants. Appraisals of an ethnographic/field study's accuracy (credibility) may be linked to how well values such as these appear to have been upheld.

Similarly, the ultimate goal of grounded theory-influenced evaluative criteria was summarized by Glaser and Strauss (1967) as: *fit*, *grab*, *work*, and *modifiability* (Box 6.15).

The pedagogic, semiotic/language-oriented approach to phenomenology of van Manen (1990/1997) is reflected in his four conditions or evaluative criteria of any human science text. The text must be *oriented*, *strong*, *rich*, and *deep* (Box 6.16).

These are just a few examples of how active researchers working within specific traditions have conceptualized their craft. Because there is such diversity in qualitative inquiry, no single set of criteria can serve all qualitative approaches equally well. But there have been efforts to articulate criteria that may more generally apply to diverse qualitative research approaches (Creswell, 2007; Flick, 2006; Marshall & Rossman, 2011). The method-specific criteria to some extent drive these general criteria. However, the primary driver for the variety of attempts to develop general criteria has been perceived as communication gaps between qualitative and quantitative researchers whose use of language and world views often differ. Despite these attempts, there is no agreement among qualitative researchers about how or whether it is appropriate to use the general appraisal criteria.

> ### Box 6.16   Van Manen's Evaluative Criteria for a Phenomenological Study
>
> ◆ **Oriented:** Answers a question of how one stands in relation to life and how one needs to think, observe, listen, and relate
> ◆ **Strong:** Clear and powerful
> ◆ **Rich:** Thick description/valid, convincing interpretations of concrete experiences
> ◆ **Deep:** Reflective/instructive and meaningful

General Criteria for Evaluating Qualitative Studies

Examples of general evaluative criteria are those proposed by Lincoln and Guba (1985) that offer qualitative equivalents to quantitative concepts of validity and reliability. These help explain the scientific rigor of qualitative methods to quantitatively oriented persons. But it has been argued that by framing discussion on the basis of the belief structures of quantitative researchers and drawing attention away from other criteria of equal importance, the criteria fail to address paradigmatic differences. The differences reflected by qualitative researchers' world views are in the ways they perceive reality as subjective and multiple, ontological differences; the way they view the relationship between the researcher and the researched as close and collaborative, epistemologic differences; the belief that all research is value laden, and biases that are naturally present need to be dealt with openly, axiologic differences; the conviction that effective use of personal and literary writing styles arc kcy to meaningful representation of research results, rhetorical differences; and the ways in which inductive logic is used to draw out and encourage development of emerging understanding of what the data mean, methodological differences (Creswell, 2007).

Trustworthiness Criteria

When appraising qualitative research, applying Lincoln and Guba's (1985) trustworthiness criteria can be helpful. These criteria include *credibility*, *transferability*, *dependability*, and *confirmability* (Box 6.17). These four criteria parallel the quantitative criteria for good research, namely internal validity, external validity, reliability, and objectivity.

Credibility. Credibility is demonstrated by accuracy and validity that are assured through documentation of researcher actions, opinions, and biases; negative case analysis (e.g., accounting for outliers/exceptions); appropriateness of data (e.g., purposeful sampling); adequacy of the database (e.g., saturation); and verification/corroboration by use of multiple data sources (e.g., triangulation), validation of data and findings by informants (e.g., member checks), and consultation with colleagues (e.g., peer debriefing).

Much like internal validity in quantitative methods (the extent to which you can infer causality), there are some caveats about the above indicators of credibility that merit mentioning. Member checks can be problematic when researchers' findings uncover implicit patterns or meanings of which informants are unaware. Thus, they may not be able to corroborate findings and may need to reexamine the situation and "check out results for themselves" (Morse, 1994, p. 230).

When reading a qualitative report, member checks may or may not be present. Also, they are seldom useful for corroborating reports that are a synthesis of multiple perspectives, because individuals are not positioned well to account for perspectives beyond their own. Therefore, member checks should be seen as an ongoing process for assuring that informants' recorded accounts accurately and fairly reflect their perceptions and experiences. But as an ultimate check on the final interpretation of data, they are not required; it is up to the researcher to decide when and how they may be useful (Morse, 1998a; Sandelowski, 1993, 1998a).

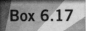 **Box 6.17**

Lincoln and Gubas' Evaluative Criteria: Trustworthiness Criteria

◆ Credibility
◆ Dependability
◆ Transferability
◆ Confirmability

Peer debriefing involves seeking input (substantive or methodological) from knowledgeable colleagues as consultants, soliciting their reactions as listeners, and using them as sounding boards for the researcher's ideas. It is up to the researcher to decide when and whether peer debriefing will be useful. It is important to distinguish peer debriefing from quantitative researchers' use of multiple raters and expert panels. In qualitative research, it is not appropriate to use individuals outside of the research to validate the researcher's analyses and interpretations because these are arrived at inductively through closer contact and understanding of the data than an outside expert could possibly have (Morse, 1994, 1997b, 1998a; Sandelowski, 1998a). Because peer debriefing may not always be useful, the reader should not expect to encounter this credibility criterion in every qualitative report.

Transferability. Transferability is demonstrated by information that is sufficient for a research consumer to determine whether the findings are meaningful to other people in similar situations (analytic or theoretical vs. statistical generalizability). Statistical generalization and analytic or theoretic generalization are *not* the same thing. In quantitative traditions, external validity has concerned with *statistical generalization,* which involves extending or transferring implications of study findings to a larger population by using mathematically based probabilities. *Analytic or theoretic generalization,* on the other hand, involves extending or *transferring* implications of study findings to a larger population by logically and pragmatically based possibilities, which is appropriate for qualitative research.

The practical usefulness of a qualitative study is judged by its:

◆ Ability to represent how informants feel about and make sense of their experiences
◆ Effectiveness in communicating what that information means and the lessons that it teaches

Dependability. Dependability is demonstrated by a research process that is carefully documented to provide evidence of how conclusions were reached and whether, under similar conditions, a researcher might expect to obtain similar findings (i.e., the concept of the audit trail). In quantitative traditions, reliability refers to consistency in findings across time. This is another example of what is called parallelism—parallel concepts within the qualitative and quantitative traditions; however, these concepts are entirely different in meaning and application.

Confirmability. Confirmability is demonstrated by providing substantiation that findings and interpretations are grounded in the data (i.e., links between researcher assertions and the data are clear and credible). The parallel concept of objectivity in quantitative traditions speaks to reduction of bias through data-driven results.

Other general criteria are linked to concepts of credibility and transferability but relate more to the effects that various portrayals of the research may have. For example, a second set of criteria developed by Guba and Lincoln (1989) have overtones of a critical theory view that when the goal of research is to provide deeper understanding and more informed insights into human experiences, it may also prove to be empowering (Guba & Lincoln, 1994).

Authenticity Criteria

Box 6.18 lists Guba and Lincoln's (1989) evaluative *authenticity criteria.* Ontological and educative authenticity, in particular, is at the heart of concerns about how to represent research results. That is, to transfer a deeper understanding of a phenomenon to the reader, researchers may strive for literary styles of writing that make a situation seem more "real" or "alive." This is also called making use of *verisimilitude,* an important criterion of traditional validity (Creswell, 2007; Denzin, 1997) and describes when the readers are drawn *vicariously into the multiple realities of the world that the research reveals,* from perspectives of both the informant and researcher.

Evaluation Standards

The authenticity criteria (Guba & Lincoln, 1989) are not as well recognized or cited as regularly by many quantitative researchers and practitioners as Lincoln and Guba's (1985) trustworthiness criteria, which

> | Box 6.18 | Guba and Lincoln's Evaluative Criteria: Authenticity Criteria |
>
> ◆ **Fairness:** Degree to which informants' different ways of making sense of experiences (i.e., their "constructions") are evenly represented by the researcher
> ◆ **Ontological authenticity:** Scope to which personal insights are enhanced or enlarged
> ◆ **Catalytic authenticity:** How effectively the research stimulates action
> ◆ **Tactical authenticity:** Degree to which people are empowered to act
> ◆ **Educative authenticity:** Extent to which there is increased understanding of and appreciation for others' constructions

are understandable and seek to impose a sense of order and uniformity on a field that is diverse and difficult to understand. Thus, some readers have greater confidence in qualitative reports that use the classic trustworthiness criteria terminology to explain what researchers did to assure *credibility*, *transferability*, *dependability*, and/or *confirmability*.

However, it does not mean that reports that do not do so are necessarily deficient. Many qualitative researchers and practitioners resist using words that mirror the concepts and values of quantitative research (e.g., our example of the parallel concepts of internal validity and credibility) because they think that it may detract from better method-specific explanations of their research (a matter of training and individual preference). Some also think, as a matter of principle, that it could undermine the integrity of qualitative methods themselves. Furthermore, they know that examples of procedures to ensure quality and rigor are more or less appropriate for different kinds of qualitative studies and, therefore, attempts to talk about the general properties of qualitative designs and findings pose many constraints. As a result, there is a threat to integrity if general criteria come to be viewed as rigid rules that must apply in every instance. Therefore, it is incumbent upon nonqualitative researchers and practitioners to assimilate more details about the differences, similarities, and nuances of this large field of research than they might at first prefer in order to conduct a fair and accurate appraisal of qualitative reports.

WALKING THE WALK AND TALKING THE TALK: CRITICAL APPRAISAL OF QUALITATIVE RESEARCH

We began by comparing critical appraisal of individual research reports with separation of the wheat from the chaff. Separating out the chaff involves applying the reader's understanding of the diversity within qualitative research to the content of the report. Next, extracting what is good and useful involves applying the appropriate method-specific and general evaluative criteria to the research report. A degree of familiarity with the diversity of characteristics, language, concepts, and issues associated with qualitative research is necessary before using the guide in Box 6.1 to appraise qualitative research studies.

The guide adopts the EBP format of basic quick appraisal questions followed by more specific questions, but there are caveats. One is that no individual study contains the most complete information possible about everything in the appraisal guide. Sometimes, as in quantitative reports, the information is available and built into the design itself, but is dependent on the reader's knowledge of the method. At other times, because the volume of data and findings may require a series of reports that focus on different aspects of the research, authors sometimes direct readers to introductory articles that are more focused on the methods and broad overviews of the study. The final caveat is that space limitations and a journal's priorities determine the amount of detail that an author may provide in any given section of the report.

....

That inner voice has both gentleness and clarity. So to get to authenticity, you really keep going down to the bone, to the honesty, and the inevitability of something.
—Meredith Monk

....

Putting Feet to Knowledge: Walking the Walk

It is time to put feet to the knowledge the reader has gained through this chapter. The reader is encouraged to use Appendix D that demonstrates a rapid critical appraisal application of the appraisal guide for qualitative evidence. The appendix contains exemplars of qualitative research reports. The range of topics appearing in the literature confirms that clinical researchers across professions and specialty areas are "walking the walk and talking the talk" and using a variety of qualitative approaches with attendant methodologies, terms, and concepts as described earlier.

Choice of exemplars presented here was guided by the following criteria:

◆ A mix of articles representing a variety of concerns across different areas of clinical interest
◆ A range of qualitative research designs that illustrate the achievement of valid results
◆ A range of research purposes that illustrate a variety of ways in which results may help readers care for their patients

The source of these studies is *Qualitative Health Research*, an interdisciplinary journal that addresses a variety of healthcare issues and is an excellent resource for individuals seeking good examples of qualitative methods. Factors that may affect reader response to the appraisal of articles using the rapid critical appraisal format are:

1. Individual preference: In the real world, people choose the topics that interest them.
2. The ease with which the report submits to appraisal: Appreciation and understanding of qualitative reports depend on individual reading of and engagement with the report in its entirety. Therefore, the articles lose some of their communicative and evocative qualities when parsed apart and retold.

The results of the appraisal process combined with individual preference may affect the studies' initial appeal. Because in every case evaluations of an article's plausibility and generalizability (transferability) require the use of independent reader judgments, firsthand reading is recommended.

....

Changes may not happen right away, but with effort even the difficult may become easy.
—Bill Blackman

....

KEEPING IT TOGETHER: SYNTHESIZING QUALITATIVE EVIDENCE

Synthesizing qualitative evidence is not a new endeavor, given the history of the *meta-study* in the social sciences. A meta-study is not the same as a critical literature review or a secondary analysis of an existing data set. Instead, meta-studies involve distinct approaches to the analysis of previously published research findings in order to produce new knowledge (a synthesis of what is already known).

In quantitative research, *meta-analysis* is the research strategy designed to ask a new question on multiple studies that address similar research hypotheses using comparable methodologies, reanalyzing, and combining their results to come to a conclusion about what is known about the issue of interest. In qualitative research, various strategies for performing *meta-synthesis* have been proposed.

In an article by Thorne, Jensen, Kearney, Noblit, and Sandelowski (2004), these scholars presented their distinct perspectives on meta-synthesis methodology in order to underscore what it is not (i.e., it is not an integrative critical literature review) and to explore the various methodological conventions they used and/or recommended.

The result of various approaches to qualitative meta-synthesis can be a formal theory or a new refined interpretive explanation of the phenomenon. For example, Kearney (2001), using a grounded formal theory approach, analyzed 13 qualitative research reports and synthesized a middle-range theory of women's responses to violent relationships. She found that "within cultural contexts that normalized relationship violence while promoting idealized romance, these women dealt with the incongruity of violence in their relationships as a basic process of enduring love" (p. 270).

Thorne et al. (2002) presented insights about a body of qualitative evidence related to the experience of chronic illness gained through use of general meta-method approaches developed within sociology and anthropology. Their findings uncovered a tension between conceptualizations of chronic illness (e.g., loss vs. opportunity for growth) that suggested the need for "a functional model of chronic illness...to account for both possibilities, focusing its attention on, for example, how we might know which conceptualization to engage in any particular clinical encounter" (p. 448). The methodological approach that was used is described in greater detail in *Meta-Study of Qualitative Health Research: A Practical Guide to Meta-Analysis and Meta-Synthesis* (Paterson, Thorne, Canam, & Jillings, 2001).

Sandelowski and Barroso (2003) used meta-summary and meta-synthesis techniques in an ongoing study of research conducted on HIV-positive women. Their findings in this report, in part, revealed that "motherhood itself positioned these women precariously between life as a normal woman and life as a deviant one" (p. 477). Women's response to "mortal and social threats of HIV infection and the contradictions of Western motherhood embodied in being an HIV-positive mother...was to engage in a distinctive maternal practice [described as] *virtual motherhood*" (p. 476). A detailed description of how to perform qualitative research synthesis, including illustrative examples from this research, is provided in their *Handbook for Synthesizing Qualitative Research* (Sandelowski & Barroso, 2007).

Further examples of meta-synthesis include Hammell's (2007a, 2007b) meta-synthesis of qualitative findings on the experience of rehabilitation and factors contributing to or detracting from the quality of life after spinal cord injury, and a meta-ethnographic approach to the synthesis of qualitative research on adherence to tuberculosis treatment by Atkins et al. (2008).

Despite the lack of a single set of agreed-upon techniques for synthesizing qualitative studies, there is an appreciation for the basic definition and underlying purposes of meta-synthesis and the general procedural issues that any approach to it will need to address. Basically, meta-synthesis is a holistic translation, based on comparative analysis of individual qualitative interpretations, which seeks to retain the essence of their unique contributions. Although individual studies can provide useful information and insights, they cannot give the most comprehensive answers to clinical questions. A benefit of meta-synthesis methods is that they provide a way for researchers to build up bodies of qualitative research evidence that are relevant to clinical practice.

Specific approaches to meta-synthesis need to address issues of:

- How to characterize the phenomenon of interest when comparing conceptualizations and interpretations across studies
- How to establish inclusion criteria and sample from among a population of studies
- How to compare studies that have used the same or different qualitative strategies
- How to reach new understandings about a phenomenon by seeking consensus in a body of data where it is acknowledged that there is no single "correct" interpretation (Jensen & Allen, 1996)

Appraisal of meta-synthesis research reports requires an appreciation for the different perspectives that may be guiding the analysis. Mechanisms described by Sandelowski and Barroso (2007) for promoting valid study procedures and outcomes include:

- Using all search channels of communication and maintaining an audit trail (Rodgers & Cowles, 1993) tracking search outcomes as well as procedural and interpretive decisions

- Contacting primary study investigators
- Consulting with reference librarians
- Independent search by at least two reviewers
- Independent appraisal of each report by at least two reviewers
- Ensuring ongoing negotiation of consensual validity (Belgrave & Smith, 1995; Eisner, 1991) facilitated by collaborative efforts by team members to establish areas of consensus and negotiate consensus in the presence of differing points of view
- Securing expert peer review (Sandelowski, 1998a) by consultation with experts in research synthesis and with clinical experts

Written reports will vary in their use or mention of these approaches and in their detailing of research procedures. Readers will have to be alerted about references to a named methodology; explanation of the search strategy that was used; clarity in the manner in which findings (data that comprise the study sample) are presented; and the originality, plausibility, and perceived usefulness of the synthesis of those findings.

....

You will come to know that what appears today to be a sacrifice [learning to appraise qualitative evidence is hard work!] will prove instead to be the greatest investment that you will ever make.
—Gorden B. Hinkley

....

EBP FAST FACTS

- Qualitative evidence has an impact on clinical decision making, providing relevant, influential information for patients, families, and systems.
- Qualitative studies help to answer clinical questions that address the how of healthcare interventions.
- Unique language and concepts are encountered in the qualitative literature, including such terms as purposive sampling, saturation, and participant observation.
- Qualitative evidence requires a different approach to appraisal than quantitative evidence.
- Intentional understanding of the appropriate evaluative criteria for qualitative evidence is required to avoid misuse of appraisal of studies and subsequent erroneous conclusions.

References

Atkins, S., Lewin, S., Smith, H., Engel, M., Fretheim, A., & Volmink, J. (2008). Conducting a meta-ethnography of qualitative literature: Lessons learnt. *BMC Medical Research Methodology, 8,* 21.

Atkinson, P. (1992). *Understanding ethnographic texts.* Newbury Park, CA: Sage.

Baker, T. A., & Wang, C. C. (2006). Photovoice: Use of a participatory action research method to explore the chronic pain experience in older adults. *Qualitative Health Research, 16,* 1405–1413.

Beck, C. T. (2007). Teetering on the edge: A continually emerging theory of postpartum depression. In P. L. Munhall (Ed.), *Nursing research: A qualitative perspective* (4th ed., pp. 273–292). Sudbury, MA: Jones & Bartlett.

Beck, C. T., & Watson, S. (2008). Impact of birth trauma on breast-feeding. *Nursing Research, 57,* 228–236.

Belgrave, L. L., & Smith, K. J. (1995). Negotiated validity in collaborative ethnography. *Qualitative Inquiry, 1,* 69–86.

Bingley, A. F., Thomas, C., Brown, J., Reeve, J., & Payne, S. (2008). Developing narrative research in supportive and palliative care: The focus on illness narratives. *Palliative Medicine, 22,* 653–658.

Bryant, A., & Charmaz, K. (Eds.). (2007). *The SAGE handbook of grounded theory.* London: Sage.

Charmaz, K. (2006). *Constructing grounded theory: A practical guide through qualitative analysis.* London: Sage.

Cheek, J. (2004). At the margins? Discourse analysis and qualitative research. *Qualitative Health Research, 14,* 1140–1150.

Chenitz, W. C., & Swanson, J. M. (1986). *From practice to grounded theory.* Menlo Park, CA: Addison-Wesley.

Clabo, L. M. L. (2007). An ethnography of pain assessment and the role of social context on two postoperative units. *Journal of Advanced Nursing, 61*, 531–539.

Copeland, D. A., & Heilemann, M. V. (2008). Getting "to the Point": The experience of mothers getting assistance for their adult children who are violent and mentally ill. *Nursing Research, 57*, 136–143.

Corbin, J., & Strauss, A. (2008). *Basics of qualitative research: Techniques and procedures for developing grounded theory* (3rd ed.). Thousand Oaks, CA: Sage.

Creswell, J. W. (2007). *Qualitative inquiry & research design: Choosing among five approaches* (2nd ed.). Thousand Oaks, CA: Sage.

Cricco-Lizza, R. (2007). Ethnography and the generation of trust in breastfeeding disparities research. *Applied Nursing Research, 20*, 200–204.

Denzin, N. K. (1997). *Interpretive ethnography: Ethnographic practices for the 21st century.* Thousand Oaks, CA: Sage.

Dickson-Swift, V., James, E. L., Kippen, S., & Liamputtong, P. (2006). Blurring boundaries in qualitative health research on sensitive topics. *Qualitative Health Research, 16*, 853–871.

Edwards, S., & Gabbay, M. (2007). Living and working with sickness: A qualitative study. *Chronic Illness, 3*, 155–166.

Eisner, E. W. (1991). *The enlightened eye: Qualitative inquiry and the enhancement of educational practice.* New York: Macmillan.

Ellingson, L. L. (2006). Embodied knowledge: Writing researchers' bodies into qualitative health research. *Qualitative Health Research, 16*, 298–310.

Etowa, J. B., Bernard, W. T., Oyinsan, B., & Clow, B. (2007). Participatory action research (PAR): An approach for improving Black women's health in rural and remote communities. *Journal of Transcultural Nursing, 18*, 349–357.

Evans, M. J., & Hallett, C. E. (2007). Living with dying: A hermeneutic phenomenological study of the work of hospice nurses. *Journal of Clinical Nursing, 16*, 742–751.

Fawcett, J., Watson, J., Neuman, B., Hinton-Walker, P., & Fitzpatrick, J. J. (2001). On theories and evidence. *Journal of Nursing Scholarship, 33*, 115–119.

Fineout-Overholt, E., Melnyk, B., & Schultz, A. (2005). Transforming health care from the inside out: Advancing evidence-based practice in the 21st century. *Journal of Professional Nursing, 21*(6), 335–344.

Flick, U. (2006). *An introduction to qualitative research* (3rd ed.). London: Sage.

Fochtman, D. (2008). Phenomenology in pediatric cancer nursing research. *Journal of Pediatric Oncology Nursing, 25*, 185–192.

Foster, K., McAllister, M., & O'Brien, L. (2005). Coming to autoethnography: A mental health nurse's experience. *International Journal of Qualitative Methods, 4*, 1–13.

Furman, R. (2006). Poetic forms and structures in qualitative health research. *Qualitative Health Research, 16*, 560–566.

Geertz, C. (1973). *The interpretation of cultures.* New York: Basic Books.

Glaser, B. G. (1978). *Theoretical sensitivity.* Mill Valley, CA: Sociology Press.

Glaser, B. G. (1992). *Emergence vs. forcing: Basics of grounded theory analysis.* Mill Valley, CA: Sociology Press.

Glaser, B. G., & Strauss, A. L. (1967). *The discovery of grounded theory: Strategies for qualitative research.* New York: Aldine.

Grace, J. T., & Powers, B. A. (2009). Claiming our core: Appraising qualitative evidence for nursing questions about human response and meaning. *Nursing Outlook, 57*(1), 27–34.

Graffigna, G., & Bosio, A. C. (2006). The influence of setting on findings produced in qualitative health research: A comparison between face-to-face and online discussion groups about HIV/AIDS. *International Journal of Qualitative Methods, 5*(3), Article 5. Retrieved, September 16, 2008, from http://www.ualberta.ca/~iiqm/backissues/5_3/pdf/graffigna.pdf

Guba, E. G., & Lincoln, Y. S. (1989). *Fourth generation evaluation.* Newbury Park, CA: Sage.

Guba, E. G., & Lincoln, Y. S. (1994). Competing paradigms in qualitative research. In N. K. Denzin & Y. S. Lincoln (Eds.), *Handbook of qualitative research* (pp. 105–117). Thousand Oaks, CA: Sage.

Guell, C. (2007). Painful childhood: Children living with juvenile arthritis. *Qualitative Health Research, 17*, 884–892.

Hammell, K. W. (2007a). Experience of rehabilitation following spinal cord injury: A meta-synthesis of qualitative findings. *Spinal Cord, 45*, 260–274.

Hammell, K. W. (2007b). Quality of life after spinal cord injury: A meta-synthesis of qualitative findings. *Spinal Cord, 45*, 124–139.

Homans, G. C. (1955). *The human group.* New York: Harcourt Brace.

Hsieh, H. F., & Shannon, S. E. (2005). Three approaches to qualitative content analysis. *Qualitative Health Research, 15*, 1277–1288.

Jensen, L. A., & Allen, M. N. (1996). Meta-synthesis of qualitative findings. *Qualitative Health Research, 6*, 553–560.

Kayser-Jones, J. (2002). The experience of dying: An ethnographic nursing home study. *The Gerontologist, 42,* 11–19.

Kayser-Jones, J., Schell, E., Lyons, W., Kris, A. E., Chan, J., & Beard, R. L. (2003). Factors that influence end-of-life care in nursing homes: The physical environment, inadequate staffing, and lack of supervision. *The Gerontologist, 43,* 76–84.

Kearney, M. H. (2001). Enduring love: A grounded formal theory of women's experience of domestic violence. *Research in Nursing & Health, 24,* 270–282.

Kleinman, A. (1988). *The illness narratives: Suffering, healing & the human condition.* New York: Basic Books.

Kontos, P. C., & Naglie, G. (2006). Expressions of personhood in Alzheimer's: Moving from ethnographic text to performing ethnography. *Qualitative Research, 6,* 301–317.

Kontos, P. C., & Naglie, G. (2007). Expressions of personhood in Alzheimer's disease: An evaluation of research-based theatre as a pedagogical tool. *Qualitative Health Research, 17,* 799–811.

Krueger, R., & Casey, M. (2000). *Focus groups: A practical guide for applied research* (3rd ed.). Thousand Oaks, CA: Sage.

Lincoln, Y. S., & Guba, E. G. (1985). *Naturalistic inquiry.* Beverly Hills, CA: Sage.

Mantzoukas, S. (2004). Issues of representation within qualitative inquiry. *Qualitative Health Research, 14,* 994–1007.

Marshall, C., & Rossman, G. B. (2011). *Designing qualitative research* (5th ed.). Thousand Oaks, CA: Sage.

Melia, K. M. (1996). Rediscovering Glaser. *Qualitative Health Research, 6,* 368–378.

Milton, C. L. (2007). Evidence-based practice: Ethical questions for nursing. *Nursing Science Quarterly, 20,* 123–126.

Mordoch, E., & Hall, W. A. (2008). Children's perceptions of living with a parent with a mental illness: Finding the rhythm and maintaining the frame. *Qualitative Health Research, 18,* 1127–1144.

Morse, J. M. (1994). Designing funded qualitative research. In N. K. Denzin & Y. S. Lincoln (Eds.), *Handbook of qualitative research* (pp. 220–235). Thousand Oaks, CA: Sage.

Morse, J. M. (1997a). Learning to drive from a manual? *Qualitative Health Research, 7,* 181–183.

Morse, J. M. (1997b). "Perfectly healthy, but dead": The myth of inter-rater reliability. *Qualitative Health Research, 7,* 445–447.

Morse, J. M. (1998a). Validity by committee. *Qualitative Health Research, 8,* 443–445.

Morse, J. M. (2000). Determining sample size. *Qualitative Health Research, 10,* 3–5.

Morse, J. M. (2007). Quantitative influences on the presentation of qualitative articles. *Qualitative Health Research, 17,* 147–148.

Morse, J. M., Stern, P. N., Corbin, J., Bowers, B., Charmaz, K., & Clarke, A. (Eds.). (2009). *Developing grounded theory: The second generation.* Walnut Creek, CA: Left Coast Press.

Paterson, B. L., Thorne, S. E., Canam, C., & Jillings, C. (2001). *Meta-study of qualitative health research: A practical guide to meta-analysis and meta-synthesis.* Thousand Oaks, CA: Sage.

Perkins, P., Barclay, S., & Booth, S. (2007). What are patients' priorities for palliative care research? Focus group study. *Palliative Medicine, 21,* 219–225.

Porter, E. J., Ganong, L. H., Drew, N., & Lanes, T. I. (2004). A new typology of home-care helpers. *Gerontologist, 44,* 750–759.

Powers, B. A. (2001). Ethnographic analysis of everyday ethics in the care of nursing home residents with dementia: A taxonomy. *Nursing Research, 50,* 332–339.

Powers, B. A. (2005). Everyday ethics in assisted living facilities: A framework for assessing resident-focused issues. *Journal of Gerontological Nursing, 31,* 31–37.

Powers, B. A., & Knapp, T. R. (2011a). Evidence and best evidence. In B. A. Powers & T. R. Knapp (Eds.), *A dictionary of nursing theory and research* (4th ed., pp. 56–57). Thousand Oaks, CA: Sage.

Powers, B. A., & Knapp, T. R. (2011b). Evidence-based practice (EBP). In B. A. Powers & T. R. Knapp (Eds.), *A dictionary of nursing theory and research* (4th ed., pp. 57–58). Thousand Oaks, CA: Sage.

Richardson, L. (1990). *Writing strategies: Reaching diverse audiences.* Newbury Park, CA: Sage.

Rodgers, B. L., & Cowles, K. V. (1993). The qualitative research audit trail: A complex collection of documentation. *Research in Nursing & Health, 16,* 219–226.

Sandelowski, M. (1991). Telling stories: Narrative approaches in qualitative research. *Image: Journal of Nursing Scholarship, 23,* 161–166.

Sandelowski, M. (1993). Rigor or rigor mortis: The problem of rigor in qualitative research revisited. *Research in Nursing & Health, 16,* 1–8.

Sandelowski, M. (1995). Sample size in qualitative research. *Research in Nursing & Health, 18,* 179–183.

Sandelowski, M. (1998a). The call to experts in qualitative research. *Research in Nursing & Health, 21,* 467–471.

Sandelowski, M. (1998b). Writing a good read: Strategies for re-presenting qualitative data. *Research in Nursing & Health, 21,* 375–382.

Sandelowski, M. (2000a). Combining qualitative and quantitative sampling, data collection, and analysis techniques in mixed-method studies. *Research in Nursing & Health, 23,* 246–255.

Sandelowski, M. (2000b). Whatever happened to qualitative description? *Research in Nursing & Health, 23,* 334–340.

Sandelowski, M. (2004). Counting cats in Zanzibar. *Research in Nursing & Health, 27,* 215–216.

Sandelowski, M. (2007). Words that should be seen but not written. *Research in Nursing & Health, 30,* 129–130.

Sandelowski, M., & Barroso, J. (2003). Motherhood in the context of maternal HIV infection. *Research in Nursing & Health, 26,* 470–482.

Sandelowski, M., & Barroso, J. (2007). *Handbook for synthesizing qualitative research.* New York: Springer.

Sandelowski, M., Trimble, F., Woodard, E. K., & Barroso, J. (2006). From synthesis to script: Transforming qualitative research findings for use in practice. *Qualitative Health Research, 16,* 1350–1370.

Scott, S. D., & Pollock, C. (2008). The role of nursing unit culture in shaping research utilization behaviors. *Research in Nursing & Health, 31,* 298–309.

Smith, C. A. M., & Gallo, A. M. (2007). Applications of performance ethnography in nursing. *Qualitative Health Research, 17,* 521–528.

Starks, H., & Trinidad, S. B. (2007). Choose your method: A comparison of phenomenology, discourse analysis, and grounded theory. *Qualitative Health Research, 17,* 1372–1380.

Stewart, L., & Usher, K. (2007). Carspecken's critical approach as a way to explore nursing leadership issues. *Qualitative Health Research, 17,* 994–999.

Straus, S. E., Richardson, W. S., Glasziou, P., & Haynes, R. B. (2005). *Evidence-based medicine: How to practice and teach EBM* (3rd ed.). Edinburgh: Elsevier.

Strauss, A. L., & Corbin, J. (1990). *Basics of qualitative research: Grounded theory procedures and techniques.* Newbury Park, CA: Sage.

Strauss, A. L., & Corbin, J. (1998). *Basics of qualitative research: Techniques and procedures for developing grounded theory* (2nd ed.). Thousand Oaks, CA: Sage.

Thomas, J. (1993). *Doing critical ethnography.* Newbury Park, CA: Sage.

Thorne, S., Jensen, L., Kearney, M. H., Noblit, G., & Sandelowski, M. (2004). Qualitative metasynthesis: Reflections on methodological orientation and ideological agenda. *Qualitative Health Research, 14,* 1342–1365.

Thorne, S., Paterson, B., Acorn, S., Canam, C., Joachim, G., & Jillings, C. (2002). Chronic illness experience: Insights from a metastudy. *Qualitative Health Research, 12,* 437–452.

Tutton, E., Seers, K., & Langstaff, D. (2007). Professional nursing culture on a trauma unit: Experiences of patients and staff. *Journal of Advanced Nursing, 61,* 145–153.

Van Maanen, J. (1988). *Tales of the field.* Chicago: University of Chicago Press.

van Manen, M. (1990/1997). *Researching lived experience.* London, Ontario: University of Western Ontario & State University of New York Press.

van Manen, M. (2002). *Writing in the dark: Phenomenological studies in interpretive inquiry.* London, Ontario: University of Western Ontario.

Varcoe, C. (2001). Abuse obscured: An ethnographic account of emergency nursing in relation to violence against women. *Canadian Journal of Nursing Research, 32,* 95–115.

Wolcott, H. (2001). *Writing up qualitative research* (2nd ed.). Thousand Oaks, CA: Sage.

Wolcott, H. (2002). Writing up qualitative research … better. *Qualitative Health Research, 12,* 91–103.

Wolf, Z. R. (2007). Ethnography: The method. In P. L. Munhall (Ed.), *Nursing research: A qualitative perspective* (4th ed., pp. 293–330). Sudbury, MA: Jones & Bartlett.

Woodgate, R. L., Ateah, C., & Secco, L. (2008). Living in a world of our own: The experience of parents who have a child with autism. *Qualitative Health Research, 18,* 1075–1083.

Wuest, J. (2007). Grounded theory: The method. In P. L. Munhall (Ed.), *Nursing research: A qualitative perspective* (4th ed., pp. 239–271). Sudbury, MA: Jones & Bartlett.

Making EBP a Reality by Reducing Patient Falls Through Transdisciplinary Teamwork

Marcia Belcher, MSN, BBA, RN, CCRN-CSC, CCNS and Michelle Simon, BSN, RN, CCRN

Staff Nurse
The Ohio State University Wexner Medical Center Richard M. Ross Heart Hospital

Step 0: The Spirit of Inquiry Ignited

Each year, an estimated 700,000 and 1,000,000 patients in the United States fall in the hospital. "A patient fall may be defined as an unplanned descent to the floor with or without injury to the patient" (National Center for Health Services Research, 2013). Falls may result in fractures, lacerations, or internal bleeding that may lead to increased healthcare utilization. As of 2008, the Centers for Medicare and Medicaid Services (CMS) do not reimburse hospitals for certain types of traumatic injuries that occur while a patient is in the hospital; many of these injuries could occur after a fall. The National Center for Health Sciences Research National Patient Safety Goal 9 states "Reduce the risk of patient harm resulting from falls" (2013). Falls are a major cause of morbidity and mortality, especially in elderly patients with medications serving as a contributing factor due to their potential to cause sedation, dizziness, orthostatic hypotension, altered gait and balance, or impaired cognition (Lim, Fink, Blackwell, Taylor, & Ensrud, 2009, p. 862)

Staff nurses at a large academic research medical center's heart hospital are challenged on a daily basis to care for patients receiving numerous fall-risk-increasing drugs (FRIDs). Research shows that medication use is one of the most modifiable risk factors for falls and fall-related injuries (Shuto et al., 2010, p. 536). This hospital's 30-bed heart failure unit had experienced an increased rate of falls and fall-related injuries. The majority of the falls occurred between the hours of 3 AM and 7 AM when the maximum effect of the diuretic would be experienced. A multidisciplinary team including physicians, staff nurses, pharmacist, and patient care assistants was assembled with a clinical nurse specialist as an evidence-based practice (EBP) mentor. An audit was conducted by the pharmacy department titled, "Evaluation of the Modification Fall Risk Scoring System to Identify Patients at Risk for Medication Related Falls and Opportunity for Pharmacist Intervention" to establish a baseline.

Step 1: The PICOT Question Formulated

In adult hospitalized patients (P), how does a nonstandard dosing time for diuretics (I) versus standard dosing time for diuretics (C) affect the rate of patient falls (O) during their hospital stay (T)?

Step 2: Search Strategy Conducted

Keywords that were utilized in the search strategy included diuretics, falls, fall risk, fall injury, medications, dosing times, inpatient, and hospitalized patient. Because this unit's patient population consisted primarily of heart failure and readmitted ventricular assist devices patients, the unit wanted to narrow its search to research that specially addressed diuretic administration versus including other medications, such as sedatives. Databases that were searched included PubMed, Cochrane, and Cumulative Index to Nursing and Allied Health Literature (CINAHL). A total of 10 articles were ultimately selected that addressed the PICOT question.

Step 3: Critical Appraisal of the Evidence Performed

Each of the articles was critically appraised; two articles were level II evidence (i.e., randomized controlled trials with large samples), rendering strong evidence to support that certain medications placed patients at risk for falls based on the time of day the medication was administered. Five other articles were **level III evidence** (i.e., case–control studies that addressed the correlation between certain medications, such as diuretics and an increased incidence of falls and fall-related injuries). There were three articles that were level V, descriptive studies that reinforced the relationship between the risk of falling and medications. Leveling of the studies using an evidence hierarchy and critical appraisal tools to determine the strength of each study and creation of synthesis tables provided a systematic approach to critically appraise the body of evidence to address the PICOT question (Melnyk & Fineout-Overholt, 2011).

Step 4: Evidence Integrated with Clinical Expertise and Patient Preferences to Inform a Decision and Practice Change Implemented

After careful critical appraisal of the body of evidence, the transdisciplinary team met to determine next steps. An informal survey of patients on the unit was conducted to determine the time that they took their diuretics at home. Interestingly, it was discovered that 50% of the patients surveyed stated that they took their morning dose of diuretic between 5 AM and 6 AM. The other 50% of the patients surveyed reported random morning dosing times. The daily dosing time that the electric medical record (EMR) system automatically assigned was at 9 AM; BID dosing times were 9 AM and 5 PM; and TID dosing times assigned were 9 AM, 2 PM and 9 PM. In order to impact the fall rate related to patient's toileting in the middle of the night, a new approach to diuretic administration was deemed the starting point of this EBP change project. With assistance from the pharmacy department and the support of the physicians, new dosing times were proposed. The new dosing times were as follows: daily dosing would remain at 9 AM, BID dosing would be at 7:45 AM and 4 PM, and TID dosing time would be at 7:45 AM, 11 AM, and 4 PM so that no diuretic was administered after 4 PM.

Prior to the implementation of this practice change, a formal letter was sent to the attending physicians outlining the background of the problem, the evidence to support the practice change, and the proposed practice (ordering) change to be implemented. A poster was presented to the nursing staff (staff nurses as well as patient care assistants) that outlined the problem, the evidence to support the change, and the practice change to be implemented. In addition, all staff was in-serviced regarding the problem as well as what and why an EBP change was being implemented.

Other fall reduction strategies were implemented at the same time in an effort to address the problem of falls and fall-related injuries. Orthostatic blood pressures were performed on all heart failure patients at 11 AM and on a daily basis. Bedside commodes were placed in all rooms to make toileting easier. Daily patient assignment sheets for the nursing staff indicated patients at high risk for falls. New signage was placed in all patient rooms that stated "Please Call, Don't Fall," which could be easily seen by the patients and their families. Bed exit alarms were set on high between the hours of 11 PM and 7 AM. PCA shifts were changed to create an overlap so that the off-going shift obtained vital signs prior to their departure, allowing the oncoming PCA to beginning assisting patients to the bathroom at the beginning of their shift. All of these changes were embraced by the staff and implemented successfully.

Step 5: Outcomes Evaluated

Six months after the EBP change, the rate of falls decreased by over 60% with no fall-related injuries. Education to the nurses and physicians is an ongoing process to accommodate new physicians, nurses, and PCAs joining the staff.

Step 6: Project Outcomes Successfully Disseminated

The success of this EBP change project has been presented to nursing leadership and shared-governance councils, including the Evidence-based Practice Council, Clinical Practice Councils, and Unit Leadership Councils. It has also been presented to the system-wide Critical Care Quality and the system-wide Patient Safety and Quality Committee. This EBP change initiative has also been highlighted on the hospital's intranet that is available to all staff in the entire system and plans to submit the project for national presentations and publication are underway.

References

Berry, S., Mittleman, M., Zhang, Y., Soloman, D., Lipsitz, L., Mostofsky, E., … Kiel, D. (2012). New loop diuretic prescriptions may be an acute risk factor for falls in the nursing home. *Pharmcoepidemiology and Drug Safety, 21*, 560–563.

Huang, A., Mallett, L., Rochefort, C., Equale, T., Buckeridge, D., & Tamblyn, R. (2012). Medication-related falls in the elderly: Causative factors and preventative strategies. *Drugs & Aging, 29*(5), 359–376.

Lim, L., Fink, H., Blackwell, T., Taylor, B., & Ensrud, K. (2009). Loop diuretic use and rates of hip bone loss and risk of falls and fractures in older women. *Journal of American Geriatric Society, 57*, 855–862.

Melnyk, B. M., & Fineout-Overholt, E. (2011). *Evidenced-based practice in nursing and healthcare: A guide to best practice* (2nd ed.). Philadelphia, PA: Wolters Kluwer/Lippincott Williams and Wilkins.

National Center for Health Sciences Research. (2013). *Preventing falls in hospitals: A toolkit for improving quality of care*. Washington, DC: RAND, Corp, January 2013, pp. 1–202.

Shuto, H., Imakyure, O., Matsumoto, J., Egawa, T., Jiang, Y., Hirakawa, M., … Yanagawa, T. (2010). *British Journal of Clinical Pharmacology, 69*(5), 532–542.

Woolcott, J., Richardson, K., Wiens, M., Patel, B., Marin, J., Khan, K., & Marra, C. (2009). Met analysis of the impact of 9 mediation classes on falls in elderly person. *Archives of Internal Medicine, 169*(21), 1952–1960.

Ziere, G., Dieleman, J. P., Hofman, A., Pols, H., van der Cammen, T., & Stricker, B. (2005) Polypharmacy and falls in the middle age and elderly population. *British Journal of Clinical Pharmacology, 61*(2), 218–223.

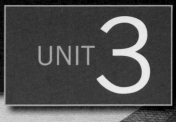

Steps Four and Five: Moving From Evidence to Sustainable Practice Change

Chapter 7

Integration of Patient Preferences and Values and Clinician Expertise Into Evidence-Based Decision Making

Lisa English Long, Lynn Gallagher-Ford, and Ellen Fineout-Overholt

Evidence-based practice (EBP) is the integration of patient preferences and values, clinical expertise, and rigorous research to make decisions that lead to improved outcomes for patients and families (Figure 7.1). In order to improve outcomes for patients and families, transdisciplinary healthcare professionals must collaborate with patients and families as they enter into decision-making processes. The assumption is that clinicians combine external evidence with patient preferences and clinical expertise. While there has been a health industry-wide focus on gathering, appraising, and synthesizing evidence to make recommendations for practice change, the question remains: How often are **patient preferences** and **clinician expertise** factored into the decisions that affect the best interest of the patient and family? Furthermore, these decisions are best achieved through a context of caring, which prompts the question: How is this context fostered and monitored? This chapter discusses the importance of engaging patients and families in the decision-making process to achieve their best outcomes.

Gillian has just started her shift at 7 AM. She receives report that the new mom, Mrs. Blum, in room 26B has a moderately distended bladder, cannot void, and will need to be catheterized; however, the patient has not been out of bed yet after her vaginal delivery at 5 AM. Gillian pops her head in 26B and tells the patient she will be in shortly to do her catheterization. Gillian focuses on gathering her supplies to do a straight catheterization and, since she has not done a lot of these procedures, goes over it in her mind several times. She walks into Mrs. Blum's room and notes that she is crying. Gillian realizes that her assessment has not been complete. She puts down her materials and lets Mrs. Blum know she is here to help. Mrs. Blum informs Gillian that all night the nurse caring for her and the resident who came in this morning were all focused on her going to the bathroom. No one asked about her baby, and she is concerned since the night nursery nurses did not bring her back for her early morning feeding. Gillian further assesses Mrs. Blum's bladder and asks her if she thinks she can void if she goes to the bathroom and sits on the toilet. She further informs Mrs. Blum that after she voids, they will go to the nursery to see her daughter. Mrs. Blum agrees and, after assessing Mrs. Blum's balance, together they walk to the bathroom. Mrs. Blum expresses appreciation for being able to sit on the toilet as the bedpan "is just unbearable." She promptly voids 450 cc of amber urine. Gillian then helps her to clean up and gets a wheelchair to reserve her energy so she can focus on her daughter. Upon arrival at the nursery, Mrs. Blum is visibly relieved and pleased to see and hold her daughter. She indicates to Gillian that she cannot thank her enough for taking the time to treat her "like a person versus a procedure."

In this scenario and many others like it across multiple disciplines, clinicians actualize on a daily basis what the American Nurses Association's (ANA) (2008) official position statement on professional role competence states, that the public has a right to expect clinicians to demonstrate professional competence, and each clinician is "individually responsible and accountable for maintaining professional competence." Health professions are also responsible to the public to shape and guide any process that will assure clinician competence. The competent clinician is expected to deliver the best care possible, which, as demonstrated by patient outcomes, is care that is supported by evidence. However, evidence from research and clinician assessment is not the only influence on clinical decision making. What do patients and their families want from the healthcare experience?

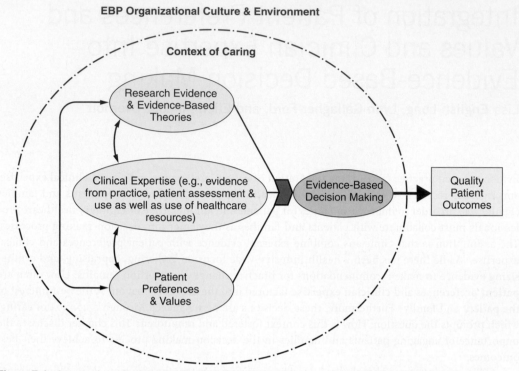

Figure 7.1: Integration of external evidence, clinical expertise (wisdom and judgment), and patient preferences and values into evidence-based decision making. (© 2003 Melnyk & Fineout-Overholt, used with permission.)

Within a **context of caring**, integration of the concepts of patient preferences and values and clinical expertise in combination with evidence from well-conducted studies are part of everyday decision making—whether inserting a urinary catheter or simply holding a hand during a painful procedure. This principle is wonderfully illustrated in a *New York Times* article entitled "When Doctors Say Don't and the Patient Says Do" (Siegel, 2002). Marc Siegel describes a determined 93-year-old woman who is a tap dancer. A former teacher of dance at Julliard, she has, for the past 50 years since her retirement, been an avid tap dancer at amateur shows and recitals, until it was discovered that she had a "bulging disc in her neck, tissue so inflamed that it encroached on the space intended for the spinal cord, the crucial super-highway of the nervous system." All scientific evidence on prognosis for someone of her age undergoing spinal surgery unanimously showed that the risks outweighed the benefits, even though this particular patient's heart was in excellent health and she was also in excellent physical condition. When Siegel enumerated the risks of having the surgery, and the almost certain continued pain and incapacitation without the surgery, she asked, "Can the surgery make me dance again?" To which he replied, "It's possible." "Then," she responded, "I'll take my chances." Dr. Siegel was able to find a neurosurgeon willing to do the surgery, and when the patient returned to Dr. Siegel's office, she appeared a vigorous woman whose vitality was returning. Her walking had already progressed beyond her presurgical capacities. And several weeks later Dr. Siegel received an invitation to her first postsurgical tap dancing recital. She explained to Dr. Siegel: "You see," she said, "we patients are not just statistics. We don't always behave the way studies predict we will."

In this story, many processes were occurring simultaneously that reflect integration of research evidence, patient preferences and values, and clinical expertise throughout the patient and healthcare professional's relationship. Evidence-based decision makers don't have a magic formula that guides them; rather, their care is delivered with careful discernment about how to integrate their best knowledge and expertise with what researchers have found to be best practice and what patients have identified as their preferences in a particular healthcare encounter. To successfully engage in evidence-based decision making, one must first understand the meaning of evidence, from both practical and theoretical perspectives (also see Chapters 4 to 6), as well as actively participate in decision making with patients and families.

EVIDENCE: WHAT IT IS AND HOW GOOD IT IS

Evidence is generically defined in the dictionary as "that which tends to prove or disprove [support or not support] something: grounds for beliefs; truth, proof [and] something that makes plain or clear; an indication or sign" (Dictionary.com, 2013). In some disciplines, the term evidence refers to information solely derived from experimental research designs, with randomized controlled trials (RCTs) being the most rigorous of designs and, therefore, rendering what is considered the most valued information. However, the term evidence in the healthcare domain refers to a more complex concept because healthcare professionals seek evidence related to a wide range of interventions and situations involving human beings in which research designs such as an RCT may not be realistic or ethical to perform. Evidence in health care encompasses more than research; however, research (i.e., external evidence) is a central source of evidence in clinical decision making. The implications for researchers (i.e., evidence-generators) are that the design a researcher uses is driven by the type of particular healthcare concern being examined. The implication for clinicians (i.e., evidence-user) is that the broad range of research methodologies allows clinicians to have the most meaningful external evidence possible. As a result, external evidence used in health care is based on a wide-range of methodologies that reflect our best knowledge of interventions and human experiences that impact healthcare outcomes.

Clinicians use the range of evidence (i.e., external and internal) that reflects knowledge derived from a variety of sources including psychosocial and basic sciences (e.g., psychology, physiology, anatomy, biochemistry, pharmacology, genetics), reasoning across time about the patient's transitions and history (i.e., experience), an understanding of the patient's particular concerns, as well as research drawn from appraisal of a range of methodologies, not just RCTs. Evidence must always be understood by clinicians in light of the their interpretations of the patient's concerns, history, family and cultural context, and disease trajectory as well as what they know about the way the evidence was obtained. It is a dangerous simplification to imagine that evidence from clinical trials could apply directly to a particular patient care decision without evaluating the validity and reliability of the clinical trial and its relevance for that particular patient (see Chapter 5). This process of evaluation, called **critical appraisal**, applies to single studies and summaries of comparative evidence.

As part of critical appraisal, it is important for clinicians to consider possible flaws in the research before they apply study findings. For example, were there biased commercial influences in the design, presentation, or dissemination of the research, or is the study credible, or how well can a study be directly applied to particular patients? Sometimes research is robust and convincing; at other times, it is weaker and more conflicted. Still at other times, the clinical trial that would address the issue for a particular patient has not yet been done. As part of the evaluation process, it is important to constantly clarify practice patterns, skills, and clinical insights (i.e., thoughtful questioning and reflection about particular patient outcomes and a careful review of the basic science supporting associated interventions and its effectiveness).

Evidentialism: It's About How You Think About Decisions

As clinicians, it is important to understand how we establish the credibility of the information we use in making clinical decisions. We will introduce a framework called **evidentialism** that helps in this understanding. While that may seem like an abstract word, it is important to consider given that one of the most important underpinnings for evidence-based decision making is the degree to which clinicians consider evidence as a foundational part of how they make decisions about the care they provide. In EBP, the evidence is categorized in two ways—(1) the sources of information, ranging from highly reliable sources to opinions of experts (i.e., levels of evidence) and (2) the quality of the information produced by these sources. Evidentialism provides a framework for understanding how the evidence as well as the process a clinician undertakes in considering that evidence influences subsequent decisions.

Conee and Feldman (2004) spoke to a theory that explains what is required for an individual to have a justified belief about something (e.g., a clinical decision) called evidentialism. The authors call this "epistemic justification," which means that the information that you currently have justifies your decision at a particular time. Conee and Feldman suggested that epistemic justification is determined by the "quality of the believer's evidence" (i.e., credibility of the evidence) (p. 63). This is why it is so important to establish the validity, reliability, and applicability (i.e., the credibility) of the evidence being applied to a clinical issue. In addition, the relevance of current evidence to a clinical issue reinforces the importance of continually learning throughout one's career (i.e., life-long learning). The authors' central point is that the decision a person makes is justified because it fits the person's evidence at a particular time. Should the evidence change or circumstances change, the same decision may not be justified if the evidence that supported the previous decision is not relevant at this time.

The central themes of evidentialism that are most relevant and support the use of evidence in clinical practice include:

◆ Evidence is mental information, which means that I must be aware of or know about the information upon which I make decisions.
◆ Beliefs are based on current evidence, which means my beliefs are based on what I know at this moment; given this, there is no requirement that a person pursues more evidence at a particular moment without a reason.
◆ Experiences that a person has had can be counted as evidence.

There are assumptions in evidentialism that underpin the role of clinical wisdom and judgment in evidence-based decisions, including:

◆ Only decisions that result from thoughtfully responsible behavior are justified.
◆ External evidence that supports a conclusion about patient care may not be sufficient to make that conclusion clinically meaningful.
◆ As available external evidence changes, the decision maker's responses should change too.
◆ Decisions made from some set of external evidence depend on the validity, reliability, and applicability (i.e., credibility) of the actual evidence and the subject's grasp of the evidence, which is clinical wisdom.
◆ Having a belief without supportive external evidence is unwise, and therefore, that belief is unjustified. Not only will such a belief have an impact on decisions that are based on that belief, it will affect all decisions connected to that unjustified belief.

These assumptions support why **clinical wisdom and judgment** are critical to evidence-based decisions and how their integration with external evidence is imperative. Aikin, a philosopher, published a modified version of the theory of evidentialism, which he called "modest evidentialism" (2006). Aikin's modification strengthened the alignment of evidentialism with clinical practices because it emphasized that what we base our clinical decisions on does reflect our values and beliefs that help us to minimize the occurrence of adverse events. This makes sense when considering how healthcare professionals engage patients and subsequently integrate their values and preferences into their care. Furthermore, Aikin discussed the obligation that clinicians bear related to evidence, beliefs, and decisions with patients. Healthcare providers are required to know how to obtain and evaluate current evidence that is relevant to their patient care as well as understand its importance to fulfilling their professional, social obligation to the people for whom they care. Patients rely on healthcare providers to be expert in their work and knowledgeable of current best practices. When healthcare providers do not meet this expectation, they fail the patient care community. Consider that a health professions student who read the textbook for a prerequisite history class 10 years ago was asked a question today about the U.S. Civil War. That student would rationally base her response on the information from the 10-year-old textbook. However, if she has changed her major to history and was considered *an expert* on the U.S. Civil War, or if *her job required her to be well informed about this topic*, she necessarily would have a different obligation to have her beliefs more thoroughly grounded in the most up-to-date evidence. It would be irrational for the history expert (i.e., the authority) to solely base her beliefs, upon which others are going to rely, on a 10-year-old textbook. Ultimately, the information that is important to one's work has to be the latest, best information possible.

Aikin (2006) also addresses whether there is ever an opportunity or duty to modify or override external evidence. Aikin argues against making decisions that are thoroughly based solely on external evidence, particularly when they could cause harm to patients. In these situations, it is wise to make the prudent, pragmatic, and/or moral decision, which may or may not agree with the external evidence. In health care, it could be interpreted that this is the only kind of decisions healthcare providers make. Therefore, our decisions should never be solely based on the external evidence but should include patient preference information along with clinical wisdom and judgment and practice data that are subsumed in clinical expertise. This position means that relevant external evidence is the first requirement for decision making. However, external-evidence-only decisions should be overridden, and the more comprehensive evidence-based decision (i.e. including clinical expertise and patient preferences) be made as it demonstrates itself as a better choice for achieving outcomes. This philosophical framework provides clear support for the professional obligation of healthcare providers to shift practice from what we have known (i.e., tradition-based) to EBP, in which evidence encompasses research, clinical expertise and patient preferences and values.

CLINICAL EXPERTISE

To continuously improve practice, different clinical interventions and consequent outcomes must be compared. The goal is for practice to be self-improving through application of external evidence and experiential clinical learning (i.e., use of internal evidence and clinical expertise) that leads to correction and improvement rather than practice that is stagnant and based on tradition with the potential to repeat errors. Experiential learning and clinical inquiry are equally important to individual practitioners and organizations. Organizations cannot be self-improving without every practitioner actualizing self-improvement in the everyday course of their practice.

In the classic work by Gadamer (1976), experience is never a mere passage of time or exposure to an event. To quality as experience, a turning around of preconceptions, expectations, sets, and routines or adding some new insights to a particular practical situation needs to occur. **Experiential learning** is at the heart of improving clinical judgment and directly contributes to clinical expertise, which is a core aspect of the EBP process. Learning can be from past or present experiences that involve the examination of evidence when considering a practice change.

Although there is a considerable amount of literature that refers to and discusses clinical expertise, there is a paucity of literature that clearly describes the nature and purpose of such expertise. In general, expertise is defined as including "the possession of a specialized body of knowledge or skill, extensive experience in that field of practice, and highly developed levels of pattern recognition..." (Jasper, 1994). More specifically, McCracken and colleagues (2004), defined practitioner expertise as "a set of cognitive tools that aid in the interpretation and application of evidence. This set of tools for thinking develops over a period of extended practice such that the individual with experience in a decision area is likely to respond very differently from the novice" (p. 302). These authors suggest that practitioner expertise includes three overlapping knowledge and skill sets: clinical, technical, and organizational. The clinical set includes knowledge, skills, and experience related to direct practice with clients and includes diagnosis, assessment, engagement, relationships, communication related to warmth and genuineness as well as knowledge of theory, and mastery of skills related to specific care models and interventions (Barlow, 2004; Lambert & Barley, 2001). The technical set includes knowledge, skills, and experience related to formulating questions, conducting an electronic search, and evaluating validity and reliability of findings in order to engage evidence-based decision making (Gibbs, 2003). The organizational set includes knowledge, skills, and experience related to teamwork, organizational design and development, and leadership (McCracken & Corrigan, 2004).

The application of clinical expertise in the triad of evidence-based decision making highlights the fluid interaction that must occur in order to make the best decisions with a particular patient/family who is in unique moments and spaces. In the everyday clinical practice, individual perceptions, decisions, and actions are influenced by consideration of the foreground/current situation as well as the background knowledge/experience that one possesses. In order to deliver best practice, there must be a continuous flow of external evidence into practice and out to the patients. The notion of what counts as good practice in a particular discipline influences what is considered the best practice (i.e., what is supported by external evidence). Clinicians must develop mastery of this flow of external evidence in order to be clinical experts, in which they can effectively use their clinical judgment and integrate patient preferences to facilitate a decision-making relationship with the patient.

Clinical expertise is more than the skills, knowledge, and experience of clinicians. Rather, expertise can only develop when the clinician is able to use that knowledge and skill with external evidence in contextualized (i.e., different clinical settings), situated, clinical experiences. Clinical expertise is on a continuum of experiential learning and can be described as clinicians becoming more expert through decision making within such contextualized experiences. At any point in the experiential learning continuum, clinicians are able to perform at their best and progress in expertise as they engage in additional clinical decision-making experiences.

Much of the literature on clinical expertise is implicitly based on the assumption that expertise is based on tacit (inferred) knowledge and intuition that cannot be described. Kinchin, Cabot, and Hay (2008) suggested that although the development of expertise is highly regarded, the indicators of it have often been described as an "opaque phenomenon" (Benner, 1984; Dreyfus & Dreyfus, 1986) and labeled as intuition or implicit (i.e., not readily describable or hidden). These descriptions, according to Kinchin and colleagues, have clouded what is actually happening and that indeed expertise is not implicit or indescribable, it has simply not been described adequately with the tools and vocabulary that we have applied to other aspects of decision making. New tools, such as concept maps and other advanced technology applications, are available to explicate the multidimensionality of clinical expertise-related concepts and how they interact. Individuals can use these concepts and their interactions to describe their decision making and growth in experiential learning.

Beginning evidence-based decision makers start their experiential learning journey through perceive assessment and evaluation of simple indicators of competence (i.e., tasks), with a linear progression of assimilation of activities (e.g., how many tasks have I done on my checklist) that do not necessarily reflect clinicians' capacities to perform or excel in the inevitable uncertainties of real-world clinical practice, in which evidence-based decision making with patients is an imperative. Clinical expertise is cultivated in teaching and precepted experiences in clinical settings in which the interaction of external evidence, clinical expertise, and patient preference are demonstrated, learned, assessed, scrutinized, valued, and ultimately actualized. All clinicians can engage in evidence-based decision making; however, the ability to embrace the ambiguity in health care and anticipate the complexity in a patient situation is key to demonstrating clinical expertise.

PATIENT PREFERENCES AND VALUES

Patient-centeredness is required for the integration of patient preferences and values in evidence-based decision making. Patient-centeredness is not a new concept in the delivery of health care. Early work was in the areas of skills, attitudes, and knowledge of physicians in training, components, and drivers of patient satisfaction; dysfunction and improvement strategies in doctor–patient communication; and deeper understanding of what patients want to know and how to help them discover what they want to know (Hibbard, 2007; Korsch, 1999; Roter & Hall, 2006; Ware, Snyder, Wright, & Davies, 1983). System-wide patient-centeredness leads to patient-centered care, which is imperative for evidence-based decision making.

Patient-centered care has been defined as "Providing care that is respectful of and responsive to individual patient preferences, needs and values, and ensuring that patient values *guide* all clinical decisions" (IOM, 1999). Non-consumer-focused stakeholders are sometimes not aware of what is truly important to patients and, therefore, do not engage them in the decision-making process. The Institute for Healthcare Improvement (IHI) (2013) describes "patient-centered" as placing an intentional focus on patients' cultural traditions, values and personal preferences, family issues, social circumstances, and lifestyles. Including patient preferences and values in decision makings leads to higher level of patient engagement, and engaged patients seem to have better perceived health outcomes (Gill, 2013a, 2013b).

It is important to consider that not only individual clinicians provide patient-centered care but systems also must be focused on patient-centered health care (IAPO, 2006). An additional resource designed to catapult the incorporation of patient preferences and values into healthcare decision-making processes is the Patient-Centered Outcomes Research Institute (PCORI). The PCORI conducts research to provide information about the best available evidence to help patients and their healthcare providers make more informed decisions. Proposals for comparative effectiveness research studies must include patient preferences in their research design to be considered by PCORI. The vision of PCORI is for patients and the public to have the information they need to make decisions that reflect their desired outcomes. The work of PCORI answers clinical questions for both the healthcare professional and the consumer and shares that information with the broader healthcare community (Figure 7.2).

Studies conducted to address patient-centeredness and shared decision making provide insight into the importance of patient engagement in their care. Decisions need to be realized through the interactions of patients and transdisciplinary healthcare providers. In addition, the evidence produced through

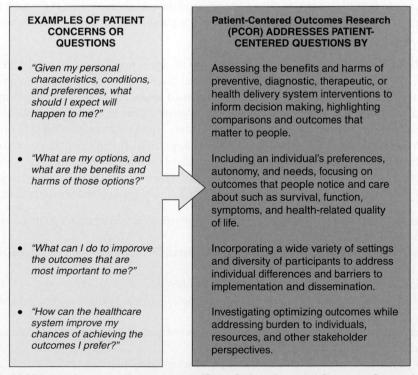

Figure 7.2: PCORI responses to patient concerns. [From Patient-Centered Outcomes Research Institute (PCORI) (2013).]

studies that address patient-centeredness and transdisciplinary collaborative care may guide future actions and outcomes for healthcare staff, patients, and families. Légaré and colleagues (2011) conducted their first mixed methods study to determine the validity of an interprofessional (IP) approach to a shared decision-making (SDM) model with stakeholders, which typically includes patients. The data were analyzed using thematic analysis of transcripts and descriptive analysis of questionnaires. Results showed that most stakeholders believed that the concepts for interprofessional shared decision making (IPSDM) and relationships between those concepts were clear. With all IP healthcare providers valuing patient preferences in their decision making, the focus can be easily turned to improving patient outcomes.

In a later study, Légaré and colleagues (2013) evaluated health professionals' intentions to engage the same IPSDM in home care and also explore factors associated with the intent for shared decision making. Researchers of the mixed methods study reported factors associated with this intention vary depending on the healthcare provider, even within the same setting. In addition, researchers described barriers and facilitators to engaging in IPSDM. The greatest barrier reported was a lack of time to engage in the process, in addition to lack of resources and high staff turnover. A third finding that could influence decision making was that perceived behavioral control ("respondent's perception of barriers and facilitators to his/her performing the behavior," Légaré and colleagues, 2013, p. 215) was most closely associated with the intention to engage in IPSDM.

Hesselink and colleagues (2012) explored barriers and facilitators to patient-centered care in the hospital discharge process in a qualitative study. Researchers identified four themes as barriers:

1. time constraints and competing care obligations interferes with healthcare providers' prioritization in discharge consultations with patients and families;
2. discharge communication ranged from instruction to shared decision making;
3. patients did not feel prepared for discharge and post discharge care was not individualized; and
4. discharge process is affected by pressure for use of available beds. Researchers suggested increased communication between providers, patients and families, the hospital, and community care providers as a future intervention. These findings lend themselves in support of the need for change in the process of shared decision making and the incorporation of patient preferences and values within the agreed upon IPSDM framework.

Berwick (2009) discusses the need for a radical change in care delivery and disruptive shift in control and power. The shift involves moving control and power out of the hands of those who give care and into the hands of those who receive care. He has proposed a new definition of patient-centered care: "the experience (to the extent the informed, individual patient desires it) of transparency, individualization, recognition, respect, dignity, and choice in all matters, without exception, related to one's person, circumstances, and relationships in health care" (Berwick, p. w560). In exploring the concept of patient-centeredness, three slogans were developed: (1) "the needs of the patient come first," (2) "Nothing about me without me," and (3) "Every patient is the only patient" (Berwick, p. w560). Based on the patient as a member of the healthcare system, Berwick proposed the following radical changes to patient care:

- Hospitals would have no restrictions on visiting—restrictions would be decided upon by the individual and/or family.
- Patients would determine what food they eat and what clothes they wear in hospitals based upon patient condition.
- Rounding would include the patient and family member(s).
- Medical records would belong to the patient—healthcare providers would need permission to access patient healthcare information.
- Operating room schedules would change with the aim of minimizing wait time for patients as opposed to schedules based on clinician choice.
- Patients physically capable of self-care would have the option to do it.

(Berwick, p. 561)

Berwick (2009), knowing the need for quality in healthcare design and systems to support patient-centeredness, suggests the following statement become a part of a healthcare providers ending interaction with each person: "Is there anything at all that could have gone better today from your point of view in the care you experienced?" (p. w563).

Evidence-Based Decision Making

As healthcare profession students learn about EBP, they often have challenges with the language—what are patient preference, **internal evidence**, **external evidence**, RCT, synthesis, expertise? This is one barrier to evidence-based decision making that must be overcome. As the reader, you have the opportunity to review and learn the glossary of terms for this book. This list is compiled from the chapters and is a great resource for laying the foundation for learning how to make evidence-based decisions. The terms used to discuss a clinical topic matter, as does how a clinician considers options for how to guide patients through a healthcare decision.

How You Think Matters

As potential healthcare clinicians enter their basic preparation, it is interesting to ask why they made their choice. As health professions educators, we often hear many indicate that they were encouraged by their parents, mentor, or teacher to pursue their career in the health professions because they "would be so good at helping people." However, we know that nursing and other healthcare professions include far more than "helping people." Developing good thinking, as Dr. John Maxwell (2009) calls it, is an imperative. Good thinking requires embracing big picture thinking, which in this discussion means to embrace the research, clinical expertise, and patient preference/values in each decision. However, focused thinking is also required, in which the perspective gained by big-picture thinking is brought to fruition.

In our example of the 93-year old tap dancer, the complexity of thinking required to make this decision with her is revealed in the challenges that the inextricable links between ethical and clinical decision-making bring as well as the problematic implications of applying population-based research findings to individual patients. Both clinician and patient had to choose to see the big picture first and then use focused thinking to make the best decision to achieve the patient's desired outcome.

Within this framework, good clinical judgment requires that the clinician discerns what is good in a particular situation. This clinical wisdom does not come without purposeful reflection on; how you are considering your learning to become a healthcare professional or your approach to your profession. Facts from science are wonderful, if they are interwoven with clinical wisdom and sound judgment that leads to careful consideration of the influence of patient preferences on a decision.

As much as clinicians like certainty, uncertainty is part of healthcare decision making (Kamhi, 2011). Patients do not represent an average statistical life to a possible medical intervention…each patient is concerned with his or her particular chances and has only the particular life they have. Every clinical judgment has ethical aspects about what are the potential benefits and potential harms in the particular situation. The clinician must act in the patient's best interests and do as little harm and as much good as possible, demonstrating a relationship grounded in clinical stewardship and patient trust. In our example, the patient presented evidence that she experienced an exceptional health and fitness level, far different from projections based on the "average" 93-year-old person. For this woman the social aspects weighed in heavily in this decision, as they do in many other clinical decisions. The patient explained that tap dancing was her life, and she literally could not imagine a life without tap dancing. She also had robust confidence in her physical and emotional ability to withstand the surgery successfully. It is her life and her choice, and in the end, her outcomes proved that she was right. This is a great example of evidence-based decision making in which science is weighed and considered and indicates one path for treatment, but, in this case, the patient's values and preferences were what really drove the decision making toward a different intervention (i.e., the evidence was "trumped"). Furthermore, evidence-based decision making includes clinicians using their judgment in helping patients make decisions that are best for them. In this example, this clinical wisdom extended to subsequently finding a surgeon to bring the patient's decision to fruition. This example has helped many people who have heard this story to understand the idea that inclusion of patient information, preferences, values, and concerns is a must for evidence-based decision making.

CONCLUSIONS

Evidence-based decision making must be contextualized by the clinician in any particular clinical setting through actualizing particular patient–provider relationships, concerns, and goals. EBP can provide guidance and intelligent dialogue that brings best practice options to particular situations; however, clinicians need to intentionally seek out EBP knowledge for this to occur successfully. It cannot be assumed that all clinicians have current scientific knowledge or that knowledge flows only from science to practice. Knowledge also results from direct experiential learning in practice. Patient/family and healthcare values and concerns, practice-based knowledge, understanding change processes, and impact on patients and families all must be central to the dialogue between patient and clinician that incorporates the patients' values, concerns, and choices. In patient care, evidence-based decision making incorporates developing expertise and use of clinical judgment in conjunction with understanding patient preferences and applying valid external evidence to provide the best possible care.

References

Aikin, S. (2006). Modest evidentialism. *International Philosophical Quarterly, 46*(3), 327–343.

American Nurses Association. (2008). *Professional role competence*. Retrieved from http://nursingworld.org/MainMenuCategories/Policy-Advocacy/Positions-and-Resolutions/ANAPositionStatements/Position-Statements-Alphabetically/Professional-Role-Competence.html on August 17, 2013.

Barlow, D. H. (2004). Psychological treatments. *American Psychologist, 59*, 869–878.

Benner, P. (1984, 2001). *From novice to expert: Excellence and power in clinical nursing practice.* Menlo Park, CA: Addison-Wesley.

Berwick, D. (2009). What "patient-centered" should mean: Confessions of an extremist. *Health Affairs, 28*(4), w555–w565.

Conee, E., & Feldman, R. (2004). *Evidentialism: Essays in epistemology.* Oxford: Clarendon Press.

Dictionary.com. (2013). *Evidence*. Retrieved August 17, 2013 from http://dictionary.reference.com/browse/evidence?s=t

Dreyfus, H. L., & Dreyfus, S. E. (1986). *Mind over machine: The power of human intuition and expertise in the era of the computer.* New York: Free Press.

Gadamer, H. G. (1976). *Truth and method.* (G. Barden & J. Cummings, Eds. and Trans.). New York: Seabury.

Gibbs, L. E. (2003). *Evidence-based practice for the helping professions.* Pacific Grove, CA: Brooks/Cole.

Gill, P. S. (2013a). Improving health outcomes: Applying dimensions of employee engagement to patients. *The International Journal of Health, Wellness and Society, 3*(1), 1–9.

Gill, P. S. (2013b). Patient engagement: An investigation at a primary care clinic. *International Journal of General Medicine, 6*, 85–98. doi:10.2147/IJGM.S42226. http://dx.doi.org/10.2147%2FIJGM.S42226.

Hesselink, G., Flink, M., Olosson, M., Barach, P., Dudzik-Urbaniak, E., Orrego, C., … Wollersheim, H. (2012). Are patients discharged with care? A qualitative study of perceptions and experiences of patients, family members and care providers. *BMJ Quality and Safety, 21*, i39–i49.

Hibbard, J. (2007). Consumer competencies and the use of comparative quality information: It isn't just about literacy. *Medical Care Research and Review, 64*(4), 379–394.

Institute for Healthcare Improvement (IHI). (2013). *Across the chasm aim #3: Health care must be patient-centered*. Retrieved from http://www.ihi.org/knowledge/Pages/ImprovementStories/AcrosstheChasmAim3HealthCareMustBePatientCentered.aspx on September 5, 2013.

Institute of Medicine (IOM). (1999). *Crossing the quality chasm: A new health system for the 21st century*. Retrieved from http://iom.edu/Reports/2001/Crossing-the-Quality-Chasm-A-New-Health-System-for-the-21st-Century.aspx on November 26, 2012.

International Alliance of Patients' Organizations (IAPO). (2006). *Declaration on patient-centred healthcare*. Retrieved from http://www.patientsorganizations.org/showarticle.pl?id=712&n=312 on August, 17, 2013.

Jasper, M. A. (1994). Expert: A discussion of the implications of the concept as used in nursing. *Journal of Advanced Nursing, 20*(4), 769–776.

Kamhi, A. (2011). Balancing certainty and uncertainty in clinical practice. *Language, Speech and Hearing Services, 42,* 88–93.

Kinchin, I. M., Cabot, L. B., & Hay, D. B. (2008). Using concept mapping to locate the tacit dimension of clinical expertise: Towards a theoretical framework to support critical reflection on teaching. *Learning in Health and Social Care, 7*(2), 93–104.

Korsch, B. M. (1999). Current issues in communication research. *Health Communication, 1*(1), 5–9.

Lambert, M. J., & Barley, D. E. (2001). Research summary on the therapeutic relationship and psychotherapy outcome. *Psychotherapy, 38,* 357–361.

Maxwell, J. (2009). *How successful people think.* New York: Center Street Press.

McCracken, S. G., & Corrigan, P. W. (2004). Staff development in mental health. In H. E. Briggs & T. L. Rzepnicki (Eds.), *Using evidence in social work practice: Behavioral perspectives* (pp. 232–256). Chicago: Lyceum.

Légaré, F., Stacey, D., Brière, N., Fraser, K., Desroches, S., Dumont, S., … Aubé, D. (2013). Healthcare providers' intentions to engage in an interprofessional approach to shared decision-making in home care programs: A mixed methods study. *Journal of Interprofessional Care, 27,* 214–222.

Légaré, F., Stacey, D., Gagnon, S., Dunn, S., Pluye, P., Frosh, D., … Graham, I. D. (2011). Validating a conceptual model for an inter-professional approach to shared decision making: A mixed methods study. *Journal of Evaluation in Clinical Practice, 17,* 554–564.

Patient Centered Outcomes Research Institute (PCORI). (2013). *Patient-centered outcomes research.* Retrieved from http://pcori.org/research-we-support/pcor/ on September 8, 2013.

Roter, D. L., & Hall, J. A. (2006). *Doctors talking with patients/patients talking with doctors: Improving communication in medical visits.* Westport, CT: Prager.

Siegel, M. (2002). When doctors say don't and the patient says do. *New York Times, (Science),* Oct. 29, p. D7.

Ware, J. E., Jr., Snyder, M. K., Wright, W. R., & Davies, A. R. (1983). Defining and measuring patient satisfaction with medical care. *Evaluation and Program Planning, 6*(3–4), 247–263.

Chapter 8

Advancing Optimal Care With Rigorously Developed Clinical Practice Guidelines and Evidence-Based Recommendations

Doris Grinspun, Bernadette Mazurek Melnyk, and Ellen Fineout-Overholt

> **Whatever you can do or dream you can, begin it. Boldness has genius, power, and magic in it.**
>
> —Johann Wolfgang von Goethe

Clinical practice variations are problematic and a well-recognized phenomenon (Melnyk, Grossman, & Chou, 2012). More than 30 years have passed since Wennberg and Gittelsohn (1973, 1982) first described the variation in treatment patterns in New England and other parts of the United States. Since then, researchers have continued to document large variations in service use and healthcare spending across geographic regions (Institute of Medicine, 2013). These remarkable practice differences in the diagnosis, treatment, and management of patients continue to permeate health care everywhere.

The Dartmouth Atlas of Health Care (Wennberg, McAndrew, & the Dartmouth Medical School Center for Evaluative Clinical Sciences Staff, 1999) has long offered many queries that can assist in graphically demonstrating the variability of healthcare services in the United States. Features allow comparisons of states and resource utilization (Table 8.1). In Canada, similar reports are available through the Institute for Clinical Evaluative Sciences (http://www.ices.on.ca). These regional variations in care and resource utilization are reflections of the many factors that influence outcomes of healthcare delivery.

One critical factor that may hold the key to reducing variation in outcomes is the availability, uptake, and consistent utilization of clinical evidence at the point of care in the form of **clinical practice guidelines** and rigorously developed evidence-based recommendations by groups such as the U.S. Preventive Services Task Force (USPSTF) and the Community Task Force. Clinical practice guidelines are statements that include recommendations for practice based on a systematic review of evidence along with the benefits and harms of interventions intended to optimize patient care and outcomes.

Practicing based on evidence includes the integration of individual clinical expertise, including **internal evidence** (i.e., practice-generated data; see Chapter 4), and patient preferences and values with the best available evidence from systematic research (Melnyk & Fineout-Overholt, 2011; Sackett, Richardson, Rosenberg, & Haynes, 1997). Evidence-based practice (EBP) requires clinicians to determine the clinical options that are supported by high-quality scientific evidence and corroborated with the internal evidence. Gaining access to up-to-date scientific clinical information can be very challenging, particularly where access to healthcare journals is limited. Synthesizing the information can be even more challenging. The U.S. National Library of Medicine (NLM) indicated that, in 2008, PubMed contained more than 18 million citations to articles from more than 5,200 journals published worldwide, making it impossible for the individual clinician to master the body of emerging evidence (NLM, 2008). The reality of information overload is especially difficult for busy point-of-care providers who find themselves already overwhelmed by competing clinical priorities.

During a landmark workshop on clinical practice guidelines organized by the American Thoracic Society and the European Respiratory Society that drew experts from more than 40 international

Table 8.1   **Example of Data That Can Be Accessed From *Dartmouth Health Atlas***

State Name	State No.	No. of Deaths*	RNs Required Under Proposed Federal Standards per 1,000 Decedents During the Last 2 Years of Life (2001–2005)
Arizona	3	15,568	38.73
Nevada	29	6,020	48.18
New Mexico	32	6,344	35.82

*No. of deaths are from 20% sample.

Source: http://www.dartmouthatlas.org/index.shtm

organizations, a vision statement was created that highlighted 10 key visions for guideline development and use (Schunemann et al., 2009). These included:

1. Globalize the evidence (i.e., make the evidence applicable on a worldwide basis)
2. Focus on questions that are important to patients and clinicians and include relevant stakeholders in guideline panels
3. Undertake collaborative evidence reviews relevant to healthcare questions and recommendations
4. Use a common metric to assess the quality of evidence and strength of recommendations
5. Consider comorbidities in guideline development
6. Identify ways that help guideline consumers (clinicians, patients, and others) understand and implement guidelines using the best available tools
7. Deal with conflicts of interest and guideline sponsoring transparently
8. Support development of decision aids to assist implementation of value- and preference-sensitive guideline recommendations
9. Maintain a collaboration of international organizations
10. Examine collaborative models for funding guideline development and implementation

GUIDELINES AS TOOLS

Overwhelming evidence, competing clinical priorities, and ever-increasing accountability highlight the importance of synthesis studies and clinical practice guidelines. **Meta-analyses** (the highest form of systematic review) and **integrative reviews** (a narrative evidence review that synthesizes research on a given topic) facilitate practitioners' ability to base their interventions on the strongest, most up-to-date, and relevant evidence, rather than engaging with the challenging task of individually appraising and synthesizing large volumes of scientific studies. Evidence-based practice guidelines (EBPGs), which are systematically developed statements based on the best available evidence, including syntheses, make recommendations in order to assist practitioners with decisions regarding the most effective interventions for specific clinical conditions across a broad array of clinical diagnoses and situations (Tricoci, Allen, Kramer, Califf, & Smith, 2009). They are also designed to allow some flexibility in their application to individual patients who fall outside the scope of the guideline or who have significant comorbidities not adequately addressed in a particular guideline. These tools are increasingly being used to reduce unnecessary variations in clinical practice.

Rigorously and explicitly developed EBPGs can help bridge the gap between published scientific evidence and clinical decision making (Davies, Edwards, Ploeg, & Virani, 2008; Grinspun, Virani, &

Bajnok, 2002; Miller & Kearney, 2004). As expected, the dramatic growth in guideline development is not without unintended consequences. The rigor of guidelines varies significantly as does the reporting on how a particular guideline is formulated. In a recent review of 53 guidelines on 22 topics by the American College of Cardiology (ACC) and the American Heart Association (AHA), Tricoci et al. (2009) found that the recommendations issued in these guidelines were largely developed from lower levels of evidence (e.g., nonrandomized trials, case studies) or expert opinion. As another example, Belamarich and colleagues found that none of the 162 verbal health advice directives from 57 policy statements by the American Academy of Pediatrics, on which pediatric healthcare providers should council patients and parents, included evidence to support the efficacy of the advice (empirical data to support that the advice produces positive outcomes). The findings from the Tricoci and Belamarich reviews indicate that the process of developing guidelines and recommendations needs to improve, and the research base from which guidelines are derived needs to be expanded. These inconsistencies in guideline development are also the reason that clinicians need to have excellent knowledge and skills in how to critically appraise clinical practice guidelines and recommendation statements.

At times, one can find guidelines with conflicting recommendations, posing dilemmas for users and potentially hindering, rather than advancing, quality patient care. For example, many professional organizations recommend routine lipid screening in children with cardiovascular risk factors when there is insufficient and less than high-quality evidence to support this recommendation (Daniels & Greer, 2008; Grossman, Moyer, Melnyk, Chou, & DeWitt, 2011). Guidelines are also often developed and written in ways that clinicians and organizations may find difficult to implement, which limits their effectiveness in influencing clinical practice and improving patient outcomes. Despite these limitations or "growing pains," the increased emphasis over the past decade on evidence-based guideline development, implementation, and evaluation is a welcome direction toward evidence-based decision making at the point of care. This chapter offers clinicians a brief overview of EBPGs and ways to access, appraise, and use these tools to improve the care and health outcomes of their patients.

HOW TO ACCESS GUIDELINES

In the past, finding EBPGs was a formidable challenge. The large number of guideline developers and topics, coupled with the various forms of guideline publication and distribution, made identification of guidelines difficult and unpredictable. Fortunately today, a two-step Google search brings forward the most commonly used EBPG sites. Use the term *practice guideline* and you will immediately access the Centre for Health Evidence (http://www.cche.net), the National Guideline Clearinghouse (NGC; http://www.guideline.gov/), the Canadian Medical Association (CMA; http://www.cma.ca), the Registered Nurses' Association of Ontario (RNAO; http://www.rnao.org), the United States Preventive Services Task Force (USPSTF) (http://www.ahrq.gov/professionals/clinicians-providers/guidelines -recommendations/uspstf/index.html) and other such reliable sources of EBPG. In addition, to make finding EBPGs easier, the term *practice guideline* can be used as a limit to define a publication type when searching NLM's PubMed database.

Access the PubMed database at **http://www.ncbi.nlm.nih.gov/pubmed**

Using the search term *practice guideline* alone, without any qualifiers, yields almost 100,000 citations. Most of these citations are not actual guidelines but studies of guideline implementation, commentaries, editorials, or letters to the editor about guidelines. Thus, once a specific site (e.g., PubMed, NGC, RNAO, USPSTF) is accessed, it is important to refine the search by adding the clinical areas or interventions of interest. Searching citation databases for EBPGs can present challenges as not all guidelines are published in indexed journals or books, making it difficult to locate them in traditional healthcare databases.

In the last decade, individual collections that distribute international, regional, organizational, or specialty-specific guidelines have matured (Box 8.1). The list of individual guideline developers is long, and the distribution venues for guidelines can be as plentiful as the number of developers.

> **Box 8.1**   Selected Guideline Databases
>
> **General**
>
> - NGC: http://www.guideline.gov
> - The USPSTF: http://www.uspreventiveservicestaskforce.org/
> - The Community Guide: http://www.thecommunityguide.org/index.html
> - Primary Care Clinical Practice Guidelines: http://medicine.ucsf.edu/education/resed/ ebm/practice_guidelines.html
> - RNAO: http://www.rnao.org
> - CMA Infobase: Clinical Practice Guidelines (CPGs): http://mdm.ca/cpgsnew/cpgs/ index.asp
> - HSTAT: http://hstat.nlm.nih.gov
> - Guidelines Advisory Committee (GAC): http://www.gacguidelines.ca
> - SIGN: http://www.sign.ac.uk/guidelines/index.html
> - NICE: http://www.nice.org.uk
> - NZGG: http://www.nzgg.org.nz
> - G-I-N: http://www.G-I-N.net
>
> **Specific**
>
> - American College of Physicians: http://www.acponline.org/clinical_information/ guidelines
> - American Cancer Society: http://www.cancer.org/docroot/home/index.asp
> - American College of Cardiology: http://www.acc.org/qualityandscience/clinical/ statements.htm
> - American Association of Clinical Endocrinologists: http://www.aace.com/pub/ guidelines/
> - American Association of Respiratory Care: http://www.aarc.org/resources/
> - American Academy of Pediatrics: http://aappolicy.aappublications.org/
> - American Psychiatric Association: http://www.psych.org/psych_pract/treatg/pg/ prac_guide.cfm
> - Ministry of Health Services, British Columbia, Canada: http://www.gov.bc.ca/health/
> - New York Academy of Medicine: http://www.ebmny.org/cpg.html
> - Veterans Administration: http://www1.va.gov/health/index.asp
> - National Kidney Foundation: https://www.kidney.org/professionals/doqi/ guidelineindex.cfm
> - American Medical Directors Association: http://www.amda.com
> - Association of Women's Health, Obstetric, and Neonatal Nurses: http://awhonn.org
> - National Association of Neonatal Nurses: http://www.nann.org
> - Oncology Nursing Society: http://www.ons.org
> - University of Iowa Gerontological Nursing Interventions Research Center: http://www .nursing.uiowa.edu/excellence/nursing_interventions/

In Canada, the RNAO disseminates its production of about 50 rigorously developed best practice guidelines (those supported by evidence from rigorous research) on its website (http://www.rnao .org). Forty of these guidelines are clinical and nine are healthy work environment ones, all are freely downloadable and widely used across Canada and internationally. In addition, the CMA maintains its InfoBase of clinical practice guidelines for physicians (http://mdm.ca/cpgsnew/cpgs/index.asp).

Guidelines are included in the CMA InfoBase only if they are produced or endorsed in Canada by a national, provincial/territorial, or regional medical or health organization, professional society, government agency, or expert panel.

In the United Kingdom, another country-specific guideline collection is the Scottish Intercollegiate Guidelines Network (SIGN) sponsored by the Royal College of Physicians (http://www.sign.ac.uk). Also, the National Institute for Health and Clinical Excellence (NICE) in England maintains a collection of guidelines to advise the National Health Service (http://www.nice.org.uk/). In New Zealand, the New Zealand Guidelines Group (NZGG) maintains a collection of guidelines developed under its sponsorship (http://www.nzgg.org.nz/).

In the United States, the USPSTF produces rigorously developed evidence-based recommendations about clinical preventive services, such as screenings, counseling services, or preventive medications that are released in an annual updated pocket guide for clinicians entitled Guide to Clinical Preventive Services (http://www.ahrq.gov/professionals/clinicians-providers/guidelines-recommendations/guide/index.html), which is an authoritative source for making decisions about preventive services. The USPSTF is comprised of 16 national experts in prevention and EBP who work to improve the health of all Americans through their evidence-based recommendations, which are based on a rigorous review of the literature and an analysis of benefits and harms of the recommended clinical practice. Similar to the Guide to Clinical Preventive Services, the Guide to Community Preventive Services is a free resource that is rigorously developed by a panel of national experts to help clinicians choose programs and policies to improve health and prevent disease in their communities (see http://www.thecommunityguide.org/index.html).

Several individual professional societies and national groups in the United States also maintain collections of guidelines specific to a particular practice, professional specialty, disease screening, prevention, or management. The ACC and the AHA have joint guideline panels and publish their guidelines in a variety of formats (http://www.acc.org/qualityandscience/clinical/statements.htm). The American Cancer Society (ACS) also convenes multidisciplinary panels to develop cancer-related guidelines and to make the guidelines available on the Internet (http://www.cancer.org/).

In addition, there is an international collaboration of researchers, guideline developers, and guideline implementers called the ADPATE Collaboration that promotes the development and use of clinical practice guidelines through adaptation of existing guidelines. This collaboration develops and validates a generic adaptation process that fosters valid and high-quality adapted guidelines (http://www.adapte.org/rubrique/the-adapte-collaboration.php).

Although it is useful to have collections of guidelines that are specific to a disease or specialty, this can make it difficult to find guidelines in more than one clinical area. In 1998, the U.S. Agency for Health Care Policy and Research, now the Agency for Healthcare Research and Quality (AHRQ), released the NGC.

    Access the NGC at http://www.guideline.gov

The NGC was developed in partnership with the American Medical Association and the American Association of Health Plans. In developing the NGC, AHRQ intended to create a comprehensive database of up-to-date English language EBPGs (Box 8.2). Today, NGC contains well over 10,000 clinical guidelines from developers all over the world. That number is exponentially higher than the 2,950 guidelines posted in 2008. The NGC also contains an archive of guideline titles that are out of date. The archived guidelines do not get circulated on the site. The database is updated at least weekly with new content and provides guideline comparison features so that users can explore differences among guidelines, facilitating critical appraisal. An important feature to the NGC is the guideline synthesis, which enables users to access comprehensive information with the best available evidence to support recommendations. Users can register to receive weekly emails listing the guideline changes on the site.

Of the various guideline collections and databases, the NGC contains the most descriptive information about guidelines. It is also the most selective about the guidelines that are included in its database. Inclusion criteria are applied to each guideline to determine whether or not they will be incorporated in

> **Box 8.2**
>
> # National Guideline Clearinghouse: http://www.guideline.gov
>
> ## Features
>
> ◆ Structured abstracts (summaries) about the guideline and its development
> ◆ Links to full-text guidelines, where available, and/or ordering information for print copies
> ◆ Palm-based PDA downloads of the Complete NGC Summary for all guidelines represented in the database
> ◆ Weekly email feature
> ◆ A guideline comparison utility that gives users the ability to generate side-by-side comparisons for any combination of two or more guidelines
> ◆ Unique guideline comparisons called Guideline Syntheses, comparing guidelines covering similar topics, highlighting areas of similarity and difference
> ◆ An electronic forum, NGC-L, for exchanging information on clinical practice guidelines, their development, implementation, and use
> ◆ Annotated bibliographies on guideline development, methodology, structure, evaluation, and implementation
> ◆ Expert commentary
> ◆ Guideline archive
>
> ## Inclusion Criteria
>
> ◆ The clinical practice guideline contains systematically developed statements that include recommendations, strategies, or information that assist healthcare practitioners and patients to make decisions about appropriate health care for specific clinical circumstances.
> ◆ The clinical practice guideline was produced under the auspices of medical specialty associations; relevant professional societies; public or private organizations; government agencies at the federal, state, or local levels; or healthcare organizations or plans.
> ◆ A systematic literature search and review of existing scientific evidence published in peer-reviewed journals was performed during the guideline development.
> ◆ The guideline was developed, reviewed, or revised within the last 5 years.

the database. Furthermore, guidelines in the NGC database reflect the most current version. In nursing, almost all of RNAO clinical guidelines are posted on the NGC.

Another website that is very helpful is NLM Gateway. The Gateway allows users to enter a search term that is then sent out to eight different NLM databases. One of these, Health Services/Health Technology Assessment Text (HSTAT), is especially practical. HSTAT is unique because it takes large guidelines, systematic reviews, and technology assessments and enables their texts to be searchable on the Internet, making them much easier to navigate electronically.

   Access the NLM Gateway at http://gateway.nlm.nih.gov/gw/Cmd

There is no shortage of guideline-related sites on the Internet. The challenge is finding the source of guidelines that is easiest to use and provides the best mechanisms for making sure the contents are up to date. Because so many guideline resources are now on the Internet, it is wise to consider the quality of the website when choosing a source. Extremely useful databases of evidence-based guidelines exist. Many of these resources provide users with the guidelines, and some also provide additional information on how guidelines are developed and used. Evaluation of guideline databases is necessary to ensure that the information is reliable and current.

FINDING THE RIGHT GUIDELINE

Locating and reviewing current guidelines on a particular subject are often overwhelming. Even after a guideline has been identified, it can be difficult to determine critical information of the guideline, such as who developed and funded it, who was on the panel, how the guideline was developed, and what dates the literature review covered. Guidelines should provide this background and be explicit in their discussion of the evidence supporting their recommendations as well as in identifying the benefits and harms of interventions (Barratt et al., 1999; Burgers, Grol, & Eccles, 2005; DiCenso, Ciliska, Dobbins, & Guyatt, 2005). Guidelines developed using evidence of established benefit and harms of treatments or interventions have the potential to improve healthcare and health outcomes as well as decrease morbidity and mortality (Grimshaw, Thomas, & MacLennan, 2004; Melnyk, Grossman, & Chou, 2012). However, guidelines of low quality may cause harm to patients and should be carefully appraised for validity and reliability of their information and supporting evidence (Shekelle, Kravitz, & Beart, 2000).

Users of guidelines need to keep in mind that "one size *does not* fit all." Haynes describes the "three Rs" of clinical practice guideline application as their application to the *right person* at the *right time* and in the *right way* (Haynes, 1993). Davis and Taylor-Vaisey (1997) suggest that the effect of clinical guidelines on improved healthcare outcomes is dependent on taking into account their nature, the nature and beliefs of the target clinicians, and environmental factors when trying to implement them. In a landmark work, Hayward, Wilson, Tunis, Bass, and Guyatt (1995) from the Evidence-Based Medicine Working Group identified three main questions to consider when using EBPGs: (a) What are the guideline recommendations? (b) Are the guideline recommendations valid? and (c) How useful are the recommendations? Lastly, in a recent article Straus and Haynes (2009) remind us that evidence alone is never sufficient to make clinical decisions. One must weigh the evidence in context, always accounting for the values and preferences of patients, with the goal to achieve optimal shared decision making. These authors add that key to supporting clinicians is ensuring that information resources are reliable, relevant, and readable.

How to Read and Critically Appraise Recommendations

The strength of a guideline is based on the validity and reliability of its recommendations. In addition, guideline usefulness is highly dependent on the meaningfulness and practicality of the recommendations. Practicality relates to the ease with which a recommendation can be implemented. The recommendations should be as unambiguous as possible. They should address how often screening and other interventions should occur to achieve optimal outcomes. In addition, the recommendations should be explicit about areas where informing the patient of choices can lead to varying decisions. Furthermore, recommendations should address clinically relevant actions. The developers' assessment of the benefits against the harms of implementing the recommendation should be part of the supporting documentation for the recommendation.

It is important to know whether the developers focused on outcomes that are meaningful to patients and whether they were inclusive in considering all reasonable treatment options for a given condition or disease. The user should consider whether the developers assigned different values to the outcomes they evaluated, taking patient preferences into consideration. Developers need to fully describe the process used to systematically search and review the evidence on which the guideline recommendations are based. When combining the evidence, it is important to note whether the developer used a rating scheme or similar method to determine the quality and strength of the studies included, both primary studies and syntheses. Developers often use letter grades or words such as *strongly recommend* to rate their assessment of the strength of the evidence for a given recommendation. In 2002, the Research Training Institute at the University of North Carolina at Chapel Hill (RTI-UNC) Evidence-Based Practice Center completed a **systematic review** of schemes used to rate the quality of a body of evidence. While there is no universal consensus on grading evidence or determining the strength of a body of evidence supporting a recommendation, there are well-established norms. The most notable process for grading recommendations is the one used by the USPSTF (Harris et al., 2001; USPSTF, 2008; Box 8.3).

As another example of grading recommendations in clinical practice guidelines, the ACC and the AHA use a system based on level of evidence and class or recommendation (see http://www.acc.org and http://www.aha.org). The **level of evidence** integrates an objective description of the existence and type of studies supporting the recommendation and expert consensus according to one of three categories, including:

(a) Level of evidence A (i.e., the recommendation is based on evidence from multiple **randomized controlled trials** or **meta-analyses**),

(b) Level of evidence B (i.e., the recommendation is based on evidence from a single randomized trial or nonrandomized studies), and

(c) Level of evidence C (i.e., the recommendation is based on expert opinion, case studies, or standards of care).

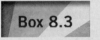

Box 8.3   The USPSTF System for Evaluating Evidence to Support Recommendations

A—The USPSTF recommends the service. There is high certainty that the net benefit is substantial. Offer or provide this service.

B—The USPSTF recommends the service. There is high certainty that the net benefit is moderate or there is moderate certainty that the net benefit is moderate to substantial. Offer or provide the service.

C—The USPSTF recommends against routinely providing the service. There may be considerations that support providing the service in an individual patient. There is at least moderate certainty that the net benefit is small. Offer or provide this service only if other considerations support the offering or providing the service in an individual patient.

D—The USPSTF recommends against the service. There is moderate or high certainty that the service has no net benefit or that the harms outweigh the benefits. Discourage the use of this service.

I—The USPSTF concludes that the current evidence is insufficient to assess the balance of benefits and harms of the service. Evidence is lacking, of poor quality, or conflicting, and the balance of benefits and harms cannot be determined. Read the clinical considerations section of the USPSTF Recommendation Statement. If the service is offered, patients should understand the uncertainty about the balance of benefits and harms.

Source: http://www.ahrq.gov/CLINIC/uspstfix.htm

The class of recommendation indicates the strengths and weaknesses of the evidence as well as the relative importance of the risks and benefits identified by the evidence. The following are definitions of classes used by the ACC and AHA:

◆ Class I: conditions for which there is evidence and/or general agreement that a given procedure or treatment is useful and effective,

◆ Class II: conditions for which there is conflicting evidence and/or a divergence of opinion about the usefulness/efficacy of a procedure or treatment,

◆ Class IIa: weight of evidence/opinion is in favor of usefulness/efficacy,

◆ Class IIb: usefulness/efficacy is less well established by evidence/opinion, and

◆ Class III: conditions for which there is evidence or general agreement that the procedure/treatment is not useful/effective and in some cases may be harmful (Tricoci et al., 2009).

Because guidelines reflect snapshots of the evidence at a given point in time, they require consistent updating to incorporate new evidence. Thus, it is critical that developers commit to a cyclical systematic review of their guidelines. In addition, developers can alert guideline users to ongoing research studies that may have an impact on the recommendations in the future. It is advisable that guidelines undergo peer review and pilot testing in actual practice before being released. Stakeholders' review allows a reality check to identify last-minute inconsistencies or relevant evidence that might have been overlooked. Pilot testing allows organizational or functional problems with implementing the guideline to be identified, including the cost of implementing the guideline. These can then be corrected or accommodated to enhance the chances of the guideline being implemented.

Will the Recommendations Help Patient Care?

Applying a guideline on management of heart failure in the ambulatory setting is not the same as using a guideline on management of heart failure in the hospital. Similarly, a guideline on management of heart failure in children is not comparable with a guideline on management of heart failure in adults. The guideline should (a) fit the setting of care and the age and gender of the patients, (b) be usable by the type of clinicians providing the care, and (c) take into consideration the presence of any comorbidities. Ultimately, both the guideline user and developer must keep in mind the role evidence plays in developing recommendations. For example, most experimental studies do not take into account the characteristics of individual patients, including comorbidities and clinical settings (Burgers et al., 2005). Although EBPGs do not always take into account multiple conditions and patients generally do not present with only one disease or condition, guidelines can help point clinicians in the right direction when looking for the right care for their patients. Practitioners have the responsibility to individualize guideline implementation for their particular patients' circumstances.

Tools for Critically Appraising Guidelines

Finding the right guideline to use is contingent on being able to critically appraise the validity and reliability of a guideline. There is ample evidence that guideline developers do not always adhere to best practices in guideline development. Two studies of guidelines developed by medical specialty societies found that a significant percentage did not adhere to accepted methodological practices in their development (Grilli, Magrini, Penna, Mura, & Liberati, 2000; Shaneyfelt, Mayo-Smith, & Rothwangl, 1999). In a landmark work, the Institute of Medicine (IOM) identified eight attributes of good guideline development, including:

1. Validity
2. Reliability and reproducibility
3. Clinical applicability
4. Clinical flexibility
5. Clarity
6. Documentation

7. Development by a multidisciplinary process
8. Plans for review (Field & Lohr, 1990, 1992)

Guidelines are complex and heterogeneous documents with many different components; therefore, evaluating them is often difficult. However, with a good guide, critical appraisal of guidelines can be accomplished (see Appendix B for rapid critical appraisal [RCA] checklists for clinical practice guidelines).

Provisional Instrument for Assessing Guidelines

Lohr and Field (1992) developed a provisional instrument for assessing clinical practice guidelines (provisional because it was in the early stages of development and the committee tested it on different kinds of guidelines). They developed the instrument because they recognized that there was a need for an explicit mechanism to appraise the validity of individual clinical practice guidelines. The instrument was a first step in trying to identify a way to appraise critical attributes of guidelines. Nonetheless, it was long and difficult to complete. It was not intended to be used by practicing clinicians but by groups or organizations wanting to adopt a guideline. The instrument was also appropriate for self-assessment by guideline developers.

Rapid Critical Appraisal Checklist

RCA of a guideline can be accomplished by applying standardized criteria when evaluating the attributes of the guideline (Box 8.4). The answer to each question in the RCA checklist supplies the end user with information that, when weighed all together, enables the clinician to decide whether the given guideline is the best match for his or her setting, patient, and desired outcomes.

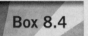

Box 8.4

Rapid Critical Appraisal Questions to Ask of Evidence-Based Guidelines

- Who were the guideline developers?
- Were the developers representative of key stakeholders in this specialty (interdisciplinary)?
- Who funded the guideline development?
- Were any of the guideline developers funded researchers of the reviewed studies?
- Did the team have a valid development strategy?
- Was an explicit (how decisions were made), sensible, and impartial process used to identify, select, and combine evidence?
- Did its developers carry out a comprehensive, reproducible literature review within the past 12 months of its publication/revision?
- Were all important options and outcomes considered?
- Is each recommendation in the guideline tagged by the level/strength of evidence upon which it is based and linked with the scientific evidence?
- Do the guidelines make explicit recommendations (reflecting value judgments about outcomes)?
- Has the guideline been subjected to peer review and testing?
- Is the intent of use provided (e.g., national, regional, local)?
- Are the recommendations clinically relevant?
- Will the recommendations help me in caring for my patients?
- Are the recommendations practical/feasible? Are resources (people and equipment) available?
- Are the recommendations a major variation from current practice? Can the outcomes be measured through standard care?

Agree Instrument for Assessing Guidelines

In 1992, the U.K. National Health Services Management Executive set in motion the development of an appraisal instrument for the National Health Services (Cluzeau, Littlejohns, Grimshaw, Feder, & Moran, 1999). This was the first attempt to formally evaluate the usefulness of a guideline appraisal instrument. Subsequently, the European Union provided funding for the development of the Appraisal of Guidelines for Research and Evaluation (AGREE) instrument.

 The AGREE instrument can be found at http://www.agreetrust.org

The AGREE instrument (Refer to Box 8.5 on page 200) was developed and evaluated by an international group of guideline developers and researchers. Since its original release in 2003, the AGREE instrument has been translated into many languages and has gained significant acceptance as the standard guideline appraisal tool. It is important to note that some studies raised serious questions regarding the interrater reliability of the AGREE instrument and suggested that the tool could benefit from further detailed appraisal (Wimpenny & van Zelm, 2007). The tool was further refined, and the AGREE II version was released in 2010.

The instrument contains 6 quality domains (areas or spheres of information) and 23 items. The domain scores remain the same as originally and are not meant to be aggregated into one overall score for the guideline. Thus, using the instrument to evaluate the robustness (strength) of clinical practice guidelines will produce individual domain scores and not an overall rating for a guideline. The revised instrument uses a 7-point Likert scale (up from the 4-point Likert scale) from 1 being "strongly disagree" to 7 being "strongly agree" depending on completeness and quality of reporting. The instrument allows the appraiser to give a subjective assessment of the guideline based on review of the individual domain scores. The AGREE instrument recommends there be more than one appraiser for each guideline—preferably four—to increase confidence in the reliability of the instrument.

Alternative appraisal instruments are being developed that address more than the guidelines along other sources of evidence. A promising example is the GRADE (Grades of Recommendations, Assessment, Development and Evaluation) instrument (Atkins et al., 2004).

National Guideline Clearinghouse and Others

The NGC produces structured summaries of each guideline in its database to aid the user in assessing the quality and appropriateness of a guideline. The summaries describe guideline attributes similar to those contained in the Lohr and Field (1992) provisional instrument, the RCA checklist, and the AGREE instrument. In addition, the Conference on Guideline Standardization (COGS) Statement recommends standardizing the development and reporting of a guideline; hence, developers can ensure the quality of their guidelines and make their implementation easier (Shiffman et al., 2003).

 More can be learned about the COGS appraisal guides at http://gem.med.yale.edu/cogs/welcome.do

HOW GUIDELINES ARE DEVELOPED

Determining when to develop guidelines should be systematically approached due to the amount of resources, skill, and time needed to accomplish these activities. In 1995, the IOM issued guidance on setting priorities for clinical practice guidelines (Field, 1995). The report emphasized the importance of considering whether the guideline had the potential to change health outcomes or costs and the availability of scientific evidence on which to develop the recommendations (Field, 1995). Other criteria used by organizations include the following:

- The topic is clinically important, affecting large numbers of people with substantial morbidity or mortality (the burden of illness).
- The topic is complex and requires clinical practice clarity.
- There is evidence of substantive variation between actual and optimal care.

◆ There are no existing valid or relevant guidelines available to use.
◆ There is evidence available to support evidence-based guideline development.
◆ The topic is central to healthy public policy and serves to introduce innovation.

When it is determined that there is uncertainty about how to treat or when gaps between optimal practice and actual practice have been identified, an organization may decide to develop a clinical practice guideline. Because it is difficult and expensive to develop guidelines, many organizations would be better served by adopting or adapting existing guidelines that have already been developed. Critically appraising already developed guidelines will allow an organization to screen for the best developed and suited guidelines for their organization.

Processes and Panels

When the decision is made that a guideline will be developed, several important steps must take place. Guidelines can be developed at a central level with a good scientific basis and broad validity, or they can follow a local approach in the form of care protocols agreed upon by a department or institution. The emphasis of the latter is on practical feasibility and support of care processes (Burgers et al., 2005). These local guidelines can be developed using informal consensus, formal consensus, evidence-based methodologies, and explicit methodologies, either alone or in any combination. However, it is highly recommended that development focus on more formal and explicit processes so that another developer using similar techniques would likely come to the same conclusions.

Next, the guideline panel must be identified. The process for development of the panel should include multidisciplinary major stakeholders for the guideline, including users and patients (Field & Lohr, 1990; Shekelle, Woolf, Eccles, & Grimshaw, 1999; Scottish Intercollegiate Guideline Network [SIGN], 2008). Guideline panels should be composed of members who can adequately address the relevant interventions and meaningful outcomes and can weigh benefits and harms. To increase the feasibility of implementation, it is advisable that panels be composed of subject experts who bring the different perspectives of research, clinical practice, administration, education, and policy (Grinspun et al., 2002; McQueen, Montgomery, Lappan-Gracon, Evans, & Hunter, 2008). Variations in the composition of the guideline development panel, the developing organization, and the interpretation of the evidence are often the source of differing recommendations on the same clinical topic across guidelines (Berg, Atkins, & Tierney, 1997; Burgers et al., 2005; DiCenso & Guyatt, 2005; Lohr, 1995).

Review Questions

The next step in guideline development is the formal assessment of the clinical questions to be reviewed. This can be aided by the development of an analytic framework or causal pathway (Harris et al., 2001). These diagrams provide a roadmap for the precise description of the target population, setting of care, interventions, and intermediate as well as final health outcomes. They also help focus the most meaningful questions that will guide the literature review and subsequent recommendations. Figure 8.1 shows an analytic framework for prevention screening used by the USPSTF (Harris et al., 2001).

The numbers in the diagram relate to the key questions that will be considered. For example, (1) relates to whether the screening test actually reduces morbidity and/or mortality; and (5) asks the important question of whether treatment of clinically diagnosed patients results in reduced morbidity and/or mortality.

Literature Search and Review

After the key questions have been identified, a formal search and review of the literature take place. It is easiest if a systematic review has already been identified by searching databases such as the Cochrane Library, MEDLINE, CINAHL, and EMBASE. If an already completed systematic review is not found, it is necessary to develop one. The first step is to determine what types of evidence will be considered, including study design, dates of publication, and language. A search strategy of relevant citation databases

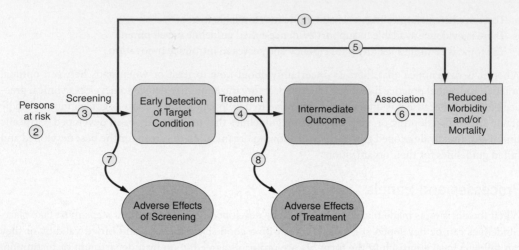

Figure 8.1: Example of an analytic framework with key questions for prevention screening evidence-based recommendations used by the United States Preventive Services Task Force. (From Harris, R. P., Helfand, M., Woolf, S. H., Lohr, K. N., Mulrow, C. D., Teutsch, S. M., ... Methods Work Group, Third US Preventive Services Task Force. [2001]. Current methods of the U.S. Preventive Services Task Force: A review of the process. *American Journal of Preventive Medicine, 20*[3 Suppl], 21–35.)

should be developed, preferably with the assistance of a medical librarian familiar with electronic searches. Once the search is completed, a process for screening titles and abstracts for relevance is conducted. The remaining titles are retrieved for evaluation. These articles are then screened, and data are extracted from the studies. The individual articles are reviewed for internal and external biases, and their quality is often rated based on standardized criteria. Once data are extracted from the individual studies, the results are summarized, sometimes using meta-analysis to combine results from similar studies.

Evidence-Based Recommendations

The formal search, review, and appraisal of the literature lead to developing recommendations based on the strength of the evidence for each of the questions that were identified in the analytic framework. Some guideline panels choose to make recommendations based solely on evidence, whereas others will use expert opinion when the evidence is poor or lacking. When expert opinion is used, it should be identified as such and be gathered using formal, explicit methods (Grinspun et al., 2002).

Peer Review and Dissemination

After the guideline recommendations are formulated, the guideline should be subjected to peer review to uncover any omissions or misinterpretations. In some cases, pilot testing will uncover that it is not feasible to implement a certain guideline or will offer tips to facilitate contextual modifications that ease adoption. Following the peer review and pilot testing, if necessary, the guideline is revised. Then, it is published and broadly disseminated.

IMPLEMENTING EVIDENCE-BASED GUIDELINES

It is important to understand that evidence and the quality of a guideline are vital, but two of many factors influencing guidelines' utilization. Implementing evidence-based guidelines into daily clinical practice requires a multifaceted and sustained approach with individual and systemic interventions.

Indeed, despite the increasing availability of high-quality guidelines, their utilization remains low (Melnyk, Grossman, & Chou, 2012). Thus, the process for implementation is as important as that for selecting a robust guideline, and it must be purposeful and well thought out.

Assessing organizational readiness for best practice guidelines implementation is a critical step, and it must include all levels of administrative leadership and clinical practice staff. Studies report successful results and improvements in clinical practice and patients' outcomes following well-thought-out multilevel and multibundled interventions (Devlin, Czaus, & Santos, 2002; O'Connor, Creager, Mooney, Laizner, & Ritchie, 2006; Ploeg et al., 2010). Critical elements that assist in uptake and translation of evidence into day-to-day practice include (a) facilitating staff to utilize best practice guidelines; (b) creating a positive milieu and securing structures and processes that inspire EBP (Gifford, Davies, Edwards, & Graham, 2006); (c) interactive education with skills building practice sessions and attention to patient education (Davies et al., 2008; Straus et al., 2011); (d) use of reminders (Cheung et al., 2012); (e) electronic gathering and dissemination systems offering real-time feedback and access to guidelines (Davies et al., 2008; Doran et al., 2009); (f) changing organizational policies and procedures to reflect best clinical practices and making staff aware of these changes (St-Pierre, Davies, Edwards, & Griffin, 2007); and (g) organizational and unit-based champions, EBP mentors, teamwork and collaboration, professional association's support, interorganizational collaboration, networks, and administrative leadership (Melnyk & Fineout-Overholt, 2011; Ploeg, Davies, Edwards, Gifford, & Miller, 2007). Gifford, Davies, Edwards, Griffin, and Lybanon (2007) and Sandström, Borglin, Nilsson, and Willman (2011) discuss in detail the pivotal role that managerial leadership plays in securing uptake of research evidence by point-of-care clinical staff.

Several strategies are available to facilitate knowledge transfer (Thompson, Estabrooks, & Degner, 2006). An effective example is the use of best practice champions (Ploeg et al., 2010; Santos, 2008). Best practice champions are nurses who promote, support, and influence the utilization of nursing best practice guidelines (RNAO, 2008). In addition, EBP mentors as first proposed in the Advancing Research and Clinical practice through close Collaboration (ARCC) Model (Melnyk & Fineout-Overholt, 2002) are also a promising strategy for implementation and sustainability of evidence-based guidelines and care (Melnyk, 2007). EBP mentors, typically advanced practice nurses who have in-depth knowledge and skills in EBP as well as individual and organizational change strategies, work with direct care staff in promoting evidence-based care.

A review of guidelines conducted by Gagliardi, Brouwers, Palda, Lemieux-Charles, and Grimshaw (2011) shows that guideline producers do not for the most include implementability content. Excellent toolkits exist however that can facilitate the implementation process (DiCenso et al., 2002; Dobbins, Davies, Danseco, Edwards, & Virani, 2005; RNAO, 2012). Implementation in nursing education is also of critical importance in preparing future nurses to "think evidence." Workshops with clinical instructors have been shown to be an effective way to assist faculty in initiating integration of practice guidelines in undergraduate nursing education (Higuchi, Cragg, Diem, Molnar, & O'Donohue, 2006). Quality measurement and feedback mechanisms can help determine whether the guideline is actually being used in practice. Lastly, to implement guidelines at the system level is a major undertaking that requires a whole systems thinking approach. Edwards and Grinspun (2011) explain that to produce whole systems change requires the engagement of institutional, political, and educational stakeholders at the micro, meso, and macro levels of the system. In Canada, such a whole system change approach for cross-country clinical practice guidelines implementation is being spearheaded since 2011 by the Council of the Federation (2012).

Once best practice guidelines are successfully implemented, it is vital to ensure that utilization is sustained over time. This is critical to ensure long-lasting practice changes, improved clinical outcomes for patients, as well as organizational and system effectiveness. Ongoing administrative support and staff engagement are critical elements, as is embedding the evidence in policies, procedures, and plans of clinical care. Organizational learning theory provides a complementary perspective to understanding the sustainability of practice changes. A critical aspect of this approach is that of "organizational memory," which refers to the various ways knowledge is stored within organizations for current and future use (Virani, Lemieux-Charles, Davis, & Berta, 2008).

Do Context and Culture Matter?

The ability of practitioners to implement a guideline's recommendations is highly dependent on **context** (i.e., the milieu or environment) and culture of an organization. A teaching hospital that has multiple clinical supports in the United States or urban Canada may differ greatly from a hospital with fewer supports in rural and remote areas in the same countries, let alone in developing nations. The level of staffing and skill mix impact guideline implementation as well as the organizational model of care delivery. A critical success factor is the continuity of the care provider within the model of care delivery.

Practice guidelines can serve to build capacity and improve clinical practice across all sectors of care. However, strategies to promote uptake may be different in public health, hospital care, nursing homes, or home healthcare agencies.

Despite the need to account for practice context and culture, most practice guidelines focus only on clinical recommendations and overlook the critical role that work environments play, leaving it to individuals to determine the appropriate method for implementation. However, there are some guidelines that are improving on this development process. For example, RNAO's best practice guidelines contain clinical, work environment, and educational recommendations making them easier to implement into practice (Grinspun et al., 2002; Nelligan et al., 2002; RNAO, 2012).

IMPLICATIONS FOR PATIENT CARE

Evidence-based clinical practice guidelines have the potential to dramatically improve patient care, health outcomes, and organizational/system performance. When developed rigorously and implemented consistently, they can achieve their purpose of improving healthcare quality and patient outcomes. Guidelines can be an important vehicle for translating complex research findings into recommendations that can be acted upon. Because organizations still struggle with the best mechanisms to implement research into practice, guideline developers need to continue to strive toward collaboration and avoidance of duplication. Increasing collaboration between developers and implementers will result in practice recommendations that are readily usable by point-of-care practitioners as well as more easily utilized in electronic health records and clinical decision support tools. An encouraging sign is that developers are also condensing guidelines for download onto today's technology devices (e.g., RNAO, NGC). Collaboration among healthcare providers and joint clinical decision making are also central to improving patients' clinical outcomes (Grinspun, 2007). Moreover, transdisciplinary EBPGs can serve as a catalyst for positive team work.

In 2002, a new international organization, the G-I-N (http://www.G-I-N.net) was formed. This not-for-profit organization is made up of 93 guideline developers from throughout the world. Its mission is to improve the quality of healthcare by promoting systematic development of EBPGs and their application into practice by supporting international collaboration. The presence of G-I-N is indicative of the move toward globalizing evidence while still promoting localized decision making. Given the complexity and expense of developing EBPGs, this type of initiative is essential. Moreover, this collaboration signifies a universal awareness that clinical decisions can no longer be made without being informed by the best available evidence.

NEXT FRONTIERS: CLINICAL DECISION TOOLS AND EVALUATION

The next 10 years will bring new developments to the area of EBPGs. Most notable are clinical decision tools derived from EBPGs and available application into electronic medical records to support decision making and documentation at the point of care and outcome evaluation of EBPGs.

The RNAO is a leading organization in these two fields. RNAO's Nursing Order Sets are designed to be embedded within clinical information and decision support systems. These Nursing Order Sets are derived from RNAO's clinical BPGs and are coded using standardized terminology language based on the International Classification for Nursing Practice (ICNP).

RNAO is also heavily engaged in outcomes evaluation. The launching in 2012 of Nursing Quality Indicators for Reporting and Evaluation® (NQuIRE®) indicates the maturity of RNAO's EBPG Program. NQuIRE collects, analyzes, and reports comparative data on nursing-sensitive indicators reflecting the structure, process, and outcomes of care arising from EBPG implementation. For now, NQuIRE focuses only on Best Practice Spotlight Organizations (BPSOs). These are organizations that have a formal agreement with RNAO to systematically implement, sustain, and evaluate RNAO's guideline—about 300 sites in Canada, the United States, Chile, Colombia, Spain, and Australia. These healthcare organizations are using NQuIRE data to inform where and how nursing is providing valuable benefits to patient, organization, and system outcomes by using evidence-based decision making to optimize safe, quality health care (https://nquire.rnao.ca/2013; Van De Velde-Coke et al., 2012).

> **To think is easy. To act is hard. But the hardest thing in the world is to act in accordance with your thinking.**
> **—Johann Wolfgang von Goethe**

EBP FAST FACTS

◆ Clinical practice guidelines are statements that include recommendations for practice based on a systematic review of evidence along with the benefits and harms of interventions intended to optimize patient care and outcomes.

◆ Clinical practice guidelines that are rigorously developed reduce variations in care and enhance healthcare quality and patient outcomes.

◆ Not all clinical practice guidelines that are published follow rigorous methods in their development, which is why critical appraisal of guidelines before adopting them for implementation in clinical practice settings is necessary.

◆ An excellent exemplar of the process used to develop rigorous evidence-based clinical recommendations can be found in the procedure manual used by the U.S. Preventive Services Task Force (see http://www.uspreventiveservicestaskforce.org/uspstf08/methods/procfig3.htm).

◆ Implementing evidence-based guidelines into daily clinical practice requires a multifaceted and sustained approach with individual and systemic interventions, including individual skills building along with factors such as developing a culture and context that supports EBP, providing EBP champions and mentors, and administrative support that includes the provision of tools that support implementation of evidence-based guidelines and recommendations.

References

AGREE Collaboration. (2001). *Appraisal of Guidelines for Research & Evaluation (AGREE) Instrument.* Retrieved from http://www.agreecollaboration.org

Atkins, D., Eccles, M., Flottorp, S., Guyatt, G. H., Henry, D., Hill, S., ... Williams, J. W. (2004). Systems for grading the quality of evidence and the strength of recommendations: Critical appraisal of existing approaches. The Grade Group. *BMC Health Services Research, 4*(38), 1–7.

Barratt, A., Irwig, L., Glasziou, P., Cumming, R. G., Raffle, A., Hicks, N., ... Guyatt, G. H. (1999). Users' guides to the medical literature: XVII. How to use guidelines and recommendations about screening. *JAMA, 281,* 2029–2034.

Berg, A. O., Atkins, D. J., & Tierney, W. (1997). Clinical practice guidelines in practice and education. *Journal of General Internal Medicine, 12*(Suppl 2), S25–S33.

Burgers, J., Grol, R., & Eccles, E. (2005). Clinical guidelines as a tool for implementing change in patient care. In R. Grol, M. Wensign, & M. Eccles (Eds.), *Improving patient care: The implementation of change in clinical practice* (pp. 71–93). Edinburgh: Elsevier.

Cheung, A., Weir, M., Mayhew, A., Kozloff, N., Brown, K., & Grimshaw, J. (2012). Overview of systematic reviews of the effectiveness of reminders in improving healthcare professional behavior. *Systematic Review, 1*, 36.

Cluzeau, F. A., Littlejohns, P., Grimshaw, J. M., Feder, G., & Moran, S. E. (1999). Development and application of a generic methodology to assess the quality of clinical guidelines. *International Journal of Quality Health Care, 11*(1), 21–28.

Council of the Federation. (2012). *From innovation to action: The first report of the health care innovation working group.* Author. Retrieved from http://www.conseildelafederation.ca/en/featured-publications/75-council-of-the-federation-to-meet-in-victoria

Daniels, S. R., & Greer, F. R. (2008). Lipid screening and cardiovascular health in childhood. *Pediatrics, 122*(1), 198–208.

Davies, B., Edwards, N., Ploeg, J., & Virani, T. (2008). Insights about the process and impact of implementing nursing guidelines on delivery of care in hospitals and community settings. *BMC Health Services Research, 8*(29), 1–44.

Davis, D. A., & Taylor-Vaisey, A. (1997). Translating guidelines into practice: A systematic review of theoretic concepts, practical experience and research evidence in the adoption of clinical practice guidelines. *Canadian Medical Association Journal, 157*(4), 408–416.

Devlin, R., Czaus, M., & Santos, J. (2002). Registered Nurses Association of Ontario's Best Practice Guideline as a tool for creating partnerships. *Hospital Quarterly, 5*(3), 62–65.

DiCenso, A., Ciliska, D., Dobbins, M., & Guyatt, G. (2005). Moving from evidence to actions using clinical practice guidelines. In A. DiCenso, G. Guyatt, & D. Ciliska (Eds.), *Evidence-based nursing: A guide to clinical practice* (pp. 154–169). Philadelphia, PA: Elsevier Mosby.

DiCenso, A., & Guyatt, G. (2005). Interpreting levels of evidence and grades of health care recommendation. In A. DiCenso, G. Guyatt, & D. Ciliska, D. (Eds.), *Evidence-based nursing: A guide to clinical practice* (pp. 508–525). Philadelphia, PA: Elsevier Mosby.

DiCenso, A., Virani, T., Bajnok, I., Borycki, E., Davies, B., Graham, I., … Scott, J. (2002). A toolkit to facilitate the implementation of clinical practice guidelines in healthcare settings. *Hospital Quarterly, 5*(3), 55–59.

Dobbins, M., Davies, B., Danseco, E., Edwards, N., & Virani, T. (2005). Changing nursing practice: Evaluating the usefulness of a best-practice guideline implementation toolkit. *Nursing Leadership, 18*(1), 34–45.

Doran, D., Carryer, J., Paterson, J., Goering, P., Nagle, L., Kushniruk, A., … Srivastava, R. (2009). Integrating evidence-based interventions into client care plans. *Nursing Leadership, 143*, 9–13.

Edwards, N., & Grinspun, D. (2011). *Understanding whole systems change in healthcare: The case of emerging evidence-informed nursing service delivery models.* Canadian Health Services Research Foundation. Ottawa, Ontario.

Field, M. J. (Ed.). (1995). *Setting priorities for clinical practice guidelines.* Washington, DC: National Academy Press.

Field, M. J., & Lohr, K. N. (Eds.). (1990). *Clinical practice guidelines: Directions for a new program.* Washington, DC: National Academy Press.

Field, M. J., & Lohr, K. N. (Eds.). (1992). *Guidelines for clinical practice: From development to use.* Washington, DC: National Academy Press.

Gagliardi, A. R., Brouwers, M. C., Palda, V. A., Lemieux-Charles, L., & Grimshaw, J. M. (2011). How can we improve guideline use? A conceptual framework of implementability. *Implementation Science, Mar 22, 6*, 26.

Gifford, W. A., Davies, B., Edwards, N., & Graham, I. (2006). Leadership strategies to influence the use of clinical practice guidelines. *Nursing Research, 19*(4), 72–88.

Gifford, W. A., Davies, B., Edwards, N., Griffin, P., & Lybanon, V. (2007). Managerials leadership for nurses' use of research evidence: An integrative review of literature. *Worldviews on Evidence-Based Nursing, 4*(3), 126–145.

Grilli, R., Magrini, N., Penna, A., Mura, G., & Liberati, A. (2000). Practice guidelines developed by specialty societies: The need for a critical appraisal. *Lancet, 355*, 103–105.

Grimshaw, J. M., Thomas, R. E., & MacLennan, G. (2004). Effectiveness and efficiency of guidelines dissemination and implementation strategies. *Health Technology Assessment, 8*(6), 1–84.

Grinspun, D. (2007). Healthy workplaces: The case for shared clinical decision making and increased full-time employment. *Healthcare Papers, 7*, 69–75.

Grinspun, D., Virani, T., & Bajnok, I. (2002). Nursing best practice guidelines: The RNAO Project. *Hospital Quarterly, Winter*, 54–58.

Grossman, D. C., Moyer, V. A., Melnyk, B. M., Chou, R., & DeWitt, T. G. (2011). The anatomy of a US Preventive Services Task Force recommendation: Lipid screening for children and adolescents. *Archives of Pediatrics and Adolescent Medicine, 165*(3), 205–210.

Harris, R. P., Helfand, M., Woolf, S. H., Lohr, K. N., Mulrow, C. D., Teutsch, S. M., ... Methods Work Group, Third US Preventive Services Task Force. (2001). Current methods of the U.S. Preventive Services Task Force: A review of the process. *American Journal of Preventive Medicine, 20*(3 Suppl), 21–35.

Haynes, R. B. (1993). Where's the meat in clinical journals? *ACP Journal Club, 119,* A22–A23.

Hayward, R. S., Wilson, M. C., Tunis, S. R., Bass, E. B., & Guyatt, G. (1995). Users' guides to the medical literature. VIII. How to use clinical practice guidelines. A. Are the recommendations valid? *JAMA, 274,* 570–574.

Higuchi, K. A., Cragg, C. E., Diem, E., Molnar, J., & O'Donohue, M. S. (2006). Integrating clinical guidelines into nursing education. *International Journal of Nursing Education Scholarship, 3*(1), article 12.

Institute of Medicine (IOM). (2013). *Variation in health care spending: Target decision-making, not geography.* Washington, DC: The National Academies Press.

Lohr, K. N. (1995). Guidelines for clinical practice: What they are and why they count. *Journal of Law, Medicine and Ethics, 23*(1), 49–56.

Lohr, K. N., & Field, M. J. (1992). A provisional instrument for assessing clinical practice guidelines. In M. J. Field & K. N. Lohr (Eds.), *Guidelines for clinical practice: From development to use* (pp. 346–410). Washington, DC: National Academy Press.

McQueen, K., Montgomery, P., Lappan-Gracon, S., Evans, M., & Hunter, J. (2008). Evidence-based recommendations for depressive symptoms in postpartum women. *Journal of Obstetric, Gynecologic, & Neonatal Nursing, 37*(2), 127–135.

Melnyk, B. M. (2007). The evidence-based practice mentor: A promising strategy for implementing and sustaining EBP in healthcare systems. *Worldviews on Evidence-Based Nursing, 4*(3), 123–125.

Melnyk, B. M., & Fineout-Overholt, E. (2002). Putting research into practice. *Reflections on Nursing Leadership, 28*(2), 22–25.

Melnyk, B. M., & Fineout-Overholt, E. (2011). *Evidence-based practice in nursing & healthcare. A guide to best practice* (2nd ed.). Philadelphia, PA: Wolters Kluwer/Lippincott Williams & Wilkins.

Melnyk, B. M., Grossman, D., & Chou, R. (2012). USPSTF perspective on evidence-based Preventive Recommendations for Children. *Pediatrics, 130*(2):e399–e407.

Miller, M., & Kearney, N. (2004). Guidelines for clinical practice: Development, dissemination and implementation. *International Journal of Nursing Studies, 41*(1), 813–821.

National Library of Medicine. (2008). *Fact sheet: PubMed®: MEDLINE® retrieval on the world wide web.* Retrieved February 14, 2009, from http://www.nlm.nih.gov/pubs/factsheets/pubmed.html

Nelligan, P., Grinspun, D., Jonas-Simpson, C., McConnell, H., Peter, E., Pilkington, B., ... Sherry, K. (2002). Client centred care: Making the ideal real. *Hospital Quarterly, Summer,* 70–76.

O'Connor, P., Creager, J., Mooney, S., Laizner, A. M., & Ritchie, J. (2006). Taking aim at falls injury adverse events: Best practices and organizational change. *Healthcare Quarterly, 9*(Special Issue), 43–49.

Ploeg, J., Davies, B., Edwards, N., Gifford, W., & Miller, P. (2007). Factors influencing best-practice guideline implementation: Lessons learned from administrators, nursing staff, and project leaders. *Worldviews on Evidence-Based Nursing, 4*(4), 210–219.

Ploeg, J., Skelly, J., Rowan, M., Edwards, N., Davies, B., Grinspun, D., ... Downey, A. (2010). The role of nursing best practice champions in diffusing practice guidelines: A mixed methods study. *Worldviews on Evidence-Based Nursing, 7*(4), 238–251.

Registered Nurses' Association of Ontario. (2008). Retrieved July 21, 2013, from https://nquire.rnao.ca

Registered Nurses' Association of Ontario. (2008). *Who are best practice champions.* Retrieved October 10, 2008, from http://www.rnao.org/

Registered Nurses' Association of Ontario. (2012). *Toolkit: Implementation of clinical practice guidelines* (2nd ed.). Toronto, Ontario: RNAO.

Research Training Institute. (2002). *RTI-UNC Evidence-based practice center.* Retrieved July 29, 2009, from http://www.rti.org

Sackett, D. L., Richardson, W. S., Rosenberg, W., & Haynes, R. B. (1997). *Evidence-based medicine: How to practice and teach EBM.* New York: Churchill Livingstone.

Sandström, B., Borglin, G., Nilsson, R., & Willman, A. (2011). Promoting the implementation of evidence-based practice: A literature review focusing on the role of nursing leadership. *Worldviews on Evidence-Based Nursing, 8*(4), 212–223.

Santos, J. (2008). Promoting best practices in long-term-care. *Perspectives, 31*(2), 5–9.

Schunemann, H. J., Woodhead, M., Anzueto, A., Buist, S., MacNee, W., Rabe, K. F., & Heffner, J. (2009). A vision statement on guideline development for respiratory disease: The example of COPD. *Lancet, 373,* 774–779.

Scottish Intercollegiate Guideline Network. (2008). *SIGN 50: A guideline developers' handbook. An introduction to SIGN methodology for the development of evidence-based clinical guidelines.* Edinburgh, Scotland: Author.

Shaneyfelt, T. M., Mayo-Smith, M. F., & Rothwangl, J. (1999). Are guidelines following guidelines? The methodological quality of clinical practice guidelines in the peer-reviewed medical literature. *JAMA, 281,* 1900–1905.

Shekelle, P. G., Kravitz, R. L., & Beart, J. (2000). Are nonspecific practice guidelines potentially harmful? A randomized comparison of the effect of nonspecific versus specific guidelines on physician decision making. *Health Services Research, 34*(2), 1429–1448.

Shekelle, P. G., Woolf, S. H., Eccles, M., & Grimshaw, J. (1999). Clinical guidelines: Developing guidelines. *British Medical Journal, 318*(7183), 593–596.

Shiffman, R. N., Shekelle, P., Overhage, J. M., Slutsky, J., Grimshaw, J., & Deshpande, A. M. (2003). A proposal for standardized reporting of clinical practice guidelines: The COGS statement. *Annals, 139*(6), 493–500.

St-Pierre, I., Davies, B., Edwards, N., & Griffin, P. (2007). Policies and procedures: A tool to support the implementation of clinical guidelines. *Nursing Research, 20*(4), 63–78.

Straus, S. E., Brouwers, M., Johnson, D., Lavis, J. N., Légaré, F., Majumdar, S. R., … KT Canada Strategic Training Initiative in Health Research (STIHR). (2011). Core competencies in the science and practice of knowledge translation: Description of a Canadian strategic training initiative. *Implementation Science, 6*, 127.

Straus, S., & Haynes, B. (2009). Managing evidence-based knowledge: The need for reliable, relevant and readable resources. *Canadian Medical Association Journal, 180*(9), 942–945.

Thompson, G. N., Estabrooks, C. A., & Degner, L. F. (2006). Clarifying the concepts in knowledge transfer: A literature review. *Journal of Advanced Nursing, 53*(6), 691–701.

Tricoci, P., Allen, J. M., Kramer, J. M., Califf, R. M., & Smith, S. C. (2009). Scientific evidence underlying the ACC/AHA Clinical Practice Guidelines. *JAMA, 301*(8), 831–841.

U.S. Preventive Services Task Force. (2008). *The guide to clinical preventive services.* Rockville, MD: The Agency for Healthcare Research and Quality.

Van De Velde-Coke, S., Doran, D., Grinspun, D., Hayes, L., Sutherland-Boal, A., Velji, K., & White, P. (2012). Measuring outcomes of nursing care, improving the health of Canadians: NNQR(C), C-HOBIC, and NQuIRE. *Canadian Journal of Nursing Leadership, 25*(2), 26–37.

Virani, T., Lemieux-Charles, L., Davis, D., & Berta, W. (2008). Sustaining change: Once evidence-based practices are transferred, what then? *Hospital Quarterly, 12*(1), 89–96.

Wennberg, J., & Gittelsohn, A. (1973). Small area variations in health care delivery. *Science, 182*(117), 1102–1108.

Wennberg, J., & Gittelsohn, A. (1982). Variations in medical care among small areas. *Scientific American, 246*(4), 120–134.

Wennberg, J. E., McAndrew, C., & the Dartmouth Medical School Center for Evaluative Clinical Sciences Staff. (1999). *The Dartmouth atlas of health care.* Washington, DC: The American Hospital Association.

Wimpenny, P., & van Zelm, R. (2007). Appraising and comparing pressure ulcer guidelines. *Worldviews on Evidence-Based Nursing, 4*(1), 40–50.

Box 8.5   AGREE Instrument

Scope and Purpose

Item 1. The overall objective(s) of the guideline is (are) specifically described.

Item 2. The clinical question(s) covered by the guideline is (are) specifically described.

Item 3. The patients to whom the guideline(s) is (are) meant to apply are specifically described.

Stakeholder Involvement

Item 4. The guideline development group includes individuals from all relevant professional groups.

Item 5. The patients' views and preferences have been sought.

Item 6. The target users of the guideline are clearly defined.

Item 7. The guideline has been piloted among target users.

Rigor of Development

Item 8.   Systematic methods were used to search for evidence.

Item 9.   The criteria for selecting the evidence are clearly described.

Item 10. The methods used for formulating the recommendations are clearly described.

Item 11. The health benefits, side effects, and risks have been considered in formulating the recommendations.

Item 12. There is an explicit link between the recommendations and the supporting evidence.

Item 13. The guideline has been externally reviewed by experts prior to its publication.

Item 14. A procedure for updating the guideline is provided.

Clarity and Presentation

Item 15. The recommendations are specific and unambiguous.

Item 16. The different options for management of the condition are clearly presented.

Item 17. The key recommendations are easily identifiable.

Item 18. The guideline is supported with tools for application.

Application

Item 19. The potential organizational barriers in applying the recommendations have been discussed.

Item 20. The possible cost implications of applying the recommendations have been considered.

Item 21. The guideline presents key review criteria for monitoring and/or audit purposes.

Editorial Independence

Item 22. The guideline is editorially independent from the funding body.

Item 23. Conflicts of interest of guideline development members have been recorded.

From Cluzeau, F. A., Littlejohns, P., Grimshaw, J. M., Feder, G., & Moran, S. E. (1999). Development and application of a generic methodology to assess the quality of clinical guidelines. *International Journal of Quality Health Care, 11*(1), 21–28.

Chapter 9

Implementing Evidence in Clinical Settings

Marilyn J. Hockenberry, Terri L. Brown, and Cheryl C. Rodgers

I never worry about action, only inaction.

—Winston Churchill

It is not enough to have knowledge of the best evidence to guide clinical practice; that knowledge must be translated into clinical practice to improve patient care and outcomes. Because evidence-based practice (EBP) is known to improve the quality of healthcare and patient outcomes as well as decrease healthcare costs, there is currently an increased emphasis in clinical settings on promoting EBP. However, the understanding of care based on evidence is often far removed from clinical practice (Hockenberry, Wilson, & Barrera, 2006; Rycroft-Malone et al., 2004). This chapter describes essential concepts for developing an environment that fosters a culture of EBP and key strategies for successful implementation of EBP in clinical settings. We will discuss the essential mechanisms for creating an evidence-based clinical environment, which include vision, engagement, integration, and evaluation (Figure 9.1; Hockenberry, Walden, Brown, & Barrera, 2007).

A VISION FOR EVIDENCE-BASED PRACTICE

Healthcare institutions with successful EBP programs begin with a vision and an understanding of the goals to be accomplished. A clear vision gives substance to the actions needed to transform a healthcare setting into an EBP environment. The EBP vision provides a compelling and motivating image of desired changes that result in achievement of excellence in clinical practice throughout the healthcare organization. An image of the future, defined as a shared mental framework, is created to begin the transformation process (Box 9.1).

Reasons for transforming a clinical culture into an EBP environment are numerous, depending on the type of clinical setting and its mission. For many institutions, the vision for EBP is based on regulatory initiatives and insurance-mandated outcomes. One such regulation is the Centers for Medicare and Medicaid Services' (CMS's) decision to stop paying for "preventable complications" in hospitalized patients. Numerous hospital-acquired conditions that have current evidence-based guidelines for prevention were among the list that CMS ruled as nonreimbursable in late 2008. These complications that resulted from medical errors or improper care could have reasonably been avoided through the application of evidence-based guidelines (Rosenthal, 2007).

To provide further perspective on the importance of creating a vision for transforming health care, in March 2011, the U.S. Department of Health and Human Services (DHHS) released the inaugural report to Congress on the National Strategy for Quality Improvement in HealthCare (National Strategy for Quality Improvement in Health Care, 2012). The National Quality Strategy focuses on three aims:

1. *Better Care*: Improve the overall quality of care by making health care more patient-centered, reliable, accessible, and safe.
2. *Healthy People/Healthy Communities*: Improve the health of the U.S. population by supporting proven interventions to address behavioral, social, and environmental determinants of health in addition to delivering higher-quality care.
3. *Affordable Care*: Reduce the cost of quality health care for individuals, families, employers, and government.

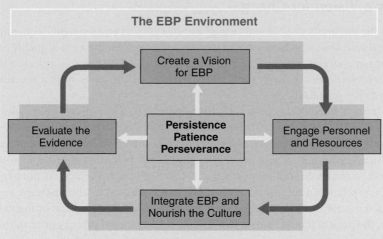

Figure 9.1: EBP environment model (With permission from Hockenberry, M., Walden, M., Brown, T., & Barrera P. [2007]. Creating an evidence-based environment: One hospital's journey. *Journal of Nursing Care Quality, 22*[3]:223.)

Box 9.1

A shared mental framework exemplifies an institution's most closely held values and ideals that inspire and motivate administrators, researchers, and clinicians to participate in practice changes.

It serves as the catalyst for change within the organization. With increasing emphasis on quality patient care and outcome metrics, a new image is emerging at hospitals that places tremendous value in providing excellence in care throughout the organization. A new, shared mental framework is established by administration's willingness to increase resources for quality initiatives and EBP programs.

This strategy calls clinical institutions into action to develop and share methods for data collection, measurement, and reporting that support measurement and improvement efforts of both public and private sector stakeholders at the national and community level (National Strategy for Quality Improvement in Health Care, 2012).

The Magnet Recognition Program also provides specific expectations for transforming a nursing culture into an environment that promotes superior performance through EBP (American Nurses Credentialing Center [ANCC], 2013). This program recognizes hospitals that demonstrate quality patient care, nursing excellence, and innovations in practice. Magnet hospitals must promote quality and disseminate best practices throughout nursing, which are attainable only through the pursuit of an EBP environment. Magnet recognition requirements include specific demonstration of expected outcomes for 2 years prior to submission of the Magnet application (ANCC). To acquire this type of evidence over time for nursing practice, an environment must promote staff use of an EBP approach to the care that is provided every day.

Developing a Vision for Change

Understanding the importance of cultural change within a clinical environment frequently begins with a few passionate individuals who have a shared mental framework for the kind of quality care they want to provide their patients and families. The vision of a dedicated EBP team is critical to the success of implementation projects (Hockenberry et al., 2007). Chapter 12 elaborates further on creating a vision and motivating a change to EBP.

Early involvement of clinical experts and EBP mentors (i.e., clinicians who have advanced knowledge and skills in EBP as well as individual and organizational change strategies [Melnyk, 2007]) shapes the future vision for EBP at any institution. While increased knowledge and understanding are important to any EBP initiative, a key to changing actual behaviors is ownership of change. An effective method to obtain clinical support is to include experts or mentors at the beginning of an EBP project, preferably when the vision for change is first established. Administrative support for the vision is obtained as soon as those involved have organized their shared vision or mental framework. When possible, the project should be designated as an organizational priority prior to the first formal meeting (Box 9.2).

 Box 9.2

Creating a Vision for Change: Pain Prevention for Hospitalized Children

The first formal EBP initiative at the Texas Children's Hospital involved developing an EBP pain prevention protocol for use throughout the hospital. A procedural pain leadership group consisting of clinical nurse specialists from Acute Care, the Pediatric Intensive Care Unit (PICU), the Neonatal Intensive Care Unit (NICU), the Cancer Center, the chair of the Clinical Practice Council, a nurse researcher, and research assistant was established.

◆ **Small steps toward change**
- The pain prevention initiative began with small steps toward change. Leaders of this initiative recognized that the vision for change needed to first start within nursing.
- Specific nursing interventions that commonly cause pain for children were selected, and an intensive evidence review provided the strategies for improving pain management.
- Changes in practice began as a purposeful, selected focus rather than an attempt to transform pain management across all disciplines at once.

◆ **Focusing awareness**
- The evidence-based pain prevention initiative first began by increasing awareness that pain remains a major problem for hospitalized children.
- Many clinicians believed that pain intervention was not necessary for common nursing procedures and routinely performed painful procedures without intervention for a number of reasons because the painful period of time was limited for the child, or the clinician felt like such an expert at performing the procedure that the pain experienced was minimal.
- Since the procedural pain leadership group had completed an extensive review of the evidence and found that pain experiences of hospitalized children are significant and long lasting, regardless of the length of procedure or expertise of the provider, a new awareness of pain practices throughout the hospital was an essential first step for the EBP pain prevention program's vision.

Table 9.1   EBP Vision: Transforming a Clinical Environment

Objective	Strategies
Develop a mental framework	• Develop a written summary of what you want to accomplish • Brainstorm with colleagues regarding the environment you want to create
Establish a motivating image for change	• Use creativity to capture attention of the clinical staff • Take advantage of real clinical scenarios to stress the need for changes in practice
Create specific goals	• Focus on short-term, attainable goals • Establish only two to three goals at a time
Gain administrative support	• Contact administrators responsible for clinical practice • Create a presentation that reflects the need for transforming the culture into an EBP environment • Seek administration support for the project to be identified as an organizational priority
Establish a leadership team	• Identify key personnel with a passion for EBP • Conduct small focus group meetings
Involve experts and EBP mentors in clinical practice	• Identify clinical experts and EBP mentors focused on the area • Engage clinical expert support

Keys to accomplishing a successful vision include preparation and planning. The old saying "begin with the end in mind" serves vision planners well at this stage of an EBP initiative. Selecting strategies that promote small changes over time is known to be more effective than conducting large-scale initiatives. Effective programs capture the momentum by acting quickly to disseminate the vision and by emphasizing small goals that are easily attainable (Table 9.1). Small goals with measurable outcomes provide concrete examples of motivating the vision for change.

Sharing the vision for excellence in practice is perhaps the most essential catalyst for promoting EBP. Initiatives that are most effective in changing the environment engage strategies that share the vision for change as early as possible. Expert clinicians may be less aware of the need for change than their nonexperienced colleagues. Emphasizing the need for change must be direct and to the point. Recognizing that one's own patient care is less than excellent is often painful for clinicians to realize (Box 9.3). Establishing the direction for EBP in a clinical environment sets the stage for an organized approach for all future initiatives. While process toward change takes time, establishing a clear direction for change provides focus toward a common goal—improved patient outcomes.

PROMOTE ENGAGEMENT

A 2013 Hastings Center Report stresses the importance of learning healthcare systems committed to carrying out activities that promote quality clinical care. As healthcare systems continue to evolve, it is evident that clinical practice cannot be of the highest quality if it is independent of its connection with engagement in ongoing, systematic learning. Learning healthcare systems, described in the Hastings Center Report, view staff engagement as essential and clinical practice as an ongoing source of data to be used for continuously changing and improving patient care (Kass et al., 2013). This requires that staff at all levels must be engaged in high-priority clinical issues to develop a successful, supportive

---

Box 9.3   Sharing the Vision for Change

To develop a vision for needed changes in pain management, the project at the Texas Children's Hospital began by increasing awareness that hospitalized infants and children commonly experience pain.

◆ A video was used to create a dramatic image and raise nurses' emotions regarding the need for change.

◆ The video demonstrated two infants undergoing a heel stick; one infant was given a sucrose/pacifier intervention and the other infant underwent the heel stick without pain intervention.

◆ The video showed dramatic differences in infant behavior during the heel stick procedure. The infant who received standard care without pain intervention cried, moved, and thrashed his arms and legs throughout the entire procedure. The infant who received the pain intervention quietly sucked on the pacifier without movement during the entire heel stick.

◆ While a written summary of the evidence supporting sucrose as a pain intervention for young infants was given to all staff, the video was much more powerful in creating a needed change in our mental framework for managing pain.

◆ After viewing the video, numerous staff began using the sucrose/pacifier intervention prior to heel sticks as well as for other painful procedures.

---

environment (Table 9.2). Clinical staff are best positioned to identify variations in practice and ineffective processes, as they often have a vested interest in streamlining inefficiencies. Administrators who are responsible for the clinical areas where changes will occur and who engage early in the planning process are likely to share ownership. A key strategy for success is involvement of staff and leaders of all disciplines who are directly affected by the potential change, including likely early adopters as well as those who may have difficulty accepting the change.

Assess and Eliminate Barriers

Barrier assessment is an integral component throughout both the engagement and integration phases of EBP implementation (Mohide & King, 2003). Change, even when welcome, is stressful to everyone. Chapter 12 provides additional information on organizational change concepts that support processes for moving a culture toward EBP. Stakeholder resistance to change must be explored early, since it frequently results from numerous factors including hesitation to break traditional practice, unfamiliarity with how evidence will improve patient outcomes, or misconceptions regarding time and effort needed to implement practice change (Box 9.4).

Common barriers to EBP implementation include inadequate knowledge and skills, weak beliefs about the value of EBP, poor attitudes toward EBP, lack of **EBP mentors**, social and organizational influences, and economic restrictions (Gale & Schaffer, 2009; Grol & Wensing, 2004; Melnyk et al., 2004; Melnyk, Fineout-Overholt, & Mays, 2008; Parkosewich, 2013).

Lack of knowledge can create barriers to daily evidence-based care due to inadequate understanding of EBP principles, unfamiliarity with how evidence will improve patient outcomes, and lack of specific skills and knowledge needed to implement change. The best evidence-based policies are of no value to the patients when the staff lack knowledge of how to implement them in practice; the right information must be in the right place at the right time and presented in a meaningful way (Feifer et al., 2004).

Table 9.2　Promoting Engagement in EBP

Objective	Strategies
Engage staff and stakeholders in assessing and eliminating barriers	• Engage stakeholders to identify educational content and strategies to learn about the practice change • Seek information about attitudes toward the affected practice directly from staff • Involve influential staff and leaders in conducting discussions with colleagues
Prioritize clinical issues	• Select clinical issues of direct interest and responsibility of clinician stakeholders • Choose issues with solid empiric evidence to begin an organizational area's EBP endeavors
Evaluate the infrastructure	• Determine the individuals and committees who have decision-making authority • Gain administrative support for adequate time and personnel for the initiative • Enlist experts to lead EBP initiatives • Ensure access to databases, search engines, and full-text articles
Develop experts in the evidence-based process	• Utilize leaders within the organization or form an academic partnership to provide expertise in research, EBP design, and evaluation • Provide formal classes and/or small-group sessions on finding and evaluating evidence • Mentor staff in critically appraising research studies and formulating practice recommendations

Box 9.4　Engage Staff and Stakeholders of All Levels

◆ Staff clinicians
◆ Leadership team members (e.g., executives, administrators)
◆ Advanced practice registered nurses
◆ Stakeholders of all disciplines directly impacted
◆ Physicians
◆ Family advisory board
◆ Allied-health professionals
◆ Doctorally prepared nurse researchers
◆ EBP mentors

Weak beliefs about the value of EBP and attitudinal barriers can be more difficult to overcome than knowledge barriers. Negative attitudes about clinical research can make it difficult for staff to become engaged in EBP (Parkosewich, 2013). Focus group discussions and anonymous electronic surveys can be valuable in identifying beliefs and attitudes about current and proposed practice changes. Traditional educational techniques (e.g., lectures and web-based training), when used alone, are usually ineffective in changing attitudes. Interactive discussions with influential colleagues, seeing the positive impact of change, and removal of perceived barriers can be powerful in overcoming resistance. Box 9.5 provides an example of barrier assessment and strategies used for elimination during an EBP procedural pain initiative.

Findings from research have indicated that a lack of EBP mentors in the environment can also be a barrier to implementing EBP by point-of-care staff (Melnyk et al., 2004). Mentors who have in-depth knowledge and skills in both EBP and individual and organizational change strategies are also a key strategy for sustaining change once it is realized. Chapter 15 expands upon the role of the EBP mentor in advancing best practice in clinical settings.

Box 9.5   Assessing and Eliminating Barriers

In the procedural pain initiative at the Texas Children's Hospital, staff members identified several barriers to prevent pain prior to performing venipunctures. The project team members implemented multiple solutions to eliminate the barriers at the organizational level.

Assessing Barriers

◆ Prolonged time to obtain orders and medications and implement interventions
◆ Lack of knowledge about what is in the hospital formulary
◆ Attitude: "Even if pain medication is used, children are already stressed out/crying"; perception that meds cause vasoconstriction which leads to multiple sticks; "I'm good so it only hurts for a moment"
◆ Unit culture: unaccustomed to medicating prior to needlesticks

Eliminating Barriers

◆ Time demands were reduced through the development of a procedural pain protocol that bundled multiple medications with varying onset times: immediate (oral sucrose, vapocoolant spray), 12 minutes (buffered lidocaine injection), 10 minutes (lidocaine iontophoresis), and 30 minutes (lidocaine cream). Nurses could select floor stock medications within the protocol that were appropriate for the child's age, procedural urgency, and developmental considerations. A pharmacist reviewed and entered the protocol into the patient's medication profile upon admission to the hospital.
◆ Additional medications were brought into formulary to accommodate urgent needs. Bundling the medications into a protocol increased the knowledge about what was available to prevent venipuncture pain. Educational modules and skills sessions were conducted to familiarize staff nurses with new and unfamiliar medications and administration techniques.
◆ A multifaceted approach was used to change individual attitudes and unit cultures. Videos of infants receiving heelsticks with and without sucrose and of older children talking about their venipuncture experiences with and without lidocaine premedication were shown. Results of published research studies on the intermediate and long-term effects of unrelieved pain during procedures were disseminated through online modules. A commitment to evaluate the medication in several children was obtained from several unit IV experts. Unit administrators communicated support for the practice in staff meetings and with individual nurses. Champions for change routinely asked colleagues what medications were used when starting IVs.

Social and organizational barriers to change include lack of support by leaders, disagreement among clinicians, and limited resources to support change (Grol & Wensing, 2004). Effective barrier assessment includes discerning knowledge, attitudes, and beliefs of mid-level and upper-level administrators surrounding practice change and their perceived roles in communicating support for this change. Peer group discussions can be very influential, and informal leaders may weigh in even stronger than formal leaders on whether practice change will actually occur. Overlooked process details can impede a well-accepted practice change, including anticipated economic and workload implications. Exploring the economic and workload impact of a practice change early in a project and securing administrative support when there may be potential increase in cost or workload can prevent these barriers from impeding progress. Economic considerations must include that an increase in one type of cost may be readily offset with savings in time (i.e., workload), satisfaction, or the additional expense of patient complications when best practices are not implemented.

Prioritize Clinical Issues

In order to spark EBP, it is best to start with a clinical issue of direct interest to clinicians, since changing one's own practice can be much easier than changing the practice of another discipline or specialty. Box 9.6 provides an example of prioritizing clinical issues for EBP initiatives. Initial efforts should be focused on maximizing the likelihood of success (Graham & Harrison, 2005). EBP changes are most likely to be successful when they are based on solid **external** as well as **internal evidence**, provide clear steps for change, and fit within the parameters of the clinician's routine practice. When an organization's readiness for change is assessed, regardless of whether the change will have a large or small impact, an easy win is more likely to occur. A practice issue that aligns with the organization/administrators' key priorities or is a focus

---

Box 9.6	Prioritize Clinical Issues

Procedures that nurses most often perform were selected as the first phase of the procedural pain initiative at the Texas Children's Hospital. Peripheral IV access, venipuncture for specimens, port access, and injections were identified as the highest priority procedures for pain prevention. Nasogastric (NG) tube and urinary catheter insertions were also considered but dropped early in the initiative. These two procedures were performed less frequently than needlesticks, and there was scant and conflicting evidence on pain prevention techniques. While important, they would have delayed protocol implementation and have a weaker evidence foundation than the other procedures.

Narrow Focus Through PICO Questions

◆ In children, how does EMLA compared to LMX affect join pain during peripheral intravenous (PIV) access, venipuncture, and injections?
◆ In children, how does lidocaine iontophoresis compared to usual care affect pain during PIV access?
◆ In infants 16 months old, how does 24% sucrose compared to 50% or 75% sucrose affect crying time during and after PIV insertion?
◆ In children, how does buffered lidocaine compared to usual care affect pain during PIV insertion?
◆ In children, how does ethyl chloride compared to usual care affect pain during PIV access and venipuncture?
◆ In children, how does ethyl chloride compared to usual care affect pain during port access?

of quality initiatives mandated by regulatory agencies, such as the Joint Commission or the Institute for Healthcare Improvement, is likely to gain administrative support more readily than an isolated initiative.

Evaluate the Infrastructure

Organizational leaders must dedicate resources, including time, to provide support for staff and their EBP mentors to ask clinical questions; search for and critically appraise evidence; analyze internal evidence; develop practice recommendations; plan changes; and develop, implement, and evaluate the EBP project. Although administrative support is crucial, it is only one of the starting points and will not lead to success on its own. Administrators should seek guidance from expert clinicians, EBP mentors, and researchers within the organization while providing authoritative as well as financial support for the EBP initiative.

Resources that support the ability to locate and critically appraise relevant literature are essential for EBP implementation (Klem & Weiss, 2005). Access to an academic medical library, databases, search engines, and full-text articles needs to be available for the EBP team to be successful in securing evidence to support practice change. While PubMed and the Cochrane Library are free to search and view abstracts, to access electronic full-text articles require a subscription to electronic journals, some of which can be accessed only through specific databases. Chapter 3 provides sources and strategies for finding relevant evidence.

Working within already-established committees and councils can be an effective strategy to gain momentum for an EBP environment. Team members should be engaged in identifying how an EBP project fits within the committee's responsibilities, priorities, and agenda. Involving multiple approval bodies within the organizational hierarchy in the engagement phase can increase the number of individuals and teams eager to ensure an EBP project's success. To allow extended time for topic exploration, focus groups may need to be formed within existing committees.

Gaining consensus for a shared vision to improve patient outcomes can help break down process silos (processes separated by departments or other divisions within a healthcare institution with different departments fixing just their part) and communication barriers. Agreement that practice changes should be based on evidence, rather than individual preferences or tradition, is a critical component that EBP teams may need to revisit several times during small-group discussions (Mohide & King, 2003).

Develop Experts in the Evidence-Based Practice Process

Expertise available to lead an EBP team may exist within an organization or may require a partner from an academic or other healthcare setting. Expertise in critically appraising and synthesizing the research literature is crucial. Education related to all steps of the EBP process through formal classes and/or small-group skill-building sessions can expand the pool of EBP experts and mentors. Staff and clinical experts may be inexperienced at critically appraising research studies and evaluating evidence. With education and mentorship, clinicians who are novices in the EBP process can learn to analyze evidence and formulate practice recommendations within a structured environment (Benner, 1984). Gaining understanding of the concepts of EBP prior to the actual practice change is essential. Mentoring clinical staff eager to learn the steps of the EBP process is an important strategy that eventually develops EBP clinical experts throughout the institution (Penz & Bassendowski, 2006).

EVIDENCE-BASED PRACTICE INTEGRATION

Ideas without action are worthless.
—Helen Keller

Integrating EBP into clinical practice is one of the most challenging tasks faced by clinicians and leaders in healthcare settings (Mohide & King, 2003; Rycroft-Malone et al., 2004). Evidence-based education and mentoring initiated during the engagement phase should continue during the integration phase, which is now directed toward overcoming knowledge and skill deficits along with stakeholder skepticism in order to enhance the likelihood of a positive EBP change (Rycroft-Malone et al., 2004). Bridging the gap between evidence and practice is essential to bring about cultural change within a clinical environment (Billings & Kowalski, 2006). Education alone will not change behavior. Interventions need to be tailored to target groups and settings and include individual, team, and organizational approaches (Grol & Grimshaw, 2003). Successful integration occurs when evidence is robust (i.e., being strong enough to withstand intellectual challenge), the physical environment is receptive to change, and the change process is appropriately facilitated (Table 9.3).

Table 9.3   Integrating EBP Into the Clinical Environment

Objective	Strategies
Establish formal implementation teams	• Integrate experts in change theory at the systems level, such as advanced practice registered nurses • Include expert staff members to ensure clinical applicability, feasibility, and adoption into practice • Exhibit passion for the practice change • Enlist local opinion leaders who can attest to the need for practice change • Bring in outside speakers who have the potential to connect and inspire key stakeholders • Create discomfort with the status quo
Disseminate evidence	• Utilize multifaceted strategies to overcome knowledge deficits, skill deficits, and skepticism • Promote experience sharing to emphasize the need for change and positive outcomes of change • Provide time to assimilate new practices
Develop clinical tools	• Anticipate tools and processes that the staff will need to transform practice • Revise patient care documentation records • Ensure easy access to clinical resources • Integrate alerts and reminders into workflow processes at the point of care • Repeatedly expose the staff to evidence-based information
Pilot test	• Choose pilot sites with consideration to unit leadership strength, patient population diversity, acuity, and geographic location • Address the root causes of problems • Decide to adopt, adapt, or abandon at the end of the pilot
Preserve energy sources	• Engage support personnel • Implement smaller, more manageable projects • Anticipate setbacks and have patience and persistence
Allow enough time	• Develop incremental project steps • Establish a timeline
Celebrate success	• Acknowledge the staff instrumental in process • Ensure recognition by supervisors and administration • Recognize the staff in presentations

Establish Formal Implementation Teams

Establishing a formal EBP project implementation team early in the process is an essential key to success. This leadership team should be appointed to guide EBP changes, and informal and formal coordinators must be engaged at the unit level to champion EBP (Rycroft-Malone et al., 2004). Advanced practice registered nurses are change agents adept at systems-level project design and often have the advantage of clinical experience with practice variations and outcomes evaluation (Ahrens, 2005; Melnyk, Fineout-Overholt, Williamson, & Stillwell, 2009). A leadership team that includes masters and/or doctorally pre-pared nurses and expert staff nurses is essential for determining the clinical applicability and feasibility of practice change recommendations and the likelihood of integrating evidence into practice and evaluating patient outcomes (Thompson, Cullum, McCaughan, Sheldon, & Raynor, 2004).

Build Excitement

One of the key factors to success of any EBP change is building excitement during implementation. Team members who exhibit passion can ignite a fire in their colleagues. Recognized national experts lend stature and credibility to the idea of implementing a practice change, whereas experts within the organization local leaders can attest to the relevance of the practice in local settings and add synergy for change. It is essential to engage the staff by demonstrating the link between proposed EBP changes and desired patient outcomes (Feifer et al., 2004). Building a "burning platform" (i.e., a passionate, compelling case to drive change) to drive change at this time can be strengthened with baseline practice-based data (e.g., quality and performance improvement data). Creating a level of discomfort with the status quo by sharing evidence of better outcomes at other healthcare settings can create a readiness for change. Fostering enthusiasm by unit/service-based staff and leaders can lead to a shared ownership in the success of an EBP initiative.

Disseminate Evidence

Passive educational approaches such as dissemination of clinical practice guidelines and didactic edu-cational sessions are usually ineffective and unlikely to result in practice change (Fineout-Overholt, Melnyk, & Schultz, 2005). Education should be planned to overcome knowledge deficits, skill deficits, and skepticism. Eliminating knowledge deficits includes not only communicating what should be done (how to change) but also why a change will be beneficial (i.e., the outcome) and the evidence to support the change. It is important to share positive outcomes of the change including external evidence, internal evidence (e.g., quality improvement data), actual patient experiences, and stories from authentic voices (i.e., practitioners using the recommended practice). Raising the level of emotion through sharing expe-riences is a powerful way to increase motivation of others toward the practice change. Stories provide not only powerful images of the need for change but also a mechanism to communicate the outcomes associated with change. The impetus for change is different for each individual; therefore, multifaceted interventions for disseminating evidence are more likely to produce change than a singularly focused endeavor (e.g., education only Grol & Grimshaw, 2003).

Strengthening beliefs about the value of EBP, an important strategy for increasing EBP implementa-tion (Melnyk et al., 2008), and changing attitudes can be more challenging than imparting knowledge. A shared understanding of the problem and identified gaps in outcomes can be a foundation to valuing the change in practice. Evidence summaries should be shared with practitioners, along with persons who would be involved in consensus building. Perceived barriers need to be removed, and processes may need to be streamlined to create time and support for the new practice.

Develop Clinical Tools

To enact change, the EBP implementation team must anticipate new processes and tools that the staff will need to transform practice. Development of resources that match interventions and overall strategies

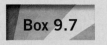

Box 9.7 | Example of an EBP Critical Appraisal Template

Ask the question	**Question:**
	Background summary
Search for the evidence	**Search strategies:**
	Dates/search limits
	Key words/terms/controlled vocabulary

Rapidly Critically Appraise, Evaluate, and Synthesize the Evidence

Summary of findings

Integrate the Evidence

Recommendation for practice, research, or education

References

Cite all references

can greatly facilitate changes in clinical practices (Kresse, Kuklinski, & Cacchione, 2007). Clinical tools to enhance appropriateness and consistency of care may include guidelines, EBP summaries, order sets, decision support embedded within the electronic medical record, clinical pathways, and algorithms (Box 9.7). Availability and ease of use are key components to the successful adoption of any of these resources.

Alerts and reminders can be helpful if well integrated into workflow processes. Whether electronic or paper, optimal timing and placement of reminders in relation to decision making about the care practices are essential. Guideline prompts at the point of care can be programmed into an electronic medical record, medication administration record, or even "smart" infusion pumps. Clinical decision support systems that provide electronic links to EBP information within an electronic health record or organizational website can positively influence an evidence-based practitioner's use of recommended practice changes.

Pilot Test the Evidence-Based Practice Change

Implementing a new EBP change requires restructuring of the flow of daily work so that routine processes make it natural for the clinician to give care in a new way. Even educated and motivated providers can have difficulty practicing in the desired manner without daily environmental supports. Piloting small tests of change with a commitment to modify and improve the practice change with staff feedback can promote positive attitudes along with engagement in the new practice. Plan to quickly respond to questions and concerns and address the root causes of problems during the pilot phase. Early evaluation results should be shared with staff at the end of each pilot cycle, and a decision should be made to adopt, adapt, or abandon the proposed practice.

Pilot testing in a select number of patient care areas before moving to widespread implementation can be useful in identifying issues of clinical applicability and feasibility that will have an impact on future efforts at successful EBP implementation (Rosswurm & Larrabee, 1999; Titler et al., 2001).

Leadership capacity, populations served, patient acuity, and geographic location are some of the initial considerations for choosing a pilot site. In addition, sites that are known to have early adopters as well as those known to be difficult or resistant implementation sites are important to consider in choosing the site to conduct a pilot project. Early adopters can serve as training sites for later adopters. Well-managed programs with a long history of successful implementation of initiatives are likely to establish practice change early in the pilot phase. However, establishing an EBP change on a struggling unit can communicate to others that change can occur even in difficult clinical settings.

Preserve Energy Sources

Change in a dynamic healthcare environment places adds stress and strain on clinicians in the care setting. When implementing EBP changes, it is important to develop strategies to maintain excitement and preserve energy resources. Implementing smaller, more manageable projects in phases rather than introducing a single large EBP project may reduce fatigue and build confidence that the recommended change is achievable and sustainable given adequate time and resources (Box 9.8). Integrating additional "champions for change" during new phases of a project can bring new energy and ownership to a project (Kirchner et al., 2012). Project leaders and teams should anticipate setbacks with patience and persistence. Periodically sharing small successes along the way can foster continued excitement for the project and reduce fatigue that is often associated with lagging outcomes.

Box 9.8 Small Steps of Change

During the engagement phase of the procedural pain initiative at the Texas Children's Hospital, many nurses became uncomfortable with the status quo and were eager to have broader access to pain prevention medications. The protocol was anticipated to take several months to allow for critically appraising evidence, building algorithms, gaining consensus, and piloting.

Sucrose had been used for years in the hospital's NICU, but young infants admitted to other areas were not given sucrose.

◆ The first step of change was to establish an upper age limit for sucrose and permit its use anywhere in the organization.
◆ The second step was to remove a time barrier by adding sucrose and LMX (4% lidocaine cream) to floor stock in many areas. Additional medications were added to formulary and available for use by individual order as the third step of the initiative.
◆ The final step was to implement the procedural pain protocol, a group of medications for multiple procedures, and expand floor stock availability.

Protocol
Additional medications to prevent the pain caused by needlesticks brought in to hospital formulary

Sucrose and LMX as floor stock

Sucrose use outside the NICU

Sucrose use within the NICU

Timeline for Success

Planning practice changes for an EBP project includes evaluating current practice, identifying gaps in "what is" and "what is desired," establishing incremental steps of the project, and setting timelines. Competing priorities within an area or organization can influence the timing needed to embark upon a successful EBP project. When conducting a large change, often it is easier to accomplish it when customarily busy periods are over or when leaders are as free as possible from competing responsibilities. Project timelines for EBP changes are extremely variable and can be influenced by many environmental issues, such as the size of the project, staff time commitment, EBP expertise, expediency of decision making, and the urgency of the need for practice change (Box 9.9).

Celebrate Success

Celebrate success early in the development phases of practice change recommendations. It is important to acknowledge members of the project team who are instrumental in the planning and implementation

---

Box 9.9   Sample EBP Implementation Project Plan

Project timelines for EBP changes are highly variable. Several project components may overlap or occur simultaneously.

Project component	Timeframe
Develop a vision for change	Variable
Identify and narrow practice topic	1–3 weeks
Evaluate current practice and analyze recent quality data	4–6 weeks
Engage staff and stakeholders	4 weeks
Evaluate the infrastructure and establish formal teams	4 weeks
Develop and refine PICO questions	2–4 weeks
Develop search strategy and conduct search	4–6 weeks
Critically appraise, evaluate, and synthesize the evidence	4–8 weeks
Formulate practice recommendations	2 weeks
Celebrate success of progress to date!	Ongoing
Gain stakeholder support	2–4 weeks
Assess and eliminate barriers	Variable
Develop clinical tools	Variable
Conduct rapid cycle pilot	Variable
Celebrate success of progress to date!	Ongoing
Gain approval for change	Variable
Disseminate evidence and educate staff	4 weeks
Implement practice change	1 week
Celebrate success of progress to date!	Ongoing
Measure clinical outcomes	Ongoing
Analyze measurement data and refine practice and processes	Ongoing
Celebrate success!	Ongoing

process in meetings where the practice is discussed, in hospital newsletters, or in any venue in which materials related to the project are presented. Recognize individuals and teams who adopt and implement the new practice. Positive outcomes from preliminary measurements of success should be shared with all point-of-care providers as well as other key stakeholders. Clinicians and administrators who see the positive results of an EBP project will be more likely to engage in and support future EBP initiatives. Leaders and point-of-care providers who are responsible for promoting EBP change should be encouraged to share their findings through presentations and publications so other professionals and institutions may benefit from their EBP endeavors.

EVALUATION: LINKING EVIDENCE-BASED PRACTICE TO CLINICAL OUTCOMES

One of the most difficult aspects of EBP is assuring that change has occurred and, even more importantly, has resulted in positive, sustained outcomes. All too frequently, patient care outcomes in clinical settings indicate a need for changes that demand immediate action by administrators and leaders, which may place clinicians in a practice environment that is shaped by practice standards and initiatives that are not well thought out or evaluated for successful outcomes. This crisis orientation to clinical practice change results in less than impressive results. Well-intentioned administrators often demand changes without considering the time taken to change a culture. Policy changes that make it difficult for the clinician to provide quality care in a timely manner will never succeed. For example, EBP that requires supplies and resources that are not readily available to the clinicians will not produce positive clinical outcomes because the clinicians will not integrate changes in their practice that are difficult or impossible to perform. For sustainable change to occur, time must be taken to evaluate influence of EBP on patient care processes.

Evaluating outcomes produced by clinical practice changes is important at the patient, clinician, and organization or system level. Outcomes reflect the impact that is being made with the change to best practice. When an effective intervention from research is translated into real-world clinical practice where confounding variables are not controlled and the patients are not the same as those involved in research, the outcomes may be different. Evaluating outcomes of an EBP change is important to determine whether the findings from research are similar when translated into the real-world clinical practice setting. It is important to measure outcomes before (i.e., baseline), shortly after (i.e., short-term follow-up), and for a reasonable length of time after (i.e., long-term follow-up) the practice change. Each of these points in time provides data on the sustainable impact of the EBP change.

The complexity of health-related outcomes associated with clinical practice presents an opportunity to evaluate the impact of EBP in the environment from multiple perspectives. Six areas of evidence are presented as important EBP evaluation indicators.

1. Outcome measures
2. Quality care improvement
3. Patient-centered quality care
4. Efficiency of processes
5. Environmental changes
6. Professional expertise

These indicators reflect evidence in the environment that demonstrates effective changes in clinical practice (Table 9.4). Health outcome measures must be a part of the EBP environment to determine whether healthcare interventions actually make a difference.

Table 9.4   EBP Evaluation in the Clinical Environment

Objective	Measurement Description
Outcome measures	Outcome measures quantify medical outcomes such as health status, death, disability, iatrogenic effects of treatment, health behaviors, and the economic impact of therapy and illness management
Quality care improvement	Managing common symptoms such as pain, fatigue, nausea and vomiting, sleep disturbances, appetite changes, and depression caused by many acute and chronic diseases
Patient-centered quality care	Measures include effective communication with healthcare personnel; open, unrushed interactions; presentation of all options for care; open discussion of the illness or disease; sensitivity to pain and emotional distress; consideration of the cultural and religious beliefs of the patient and family; being respectful and considerate; nonavoidance of the specific issues; empathy; patience; and a caring attitude and environment
Efficiency of processes	Appropriate timing of interventions, effective discharge planning, and efficient utilization of hospital beds are exemplars of efficiency of processes indicators
Environmental changes	Evaluation of policy and procedure adherence, unit resource availability, and healthcare professional access to supplies and materials essential to implement best practices
Professional expertise	Knowledge and expertise of clinical staff

Outcome Measures

Outcome measures have been defined as those healthcare results that can be quantified, such as health status, death, disability, iatrogenic (undesirable or unwanted) effects of treatment, health behaviors, and the economic impact of therapy and illness management (Bethel, 2000; IOM, 2000; Titler et al., 2001). Health outcome measures are used to evaluate changes in clinical practice, support healthcare decision making, and establish new policies or practice guidelines. Outcome-based healthcare reimbursement has become a reality in the Affordable Care Act and provides support for the importance of using appropriate clinical measures.

Important questions to ask regarding measurement of outcomes from an EBP implementation project include the following:

◆ Are the outcomes of high importance to the current health care system?
◆ Are the outcomes of interest sensitive to change over time?
◆ How will the outcome(s) of interest be measured (e.g., subjectively through self-report and/or objectively by observation)?
◆ Are there existing valid and reliable instruments to measure the outcomes of interest?
◆ Who will measure the outcomes, and will training be necessary?
◆ What is the cost of measuring the outcomes?

Identifying these aspects of measurement of outcomes will assist in the quality of outcomes obtained.

Quality Care Improvement

Quality care improvement measures complement established health outcome measures by further quantifying how interventions affect the quality of patients' and families' lives (Titler et al., 2001). Quality care improvement indicators are often used to demonstrate the effectiveness of symptom management interventions. Effectively managing common symptoms caused by many acute and chronic diseases can provide specific data to demonstrate quality care improvement in clinical practice. Often, quality indicators demonstrate the existence of a clinical issue as well as provide information about successful evidence implementation and change.

Patient-Centered Quality Care

Increasing emphasis has been placed on **patient-centered quality care measures.** These measures are defined as the value patients and families place on the health care received. Patient-centered quality care requires a philosophy of care that views the patient as an equal partner rather than a passive recipient of care, much like the EBP paradigm, in which patient preferences must be part of the decision making (Box 9.10). Commonly, patient-centered quality care measures have been described as "soft" indicators and received limited attention. Policy makers, healthcare organizations, and healthcare professionals now recognize the importance of organizing and managing health systems to ensure patient-centered quality care (Rosswurm & Larrabee, 1999).

Efficiency of Processes

As healthcare organizations become more sophisticated in evaluation strategies, it becomes essential to evaluate the efficiency of healthcare delivery processes. Information technology provides numerous EBP strategies to improve care delivery methods at every level in the organization. Efficiency in providing

---

Box 9.10 Patient-Centered Quality Care

Crucial to promoting patient-centered quality care is open, honest discussion of the illness or disease.

◆ Consideration of the cultural and religious beliefs of the patient and family, being respectful and considerate, nonavoidance of the specific issues, empathy, patience, and a caring attitude and environment are all important.
◆ Use of measures that critically evaluate key aspects of patient-centered quality care within a healthcare organization can provide crucial evidence that differentiates a good healthcare setting from an outstanding one.
◆ Busy hospital environments often prevent family coping strategies from effectively being utilized even though evidence supports the importance of family presence.
◆ Time constraints often prevent patient-centered quality care.

One family at the Texas Children's Hospital felt strongly that they needed to place a prayer rug under their child and to say a prayer over the child immediately before anesthesia. While this activity added a few more minutes to the preanesthesia preparation, it resulted in the child being relaxed and fully cooperating with the anesthesiologist once the prayer was completed. The child went to sleep without a struggle lying on the prayer rug. Parents left the anesthesia induction room feeling that their needs were met and patient/family-centered care was provided.

Box 9.11   Barriers That Influence Efficiency of Process Changes

Obstructive barriers to EBP implementation often impede measurable clinical outcomes.

◆ Implementation of an evidence-based guideline for managing bronchiolitis demonstrated a resistance to change that significantly influenced the efficiency of the EBP implementation process.

◆ An EBP review revealed that earlier discharge could occur when discharge planning was initiated earlier during hospitalization.

◆ During the implementation phase of this guideline, two different healthcare disciplines refused to compromise over who would notify the physician about early discharge orders, stating it was not their role to obtain the order.

◆ Rather than evaluate what was best for the patient and family, these professionals refused to change their practice and the administrators had to intervene to persuade a compromise.

EBP care and evaluating the best possible process for implementing these practices lead to excellence in care and cost containment. Appropriate timing of interventions, effective discharge planning, and efficient utilization of hospital beds are examples of efficiency of process indicators. These indicators are directly associated with outcomes (Box 9.11).

Environmental Changes

Environmental change evaluation reflects the creation of a culture that promotes the use of EBP throughout the organization. Environmental outcome measures are uniquely different in comparison with efficiency of processes in that a process can change or patient outcomes change, yet there is no impact on the **environment**. This difference is often observed with policy and procedure changes that are carefully updated and filed into procedure manuals, yet no practice changes actually occur in the clinical setting. Examples of indicators of environmental changes include evaluation of policy and procedure adherence, unit resource availability, and healthcare professional use of supplies and materials essential to implement best practices.

Professional Expertise

Excellence in providing the best possible health care cannot occur without expert providers. Increasing sophistication in healthcare technology places significant demands on institutions to employ healthcare professionals with appropriate expertise. Professional expertise promotes excellence by establishing expectations for adherence to accepted standards of care essential for best practice. Without healthcare providers' expertise, institutions are often unable to determine why specific outcomes are not being met (Box 9.12).

IMPLEMENTING EVIDENCE IN CLINICAL SETTINGS: EXAMPLE FROM THE FIELD

The following example from the field of successful EBP implementation projects started with identification of a clinical problem as a result of a spirit of inquiry (Melnyk, Fineout-Overhold, Stillwell, & Williamson, 2010).

Box 9.12 Linking Clinical Outcomes to Professional Expertise

Placement of nasogastric (NG) tubes in infants and children is a common and often difficult nursing procedure.

◆ Using the gold standard (radiographic documentation), Ellett et al. (2005) found that more than 20% of NG tubes were incorrectly placed in 72 acutely ill children.

◆ Other studies quote misplacement as high as 43.5% in children (Ellett & Beckstrand, 1999; Ellett, Maahs, & Forsee, 1998). Displaced NG tubes can create significant morbidity and mortality.

◆ Throughout numerous children's hospitals across the country, changes in assessing NG tube placement are being implemented because there is substantial evidence that the traditional method of auscultation is not effective in determining proper placement (Westhus, 2004).

◆ A combination of measures to ensure NG placement including pH, tube length, and physical symptoms have been shown to be more effective in the assessment of NG tube placement in children (Ellett, 2004, 2006; Ellett et al., 2005; Huffman, Pieper, Jarczyk, et al., 2004; Metheny et al., 2005; Metheny & Stewart, 2002).

However, there is significant discussion throughout the country that it is difficult to change traditional nursing practice even when there is evidence to indicate that auscultation for proper NG tube placement is not safe practice. Policy changes without education and reinforcement of this new EBP approach to NG tube placement will never be effective in producing measurable change in clinical outcomes.

Lednik and colleagues (2013) report on how the EBP process was used when their organization considered a practice change to allow families to administer subcutaneous immunoglobulin (SCIg) to the patient at home. Nurses have been administering SCIg in the home setting since 2009; however, family members were increasingly interested and inquisitive about the possibility of administering the medication without the nurse (Step 0 in the EBP Process). It was identified that evidence was needed to evaluate the safety of family administration of SCIg in the home. Therefore, the following PICOT question (Step 1 in the EBP Process) was developed:

> *Among patients receiving SCIg in the home (P) does self-infusion or infusion by family caregivers (I) versus infusion by a home care nurse (C) increase adverse events (O) and increase family satisfaction (O)?*

A search for the evidence to answer the PICOT question (Step 2 in the EBP Process) revealed 21 publications, of which 7 were determined to be relevant to the question. Critical appraisal, evaluation, and synthesis of these studies (Step 3 of the EBP Process) led to the following conclusions: administration of SCIg by the patient and/or family member was (a) safe and provided no increased risk of adverse effects and (b) increased patient and family satisfaction. Therefore, a recommendation was made to allow patients and families the option for self/family-administered SCIg.

Based on the evidence, a practice change was developed (Step 4 of the EBP Process) that included disseminating the results of the evidence, sharing the recommendation with other governance councils within the organization, creating a policy allowing self or family administration of SCIg if patients met predetermined criteria, and developing guidelines for educating patients and families. At staff meetings, nurses were educated on the process of teaching and the plan for follow-up visits. The project was initially implemented (Step 5 of the EBP Process) among five of the eight SCIg patients either with a family member or self-administration of the medication. No patient had an adverse event, and all families reported an increase in satisfaction. These results were shared with organizational leaders and home care nurses, and the policy remained in place with ongoing monitoring (Step 6 of the EBP Process). In the following 2 years, the number of family- or self-administered SCIg doubled with continued high patient/family satisfaction and no adverse events.

CONCLUSIONS

An EBP environment promotes excellence in clinical care resulting in improvement of patient outcomes. Transforming a healthcare institution into a setting where an EBP culture exists requires persistence, patience, and perseverance (Hockenberry et al., 2007). Persistence—to maintain steadiness on a course of action—allows time to realize how EBP can improve clinical outcomes and is a partner with wisdom when change may create significant stress for staff. Patience—showing the capacity for endurance—provides the strength to wait for change to occur. Perseverance—adhering to a purpose—allows the team to survive the change process by resolve and dedication during a time when it is essential to stay the course and believe that EBP can transform a clinical environment (Hockenberry et al., 2007).

EBP FAST FACTS

◆ Essential components for successful EBP implementation in clinical settings include creating a vision (a shared mental framework), developing specific goals, identifying a dedicated EBP team, involving EBP experts, and promoting engagement by eliminating barriers, prioritizing clinical issues, and evaluating the infrastructure.
◆ Key factors for a successful EBP change implementation include the following:
   1. **Establish a formal implementation team:** Integrate staff nurses and masters/doctorally prepared nurses.
   2. **Build excitement:** Engage staff, raise awareness of the need for change, foster enthusiasm, encourage ownership of EBP initiative.
   3. **Disseminate evidence:** Communicate the process and rationale for the change and share experiences to increase motivation to change.
   4. **Develop clinical tools:** Written guidelines, preprinted orders, or algorithms will encourage adoption of new practices; alerts and reminders can be helpful influences for change.
   5. **Pilot test:** Evaluating changes on a small scale before moving to widespread implementation can promote positive attitudes to engage in new practices, but early evaluation results should be shared with staff promptly along with time to address questions and concerns.
   6. **Preserve energy sources:** Implementing smaller, more manageable projects in phases may reduce fatigue and build confidence; integrating new "champions for change" for each phase can bring new energy and enthusiasm.
   7. **Develop a timeline for success:** Competing priorities or environmental issues should be considered with project timelines for EBP change.
   8. **Celebrate success:** Acknowledge project team members, early adopters, and positive outcomes of the change.
◆ Evaluating clinical practice outcomes is an important but commonly overlooked step in the EBP process. It is important to measure outcomes before, shortly after, and a reasonable length of time after the practice change implementation.

References

Ahrens, T. (2005). Evidenced-based practice: Priorities and implementation strategies. *AACN Clinical Issues, 16*(1), 36–42.

American Nurses Credentialing Center. (2013). *Magnet recognition program: Application manual.* Silver Spring, MD: Author.

Benner, P. (1984). *From novice to expert: Excellence and power in clinical nursing practice.* Menlo Park, CA: Addison-Wesley.

Bethel, C. (2000). *Patient-centered care measures for the national health care quality report.* Portland, OR: Foundation for Accountability.

Billings, D. M., & Kowalski, K. (2006). Bridging the theory-practice gap with evidence-based practice. *Journal of Continuing Education in Nursing, 37*(6), 248–249.

Ellett, M. L. (2004). What is known about methods of correctly placing gastric tubes in adults and children. *Gastroenterol Nurs, 27*(6), 253–259.

Ellett, M. L. (2006). Important facts about intestinal feeding tube placement. *Gastroenterol Nurs, 29*(2), 112–124.

Ellett, M. L., & Beckstrand, J. (1999). Examination of gavage tube placement in children. *J Soc Pediatr Nurs, 4*(2), 51–60.

Ellett, M. L., Croffie, J. M., Cohen, M. D., & Perkins, S. M. (2005). Gastric tube placement in young children. *Clin Nurs Res, 14*(3), 238–252.

Ellet, M. L., Maahs, J., & Forsee, S. (1998). Prevalence of feeding tube placement errors & associated risk factors in children. *MCN Am J Matern Child Nurs, 23*(5), 234–239.

Feifer, C., Fifield, J., Ornstein, S., Karson, A., Bates D., Jones K., & Vargas, P. A. (2004). From research to daily clinical practice: What are the challenges in "translation"? *Joint Commission Journal on Quality and Safety, 30*(5), 235–245.

Fineout-Overholt, E., Melnyk, B. M., & Schultz, A. (2005). Transforming health care from the inside out: Advancing evidence-based practice in the 21st century. *Journal of Professional Nursing, 21*(6), 335–344.

Gale, B. V., & Schaffer, M. A. (2009). Organizational readiness for evidence-based practice. *Journal of Nursing Administration, 39*(2), 91–97.

Graham, I. A., & Harrison, M. B. (2005). Evaluation and adaptation of clinical practice guidelines. *Evidence-Based Nursing, 8*(3), 68–72.

Grol, R., & Grimshaw, J. (2003). From best evidence to best practice: Effective implementation of change in patients' care. *Lancet, 362*(9391), 1225–1230.

Grol, R., & Wensing, M. (2004). What drives change? Barriers to and incentives for achieving evidence-based practice. *Medical Journal of Australia, 180*(6 Suppl), S57–S60.

Hockenberry, M., Walden, M., Brown, T., & Barrera, P. (2007). Creating an evidence-based practice environment: One hospital's journey. *Journal of Nursing Care Quality, 22*(3), 221–231.

Hockenberry, M., Wilson, D., & Barrera, P. (2006). Implementing evidence-based practice in a pediatric hospital. *Pediatric Nursing, 32*(4), 371–377.

Huffman, S., Pieper, P., Jarczyk, K. S., Bayne, A., & O'Brien, E. (2004). Methods to confirm feeding tube placement: Application of research to practice. *Pediatr Nurs, 30*(1), 10–13.

Institute of Medicine. To Err is Human: Building a Safer Health System. (2000). Washington D.C.: *National Academy Press.*

Kass, N. E., Faden, R. R., Goodman, S. N., Pronovost, P., Tunis, S., & Beauchamp, T. L. (2013). The research-treatment distinction: A problematic approach for determining which activities should have ethical oversight. *Hastings Center Report, Jan–Feb,* S4–S15.

Kirchner, J. E., Parker, L. E., Bonner, L. M., Fickel, J. J. Yano, E. M., & Ritchie, M. J. (2012). Roles of managers, frontline staff and local champions, in implementing quality improvement: Stakeholders' perspectives. *Journal of Evaluation in Clinical Practice, 18,* 63–69.

Klem, M. L., & Weiss, P. M. (2005). Evidence-based resources and the role of librarians in developing evidence-based practice curricula. *Journal of Professional Nursing, 21*(6), 380–387.

Kresse, M., Kuklinski, M., & Cacchione, J. (2007). An evidence-based template for implementation of multidisciplinary evidence-based practices in a tertiary hospital setting. *American Journal of Medical Quality, 22*(3), 148–163.

Lednik, L., Baker, M., Sullivan, K., Poynter, M., O'Quinn, L., & Smith, C. (2013). Is self-administration of subcutaneous immunoglobulin therapy safe in a home care setting? *Home Healthcare Nurse, 31*(3), 134–141.

Melnyk, B. M. (2007). The evidence-based practice mentor: A promising strategy for implementing and sustaining EBP in healthcare systems. *Worldviews on Evidence-Based Nursing, 4*(3), 123–125.

Melnyk, B. M., Fineout-Overholt, E., Feinstein, N. F., Li, H., Small, L., Wilcox, L., & Kraus, R. (2004). Nurses' perceived knowledge, beliefs, skills, and needs regarding evidence-based practice: Implications for accelerating the paradigm shift. *Worldviews of Evidence-Based Nursing, 1*(3), 185–193.

Melnyk, B. M., Fineout-Overholt, E., & Mays, M. (2008). The evidence-based practice beliefs and implementation scales: Psychometric properties of two new instruments. *Worldviews on Evidence-Based Nursing, 5*(4), 208–216.

Melnyk, B. M., Fineout-Overhold, E., Stillwell, S. B., & Williamson, K. M. (2010). The seven steps of evidence based practice. *American Journal of Nursing, 110*(1), 51–53.

Melnyk, B. M., Fineout-Overholt, E., Williamson, K., & Stillwell, S. (2009). Transforming healthcare quality through innovations in evidence-based practice. In T. Porter-O'Grady & K. Malloch (Eds.), *Innovation leadership: Creating the landscape of health care* (pp. 167–191). Boston, MA: Jones and Bartlett.

Metheny, N. A., Schnelker, R., McGinnis, J., Zimmerman, G., Duke, C., Merritt, B., Banotai, M., & Oliver, D. A. (2005). Indicators of tubesite during feedings. *J Neurosci Nurs, 37*(6), 320–325.

Metheny, N. A., & Stewart, B. J. (2002). Testing feeding tube placement during continuous tube feedings. *Appl Nurs Res, 15*(4), 254–258.

Mohide, E. A., & King, B. (2003). Building a foundation for evidence-based practice: Experiences in a tertiary hospital. *Evidence Based Nursing, 6*(4), 100–103.

National Strategy for Quality Improvement in Health Care. (2012). *Annual progress report to congress.* Washington, DC: U.S. Department of Health and Human Services.

Parkosewich, J. A. (2013). An infrastructure to advance the scholarly work of staff nurses. *Yale J Biol Med, 86*(1), 63–77.

Penz, K., L., & Bassendowski, S. L. (2006). Evidence-based nursing in clinical practice: Implications for nurse educators. *Journal of Continuing Education in Nursing, 37*(6), 251–256, 269.

Rosenthal, M. B. (2007). Nonpayment for performance: Medicare's new reimbursement rule. *New England Journal of Medicine, 357*(16), 1573–1575.

Rosswurm, M. A., & Larrabee, J. H. (1999). A model for change to evidence-based practice. *Image-The Journal of Nursing Scholarship, 31*(4), 317–322.

Rycroft-Malone, J., Harvey, G., Seers, K., Kitson, A., McCormack, B., & Titchen, A. (2004). An exploration of the factors that influence the implementation of evidence into practice. *Journal of Clinical Nursing, 13*(8), 913–924.

Thompson, C., Cullum, N., McCaughan, D., Sheldon, T., & Raynor, P. (2004). Nurses, information use, and clinical decision making: The real world potential for evidence-based decisions in nursing. *Evidence Based Nursing, 7*(3), 68–72.

Titler, M. G., Kleiber, C., Steelman, V., Rakel, B. A., Budreau, G., Everett, L. Q., … Goode, C. J. (2001). The Iowa model of evidence-based practice to promote quality care. *Critical Care Nursing Clinics of North America, 13*(4), 497–509.

Westhus, N. (2004). Methods to test feeding tube placement in children. *MCN Am J Matern Child Nurs, 29*(5), 282–287.

Chapter 10

The Role of Outcomes and Quality Improvement in Enhancing and Evaluating Practice Changes

Barbara B. Brewer and Anne Wojner Alexandrov

I do believe that when we face challenges in life that are far beyond our own power, it's an opportunity to build on our faith, inner strength, and courage. I've learned that how we face challenges plays a big role in the outcome of them.

—Sasha Azevedo

It is essential to monitor outcomes in the delivery of best practices, as they determine the impact on healthcare quality, patient outcomes, and cost (Melnyk, Morrison-Beedy, & Moore, 2012). For example, if you discover a new **systematic review** which supports that a specific type of fall prevention program decreases the prevalence of falls in older adults in long-term care, and decide to implement it in your clinical setting, tracking whether the new intervention actually works to reduce falls with your patients (the outcome) will be important to provide data that the practice change was effective.

Donabedian's (1980) quality framework defines three levels of measurement: structure, process, and outcome. Healthcare providers readily accepted the charge of defining structure and measuring process, but it was not until the late 1990s that a focus on outcomes measurement and management began to take hold (Wojner, 2001). The focus of this chapter is the measurement of the results or outcomes of **evidence-based quality improvement** (EBQI) as well as the comparison of traditional practice with new interventions. Understanding the role of outcomes evaluation is important for all healthcare providers to contribute to and appreciate.

EBQI consists of systematic and continuous actions that lead to improvement in health services and the health status or health outcomes of targeted patient groups (U.S. Department of Health and Human Services, 2011). It consists of using patient data/outcomes (i.e., internal evidence) to improve clinical care. **Outcomes** are health status changes (e.g., blood pressure, anxiety) between two or more time points that are internal to the patient and are the result of the care that is provided. Conversely, **outcomes research** uses a rigorous scientific process that generates new knowledge (external evidence) about the outcomes of certain healthcare practices (e.g., a randomized controlled trial that determines the effect of using health coaches with patients being discharged from the hospital to home on patients' readmission rates to the hospital).

OUTCOMES: THE "END-RESULT IDEA"

In 1917, Ernest Codman proposed a method (considered outrageous at the time) for aligning hospitals and physicians with the capitalist financial U.S. economic framework. Simply named the "end-result idea," it was a bold suggestion that hospitals and physicians should measure the results of their healthcare processes and make them available to the general public. Those agencies with optimal outcomes would then command a leadership position within the healthcare market, while those with suboptimal performance would be challenged to improve or resign/go out of business. Sadly for Codman (1934), his suggestion was deemed as nothing short of dangerous in the context of a paternalistic medical philosophy, which held that patients were uneducated and cognitively ill equipped to participate in both health decision making and determination of medical provider excellence. Until the emergence of Donabedian's (1980) quality framework, the prospect of outcomes measurement lay dormant.

In 1988, Paul Ellwood took up the charge for outcomes measurement where Codman left off, proposing a framework for **outcomes management** (OM). Ellwood described OM as "a technology of patient experience designed to help patients, payers, and providers make rational medical care-related choices based on better insight into the effect of these choices on patient life" (p. 1549). The principles supporting OM ascribed by Ellwood included

◆ Emphasizing practice standards that providers can use to select interventions
◆ Measuring patient functional status, well-being, and disease-specific clinical outcomes
◆ Pooling outcome data on a massive scale
◆ Analyzing and disseminating outcomes, in relation to the interventions used, to appropriate decision makers and stakeholders

Ellwood's framework for OM was published in response to a new emphasis in the mid-1980s on healthcare costs in relation to service quality and was the first to provide context for use of what were then called "best practices" (Wojner, 2001). Nursing case management also emerged in the late 1980s in response to a focus on healthcare efficiency as key to controlling healthcare costs and improving quality. Case management used methods that first surfaced in psychiatric social work (Wojner, 1997b). While these methods sharpened the focus on process efficiency, which continues to be a significant aspect of the case manager role today, they did little to promote the use of evidence-based interventions and failed to detail measurement of health outcomes. Since that time, even more pressure has been placed on healthcare providers to implement practices associated with the highest quality outcomes with the advent of value-based purchasing for hospitals in October 2012. In the new program, hospitals are paid based on quality, rather than quantity of care (Department of Health and Human Services, 2011).

In 1997, the Health Outcomes Institute's OM Model (Figure 10.1) was the first to take the Ellwood framework and build in actual steps to guide measurement of the impact of new interventions on improving healthcare outcomes (Wojner, 1997a). The model includes four phases:

1. *Phase 1*: Definition of outcome measures, along with contributing structure (e.g., infrastructure of the organization, technology) and process measures (what is done and how it is done), and construction of a database to capture targeted variables. Measurement of baseline performance allows improvement to be clearly identified in relation to a shift in practice.
2. *Phase 2*: Contrasting and comparing traditional practice methods with those identified in the literature as best practices, interdisciplinary negotiation and adoption of new evidence-based initiatives, and construction of structured care methods (e.g., order sets, protocols) to ensure practice standardization for the purpose of improved outcomes. Emphasis is placed on interdisciplinary team engagement to encourage acceptance of new practice methods.
3. *Phase 3*: Implementation of new evidence-based initiatives. This step involves role modeling and teaching new practices, making clear interdisciplinary expectations for use of newly adopted practices, determining the stability and reliability of new practices to ensure uniform use, and measuring outcome targets.
4. *Phase 4*: Analysis of process and outcome targets in relation to newly adopted evidence-based initiatives. A focus on interdisciplinary evaluation and dialogue about the findings achieved is emphasized, including the ability to generate new research questions or hypotheses for testing, ultimately driving refinement of standardized processes (Wojner, 1997a).

The Health Outcomes Institute's OM Model provided a road map for transdisciplinary practitioners to define outcome targets, establish measurement methods, identify practices supported by evidence, educate and train healthcare providers in the use of these methods, and subsequently measure the impact associated with implementation of new interventions on healthcare quality (Wojner, 2001).

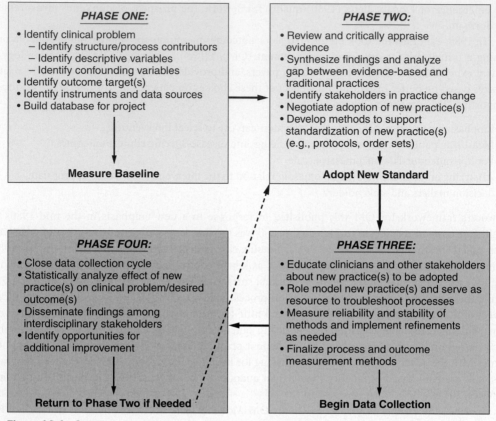

Figure 10.1: Outcomes management model. (© Health Outcomes Institute, Inc.)

QUANTIFYING THE IMPACT OF INTERVENTIONS: OUTCOMES MEASUREMENT FOR OUTCOME MANAGEMENT

The process of managing health outcomes is a natural fit for evidence-based practice (EBP), allowing for the decisions about clinical issues through outcomes measurement and the success (or not) of the implementation of an evidence-based initiative. When substandard results are achieved, new EBP should be implemented to improve outcome targets (Ellwood, 1988; Wojner, 2001).

Attitudes and beliefs that clinicians attach to traditional practices often make changing practice difficult. Measuring outcomes of practice should be viewed as a powerful change promoter. Often these powerful outcomes are measured to demonstrate EBQI (i.e., to understand the impact of evidence-based actions on patients and organizational outcomes), via data available through internal systems. Internal data are evidence that can be used to recommend practice changes aimed at standardization of evidence-based best practices. Acceptance of new evidence-based initiatives can be fostered among providers through measurement of failed outcomes achieved with traditional practices.

Healthcare organizations have a wealth of data generated by multiple individuals, often housed in multiple disparate and disconnected systems. For example, data are generated during the course of providing care to patients, as a result of tests or treatments, or by billing and financial systems. As transparency and pay-for-performance pressures have grown for providers and organizations, more and more data have been collected in response to accreditation and regulatory requirements. These types of data typically reflect evidence-based processes of care indicators that are known to produce better patient outcomes. Examples of these data include:

◆ Use of specific medications
◆ Timing of antibiotics
◆ Specific patient education
◆ Targeted discharge instructions

In addition, outcomes are also collected. Examples of these outcomes include:

◆ Fall rates
◆ Catheter-related infections
◆ Urinary tract infections
◆ Pressure ulcer rates and stage progression

The data collection for these processes and outcomes is time consuming and expensive. Therefore, before embarking on new data collection, careful consideration should be given to the usefulness of data from existing data sources for improving outcomes and demonstrating that improvement.

Sources of Internal Evidence

Internal evidence sources include quality management, finance, and human resource departments; clinical systems; administration; and **electronic health records (EHRs)**. Selected sources and examples of internal evidence discussed in the following sections are not intended to be exhaustive, as there may be data sources in other departments and systems within an organization.

Quality Management

In most organizations, quality management departments house data generated from incident reports, which may include falls, sentinel events (i.e., an unexpected event that culminates in death or serious injury), medication errors, and near misses (i.e., events that could have resulted in harm, but were corrected prior to it occurring). These types of data may be examined for trends related to types, locations, or other factors associated with care process errors, or they may be correlated with structural indicators such as staffing patterns (e.g., number of nurses scheduled to work). Other types of data that may be housed in quality management are patient satisfaction results and data collected through chart reviews submitted to regulatory or accreditation bodies.

Finance

Data housed in finance departments are frequently the most robust within an organization. Many of the data elements found within financial systems are generated by billing and registration systems and are used for billing purposes. Examples of these types of data are charges for tests, medications, equipment or supplies, patient days, readmission rates, and patient demographics such as name, age, ethnicity, gender, and nursing unit. Other data frequently housed in finance departments are codes for patient diagnosis, including Medicare-Severity Diagnosis Related Groups (MS-DRG) and International Statistical Classification of Diseases and Related Health Problems Version 9 (ICD-9) codes. These types of data are routinely used to measure patient volume, to understand care processes (types of medications used or tests done), or to risk-adjust for patient outcomes. They may also be used to evaluate incidence of errors within certain patient populations. For example, patients who have certain comorbid conditions, such as cancer or diabetes, may have a higher incidence of hospital-acquired infections. Evaluation of these data would assist in determining the severity of this association.

. . . .

We have to have a way of dealing with this that engenders confidence [and] trust, gives us every chance of getting the right outcome, and boosts both sustainability and economic return at the same time.
—John Anderson

. . . .

Human Resources

Data housed in human resource departments generally include those generated from employee and payroll systems. Data generated by employee systems include turnover and staff education levels. Frequently, if available, staff education levels reflect those at time of hire and therefore may not reflect current information. Data available from payroll systems include hours by pay category or labor category and contract labor use. In some organizations, contract labor use and expense may be housed in financial systems used for expense reporting. Hours by labor category may be used to calculate provider skill mix. Hours by pay category may be used to calculate staffing.

Clinical Systems

Clinical systems are data collection and management mechanisms that can store many kinds of data. For example, these systems may house test results such as laboratory tests or point-of-care tests. They may also house pharmacy data. Pharmacy data such as numbers of doses of a medication or types of medications may be used to evaluate care process compliance or evaluate relationships among different medications and patient outcomes. In some organizations, the clinical system is the source of data for reporting outcomes in integrated reviews, such as dashboards, which are discussed in more detail later in this chapter.

Administration

Administrative departments, such as hospital administration, may provide data related to patient complaints about care and services. Such data may be in the form of a call log or table containing information about the source, type, location, and resolution of complaints.

Electronic Health Records

For those fortunate to have access to electronic health information, the numbers and types of internal data available for use in evaluating impact are vast. Data may include patient-level information, such as vital signs and weights, non-charge-generating clinical interventions (e.g., indwelling urinary catheter use) or essentially any data elements captured through documentation of clinical care.

One caveat related to collection of data from EHRs is that data aggregation requires standardization of language in order to collect the entire group of incidences of a particular intervention, care process, or event. Many data abstracting queries (i.e., requesting information from the EHR) use a process similar to searching for articles through an electronic database. Some searches return articles based on the precise term or terms used for the search, resulting in missing articles that were filed in the database under synonyms of the search term. Searching an EHR in some systems may work the same way. Events or care processes documented using a synonym for the search term may not be included in the query results.

Measuring Outcomes to Demonstrate Impact Begins With Asking the Right Question

One of the most frustrating situations faced by clinicians who are involved with improvement activities is getting at the data that they know exist within their organization. It is not unusual to encounter barriers to getting data on the impact of current practice. Barriers to accessing needed data are usually a result of differences in language spoken by clinicians and those who "own" the data, such as the names used for the requested data elements. Other differences involve the type and form of data needed for the analysis that needs to be done, which may require patient-level data that contain data elements from multiple clinical and financial systems. For example, if a clinician wanted to evaluate glucose management over time, patient-specific data such as hospital or medical record number, name, unit, point of care and/or laboratory glucose results, time and date of sample, ICD-9 codes (for diabetes), and physician name may be needed. These data elements may be generated and housed in financial, clinical, and EHR systems in an organization. Getting these data in an integrated report may require someone with specialized skills to write a query that draws data from different databases, if an organization has a query system to achieve this kind of integration.

Clarify What You Need

Being clear about what data are needed from the outset will help avoid repeated requests for additional data elements needed to complete the analysis but not included in the original request and will facilitate the timely acquisition of data, often a challenging process. Generally, those individuals within an organization who have the report writing skills and access to the necessary databases are few in number and in high demand. As with any person who is in high demand, limited time is available to meet requests that are beyond normal workload requirements. Finding someone within the organization who is willing to mentor staff members who are novices at using internal evidence will minimize "forgotten" or unrecognized data needs, avoid repeated requests, and foster relationships with database owners, and may speed up the turnaround time for data requests.

Request Data in a Usable Format

Asking for data in a usable format is also important. When asking for a report, always inquire if the data are available in an electronic format. Many systems can run queries that will download data in a text file or in a format that can be opened and manipulated in spreadsheet software, such as Excel. Doing so can eliminate hours of data entry, which is necessary to convert a paper report of results into a format that can be used for analysis. Electronic formatted data also avoids potential data entry errors that can occur when entering data from a paper report to data analysis software (e.g., Excel or SPSS). It is very helpful if before requesting data analysis has been carefully considered so that data may be requested in a format that will require the least amount of manipulation (e.g., entry from paper) and cleaning (e.g., addressing missing information) to prepare for analysis. Once data have been prepared for analysis, statistical tests may be run using spreadsheet software, or the data file can be easily transferred to statistics software for further analysis.

When Existing Data Sources Are Not Available

All data that are required to measure the impact of evidence-based interventions on outcomes are not contained in preexisting sources, or preexisting sources of data may not be available. Therefore, it is important to discuss collection and measurement of data that are not preexisting.

Data Collection From Nonpreexisting Sources

If data are not able to be extracted from a preexisting data source, the method of data collection may be the most important aspect of evaluating the practice change. Gathering meaningful data in an efficient manner takes forethought, ingenuity, and familiarity with how data are best collected and the importance of measurement. With evidence-based initiatives, methods, and measures discovered in the evidence synthesis can be considered for use. Consideration of which patient characteristics and contextual elements might affect the outcome can increase the likelihood of collecting valid (i.e., unbiased) data. For example, if an evidence-based oral care program was initiated to reduce the incidence of ventilator-associated pneumonia (VAP), it would not be adequate to collect data solely on the frequency of oral care delivery (nonpreexisting data) and the VAP rate (possibly can be obtained from preexisting data source). Other factors, such as patient severity, preexisting pulmonary disease, or mode of suctioning (all nonpreexisting data), need to be measured because they may influence patients' risk for development of VAP. Collecting data on a unit by care providers should be done with attention to detail and in as unbiased a manner as possible to ensure data precision. As described in Phase 3 of the Health Outcomes Institute's OM Model, using methods that capture the stability of processes, such as control charts, can assist in ensuring that data are collected uniformly, resulting in accurate data.

Measurement Accuracy: Establishing Validity and Reliability

Measurement instruments, whether developed in practice or through research, should be valid and reliable so that users will be confident about the accuracy of data when collected.

Validity. Validity indicates that the measure or instrument actually measures what it is supposed to measure. For example, if you choose a valid instrument designed to measure fear, it should truly measure fear and not anxiety. There are several types of validity. For our purposes, we are going to focus on content validity, which is often reflected through an expert review of the instrument. Experts indicate whether or not they view the questions or items on the instrument as measuring the construct. For example, if a practice-developed instrument was said to measure satisfaction with the Situation-Background-Assessment-Recommendation (SBAR) communication technique, a group of experts in verbal handoffs between patients would review the instrument to indicate if the items or questions on the measure did reflect satisfaction with SBAR.

Reliability. Reliability means it will measure the construct consistently every time it is used. Often this is indicated through a statistic called *Cronbach's alpha*. A Cronbach's alpha of .80 or greater indicates an instrument that should perform reliably each time that it is used. There are many other elements of both validity and reliability of measures that go beyond the scope of this chapter. Clinicians may be tempted to develop their own instrument; however, that is ill-advised unless they have established that valid and reliable measures do not exist. If practice-developed instruments are used, it is important to take the time to establish content validity and assess reliability. Given that whole books are dedicated to understanding measurement, including establishing validity and reliability, it would be wise for those clinicians who are developing measures to obtain one and make use of liaisons with experts in the field to facilitate accurate measurement.

Making Sense of the Data

Making sense of the data is enabled through data analysis. How data are analyzed is driven by the level of data available. In larger organizations, there may be a department or portions of a department that take on this role. However, not all organizations have such resources, so we will briefly discuss data analysis. Further information on data analysis may be found in other resources that focus on that topic.

Levels of Data

There are two basic types of data, categorical and numerical. **Categorical variables** are those that are grouped due to a defined characteristic, such as gender, presence or absence of a disease, or possession of particular risk factors. Numbers are commonly used to label categorical data, but these numbers have no meaning and only facilitate grouping of cases into like data bundles. Likert scales, which allow ranking of data (e.g., not at all, somewhat, moderately so, very much so), are also categorical in nature, in that they group data by ranks. However, data analysts often consider these types of scales numerical. Generally, the statistical methods used to analyze categorical data are **frequencies** (Kellar & Kelvin, 2013).

Numeric data potentially have an infinite number of possible values, for example, measures for height, weight, mean arterial pressure, and heart rate. Unlike categorical data, the mathematical intervals that separate numeric data are equal. For example, the interval between the numbers 20 and 21 is equal to the interval between 21 and 22, namely 1.

Categorical and numeric data fall within four possible levels of measurement: nominal, ordinal, interval, and ratio. The purpose of the project and the level of the data drive the selection of the statistical methods that will be used to measure the impact of the practice change. The clinical issues that would fit within each level of measurement are discussed in the following sections.

Nominal Level Data. Data measured at the nominal level are the least sophisticated and lowest form of measurement. Nominal measurement scales assign numbers to unique categories of data, but these numbers have no meaning other than to label a group. Scales that describe the quality of a symptom by some descriptive format are nominal. For example, a nominal measure of the quality of pain may include such categories as "throbbing," "stabbing," "continuous," "intermittent," "burning," "dull," "sharp," "aching," "stinging," or "burning" (McHugh, 2003).

Ordinal Level Data. Ordinal measures use categorical data as well. Numbers assigned to categories in ordinal measures enable ranking from lowest to highest so that the magnitude of the variable can be captured. However, it is important to note that while numbers are assigned to enable sorting of findings by rank, the absolute difference in each level on an ordinal scale does not possess an equal or "true" mathematical difference in the values. Likert scales provide clinicians with ordinal-level data using selections such as "very dissatisfied," "dissatisfied," "neither dissatisfied nor satisfied," "satisfied," and "very satisfied." Clearly, each progression from very dissatisfied to very satisfied describes a greater level of satisfaction, but "very satisfied" could not be described as four times more satisfied than "very dissatisfied." When developing instruments, researchers typically use four or five categories from which to rank the variable of interest on a Likert scale.

Interval and Ratio Level Data. Interval measures are the next highest level of measurement and are purely derived from numeric data with equal and consistent mathematical values separating each discreet measurement point. While ratio-level data possess this same characteristic, the difference between these two levels of measurement is that **interval data** do not possess an absolute zero point. The best examples of interval-level data are temperature measures derived from the Fahrenheit scale that assigns $32°$ instead of zero as the point where water freezes.

Measures derived from a ruler and temperatures measured on the Centigrade scale are both examples of ratio-level data. Data measured at the interval and ratio level allow virtually all types of algebraic transformations, and therefore the greatest number of statistical options can be applied (Kellar & Kelvin, 2013). Given the significant amount of numeric variables used routinely in healthcare settings, many outcome targets, for example, those associated with objective, quantitative physiologic data, are defined at the interval or ratio level.

When defining the outcomes to be measured, clinicians must carefully consider the instruments to measure them so that they are most accurately reflected. For example, if a project were conducted to evaluate an evidence-based weight loss strategy, the outcome of weight loss could be measured at the categorical–nominal level (e.g., "BMI <25," "BMI 25–29" "BMI 30–34," "BMI 35–39," and "BMI ≥40") or at the ratio level by using actual weight loss (e.g., in pounds or kilograms). Using pounds or kilograms (i.e., ratio level) would enable those evaluating the outcome to use more powerful statistical analyses. Measurement of the impact of a practice change on outcomes denotes the need to use statistical analyses that detect a difference in the outcome target that can be attributed to the evidence-based intervention. While it is beyond the scope of this chapter to provide detailed instruction on selection and use of different forms of statistical analyses, the information presented here is meant to provide some considerations for the context of outcome measurement and analysis. Collaborating with a biostatistician is a wise decision for clinicians who are analyzing more than outcome frequencies or means.

Reporting Outcomes to Key Stakeholders

Undertaking the implementation of new interventions and ultimately the measurement of their impact requires significant work on the part of the transdisciplinary healthcare team. It is paramount that all parties involved with this process (i.e., both active and passive **key stakeholders**) be afforded an opportunity to understand the results achieved, whether positive or negative. Project coordinators need to consider which reporting methods will make the outcomes easily understood by all stakeholders to enhance dissemination of results and further knowledge associated with the clinical issues in the project. Once internal data have been gathered and analyzed, reports are generated to display results. These reports can be constructed in any way the organization chooses to present the data. Scorecards and dashboards are described here as two mechanisms for communicating data to organizational stakeholders. In a study surveying 586 hospital leaders, 81% used scorecards or dashboards for tracking outcome indicators of performance and quality (Gordon & Richardson, 2012).

Scorecards

Balanced scorecards are used to show how indicators from different areas may relate to each other. For example, relationships among financial performance indicators (e.g., hours per patient day) can be examined against clinical and safety indicators, such as patient falls or infection rates. Systematically evaluating performance from a balanced perspective allows clinicians and leaders to evaluate both intended and unintended consequences of practice change. For example, if an interdisciplinary team in the emergency department (ED) implemented an evidence-based care management program that resulted in patients who normally were admitted to the hospital for observation being discharged to home with home care, it would be prudent to ensure that the new program did not lead to higher hospital readmission rates for those patients, while at the same time evaluating whether length of stay within the ED was reduced and patient satisfaction maintained or improved. Figure 10.2 provides an example of indicators that may be used in a balanced scorecard.

Scorecard indicators can include (a) identifiers of high-level strategic initiatives, (b) objectives that are linked to the organizational strategic plan, making the outcomes relevant across the organization, (c) the measures or metrics for each outcome, and (d) indicators of how things are going, usually in relationship to given expectations or standards, often using colors. Including these components in the scorecard integrates the performance demonstrated by internal evidence with the organization's strategic plan and mission.

Using color to enhance interpretation of indicators is extremely helpful for viewing at a glance the impact of practice on outcomes. Many organizations use a red/yellow/green color scheme, where red generally indicates performance below and green indicates performance at or above goal or target. Yellow indicates performance within a certain percentage of targets, but not below or above the identified markers. Using font or background color to distinguish particular outcomes sets them apart from surrounding values. Making the scorecard easy to read and interesting to look at aids in quick overall communication of current performance. Typically, scorecards are used to indicate performance over a single year. Months or quarters may be used as reporting intervals. The decision regarding which to use is often based on frequency of data collection and preference (see Figure 10.2).

Dashboards

Dashboards are graphic displays of information that are often used at the unit level to compare performance indicators for the population being cared for on that unit. As with scorecards, color coding enables clear displays of performance indicators of excellence and of deficiencies. The same red/yellow/green color scheme can be used for dashboards to achieve the same at-a-glance overview of performance (Modern Healthcare, 2006).

Dashboards can help healthcare providers see the direct impact on performance from the care they provided. Dematteis and Werstler (2006) indicated that the use of a unit dashboard encourages active participation of staff nurses in the continued improvement of quality because they could see the results of their contributions to patient care. Performance dashboards can help build confidence in point-of-care providers that they are indeed making a difference in the outcomes of the patients for whom they care as they implement EBP.

Scorecard

Operational	Quality	Satisfaction
• Turnover • Vacancy rate • Readmission rate • Total average length of stay • Case mix index • Hours per patient day • Contract labor use • Mean wait time in ED	• Patient falls • Pressure ulcer rate • Infection rate • Compliance with evidence-based care • Mean glucose value	• Patient satisfaction • Staff satisfaction score • Medical staff satisfaction • Patient complaint rate

Figure 10.2: Balanced scorecard indicators.

Research Designs for Comparing Traditional Practice With New Interventions

When comparing a new intervention with traditional practice in a practice setting, quasi-experimental and experimental methods are typically used to generate outcomes that reflect the impact of the comparison (see Chapter 19 on generating quantitative evidence). There are both strengths and limitations associated with these methods, but each starts with ensuring that the study is adequately powered to find a difference when a true difference does exist.

An **effect size** (i.e., the extent of an intervention's impact on an outcome), calculated by subtracting the mean outcome score of one group from the mean outcome score of the other group and dividing by the average standard deviation, is often calculated when comparing a new intervention to traditional practice). It is typically used with the anticipated **power** (usually .80) and the probability (i.e., alpha) (usually $P = 0.05$) to determine exactly how many subjects are required in each study arm to find a difference in the outcome that is caused by the intervention. While it may be tempting to simply conduct a small quality study that describes the performance of an existing practice in relation to a new intervention, these studies may be less than persuasive for slow adopters to embrace new practices. Additionally, **the Health Insurance Portability and Accountability Act (HIPAA) regulations** call for ethics review boards' approval (i.e., human subject or **institutional review board [IRB]** approval of all studies involving personal health information [PHI]), and in many cases initiation of informed consent. It is also important that the knowledge learned from studies of this nature be shared, and dissemination of findings requires IRB approval prior to the beginning of the study. Because of these factors, there can be confusion about whether implementation of evidence is considered research. Chapter 22 contains more information on the confusion between EBQI and research. Either approach requires IRB review to assure participant safety and to enable the demonstration of how effective a given intervention is on outcomes within a particular setting. See Chapter 19 for information about the various types of experimental research designs that generate external evidence.

CONCLUSIONS

Demonstrating that practice change has indeed brought about improved outcomes is imperative in this era of health care when many evidence-based initiatives have been endorsed by powerful professional healthcare organizations, as well as payers, as acceptable methods to use in the treatment of specific health conditions. With steadily emerging trends, such as pay-for-performance systems supported by use of standardized evidence-based initiatives, it is important that evaluation of outcomes be conducted in a manner that is valid and reliable. These outcomes must be accessible to healthcare leadership as well as to the point-of-care providers to increase the likelihood that all those in healthcare engage in the continuous improvement of patient, provider, system, and community outcomes. Using principles of OM described in this chapter enables healthcare providers to improve healthcare practice for years to come.

EBP FAST FACTS

◆ Measurement of outcomes is essential to determine the impact that is made on healthcare quality, costs, and patient outcomes as a result of EBP changes.
◆ Value-based purchasing is a program in which hospitals are paid based on quality, rather than quantity of care.
◆ Acceptance of new evidence-based initiatives can be fostered among clinicians through measurement of failed outcomes achieved with traditional practices. Measuring outcomes of practice should be viewed as a powerful change promoter to adopt best practices.

◆ Internal evidence sources include quality management, finance, and human resource departments; clinical systems; administration; and EHRs.

◆ Data for evaluation of outcomes are available from multiple sources within healthcare organizations, including finance (billing and coding information), quality management (errors, patient satisfaction), human resources (numbers of staff), clinical systems (laboratory values, medications), administration, and EHR.

◆ Before requesting data for evaluation of outcomes, it is helpful to consider thoroughly and be clear about what is needed and how it will be analyzed in order to request all needed data in the correct format.

◆ Levels of available data (nominal, ordinal, interval, ratio) will guide analyses.

◆ Dashboards and scorecards are typically used by healthcare systems as two methods of sharing structure, process, and outcome data that indicate performance and quality.

References

Codman, E. A. (1917). The value of case records in hospitals. *Modern Hospitals, 9*, 426–428.

Codman, E. A. (1934). *The shoulder: Rupture of the supraspinatus tendon and other lesions in or about the subacromial bursa.* Brooklyn, NY: G. Miller.

Dematteis, J., & Werstler, J. (2006). Placing ownership for quality in the hands of the staff. *Critical Care Nurse, 26*(2), S38.

Department of Health and Human Services. (2011, November). *Hospital value-based purchasing program.* Retrieved from http://www.cms.gov/Outreach-and-Education/Medicare-Learning-Network-MLN/MLNProducts/downloads/Hospital_VBPurchasing_Fact_Sheet_ICN907664.pdf

Donabedian, A. (1980). *The definition of quality and approaches to its management.* Ann Arbor, MI: Health Administration.

Ellwood, P. M. (1988). Outcomes management: A technology of patient experience. *The New England Journal of Medicine, 318*, 1549–1556.

Gordon, J., & Richardson, E. (2012). Continuous improvement using balanced scorecard in healthcare. *American Journal of Health Sciences, 3*, 185–188.

Kellar, S. P., & Kelvin, E. A. (2013). *Munro's statistical methods for health care research* (6th ed.). Philadelphia, PA: Wolters Kluwer Health Lippincott Williams & Wilkins.

McHugh, M. L. (2003). Descriptive statistics, Part I: Level of measurement. *Journal for Specialists in Pediatric Nursing, 8*(1), 35–37.

Melnyk, B. M., Morrison-Beedy, D., & Moore, S. (2012). Nuts and bolts of designing intervention studies. In B. M. Melnyk & D. Morrison-Beedy (Eds.), *Designing, conducting, analyzing and funding intervention research. A practical guide for success.* New York: Springer Publishing Company.

Modern Healthcare. (2006). Ten best practices for measuring the effectiveness of nonprofit healthcare boards. *Bulletin of the National Center for Healthcare Leadership, 36*, 9–20.

U.S. Department of Health and Human Services. (2011). *Quality improvement.* Washington, DC: U.S. Department of Health and Human Services. Health Resources and Services Administration.

Wojner, A. W. (1997a). Outcomes management, from theory to practice. *Critical Care Nurse Quarterly, 19*(4), 1–15.

Wojner, A. W. (1997b). Widening the scope: From case management to outcomes management. *Case Manager, 8*(2), 77–82.

Wojner, A. W. (2001). *Outcomes management: Application to clinical practice.* St. Louis, MO: Mosby.

Chapter 11

Leadership Strategies and Evidence-Based Practice Competencies to Sustain a Culture and Environment That Supports Best Practice

Lynn Gallagher-Ford, Jackie Buck, and Bernadette Mazurek Melnyk

Today's healthcare environment is vastly complex and ever changing. Scientific knowledge continues to increase and grow at an exponential pace, yet it is well known that the integration of new knowledge into clinical practice ranges from 8 to 30 years (Sandström, Borglin, Nilsson, & Willman, 2011). Consistent implementation of evidence-based care into clinical practice, whether at the individual or organizational level, requires behavior change. Furthermore, behavior change of any kind requires more than the provision of didactic information and/or providing resources, such as computers and librarians. In order for clinicians to change their behavior and consistently implement evidence-based practice (EBP), a multitude of interventions are necessary, including

(a) EBP education combined with active repetitive skills building,

(b) EBP mentorship or facilitation and support,

(c) a culture and an environment that supports EBP,

(d) leaders and managers who support and role model EBP, and

(e) strategies to overcome system barriers to name a few (Beckette et al., 2011; Gerrish & Clayton, 2004; Majid et al., 2011; Melnyk et al., 2004; Melnyk, Fineout-Overholt, Gallagher-Ford, & Kaplan, 2011; Rycroft-Malone, Harvey, et al., 2004).

In a recent descriptive survey by Melnyk and colleagues with a random sample of over 1,000 nurses from across the United States who were members of the American Nurses Association (ANA) (2012), current barriers to EBP were identified. Although several of the barriers named by nurses were the same barriers that have been reported in previous decades, there were some new developments. The long-time barriers named by survey participants included lack of time, EBP education and resources, and availability of EBP mentors. Of particular note, agreement about the value of EBP, which had been identified as a common barrier by clinicians previously (Pravikoff, Tanner, & Pierce, 2005) was not identified in the 2011 survey. This new finding reflects that clinicians are more accepting of the idea that EBP is important and beneficial for patient care. However, a new barrier that nurses reported that had not been previously identified in the literature was resistance to EBP, not only from their peers and physicians, but also from nurse managers and leaders. Traditional organizational cultures that often upheld the philosophy of "that is the way we do it here" was also named as a barrier. Respondents to the survey expressed a need for support (as opposed to resistance) from their organizations, managers, and interdisciplinary colleagues in order to be able to implement EBP. In addition, clinicians identified relief from overwhelming workloads as an essential requirement for implementing EBP as well as education and access to EBP information (Melnyk et al., 2011).

The recent survey findings from the study by Melnyk and colleagues (2011) reinforce that implementation of EBP continues to be influenced by a multitude of factors, including

(a) beliefs and attitudes about EBP (Melnyk, Fineout-Overholt, & Mays, 2008; Rycroft-Malone, 2008),

(b) knowledge about EBP (Melnyk et al., 2004),

(c) organizational commitment to EBP (Dopson, FitzGerald, Ferlie, Gabbay, & Locock, 2002),

(d) organizational support for EBP (Hutchinson & Johnston, 2004, Rycroft-Malone, Harvey et al., 2004),

(e) a culture that is responsive to change (Gerrish & Clayton, 2004), and

(f) supported EBP ideas/initiatives.

Leaders who support colleagues and create a vision for EBP in their organizations as well as influence policy to facilitate EBP and incorporate evidence into their own leadership practices are also key in having an impact on EBP implementation (Rycroft-Malone, 2008). With all of the barriers and facilitators of EBP that have been described over the past decades, it becomes clear that a multifocal, multilayered strategy that addresses individuals as well as organizations must be developed. Strategies must be designed to facilitate change, shift practice from tradition based/provider centric care to evidence-based/patient-centered care, and create structures to embed and sustain the new paradigm. Approaching these complex challenges to deliver best healthcare practices and outcomes will require innovative thinking and courageous acts. The solutions themselves will need to be derived from an evidence-based approach and the timelines for integration of solutions into clinical practice arenas will be tight.

Despite the urgency to implement and adopt this new practice paradigm, the integration of evidence into practice continues to be perceived as challenging and burdensome and, as such, is often delegated, avoided, or ignored. Much of the distress related to implementing and sustaining EBP in organizations stems from a lack of EBP knowledge, skills and/or attitudes across the system, from executive suites to the bedside. Healthcare leaders are well poised to be held accountable to address these challenges and be at the forefront of the paradigm shift to evidence-based instead of traditional care.

RESPONSIBILITIES AND STANDARDS OF EVIDENCE-BASED LEADERSHIP

In a time when the nation is calling for EBP as standard of care, leaders must guide and support their organizations and clinicians through this challenge and opportunity. The basic definition of a leader is "one who guides or directs a group" (Dictionary.com 6/24). Leadership, on the other hand, is a process through which an individual influences a group to achieve a common goal. The definition of **evidence-based leadership** is a problem-solving approach to leading and influencing organizations or groups to achieve a common goal that integrates the conscientious use of best evidence with leadership expertise and stakeholders' preferences and values.

Evidence-based leaders are grounded in and embrace the EBP process; it is the foundation for their decision making. This requires knowledge and application of key aspects of the EBP process to leadership decisions, including

(a) clinical inquiry and formulating PICOT questions,

(b) effective searching for best evidence,

(c) critical appraisal of evidence,

(d) evaluation and synthesis of evidence/integration of evidence into decision making/implementing evidence-based changes,

(e) measuring outcomes, and

(f) disseminating findings.

Evidence-based leadership requires two levels of commitment: (1) self-actualization of EBP and public demonstration of EBP as the foundation of daily practice and decision making and (2) facilitation of the enculturation of EBP throughout the organization(s) (Rycroft-Malone, 2004).

Self-actualization and demonstration of EBP by leaders includes embracing EBP in their own practice by attaining EBP knowledge/skills, developing a pro-EBP attitude, role modeling EBP by making evidence-based leadership decisions themselves, publicly navigating EBP barriers, and recognizing EBP achievements. Beyond leaders' individual responsibilities to embrace EBP they are, by virtue of their position, power, and authority, accountable to facilitate the enculturation of EBP throughout their organizations. By embracing and role modeling EBP as well as creating a culture and environment that adopts, values, and implements EBP, evidence-based leaders build work environments and context where EBP can not only arrive but also survive and thrive.

The EBP imperative is supported by professional organizations in their scope and standards of practice statements. The ANA *Scope and Standards of Practice for the Nurse Administrator* (2010) maintains that the nurse administrator will "attain knowledge and competency reflective of contemporary current practice and integrate research findings into practice, utilize evidence and research findings, enhance the quality and effectiveness of nursing practice, nursing services administration and the delivery of services, and evaluate nursing practice against the exiting evidence and incorporate new knowledge to improve the quality of care" (ANA, 2010). The American Organization of Nurse Executives (AONE, 2010) sets forth competencies similar to ANA for healthcare leaders in executive roles. With its vision of "shaping the future of healthcare through innovative nursing leadership," the organization recognizes that nursing leaders must be proficient and competent in leadership practice to ensure excellence in patient care (AONE). Additionally, AONE emphasizes that leaders must be innovative and competent in five domains of practice: (1) communication and relationship building, (2) knowledge of the healthcare environment, (3) leadership, (4) professionalism, and (5) business skills. Competencies in all of these domains are essential for the leader to influence and cultivate a culture of innovation and EBP.

The ANCC Magnet Recognition Program, considered the highest recognition for nursing excellence, acknowledges healthcare organizations for achieving quality outcomes in patient care, innovative nursing practice, and care excellence. EBP is evident and supported throughout the Magnet model including the requirement that organizations describe components and sources of evidence that promote superior performance and excellent outcomes in their enterprise (ANCC 2008). Healthcare organizations that have achieved magnet status ensure that their clinicians are educated about EBP and research to ensure that they are able to search the literature and explore new and best practices for patient care. Leaders in Magnet organizations need to establish an infrastructure to create and sustain strong EBP and research programs. These individuals must guarantee that financial resources are secured in order to support and encourage scholarly inquiry, EBP, and research initiatives in the organization.

It is apparent that professional organizations understand the critical function that all healthcare leaders play in creating a culture of EBP. Literature from these organizations consistently conveys the expectation to leaders that they must demonstrate competency in and enact EBP on a consistent basis in order to lead the transformation needed in health care.

Organizational Structure to Promote EBP

In the majority of healthcare organizations in the U. S., there are traditional structures and hierarchies that are responsible for the delivery of services. Although titles may vary, these hierarchies generally include a chief nursing officer/executive, nursing directors, and unit-based nurse managers. Currently, organizations function within these inevitable structures and, for better or worse, they are the structures through which the EBP paradigm shift must be driven. For now, transformation to an EBP paradigm must occur though traditional structures, where both strong leadership and strong management are necessary for optimal effectiveness. As opportunities to reinvent organizational structures arise in the future, the call for leadership at each and every level of the hierarchy will need to be established for peak performance.

Contributions of Managers and Leaders

Managers and leaders make valuable contributions to the organization; however, the contributions from each is unique and different (Lunenburg, 2011). Kotter (2013) defines management as a set of processes, including budgeting and planning, organizing and staffing, controlling, and problem solving. According to Bennies, manager qualities and functions include administers, maintains, focuses on systems and structure, relies on control, holds a short range view, asks how and when, and has their eye on the bottom line and "does things right." When managers exercise their authority to ensure things are completed and advocate for consistency and maintaining the status quo, they reduce uncertainty and maintain stability of the organization on a day-to-day basis (Lunenburg, 2011). In contrast, leaders challenge the status quo and advocate for change and innovation. Leadership involves developing a vision and aligning people with that vision. The leader focuses on people; they motivate and inspire others to act by empowering them, thus building trust and commitment. They use their influence to create change in the organization in order to take it into the future (Kotter, 2013; Lunenburg, 2011).

It is clear that, in today's complex and dynamic healthcare organizations, strong leaders and managers are vital. Managers are needed to stabilize the complex organization in order to produce efficiency and reliability while leaders are needed to promote change and innovation to guide the organization into the future (Kotter, 2013). However, regardless of the title held, all clinicians within the leadership hierarchy are responsible to be evidence-based leaders. They must embrace the EBP paradigm in their own personal practice, integrate EBP into their decision making processes, and promote EBP in their sphere(s) of influence on a day to day basis.

LEADERSHIP STYLES AND THEORIES

Although many leadership theories exist, there are several that are relevant to contemporary nursing and healthcare leadership. These models of leadership focus on the relationship between the leader and the follower in order to achieve a common goal. In these relationship-based theories, the leader creates an environment where individuals are supported and recognized for their work and achievement. They feel inspired and empowered to innovate and change, resulting in positive outcomes for the organization. These attributes are critical components of an EBP culture. The theoretical models of relationship based leadership include but are not limited to innovation leadership, transformational leadership, servant leadership, and authentic leadership. While any of these leadership theories is appropriate for the healthcare leader of today, the concept of evidence-based leadership must be synergistically incorporated in tandem with the style adopted by the leader.

Innovation Leadership

Innovative leaders create an infrastructure that weaves innovation into their organization. Within a culture of innovation, employees are both empowered and encouraged to challenge the status quo and integrate new processes and technologies into the organization so that systems operate more effectively and efficiently.

Traditionally, healthcare organizations tend to avoid risk and maintain comfort where costs and outcomes are controlled and well known. Innovation and risk-taking are not traditionally viewed as positive attributes of the leader in health care. More emphasis is placed on continuing routine practices that are predictable and worked yesterday, or reworking ineffective processes, rather than taking initiative to advance innovation and move the organization to the desired future. Many contemporary leaders will challenge this traditional view of leadership in light of the looming need to transform healthcare organizations into cost-effective, efficient systems where quality and patient safety are the norm. While all leaders must maintain the necessary skills of planning, organizing, and evaluating, innovative leaders have the ability to support innovation and manage change (Porter-O'Grady & Malloch, 2010).

The innovative leader is an individual who can create the "context for innovation to occur; and create and implement the roles, decision making structures, physical space, partnerships, networks and equipment that supports innovative thinking and testing" (Malloch & Porter-O'Grady, 2009). The innovative leader is ideally suited to create the systems and structures that support implementation and sustainability of EBP, including fostering creativity and innovation to build systems and structures that support EBP; facilitating organizational changes needed to promote EBP as the foundation of all decision making; and development of partnerships and networks to hard-wire and embed EBPs and processes that will persist over time. In order to sustain an innovative culture, innovative leaders must be present and leading the organization. Malloch (2008) defines eight categories of competence for the innovative leader.

1. **Essence of Innovation**: focus is on the content of innovation
2. **Innovation Knowledge**: knowledge and experience in the concepts and processes of innovation
3. **Self-Knowledge and Competence**: understanding of one's personal strengths and limitations
4. **Collaboration**: effective collaboration is based on listening, encouraging feedback, openness, and conflict resolution
5. **Synthesis**: ability to manage considerable amount of data and information and quickly evaluate the evidence, value and outcomes
6. **Formulation**: collection of related information/evidence with subsequent identification of gaps in the information or evidence
7. **Managing Knowledge**: examine new technology from the perspective of enhancing the organization rather than a perspective focused only on the new technology
8. **Coaching**: coaches others in the principles of innovation, adult learning and change

Transformational Leadership

Transformational leadership is defined as a state in which leaders and followers "find meaning and purpose in their work, and grow and develop as a result of their relationship" (Barker, Sullivan, & Emery, 2006, p. 16). As a result of this relationship, leaders and followers become partners in pursuit of a common goal. Transformational leaders are energetic, compassionate, and enthusiastic. They have the ability to provide a vision, motive, and inspire others. As a result, followers gain trust in, admiration of, and respect for their leader. The environment created by transformational leaders is change oriented, supportive of new ideas, innovative, and open (Klainberg & Dirschel, 2010). The transformational leader is uniquely able to create and sustain environments where EBP can thrive by leveraging the deep trust-based relationships they have cultivated at multiple levels across the organization.

There are four dimensions that comprise transformational leadership: idealized influence, inspirational motivation, intellectual stimulation, and individualized consideration (Bass & Avolio, 1993). These four dimensions of transformational leadership create a synergy within a workplace where EBP can flourish and patient care quality and satisfaction excel.

- **Idealized influence**—Transformational leaders serve as role models for followers and build respect and trust. They focus on doing things right rather than ensuring that their followers do the right things (Modassir & Singh, 2008).
- **Inspirational motivation**—Transformational leaders articulate a clear vision for their followers. They are charismatic, infuse enthusiasm and optimism, and can inspire and motivate others to accomplish great achievements (Bass & Riggio, 2006; Modassir & Singh, 2008).
- **Intellectual stimulation**—Transformational leaders encourage innovation and creativity. They empower followers to explore new ways of doing things and approach problems using EBP (Doody & Doody, 2012).
- **Individualized consideration**—Transformational leaders provide support and encouragement for followers. They offer reward and recognize individuals for their unique contributions (Bass & Riggio, 2006; Modassir & Singh, 2008).

Servant Leadership

Servant leadership is both a leadership philosophy and a set of leadership behaviors. First coined by Robert K. Greenleaf in 1970, servant leadership is based on the essential elements of trust, empathy, caring, and focus on others (Greenleaf Center for Servant Leadership, 2013). Greenleaf asserted that great leadership grows out of service, and great leaders are servants first (Gersh, 2006). A servant leader shares power and focuses on the growth and well-being of their followers allowing them to reach their full potential and perform to their highest level. In that, leadership is measured not by the accumulation of exercise of power by one individual at the top of a hierarchy but rather by whether those being served develop as individuals to become more autonomous, independent, wiser, healthier, and likely to become servant leaders themselves. The servant leader can develop an EBP culture and environment by leveraging their rich relationships with individuals in the organization to build teams with strong beliefs in the value and importance of EBP. Because the servant leader is devoted to developing individuals on their teams, servant leaders are uniquely poised to cultivate committed EBP champions who perform at their highest level and encourage others to follow in their pursuit of excellence. Spears (2010) describes 10 foundational characteristics that are central to servant leadership:

- **Listening**—Traditionally, skills for all leaders have been recognized as communication and competence in decision making. Albeit these are also aptitudes for the servant leader, they are reinforced by consistently listening intently and carefully to others.
- **Empathy**—Individuals should be valued for their unique characteristics and contributions. The servant leader seeks to understand and empathize with their followers.
- **Healing**—The ability to heal relationships is a powerful strength of the servant leader. By helping others to solve problems and conflicts in relationships, the leader supports and promotes the personal growth of their followers.
- **Awareness**—Self-awareness allows the servant leader to view situations from a more holistic standpoint. This provides the leader an awareness, and better understanding of issues surrounding ethics, power, and values.
- **Persuasion**—The servant leader effectively builds consensus among followers and relies on persuasion, rather than power by authority to influence others and achieve organizational goals.
- **Conceptualization**—Thinking beyond the day to day realities requires a broader based conceptual thinking. The servant leader can see beyond the limits of the operating business and focus on long term goals.
- **Foresight**—Deeply rooted in the intuitive mind, foresight enables the servant leader the ability to learn from the past in order to understand the present and identify consequence of a decision for the future.
- **Stewardship**—Servant leadership is seen as an obligation to serving the needs of others. It stresses the use of openness and persuasion, rather than control.
- **Commitment to the growth of people**—the servant leader is committed to the personal, professional, and spiritual growth and development of each individual.
- **Building community**—A servant leader desires to develop a true community among businesses

Those who are led by servant leaders are proposed to reach their full potential and perform optimally (Greenleaf Center for Servant Leadership, 2013), thus making this theory a good fit for facilitating a culture of EBP.

Authentic Leadership

Authentic leaders are described as individuals who are confident, hopeful, optimistic, resilient, transparent, and possess high moral character. These leaders demonstrate self-awareness; they are aware of how they think and behave. They have a keen sense of who they are and where they stand on issues, values, and beliefs (Wong & Cummings, 2009).

Authentic leaders are role models and focus on the ethical and right thing to do. The development of others is a priority, and they work to ensure that their communication is transparent and comprehended as intended (Wong & Cummings, 2009). Followers perceive them as having an intense awareness of their own and others values, moral perspectives, knowledge, and strengths (Avolio, Gardner, Walumbwa, Luthans, & May, 2004). Authentic leaders are able to create and sustain high quality relationships with their followers via personal identification, which results in enhanced engagement, increased motivation, commitment, and job satisfaction (Avolio et al., 2004; Wong & Laschinger, 2013). The authentic leader is uniquely poised to lead the transition to an EBP culture through role modeling of EBP, engaging and motivating their teams to adopt best practices, and enthusiastically celebrating delivery of the best and most ethical care possible for patients.

Authentic leaders are able to build trust and healthier work environments through four types of behaviors: balanced processing, internalized moral perspective, relational transparency, and self-awareness (Avolio et al., 2004; Walumbwa, Peterson, Avolio, & Hartnell, 2010; Wong & Cummings, 2009).

◆ **Balanced processing**—The authentic leader is able to objectively analyze data in order to formulate decisions. They often solicit views that may challenge traditional ideas in order to come to a conclusion. These leaders possess the capability for accurate self-assessment and can act on these assessments without being diverted by self-protective intentions (Bamford et al., 2013; Wong, & Laschinger, 2013).

◆ **Internalized moral perspective**—The authentic leader role models high standards for moral and ethical conduct (Wong & Laschinger, 2013).

◆ **Relational transparency**—The authentic leader presents their genuine self to their followers. They share their values, emotions, and goals in a transparent manner which encourages followers to be forthcoming with their ideas and opinions (Bamford et al., 2013; Wong & Laschinger, 2013). These leaders strive to achieve trust by listening to and accepting others' opinions and views, and acting on recommendations (Wong & Cummings, 2009).

◆ **Self-awareness**—Defined as the ability to assess one's strengths and weaknesses, self-awareness is a process by which the authentic leader begins to understand their unique talents, beliefs, and desires (Wong & Cummings, 2009). Leaders with a high self-awareness use their knowledge of themselves to enhance their leadership effectiveness (Walumbwa et al., 2010).

These core behaviors resonate with competencies to promote, build, and sustain a culture of EBP. While any of these leadership styles is appropriate for the healthcare leader of today, the concept of evidence-based leadership must work in tandem with the leadership style/theory. As an evidence-based leader, role modeling, empowering others, and optimizing others to reach their full potential creates the infrastructure for best practice and positive outcomes.

UNIQUE ROLE OF LEADERS IN CHANGING THE EBP PARADIGM

Healthcare leaders must leverage their positions and power within organizational hierarchies to create organizations that are ready to integrate and sustain EBP. They should be knowledgeable about the current barriers and facilitators of EBP that clinicians articulate (Melnyk et al., 2012) and acknowledge that they have control over multiple aspects of them. Healthcare leaders must find ways to eliminate persistent barriers and advocate for clinicians to have the time, resources, and support to implement EBP. They must create and sustain work environments where the resources that clinicians need to implement EBP and provide best patient care are a reality of daily practice.

Some of the EBP barriers that healthcare leaders can address easily within their scope of authority and responsibility include:

◆ Arranging EBP education/skill building opportunities
◆ Prioritizing operational budgets to include EBP resources
◆ Revamping job descriptions and performance evaluation tools to reflect EBP expectations
◆ Integrating EBP deliverables into clinical ladder requirements
◆ Rewriting the organizational mission statement with clear EBP language included
◆ Reorganizing traditional reporting structures to better align the organization with the EBP paradigm
◆ Creating dedicated EBP mentor positions and hiring individuals with robust EBP knowledge and skills in the steps of EBP as well as change theory

There are other barriers to EBP that are more challenging for healthcare leaders to address; however, it is imperative that they be faced. Some of these barriers include allotting more time for clinicians to implement EBP and assuring that managers and leaders support EBP activities. Examples of strategies to address barriers to implementing and sustaining a culture of EBP are shown in Table 11.1.

Table 11.1 Leadership Strategies to Address EBP Barriers

Strategy	Activities	Measures
EBP education and skills building	• Develop EBP content and skill building programs targeted to clinicians at various levels of practice including; staff, managers and directors • Include EBP content and EBP competencies in onboarding/orientation and residency programs designed for new hires.	• Number of education programs developed with outcomes • Number of education programs delivered • Number of new hires oriented to EBP content • EBP knowledge, beliefs and implementation scores (pre/post) for all groups
Operational budgets for EBP resources	• Purchase computers dedicated for EBP work • Allot/budget time for EBP project work	• Number of dedicated EBP workstations • Number of hours allotted per EBP project reported with EBP project outcomes
Library services support	• Access to Library with adequate clinical databases and journals available • Support from librarians knowledgeable in EBP steps and processes	• Number of databases available • Number of journals available • Number of librarian referrals • Number of librarian searches provided to staff
Job descriptions and performance evaluation tools	• Write or revise job descriptions with EBP competencies/expectations articulated • Write or revise performance appraisal tools with EBP outcomes/deliverables articulated	• Revised staff job descriptions • Revised staff performance appraisal tools
Clinical ladder requirements	• Write or rewrite clinical ladder application with progressive EBP requirements at each level	• New clinical ladder with EBP requirements for each level
Organizational mission, vision and values statements	• Write or rewrite organizational and departmental mission, vision and values statements with EBP language integrated	• Organizational mission, vision and values statements written with EBP language integrated • Number of departmental mission, vision and values statements written with EBP language integrated

Strategy	Activities	Measures
EBP mentors aligned within the organization	• Structure EBP mentors/ champions centrally within the organization to promote, support and sustain a unified message and vision of EBP • Designate a dedicated, knowledgeable EBP leader to oversee EBP activities and create and inspire the EBP culture.	• EBP mentors reporting to a centralized leader • Organizational chart reflecting centralized EBP structure • Knowledgeable EBP leader designated
EBP mentor positions	• Create designated EBP mentor positions with specific job descriptions • Align EBP mentors centrally in the organization • Hire individuals with robust knowledge and skills in the steps of EBP as well as behavioral motivation and change theory to fill EBP mentor positions	• EBP mentor job description created • % of EBP mentor positions filled
Manager and leader accountability	• Write or rewrite leadership job descriptions with EBP expectations articulated • Write or revise performance appraisal tools with EBP outcomes/deliverables required	• Revised leadership job descriptions • Revised leadership performance appraisal tools

In addition, healthcare leaders need to design spaces and systems that promote EBP at the bedside, justify positions that support EBP in their personnel budgets, and provide a professional practice work environment where clinicians have autonomy and control over their practices. Regardless of how difficult these challenges may be, it is the ethical and professional responsibility of health care leaders to enact bold actions to promote the EBP shift in nursing and health care to assure best practices and, ultimately, best care for patients. Finally, healthcare leaders must use best evidence in making their own leadership decisions, thereby modeling EBP behaviors, making the best decisions possible, and providing the best practice environment for their staff and patients.

Healthcare leaders influence EBP through their roles and positions in organizations. Adams and Erickson (2011) have explored the definition and scope of influence related to nursing leadership specifically. In their work, influence is framed as "critical to chief nursing executives," and posited as a nurse leader competency (p. 186). In addition, the American Organization of Nurse Executives has included influence as an essential component of nurse executive competency (AONE, 2005), and the ANA identifies influence in its nurse administrator *Scope and Standards for Nursing Administration* (American Clinicians Association, 2001, 2010). Adams and Erickson also state that although healthcare leaders recognize the importance of influence related to affecting change in their organizations, they are not "familiar with how influence is acquired, enhanced, and strategically applied" (p. 186). The *Adams Influence Model* (AIM) is a framework designed to promote understanding of the factors, attributes, and process of influence and it is intended for use by healthcare leaders "as a guide to maximizing their individual influence and that of the profession" (Adams & Erickson, 2011, p. 186). The AIM recognizes that the healthcare leaders' influence in a given situation is a combination of their individual influence characteristics such as authority, communication style, and knowledge as well as the particular situation being addressed. The model posits that, beyond the personal influence attributes of the nurse leader, interpersonal and social system characteristics are interrelated and affect the level of influence of the nurse leader. The AIM Model was conceptualized to provide a systematic tool for nurse executives to "consider when developing an influence strategy" (Adams & Erickson, p. 187) and, as such, is an excellent tool for healthcare leaders to become familiar. The application of similar frameworks can help healthcare leaders build, assess, and enhance their personal influence capacity to positively influence their staff and their organizations, both in a general sense and as it relates to the shift toward an EBP paradigm. Having a better understanding of their influence and power will enable nurse executives to more effectively promote and sustain EBP. Leaders in health care are uniquely poised and directly responsible to implement evidence-based leadership and influence their organizations to promote best care and deliver best outcomes. By embracing and supporting EBP, leaders make a conscientious and active choice to achieve these goals.

EVIDENCE-BASED PRACTICE COMPETENCIES AS A KEY STRATEGY FOR SUSTAINING EVIDENCE-BASED CARE

Competencies are used across a variety of health professions as a mechanism for clinicians to provide high-quality safe care. The measurement of competencies related to various patient care activities is a standard ongoing activity in a multitude of healthcare organizations across the nation. For example, general competencies for nursing have been developed by the Quality and Safety Education for Nurses (QSEN) Project, which is a global nursing initiative whose purpose was to develop competencies that would "prepare future nurses who would have the knowledge, skills and attitudes necessary to continuously improve the quality and safety of the healthcare systems within which they work" (QSEN, 2013). This project has developed competency recommendations that address the following practice issues, these are the 6 QSEN competencies. (a) patient-centered care, (b) teamwork and collaboration, (c) EBP, (d) quality improvement, (e) safety, and (f) informatics.

Through a consensus-building process by a panel of seven national experts who developed an initial set of EBP competencies for practicing registered nurses (RNs) and advanced practice nurses (APNs) followed by two rounds of a Delphi survey with 80 EBP mentors across the United States to establish consensus, a final set of 13 competencies for practicing RNs and APNs in real-world healthcare settings now exists (see Table 11.2) (Melnyk, Gallagher-Ford, Long, & Fineout-Overholt, 2014).

Leaders can incorporate these EBP competencies into healthcare system expectations, orientation programs for new clinicians, performance appraisals, and job descriptions. These competencies also can be used for clinical ladder promotions processes in order to drive higher quality, reliability, and consistency of health care as well as to reduce costs.

In summary, healthcare leaders must take an evidence-based approach to decision making in their organizations and provide resources that support EBP. In addition, they must create cultures and environments in which clinicians can implement and sustain EBP for the ultimate purpose of improving healthcare quality and patient outcomes as well as reducing costs. Creating a vision, mission, and goals for the organization that include EBP along with adopting EBP competencies and incorporating them into role expectations and job performance requirements will communicate high prioritization of EBP within the institution.

Table 11.2 EBP Competencies

Evidence-Based Practice Competencies for Practicing Registered Nurses

1. Questions clinical practices for the purpose of improving the quality of care.
2. Describes clinical problems using internal evidence.* (*internal evidence = evidence generated internally within a clinical setting, such as patient assessment data, outcomes management, and quality improvement data)
3. Participates in the formulation of clinical questions using PICOT* format. (*PICOT = Patient population; Intervention or area of Interest; Comparison intervention or group; Outcome; Time).
4. Searches for external evidence* to answer focused clinical questions. (*external evidence = evidence generated from research)
5. Participates in critical appraisal of pre-appraised evidence (such as clinical practice guidelines, evidence-based policies and procedures, and evidence syntheses).
6. Participates in the critical appraisal of published research studies to determine their strength and applicability to clinical practice.
7. Participates in the evaluation and synthesis of a body of evidence gathered to determine its' strength and applicability to clinical practice.
8. Collects practice data (e.g., individual patient data, quality improvement data) systematically as internal evidence for clinical decision making in the care of individuals, groups and populations.
9. Integrates evidence gathered from external and internal sources in order to plan evidence-based practice changes.
10. Implements practice changes based on evidence and clinical expertise and patient preferences to improve care processes and patient outcomes.
11. Evaluates outcomes of evidence-based decisions and practice changes for individuals, groups and populations to determine best practices.
12. Disseminates best practices supported by evidence to improve quality of care and patient outcomes.
13. Participates in strategies to sustain an evidence-based practice culture.

Evidence-Based Practice Competencies for Advanced Practice Nurses

All competencies of RNs AND:

14. Systematically conducts and exhaustive search for external evidence* to answer clinical questions. (*external evidence = evidence generated from research)
15. Critically appraises relevant pre-appraised evidence (i.e., clinical guidelines, summaries, synopses, syntheses of relevant external evidence) and primary studies, including evaluation and synthesis.
16. Integrates a body of external evidence from nursing and related fields with internal evidence* in making decisions about patient care. (*internal evidence = evidence generated internally within a clinical setting, such as patient assessment data, outcomes management, and quality improvement data)
17. Leads transdisciplinary teams in applying synthesized evidence to initiate clinical decisions and practice changes to improve the health of individuals, groups, and populations.
18. Generates internal evidence through outcomes management and EBP implementation projects for the purpose of integrating best practices.
19. Measures processes and outcomes of evidence-based clinical decisions.
20. Formulates evidence-based policies and procedures.
21. Participates in the generation of external evidence with other healthcare professionals.
22. Mentors others in evidence-based decision making and the EBP process.
23. Implements strategies to sustain an EBP culture.
24. Communicates best evidence to individuals, groups, colleagues, and policy-makers.

© Melnyk & Gallagher-Ford, 2013.

EBP FAST FACTS

◆ In order for clinicians to change their behavior and consistently implement EBP, a multitude of interventions are necessary, including: EBP education combined with active repetitive skills building, EBP mentorship or facilitation and support, a culture and an environment that supports EBP, leaders and managers who support and role model EBP, and strategies to overcome system barriers.

◆ Leaders in healthcare systems must engage in evidence-based leadership, which is a problem-solving approach to leading and influencing organizations or groups to achieve a common goal that integrates the conscientious use of best evidence with leadership expertise and stakeholders' preferences and values.

◆ Leaders in healthcare organizations must role model evidence-based decision making if they expect their staff to consistently deliver evidence-based care.

◆ Leaders must create and sustain work cultures and environments where the resources clinicians need to implement EBP and provide best patient care are a reality of daily practice.

◆ Incorporation of EBP competencies into role performance expectations, evaluations, and clinical ladder systems is essential in creating an evidence-based organization.

References

Adams, J. M., & Erickson, J. I. (2011). Applying the Adams influence model in nurse executive practice. *The Journal of Nursing Administration, 41*, 186–192.

American Nurses Association. (2001, 2010). *Code of ethics for nurses with interpretive statements.* Silver Spring, MD: nursesbooks.org.

American Nurses Association. (2010). *Nursing: Scope and standards of practice.* Silver Springs, MD: nursesbooks. org.

American Organization of Nurses Executives. (2005). AONE nurse executive competencies. *Nurse Leader, 3*(1), 50–56.

American Nurses Credentialing Center. (2008). *The magnet model components and sources of evidence: Magnet recognition program.* Silver Springs, MD: American Nurses Credentialing Center

American Organization of Nurses Executives. (2010). *AONE guiding principles: For the role of the nurse in future patient care delivery.* Retrieved from http://www.aone.org/resources/PDFs/AONE_GP_for_Role_of_Nurse _Future

Avolio, B., Gardner, W., Walumbwa, F., Luthans, F., & May, D. (2004). Unlocking the mask: A look at the process by which authentic leaders impact follower attitudes and behaviors. *The Leadership Quarterly, 15*, 801–823.

Bamford, M., Wong, C. A., & Laschinger, H. (2013). The influence of authentic leadership and areas of worklife on work engagement of registered nurses. *Journal of Nursing Management, 21,* 529–540.

Barker, A. M., Sullivan, D. T., & Emery, M. J. (2006). *Leadership competencies for clinical managers: The renaissance of transformational leadership.* Jones & Bartlett Learning.

Bass, B., & Avolio, B. (1993). Transformational leadership and organizational culture. *Public Administration Quarterly, 17*(1), 112–121.

Bass, B. M., & Riggio, R. E. (2006). *Transformational Leadership* (2nd ed.). New York: Psychology Press.

Beckette, M., Quiter, E., Ryan, G., Berrebi, C., Taylor, S., Cho, M., … Kahn, K. (2011). Bridging the gap between basic science and clinical practice: The role of organizations in addressing clinician barriers. *Implementation Science, 6*(35). doi:10.1186/1748-5908-6-35.

Bennis, W. (1991). Managing the dream: Leadership in the 21st century. *The Antioch Review, 49*(1), 22.

Doody, O., & Doody, C. M. (2012). Transformational leadership in nursing practice. *British Journal of Nursing, 21*(20), 1212–1218.

Dopson, S., FitzGerald, L., Ferlie, E., Gabbay, J., & Locock, L. (2002). No magic targets! Changing clinical practice to become more evidence based. *Healthcare Management Review, 27*(3), 35–47.

Gerrish, K., & Clayton, J. (2004). Promoting evidence based practice: An organizational approach. *Journal of Nursing Management, 12*, 114–123.

Gersh, M. R. (2006). Servant-Leadership: A philosophical foundation for professionalism in physical therapy. *Journal of Physical Therapy Education, 20*(2), 12.

Greenleaf Center for Servant Leadership. (2013). Retrieved from http://www.greenleaf.org

Hutchinson, A., & Johnston, L. (2004). Bridging the divide: A survey of nurses' opinions regarding barriers to, and facilitators of, research utilization in the practice setting. *Journal of Clinical Nursing, 13*, 304–315.

Klainberg, M., & Dirschel, K. (Eds.). (2010). *Today's nursing leader: Managing, succeeding, excelling*. Jones & Bartlett Learning.

Kotter, J. (2013). *Management is (still) not leadership*. Retrieved from http://blogs.hbr.org/kotter/2013/01/management-is-still-not-leadership.html

Leader. (n.d.). In *dictionary.refence.com online dictionary*. Retrieved from http://www.dictionary.reference.com/leader

Lunenburg, F. C. (2011). Leadership versus management: A key distinction—at least in theory. *International Journal of Management, Business, and Administration, 14*(1), 1–4.

Malloch, K. (2008). Empowered for action: Innovation leaders making a difference in health care organizations. *Voice of Nursing Leadership, AONE*, 12–13.

Malloch, K., & Porter-O'Grady, T. (2009). *Introduction to evidence based practice in nursing and healthcare*. Sudbury, MA: Jones and Bartlett.

Melnyk, B. M., Fineout-Overholt, E., Fischbeck Feinstein, N., Li, H., Small, L., Wilcox, L., & Kraus, R. (2004). Nurses perceived knowledge, beliefs, skills, and needs regarding evidence based practice: Implications for accelerating the paradigm shift. *Worldviews on Evidence Based Nursing, 1*, 185–193.

Melnyk, B. M., Fineout-Overholt, E., Gallagher-Ford, L., & Kaplan, L. (2011). The state of evidence-based practice in U.S. nurses: Critical implications for nurse leaders and educators. *Journal of Nursing Administration, 42*(9), 410–417.

Melnyk, B. M., Fineout-Overholt, E., & Mays, M. Z. (2008). The evidence-based practice beliefs and implementation scales: Psychometric properties of two new scales. *Worldviews on Evidence Based Nursing, 5*, 208–216. doi:10.1111/j.1741-6787.2008.00126.x.

Melnyk, B. M., Gallagher-Ford, L., Long, L. A., & Fineout-Overholt, E. (2014). The establishment of evidence-based practice competencies for practicing registered nurses and advanced practice nurses in real world clinical settings: Proficiencies to improve healthcare quality, reliability, patient outcomes and costs. *Worldviews on Evidence-Based Nursing*. doi 10.1111/wvn.12021 WVN 2014;00:1–11.

Melnyk, B. M., Grossman, D. C., Chou, R., Mabry-Hernandez, I., Nicholson, W., Dewitt, T. G., … US Preventive Services Task Force. (2012). USPSTF perspective on evidence-based preventive recommendations for children. *Pediatrics, 130*(2), e399–e407.

Modassir, A., & Singh, T. (2008). Relationship of emotional intelligence with transformational leadership and organizational citizenship behavior. *International Journal of Leadership Studies, 4*(1), 3–21.

Porter-O'Grady, T., & Malloch, K. (2010). *Quantum leadership; Advancing innovation, transforming healthcare*. Sudbury, MA: Jones and Bartlett.

Pravikoff, D. S., Tanner, A. B., & Pierce, S. T. (2005). Readiness of U.S. nurses for evidence-based practice. *American Journal of Nursing, 105*(9), 40–51.

Quality and Safety Education for Nurses (QSEN). (2013). Retrieved from http://qsen.org/about-qsen/project-overview/

Rycroft-Malone, J. (2004). The PARIHS framework: A framework for guiding the implementation of evidence-based practice. *Journal of Nursing Care Quality, 19*(4), 297–304.

Rycroft-Malone, J. (2008). Evidence-informed practice: From individual to context. *Journal of Nursing Management, 16*, 404–408.

Rycroft-Malone, J., Harvey, G., Seers, K., Kitson, A., McCormack, B., & Titchen, A. (2004). An exploration of the factors that influence the implementation of evidence into practice. *Journal of Clinical Nursing, 13*, 913–924.

Rycroft-Malone, J., Seers, K., Titchen, A., Harvey, G., Kitson, A., & McCormack, B. (2004). What counts as evidence in evidence-based practice? *Journal of Advanced Nursing, 47*, 81–90.

Sandström, B., Borglin, G., Nilsson, R., & Willman, A. (2011). Promoting the implementation of evidence-based practice: A literature review focusing on the role of nursing leadership. *Worldviews on Evidence-Based Nursing, 8*(4), 212–223. doi:10.1111/j.1741-6787.2011.00216.x.

Scott-Findlay, S., & Golden-Biddle, K. (2005). Understanding how organizational culture shapes research use. *Journal of Nursing Administration, 15*, 359–365.

Spears, L. (2010). Character and servant leadership: Ten characteristics of effective, caring leaders. *The Journal of Virtues and Leadership, 1*(1), 25–30.

Walumbwa, F. O., Peterson, S. J., Avolio, B. J., & Hartnell, C. A. (2010). An investigation of the relationships among leader and follower psychological capital, service climate, and job performance. *Personnel Psychology, 63*(4), 937–963.

Wong, C., & Cummings, G. (2009). Authentic leadership: A new theory for nursing or back to basics? *Journal of Health Organization and Management, 23*(5), 522–538.

Wong, C., & Laschinger, H. (2013). Authentic leadership, performance, and job satisfaction: The mediating role of empowerment. *Journal of Advanced Nursing, 69*(4), 947–959. doi:10.1111/j.1365-2648.2012.06089.

Making EBP Real: A Success Story

Improving Outcomes for Depressed Adolescents with the Brief Cognitive Behavioral COPE Intervention Delivered in 30-Minute Outpatient Visits

Pamela Lusk, DNP, RN, PMHNP-BC

Clinical Associate Professor-The Ohio State University College of Nursing
Psychiatric/Mental Health Nurse Practitioner-Community Health Center of Yavapai County, AZ

Step 0: The Spirit of Inquiry Ignited

Major depressive disorder is a treatable medical illness. Despite a prevalence of 9% of adolescents with major depressive disorder or depressive symptoms that impair their functioning, less than 25% of depressed adolescents receive the evidence-based treatment they need. In outpatient mental health settings, advanced practice psychiatric nurses conduct comprehensive psychiatric evaluations with adolescents, spend time learning about their strengths, symptoms and struggles, and establish and implement treatment plans. For teens with symptoms of depression, their day to day life can be a painful struggle. Typically, parents come to the practice feeling helpless and wanting the best most active treatment to help their child feel less depressed and function better. We, as psychiatric advanced practice registered nurses (APRNs), know that the most robust treatment for depression in adolescents involves psychotherapy (which historically has been in 50 minute "hours") and medication (if indicated). Many psychiatric APRNs now practice in settings where there has been a shift to brief 20- to 30-minute medication visits with patients due to agency requirements to see an increasing number of patients each work day. APRNs are expected to adhere to the clinic schedule while providing the best evidence-based care to our young patients. Often we do not know how to bridge the gap between what the research indicates is best practice for treatment of depression in teens and what is happening in practice. This led me to wonder about whether it would be possible to deliver evidence-based cognitive behavioral therapy (CBT) and improve treatment outcomes for depressed adolescents within the limitation of 30-minute medication evaluation appointments. I needed to use the EBP process to find out.

Step 1: The PICOT Question Formulated

In depressed adolescents (P), how does CBT (I) compared to other psychotherapy interventions (C) improve depressive symptoms (O) over a 3-month period (T)?

Step 2: Search Strategy Conducted

The Cochrane Database of Systematic Reviews (CDSR) was searched first with the keywords adolescent, depression, treatment effectiveness evaluation, and psychotherapy. A systematic review by Watanabe, Hunot, Omori, Churchill, and Farukawa (2007) was found that reviewed studies of psychotherapy effectiveness for children and adolescents with depression. Next, MEDLINE, PsycINFO, and Cumulative Index to Nursing and Allied Health Literature (CINAHL) were searched using the same keywords. The search also included the National Guidelines Clearinghouse for practice guidelines to treat depression in adolescents (Cheung et al., 2007). Both level I and level II evidence studies (Melnyk & Fineout-Overholt, 2011) were found in the search process.

Step 3: Critical Appraisal of the Evidence Performed

Rapid critical appraisal checklists were used to evaluate the validity, reliability, and applicability to practice (Melnyk & Fineout-Overholt, 2011) for each of the studies found from the search. The systematic review by Watanabe and colleagues (2007) supported CBT and Interpersonal Psychotherapy (IPT) as effective treatments for adolescents with depression. In the search of PsycINFO and other databases, several meta-analyses of randomized controlled trials (RCTs), including one conducted by McCarty and Weisz (2007), supported CBT as an effective treatment for depressed adolescents. One of the RCTs, The Treatment of Adolescent Depression Study (TADS) by March, Hilgenberg, Silva, and TADS Team (2007) was a landmark 13 site RCT that compared (1) CBT, (2) placebo, (3) antidepressant medication (fluoxetine), and (4) a combination of fluoxetine and CBT. The study determined the superior effectiveness of the combination of CBT and fluoxetine in the acute and continuation treatment of adolescent major depression.

The **level I evidence**, the strongest level of evidence to guide practice, found a systematic review and a meta-analysis of RCTs that tested the efficacy of CBT for adolescent depression. Level II evidence was also found in the TADS RCT, which is the strongest study design for controlling extraneous or confounding variables (Melnyk & Fineout-Overholt, 2011), and supported that CBT is a very efficacious treatment for adolescent depression. In the studies included in the meta-analysis, individual CBT sessions were 60 minutes long. Group CBT programs for adolescents were also included in the meta-analysis.

Cited CBT treatment manuals for depressed adolescents in the studies were reviewed for their applicability to brief sessions. In these treatment manuals, the authors recommended individual CBT sessions of 60 minutes duration. For this project, a CBT-based intervention entitled COPE (Creating Opportunities for Personal Empowerment) (Melnyk, 2003) was selected because it included all of the components identified in the literature that comprise effective CBT interventions for depressed adolescents. The manual for each of the seven COPE sessions is concise, and the COPE intervention is usable in 30-minute sessions. The seven CBT-based skill-building sessions in COPE had been previously embedded into a 15-session healthy lifestyle intervention for adolescents that was delivered in required high school health courses, but it had not yet been evaluated in a community health setting (Melnyk et al., 2007, 2009). Therefore, the purpose of this EBP change project was to implement and evaluate the outcomes of delivering COPE to teens in a community mental health clinic.

Step 4: Evidence Integrated with Clinical Expertise and Patient Preferences to Inform a Decision and Practice Change Implemented

The plan for this project based on the evidence found was to translate evidence-based CBT into brief 30-minute sessions and assess its feasibility and outcomes with 12- to 17-year-old clinically depressed adolescents treated at a community mental health center in a small, rural town in the southwestern United States.

When adolescents are seen in community mental health practices and diagnosed with moderate to severe depression, the usual treatment is antidepressant medication. Antidepressants are an effective treatment to relieve symptoms of depression, but the evidence strongly supports the combination of antidepressant medication and CBT as the most effective treatment plan. In terms of patient preferences and values, many parents who bring their adolescents for treatment do not want medication as part of the treatment plan. However, some families feel that pharmacological treatment will provide the most rapid relief for their child's depressive symptoms. The advanced practice psychiatric nurse, with education and skills in both psychotherapy and pharmacology, can provide evidence from current literature and her own practice, and encourage parents and teens to share experiences, concerns, and questions related to the acceptability of various treatment options. Together, they can establish a mutually agreed upon treatment plan. With the implementation of this project, informed consents by parents and teen assents were signed. None of the families seen for initial psychiatric evaluation of their adolescent declined the COPE cognitive behavioral skills building intervention when it was explained, reviewed, and offered as an option.

A pre- and postintervention outcomes evaluation was used. Fifteen adolescents aged 12 to 17 years, who came for intake to the community mental health center and presented with significant depression, were enrolled in the project. All of the adolescents, along with their parents, agreed to receive COPE, which was presented in seven 30-minute sessions scheduled at weekly intervals. They also agreed to fill out project-related outcome measures both before and after the COPE seven-session intervention. The measures included the Beck Youth Inventory, which has five subscales (anxiety, anger, depression, self-concept, and destructive behavior), a personal beliefs scale, a COPE content quiz, and a form that asked for demographic data about the teen and family. The parents and teens were both given post-COPE evaluation forms to fill out anonymously to provide feedback regarding their experiences with the COPE intervention.

Step 5: Outcomes Evaluated

All 15 teens enrolled completed all seven sessions of COPE. Adolescents reported significant decreases in depression, anxiety, anger, and destructive behavior as well as increases in self-concept and personal beliefs about managing negative emotions (Lusk & Melnyk, 2011a). Evaluations indicated that COPE was a positive experience for teens and parents (Lusk & Melnyk, 2011b). It was concluded that COPE is a promising brief CBT-based intervention that can be delivered within 30-minute individual outpatient visits. With this intervention, advanced practice nurses can work within busy outpatient practice time constraints and still provide evidence-based treatment for the depressed teens they manage.

Step 6: Project Outcomes Successfully Disseminated

This project was presented at national conferences and was published. The COPE intervention is now standard practice for treating my depressed and anxious teens. Other psychiatric and pediatric advanced practice nurses in community mental health and pediatric primary care settings as well as schools across the country are now using COPE to prevent and treat depressed and anxious adolescents.

References

Cheung, A., Zuckerbrot, R., Jensen, P., Ghalib, K., Laraque, D., & Stein, R. (2007). Guidelines for adolescent depression in primary care (GLAD-PC): II. Treatment and ongoing management. *Pediatrics, 120*(5), 131.

Lusk, P., & Melnyk, B. M. (2011a). The brief cognitive-behavioral COPE intervention for depressed adolescents: Outcomes and feasibility of delivery in 30 minute outpatient visits. *Journal of the American Psychiatric Nurses Association, 17*(3), 226–236.

Lusk, P., & Melnyk, B. M. (2011b). COPE for the treatment of depressed adolescents: Lessons learned from implementing an evidence-based practice change. *Journal of the American Psychiatric Nurses Association, 17*(4), 297–309.

March, J., Hilgenberg, D., Silva, S., & TADS Team. (2007). The treatment of adolescents with depression study (TADS): Long term effectiveness and safety outcomes. *Archives of General Psychiatry, 64*(10), 1132–1143.

Majid S., Foo S., Luyt B., et al. Adopting evidence based practice in clinical decision making: nurses' perceptions, knowledge, and barriers. *Journal of the Medical Library Association*, 2011; 99 (3): 229–236.

McCarty, C., & Weisz, J. (2007). Effects of psychotherapy for depression in children and adolescents: What we can (and can't) learn from meta-analysis and component profiling. *Journal of the Academy of Child and Adolescent Psychiatry, 46*(7), 879–886.

Melnyk, B. M. (2003). *COPE (Creating Opportunities for Personal Empowerment) for Teens (revised): A 7-Session Cognitive Behavioral Skills Building Program.* Columbus, OH: COPE2Thrive.

Melnyk, B. M., & Fineout-Overholt, E. (2011). *Evidence-based practice in nursing & healthcare: A guide to best practice.* Philadelphia, PA: Wolters Kluwer/Lippincott Williams & Wilkins.

Melnyk, B. M., Jacobson, D., Kelly, S., O'Haver, J., Small, L., & Mays, M. Z. (2009) Improving the mental health, healthy lifestyle choices and physical health of Hispanic adolescents: A randomized controlled pilot study. *Journal of School Health, 79*(12), 575–584.

Melnyk, B. M., Small, L., Morrison-Beedy, D., Strasser, A., Spath, L., Kreipe, R., ... O'Haver, J. (2007). The COPE healthy lifestyles TEEN program: Feasibility, preliminary, efficacy, & lessons learned from an after school group intervention with overweight adolescents. *Journal of Pediatric Health Care, 21*(5), 315–322.

Watanabe, N., Hunot, V., Omori, I., Churchill, R., & Farukawa, T. (2007). Psychotherapy for depression among children and adolescents: A systematic review. *Acta Psychiatrica Scandinavica, 116*, 84–95.

Creating and Sustaining a Culture and Environment for Evidence-Based Practice

Chapter 12

Innovation and Evidence: A Partnership in Advancing Best Practice and High Quality Care

Kathy Malloch and Tim Porter-O'Grady

> Innovation distinguishes between a leader and a follower.
>
> —Steve Jobs

RELATIONSHIP BETWEEN INNOVATION AND EVIDENCE-BASED PRACTICE

There have been many assumptions regarding the relationship between innovation and evidence-based practice (EBP), many of them incorrect. Perhaps this is because good evidence is grounded in "hard" knowledge and research skews our notions of its relationship to innovation, which is considered much more "emergent" and "fluid." However, the truth is that there is an inherent relationship between evidence and innovation, one that is both dynamic and, at the same time, rigorous and structured. Both innovation (the introduction of something new that promises to be an improvement over the past) and evidence (data obtained from multiple sources from rigorous research to anecdotal information) are essential to each other since innovation frees evidence to alter the trajectory of our practice and evidence disciplines innovation to affirm the validity of practice (Malloch & Porter-O'Grady, 2009).

A fundamental requirement for understanding EBP is that it be seen not so much as a process, but more as a dynamic (Hovmand & Gillespie, 2010). Evidence as a dynamic suggests a high level of fluidity, mobility, and portability. In fact, EBP could simply not exist in a nondigital milieu since the power and capacity of digitalization is an essential requisite to the fluidity and flow that characterizes effective EBP (Malloch & Porter-O'Grady, 2010). The massive aggregation of data and the detailed requirements of analysis and synthesis that provide the foundation for effective choice-making, decisions, and action is not so much a corollary, but instead, a characteristic of the essential dynamics associated with the complexities of EBP (Schultz, 2009). This sort of evidentiary dynamic represents a mosaic of interacting and interfacing elements and relationships that lead to definitive and replicable patterns of behavior that reflect measures of effectiveness, efficiency, and efficacy (E3) (Porter-O'Grady & Malloch, 2010). At the same time, this evidentiary dynamic lays the floor for good practice, creating the foundations for creativity and innovation. From here, clinicians can stretch to new levels of practice and clinical behavior through use of innovative practices that helps them conceive and reach for the "ceiling" of practice excellence.

The challenges in the current healthcare environment related to continuum-based delivery models, interprofessional collaboration, patient-guided care, supportive cultures for new work, and all of the associated chaos and energy provide models to illustrate these complexities. Consider the current efforts in creating a continuum-based model of care delivery in response to the mandates of national healthcare reform. Key stakeholders in healthcare systems have recognized the need for increased collaboration, fully integrated system communication, and improved patient engagement in the delivery of health care. Working to address the redesign of the healthcare infrastructure is one of the more complex challenges faced by leaders and requires an approach that considers current evidence for effective system performance and then acknowledgement of gaps in knowledge that can be logically and systematically addressed with innovative approaches.

In order to comprehend the full range of interacting characteristics in this dynamic of evidence (evidentiary dynamics), one must understand the fluid, interacting, and cybernetic (involved with cyclical communication and control) nature of its stages/phases of movement. The concept of continuous and unending movement is critical to the complete comprehension of this evidentiary dynamic informing EBP (Tait & Richardson, 2010). The foundations of good practice are simply not established only to remain constant and changeless. The clinical history of health care certainly validates—to its detriment—the health system's addiction to a fixed approach to standards and practices through the use of a procedural and policy approach (Starr, 2011). This model for defining the foundations of practice assumed that such foundations were firm and fixed in time, quite rigid, and, most often, permanent. Good practice, in this format, meant a slavish addiction to the rules and consistently and routinely repeating procedural applications. Certainly, basic rules of good process such as safety checklists, functional protocols, and procedural routines do have significant value in providing safe and effective foundations for clinical routines that require little or no variation nor are subject to the notions of human relationships, culture, and communication. Indeed, more of these would prove a significant value in reducing both risk and resource use (Lorenz, Beyea, & Slattery, 2009). Yet, even these basic and routine mechanics, if informed by insight and innovation, can be altered and radically improved or advanced in ways that could not be anticipated with the same tools and processes that created them. In spite of the often overwhelming challenges of complex changes, it is the realities of the evidence–innovation interface that provide clarity for healthcare leaders. As Sharts-Hopko (2013) noted, tackling complex ("wicked") problems is indeed the nature of much of our work.

Such problems or challenges, described as "any complex issue which defies complete definition and for which there can be no final solution; such problems are diabolical in that they resist the usual attempts to resolve them" (Brown, Harris, & Russell, 2010, p. 302), give life to current realities and guidance as to what can or should be done to address these challenges. To be sure, the complexities of continuum of care planning and integration involve multiple individuals, multiple levels and types of knowledge, varied resources, and the ever-present reality that there is no road map to the future. While the diabolical label (wicked) seems unusually harsh in the world of caring, it is within the realm of informed professionals not only to overcome such stubborn complexity, but also to thrive in creating systems that are more dynamic, thrive in massive amounts of data in a sophisticated digital world, and skillfully move in new ways to facilitate rather than control health processes.

Sharts-Hopko (2013) noted that building evidence for practice is equally as important as creating new healthcare policies, new delivery models, and processes to assure safe and cost-effective care. Multiple initiatives from the Institute of Medicine (2001, 2011) drive the need for both evidence and creative approaches to improve the healthcare system specific to the infrastructure, providers, organizational cultures, and management of financial resources.

The evidence-based innovator both is grounded in and respects the discipline of the scientific process. The innovator understands the components of good science and is schooled in both the scientific process and the translational skills which help make its products amenable to guiding practice and behavior (Erickson, Ditomassi, & Adams, 2012). Science is indeed the link between evidence and innovation; the discovery and use of the laws of nature to answer questions about the world in which we live and to invent new solutions to problems (Heilbron, 2003).

At the same time, this innovator recognizes that the products of the scientific process simply form the ground upon which the innovator stands. The foundations established by good evidence serve as the beginning database of the subsequent creative work of translating, applying, questioning, testing, changing, and adapting. The evidence-based innovator is aware of the constancy and fluidity of the movement and interface between each element of the evidentiary journey. The innovator recognizes that within this dynamic lies the opportunity for new insight, connections, configurations, and collaborations. These, in turn, lead to new ways of seeing, defining, and doing—which can inexorably raise the bar of practice and performance (McCarthy, 2011). Moreover, the innovator is aware that this can be done at any point (gap) or at any phase or stage of the evidence-based process. New insights, information, collaboration, and wisdom can inform the data at any particular point in a way that alters the cascade of subsequent decisions or actions further down the evidence-based levels. The change at any one place along the evidence-based continuum ultimately alters the entire process.

Practice leaders need to be fluid, flexible, portable, and mobile in their own leadership capacity, role-modeling these patterns of behavior as their major contribution to creating a culture of innovation. It is difficult to expect that staff can become open, responsive, dynamic, and adaptive in their practice if their leaders are rigid and procedural in the expression of their role (Marshall, 2011). Leaders must first develop a deeper and richer understanding of professional practice, the requisites of collaboration, shared decision-making, science-based systems, and the characteristics of a culture of innovation.

Models of shared governance and leadership have provided structures, processes, and outcomes that support and reinforce professional autonomy. Councils provide forums for nurse engagement and participation in advancing evidence and innovation. Bylaws, policies, and principles in the shared governance model provide direction on how decisions are made. Most importantly, the emphasis is on metrics specific to patient outcomes, nurse satisfaction, and organizational excellence. There are numerous reports and evidence supporting a shared governance model from both qualitative and quantitative perspectives (Rundquist & Givens, 2013).

When examining current shared governance models through an evidence–innovation lens, new opportunities are uncovered. Current shared governance models were never intended to be rigid and procedural; rather, they were intended to be fluid, evidence-driven, and empowering. In light of the changing healthcare environment, traditional approaches to shared governance can now be seen as incomplete for the future. Innovation is needed to advance shared governance models from models focusing on nursing autonomy and ownership to models focusing on interdisciplinary decision-making, collaboration, and measurement. The need exists for an infrastructure that meaningfully supports the discussion and debate about full scope of practice not just for one discipline, but for all of the disciplines involved in the clarification, extension, and valuing of changes to role performance. Creating divisional level-shared governance structures as well as organizational and cross-setting structures can provide more robust frameworks for a system focused on continuum of care services. As multidisciplinary, continuum shared governance structures are created, new evidence and outcome measures will emerge that reflect their value.

A MODEL OF THE CYBERNETIC INTERFACE OF INNOVATION AND EVIDENCE

A systematic understanding about the dynamics of EBP and innovation is critical to a both scholarly and practical understanding of how evidence changes practice. A rich and detailed description of the characteristics and processes associated with EBP is presented in detail elsewhere in this book. In this chapter, we create an interface between the stages of EBP and the opportunities for innovation embedded in them.

Fluid and Cybernetic Dynamic

The existence of wide gaps between clinical knowledge and practice is well known and acknowledged (Melnyk & Fineout-Overholt, 2012). In the emerging value-driven healthcare system, it will become increasingly imperative to narrow that gap and provide a relevant intersection among knowledge creation, related research activity, and practice decision-making. A systematic and organized approach to knowledge translation application is an essential foundation upon which evidentiary processes can build. In addition, establishing a systematic and cyclical understanding of the cybernetic elements that underpin evidence-based processes is a critical first step to utilizing these processes to establish good decision-making and to advance practice (Brown, 2009). Valuable to both scholars and clinicians is the use of a model that links the evidence-based processes within a dynamic and cybernetic context which recognizes and accommodates the environmental, contextual, and complexity issues which are continuously interfacing and impacting evidence-based processes (evidentiary dynamics) (Curlee & Gordon, 2011). This model must reflect the realities of a fluid interaction between environment, organization, and persons in ways that influence priorities, resources, and decisions.

The combined influence of sociopolitical and economic environmental drivers has a constant and continuous influence on strategic direction, priorities, and choices made in health systems which ultimately influence the character and kind of decisions made in the clinical setting (Kinney, 2011). Such resource allocation priorities help determine what clinical conditions or situations will ascend and the order of priority upon which subsequent research and translational work will unfold. For example, the Centers for Medicare and Medicaid Services (CMS) priority related to hospital-acquired pressure ulcers, for which there will be no payment in the new regulations, increases the likelihood that a more intensive focus on generating data regarding approaches to adequate skin care will result in more effective approaches to care. In this scenario and others like it, a highly structured and disciplined approach to applying evidentiary processes will be used to increase the veracity and utility of the data in clinical practice decision-making. This model should exemplify knowledge creation and research; the application of practice expertise; inclusion of patient, family, and clinical care values; the cultural diversity of patients and populations; and the aggregate of each of these on patient care outcomes and changes in clinical performance. Within each of the critical stages of the evidentiary process, there are opportunities (gaps) for variance assessment and solution-seeking that will be useful in order to calibrate the process so each stage of the process can positively inform and guide subsequent stages with an alignment of these processes that can positively affect outcomes (Kolbasovsky, Zeitlin, & Gillespie, 2012).

These outcomes essentially become the new foundation for advancing evidence, driving the cybernetic trajectory of this dynamic in a cyclical fashion back to knowledge creation and research. At each of the stages with potential gaps in the evidence-based process, opportunities for innovation abound in ways that influence conceptualizing, planning, and approaching appropriate change everywhere in the evidentiary process. This disciplines the process and frees it to be open and available for creative conceptualizing, staging, deciding, and acting (Figure 12.1).

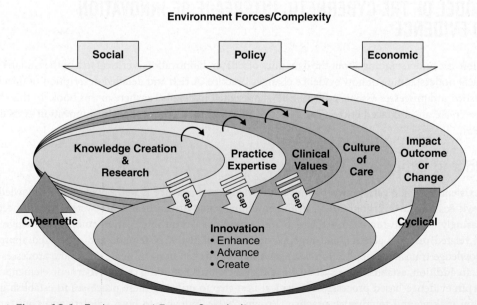

Figure 12.1: Environmental Forces: Complexity

TRANSLATIONAL INNOVATION: KNOWLEDGE CREATION AND RESEARCH

Organizations and systems attempt to "morph" knowledge and research in ways that inform practice behaviors, but face significant challenges in the interaction between innovation and evidence (Ridenour, 2010). Here, some of the foundations laid out by Everett Rogers related to diffusion of innovation, or the spread of new ideas from an individual adoption perspective, have significant applications with regard to knowledge and research adoption (Burns, 2012). While Rogers' is a relatively simple linear process, it does identify the relationship and characteristics between the social system and adopters of innovation. More complex approaches require the capacity to evaluate data, develop mechanisms for adoption, and, finally, support diffusion of appropriate practices by all affected clinicians (Topol, 2012). The role of evidentiary leadership at this stage is to confirm that the foundations of evidence are sufficiently narrow, definitive, predictive, and establish a broad enough foundation upon which rational clinical action can be taken.

Leadership and Innovation

The Nature of Leadership

The nature of leadership must now be examined to assure that values, beliefs, behaviors, and outcomes are consistent with dynamics of the evidence–innovation model. Leadership that supports the complexity of nonlinear, multiple interrelationships and directions, uncertainty, and self-organizing and emergent activities will be needed to actively support the dynamic work of the future. Traditional leadership behaviors of directing and controlling with clearly defined communication channels will obstruct the dynamic in several ways. Most notable will be the tendency to stay located in the knowledge and research stage—locking on to work that is based on high levels of evidence.

....

Courage to continually challenge exiting evidence and practices is supported by leadership principles and values steeped in the nature of complexity.
—Kathy Malloch & Tim Porter O'Grady

....

To embrace complexity leadership, leaders must engage in personal reflection and ego management, adopt a style of appreciative inquiry, develop high levels of emotional competence, use creativity and open dialogue to make decisions as a team, continually be mindful of the bigger picture in which decisions are being made, and demonstrate willingness to stretch performance (Malloch, 2010). Evidence for complexity leadership in health care is emerging slowly and will need ongoing examination and documentation of its ability to produce the desired outcomes.

Creativity in this scenario exists in several different frames. First, designing an infrastructure that makes knowledge translation a part of the architecture of practice is essential. Creating a consistent and systematic framework for knowledge management that includes knowledge generation, translation, and application is critical to successfully using evidence-based processes. Second, embedding this infrastructure into the clinical organization's "way of doing business" requires a consistent and systematic indoctrination of the established framework so that all clinical practitioners are operating using the same evidentiary set of guidelines. Third, a level of transparency around questions of translation related to the relevance, veracity, and applicability of the data within particular clinical processes is important. Clarity is essential to the comparability of the data at the outset of translation and decision-making and at the point of outcome measurement. The evidence-grounded practitioner is always looking through the lens of efficiency, effectiveness, and efficacy (Straus, Tetroe, & Graham, 2013).

Using the evidence–innovation dynamic framework, it is clear there is much evidence for selected segments of the care continuum and a lack of data supporting the integration of system segments. The design of patient care delivery models that now require integrated services across the continuum of care settings, collaboration across disciplines, value-based care, and economic sustainability is a reflection of this stage of the model. First, the evidence exists for many of the unit-based or discipline-based delivery models (Baggs, Ryan, Phelps, Richeson, & Johnson, 1992; Kohn, Corrigan & Donaldson, 2000; Salas, Sims, & Burke, 2005). The current infrastructure for healthcare delivery models focuses on the acute care experience, a physician-dominated delivery system, discipline-focused services, and control of knowledge in policy sources created by the organization. Second, the use of evidence is based on individual discipline resources and not on an integrated use of evidence from multiple disciplines focusing on the individual patient. A multidisciplinary approach to planning and coordinating patient care as a team is emerging. New evidence specific to team rounding supports the values and principles of an integrated team approach (Henneman, Kleppel, & Hinchey, 2013). Third, there is a lack of transparent and interdisciplinary evaluation of each patient's care on a routine basis related to relevance, veracity, and appropriateness. The shortcomings of these processes create gaps in existing evidence for patient care delivery models and thus opportunities for innovation.

From the current status, the gaps in the practice framework to meet the expectations and goals of IOM (2001, 2011) and other organizations focused on patient engagement and satisfaction now illuminate the need not only for a new delivery model, but also for a framework that will support meaningful change (Hast, DiGioia, Thompson, & Wolf, 2013). Innovation is needed in our complex digital system that recognizes changing patterns of interactions among individuals, environmental changes, and the introduction of new products. Creating a delivery model that is driven by the gaps in patient and family-centered care now becomes an innovation imperative. Redefining roles, values, accountabilities, and resources is necessary for transformation to improve the quality of the healthcare system and achieve optimal patient and family engagement.

Innovation is largely evidenced by systematic flexibility and individual adaptability such that when evidence indicates the need for a shift or change in practice, the structures of the system and the behaviors of the practitioners are responsive to the demand for change (Ho, 2012). Here also, the goal of innovation is to enhance effectiveness, advance practice, and create new platforms of practice excellence (MacGregor & Carleton, 2012). Innovation tools that are especially useful at this stage relate to small focused testing of evidence-based approaches with specific patient populations to determine effectiveness and the ability to replicate; technique and methodological comparisons of approach at local units of service (or against a control or standard); and, finally, comparative analysis of comprehensive EBPs with other systems and agencies serving populations with like characteristics (comparative effectiveness) (Figure 12.2).

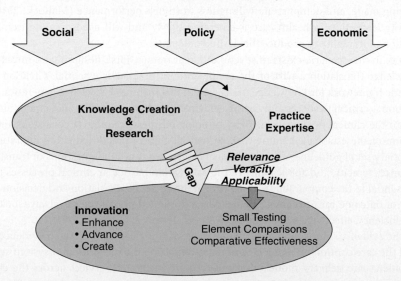

Figure 12.2: Environmental Forces: Innovation Tools

Of course, all adaptation of research and knowledge translation assumes the veracity of the science and the rigor of methodology in the research process and data retrieval. Innovation also has implications for study design and approach and provides opportunities for the creation and generation of knowledge in ways that make best use of emerging technologies that also facilitate its translation into practice. Like the evidence-based process itself, innovation is a reflection of the good use of emergent tools that are also the product of sound innovation processes. Rather than seeing innovation as a separate or nonaligned process, it is instead better seen as an embedded dynamic present in each stage of the evidence-based process and as essential to its success (Endsley, 2010). Clearly, it would be inappropriate to determine that each element of the process and the gaps emerging out of them are unaligned with subsequent stages or that such stages are iterative (building on past successful processes) or linear. Often, gaps in one stage can reach back to earlier evidence-based actions and inform changes or adjustments in them in ways imperceptible during an earlier stage in the process. Sensitivity to the "re-evidencing" process cannot be understated. Developing a strong willingness to continually challenge assumptions of current work provides incredible opportunities to advance practice excellence.

The use of Bar Code Medication Administration (BCMA) technology provides an example of good rationale to re-examine the use of this evidence-driven process. In the knowledge and research stage, significant research supported the use of BCMA to decrease medication errors with the expectation of improving medication safety by automating processes of medication checking (Hook, Pearlstein, Samarth, & Cusack, 2008). As BCMA became the standard in medication administration, Koppel, Wetterneck, Telles, and Karsh (2008) noted variations from BCMA protocols, resulting in deviations, violations, or work-arounds to the designed processes. Recently, a typology was developed that identified 15 types of BCMA-related work-arounds with 31 types of causes (Koppel et al., 2008). These deviations from the intended practice can be now considered gaps in the evidence–innovation model. It is interesting to note that Lalley (2013) acknowledges that work-arounds (work efforts that accommodate impeding structures or processes) were not all necessarily negative and could, if fact, be innovations to existing processes. The careful examination of the evidence gap now leads to the need for innovation— new ways to conduct medication administration.

Another source of an evidence gap can be identified when caregivers question current evidence. The notion that we have always done it this way is becoming less sacred in many healthcare organizations. In one organization, nurses queried why the Trendelenburg position was used and discovered that the 45-degree head down position was not a recommended position for many reasons (Makic, Rauen, & VonRueden, 2013). Multiple sources of evidence were examined, including the original use by Frederich Adolph Trendelenburg in the late 1880s. Trendelenburg, a surgeon, used the position to visualize abdominal organs for surgical procedures. Today, some clinicians use the position to treat hypotensive events to shift blood volumes and to increase brain blood flow. Interestingly, in the 1960s, researchers found that in the Trendelenburg position, patient blood pressure decreased as head and neck veins became engorged, oxygen flow decreased, and the risk for retinal detachment increased. Researchers concluded that the Trendelenburg position had little positive impact on cardiac output or blood pressure (Makic et al., 2013). This new evidence created by challenging a long-held assumption is an example of the evidence–innovation dynamic in action. New evidence now requires new thinking or innovations to quickly address hypotensive events.

Experience and Application: Practice Expertise

Evidence is an aggregating dynamic that makes it always a work in progress. The science and data process grow in veracity (inherent truth) and applicability as the information regarding episodes of care or population needs increases in volume and accuracy (precision). Multiple practice variations and provider experiences contribute to the complexity of understanding practice. In the meantime, contributing to the data generation is the sum of experience and practice patterns of colleagues with specific cases, episodes, or populations. Mechanisms for conversations, conferences, collaboration, or care planning provide the frame for the construction of practices for which there is no sufficient database upon which practices can rely (Stanhope & Lancaster, 2010).

Collaborative sessions that intentionally converge around planning and constructing models, algorithms, or approaches to care are vehicles for creating a foundation for practice for which there is yet no aggregated evidence sufficient to establish an evidentiary foundation for such practices.

Evidence for practice expertise emanates from several sources: past practices, experience, collective wisdom, and standards. Traditionally, caregivers and healthcare providers have relied on past practices and experiences to deliver care on the basis of an institutional model with distinctly separate caregiver and provider-role behaviors. The emphasis on the caregiver roles has marginalized the role of the patient or user of healthcare services. The challenges of limited communications among caregivers and providers, duplication of diagnostic tests, and delayed decision-making have been identified as a deficiency in the existing evidence—the lack of effectiveness of current collaboration models becomes a gap and opportunity for innovation and new evidence.

To address the gap is *care collaboration*, which is believed to have potential to bring stakeholders together to lower the cost and improve the quality of patient care (Tocknell, 2013). Shifting to a continuum-driven, population health model in which collaborative care is the cornerstone and expected to address current patient satisfaction challenges and the risk of readmissions, new quality measures will emerge and begin the dynamic to again identify the gap and create innovative processes. Working together to understand and facilitate each patient care episode by an informed team becomes the desired process to address the current gap. Working together in ways that create synergistic outcomes for patients rather than individual, segmented provider interventions is now the work to be done.

Another scenario within care collaboration is the nurse–physician relationship. Continuing work on nurse–physician relationships also is supported by evidence as failure to achieve effective collaboration reflects the need for innovation and more evidence to address the poor relationships that still exist. This is not necessarily a failure of nurses and physicians to get along, but also results from the lack of compelling evidence and rationale to change the current negative behaviors. Failing to support respectful and collaborative dialogue between these professionals will continue to obstruct progress in achieving higher levels of collaborative care. Overall, teamwork is the fundamental competency needed by all members of the team and becomes a gap when care is interrupted and delayed due to poor communication. Evidence clearly links collaborative practices to positive patient outcomes and staff satisfaction (Raup & Spegman, 2013).

While this seems straightforward—let's all work together for the patient—it is far from easy to achieve this complex collaboration. Increasing our understanding of care collaboration processes can be examined innovatively using social network analysis (SNA). SNA is relatively new and more available in a digital environment and provides a process to gain information about the number and strength of connections among caregiver, providers, patients, and families (Merrill, Yoon, Larson, Honig, & Reame, 2013). This type of data provides information on who is involved in the care and how many times are they involved and at different points in time. In addition, the level and length of interactions can be identified. Progress on the desired types of communication can be tracked and evaluated with interval SNA. The patterns of SNA can then be considered in light of clinical outcomes providing best practices for collaborative care processes.

Another approach to creating effective collaborative care is through patient preferences. Finding the best evidence between nursing practice and patient-centered care has been facilitated using patient preferences (Burman, Robinson, & Hart, 2013). Patient preferences serve as the focal point in linking evidence and practitioner expertise in assuring that care is respectful and responsive to patient needs, values, and engagement. Recommendations to advance collaborative care involve more than one stage of the model—much like the interconnectedness of reality! The available knowledge and research is closely linked to practitioner expertise to enact the knowledge and research in practice. To have an impact on and advance collaborative care, recommendations address healthcare redesign, decision support, an empowered organizational culture, and informed and empowered nurses (Burman et al., 2013). These recommendations further reflect the dynamic interconnectedness of the evidence–innovation model.

Similarly, new evidence that can enhance collaborative care is emerging related to nurse staffing. Having the appropriate numbers and competencies of providers is another facet of caregiver expertise.

Numerous studies link registered nurse staffing to patient outcomes, which include nurse–patient engagement (Aiken, Clarke, Sloane, Lake, & Cheney, 2008; Blegen, Goode, Spetz, Vaughn, & Park, 2011; Needleman et al., 2011). True, effective collaboration requires identifiable levels of education and certifications. Addressing gaps in staffing competencies and numbers also requires innovations to facilitate ideal staffing models.

These shared opportunities for addressing the gaps in evidence in practice provide a range of opportunities for innovation in both design and execution, facilitating the journey to a stronger evidentiary foundation for these practices. The latitude in creativity is related to methods of conception and designs of practice approaches, agreements of colleagues around roles and contributions, anecdotes about experiences and evaluation of impact, and understood knowledge of practice–impact relationships (Payne, 2011). Supplementing these opportunities with preliminary data and sources of experiences in broader categories of practice referenced from other settings or environments helps strengthen the evidence of effectiveness (Gray, Coates, & Hetherington, 2013).

In the absence of collective and historical agreement on practices, the clinician is driven to construct approaches that best validate personal experiences where replication of practices shows valuable, relevant, consistent results. In these scenarios, the evidence-driven practitioner develops a level of uncertainty and discomfort, viewing the evidence as too informal and insufficiently structured to validate the tradition of practice associated with the practitioner's work. The requisite of good evidence for practice requires the clinician to seek to connect individual practices with others' experiences in order to develop a collective database upon which to ultimately construct an evidence-grounded approach to validating practice (Mauk, 2010). Here, the discipline of innovation requires the individual practitioner to make such practices intentional and deliberate using best approaches or best practices as seen in others' practices or in the anecdotal literature. In addition, there is nothing to stop the individual clinician from designing her or his own study of practice and establishing some beginning foundations in practice evidence that can help move the practice closer to a standard of measure. This standard can be built upon and used as a part of the complex of individualized approaches to care that, when aggregated, begins to provide evidence of best practices or at least normative processes that lead in that direction (Figure 12.3).

The key to the transformation in practice and the innovations associated with it lies in creating a culture where exploration and "next steps" are permissible and encouraged. Healthcare providers need

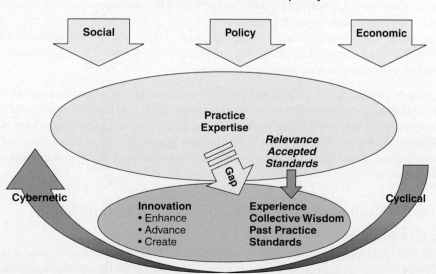

Figure 12.3: Environmental Forces: Aggregating evidence

to have clarity around expectations that (1) it is safe to take the initiative in examining individual and collective practices and (2) those practices are validated by the disciplines of research and evidence (Brynteson, 2013). Establishing the basis for particular practices that represent an approach, standard, or protocol becomes the first step in ascertaining their validity and forms the foundation for a more disciplined and structured review of the efficacies of particular practices and approaches. This culture of innovation helps support the urge for improvement, the desire to advance practice, and the goal of confirming the validity and veracity of particular approaches to patient care.

Clinical/Patient Personal and Cultural Values

In all clinical dynamics, patients bring with them a set of personal and cultural beliefs that represent grounding or traditions in faith, culture, family, and a related range of health practices (Andrews & Boyle, 2012). These beliefs can both positively and negatively affect the practice of healthy behaviors. All of these serve to bring out the patient's personal "tools" that help energize and motivate the patient towards healing and health. Some of these patient beliefs and historic and cultural norms may have some validity or evidence of value and applicability; some may not. Yet all, when integrated, may serve as a frame of reference for the patient and caring community in ways that help enable the patient to cope, confront, and address challenges and issues associated with healing and health.

Other than practices that are obviously dangerous or endangering, the provider may need to accommodate and incorporate particular personal and cultural characteristics and processes of healing into the complex of choices necessary to offer best service to particular patients and populations. The caring and insightful provider recognizes the value of incorporating culture and care, personality and practices, faith and healing, and history and experience into a mosaic that creates a positive and renewing interface between them that meets the needs of the person with the science of evidenced-based services (Giger, 2012). In the interests of evidence-driven innovation, it is important for practitioners to note that ample opportunity for linking culturally influenced and personal health practices to the evidentiary dynamic is a creative but important component of building evidentiary foundations for practices. Indeed, many nontraditional health practices may have embedded within them seeds of insight and value that can positively influence broader populations and provide for a strong foundation for effective health service (Figure 12.4). The innovation requisites would need to include:

1. Attempt to establish a cause-and-effect relationship between the cultural notions or population-specific health practices and the outcomes associated with them.
2. Enumerate a consistent historic precedence for the impact that indicates a norm of behavior or practices that demonstrate consistent approaches.
3. Make a connection between culturally delineated specific beliefs, practices, or approaches and the supporting body of scientific knowledge that correlates to it or, at least, does not contradict well-established, evidence-grounded sources of knowledge.

Respect given to cultural norms, beliefs, and practices that demonstrate an important contribution to the health of individuals and populations is important when building evidence that supports and influences positive clinical outcomes. Using evidence-based approaches and connecting them to innovative applications do not preclude the potential for broader generalizations of culturally specific health foundations; instead, it may lead to innovations that potentially advance health and improve outcomes (Dayer-Berenson, 2011).

Creating the Culture of Care Within the Culture of Innovation

Context for Innovation

In order to both generate and sustain creative and innovative behaviors, the organizational infrastructure or culture must make it possible for those behaviors to thrive (Dodgson, Gann, & Salter, 2005). Innovation does least well in organizations that are rigidly controlled, policy dominated, with a narrow

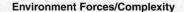

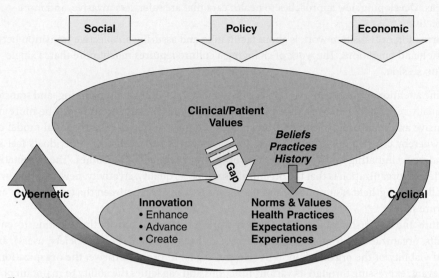

Figure 12.4: Environmental Forces: Embedding evidence

locus-of-control and an overpowering/overwhelming management authority structure. While structure is certainly a requisite for all organized human behavior, the kind of structure that advances innovation capacities and behaviors requires considerably different design. Innovation is not successfully driven from the top of any system. Instead, it is generated from the center of the system and enabled by the institutional infrastructures to move in a way that allows the innovation to grow, adapt, and succeed (Grebel, 2011). The authoritarian, hierarchal structures with rigidly defined roles, relationships, and communication pathways are no longer effective for organizations seeking to support a dynamic evidence–innovation model. It is the point of care or intersection of the healthcare user and provider that must now be the focal and driving point of action.

The cultural context for innovation is created by organizational leadership from the boardroom to the first-line manager. This culture represents an availability or openness in the organization to ideas, stimulation, questioning, and drilling deeper into issues and processes that can advance the interests of the organization (Braithwaite, Hyde, & Pope, 2010). Leadership recognizes that innovation is located everywhere in the system and that opportunities for it to arise and generate value and outcomes that are dependent on the ability of those leaders to embrace and engage individuals and opportunities in a way that brings life and energy to the enterprise. The culture of innovation suggests that the structures and systems in place be enabling rather than constraining, give deference to relationships, good ideas, and processes—rather than rules and discipline—with the rigors associated with the systematic exploration and management of them in a way that will lead to value and impact (Anderson, 2012).

While innovation is a dynamic as is EBP, it also is a discipline with elements and components, processes and stages, metrics and measures, and outcomes and impact (Leonard-Barton, 2011). Building a culture that supports the challenge to create and innovate while maintaining the rigors of good structure and process is no easy task for leadership. These challenges bring to bear the need for innovation in the organizational structure to support both rigor and creative change. The trimodal organizational model offers an approach to integrate seemingly paradoxical work processes (Malloch, 2010). The trimodal model is comprised of three major categories of work:

◆ Operations or the work of providing evidence-based patient care within a defined structure with supportive staff and resources.

◆ Innovation planning is high-intensity work with the continual introduction and evaluation of new ideas. Developing new approaches to health care that are safer, less invasive, and more cost-effective.

◆ Transformation or transition work is about facilitating and assuring an effective transition between innovation and operations. The work of changing a culture requires much more than a single education session.

With specific attention to these three work processes, operations, innovation planning, and transformation are equally represented and resourced in the organization. The organization can be more nimble and responsive and increasing able to take advantage of digital resources. The trimodal model creates a context whereby creative thinking is valued, improvement is rewarded, and individuals feel safe in recommending or initiating innovative ways of working and producing outcomes. The expectation for the fully effective organization is that the organization supports quality, creativity, new thinking, willingness to challenge long-held assumptions, and the means to transition between the current state and the desired future state.

Structure and leadership ability operate as a work in progress, constantly adjusting to environmental shifts, organizational responses to its market (for health systems; policy, society, users), and the vitality and viability of the organization itself (Howie, 2011). In order to thrive, the organization must remain relevant, expressing through its various functions and capacities the ability to maintain purpose, role, function, and impact in the broader landscape in which it lives (Ouden, 2012).

Innovation and Evidence

The core of both innovation and evidence is represented in what is often referred to as *associational thinking*. This represents an ability to find relationships and intersections between seemingly unrelated and unconnected components and processes. Indeed, the innovation embedded in evidence is represented by the clinician's capacity to look at precedence, past practices, metrics, and data and to draw insights from the data that challenge, inform, and advance new insights, connections, and responses that lead to improvement and enhancements in service and care (Mattimore, 2012).

Seeking out uncommon partners who further encourage us to challenge current assumptions, discard non-value-added work, and see the world in different ways provides new knowledge for consideration. The integration of clinical disciplines with architects has served to improve the environment of care and enhance the space for healing. Partnerships with engineers and "informaticists" provide invaluable insights into the documentation, categorization, analysis, and communication of complex health data. These uncommon partnerships enrich the evidence–innovation dynamic with the addition of knowledge from different perspectives.

The traditional notion that associates EBP with rule-defined parameters that eliminate judgment, initiative, creativity, and new insights is simply untrue. Evidence suggests an attachment to solid foundations, good science, research, validated practice precedence, and aggregated data. However, each of these simply provides the "floor" of practice, a foundation from which to discern, create, design, and construct next-step clinical approaches. These more effective approaches represent better, higher-level choices and actions. When taken together, these simple rules or practices can lead to improvements, enhancements, or entirely new approaches that result in better service, higher levels of quality, and new standards of clinical performance. In fact, without these dynamics at work, EBPs become no more than rote mechanisms that standardize and stabilize human action in a way to eliminate the vitality and initiative necessary to improve and advance. Building a culture of innovation that makes creativity, change, and improvement the "way of doing business" for the organization and its people is the essential context necessary to build a viable and sustainable culture of care (Kuratko, Hornsby, & Goldsby, 2012).

....

If you always do what you always did, you will always get what you always got.
—Albert Einstein

....

Creating the Culture of Care

The culture of care creates the necessary infrastructure in which the dynamics and processes of EBP make a lasting impact and lead to higher levels of quality service and care. This culture of care represents a fundamental commitment on the part of the organization and its people to focus in every arena, decisions, and activities in a way that advances service and care (Smith and Institute of Medicine Committee on the Learning Health Care System in America, 2012). The norms and values of the organization represent a fundamental pledge to care and exemplify that commitment in the practices and behaviors of all those who represent its interests. The culture of care falls within the context of the overriding culture of innovation. This makes it possible within the care setting to design and adapt approaches to care delivery that reflect grounding in good science, but also leads to opportunity to build approaches that reflect insights from past data, information about clinical and technological advances, the recalibration of policy and protocol, and insights from patient-related practices and experiences.

The culture of care assumes that practice unfolds within a constantly moving dynamic, ever informed by shifts in the environment, science-based evidentiary dynamics, and the dialogue and relationship between caregivers and patients. The interface of these forces represents the culture that makes possible creativity and adaptation, refinement and improvement, and advancement and enhancement of practices and processes, all of which lead to increasing intensity of relevance and value of quality care and service (Cross, 2013). The interface between the culture of innovation and care creates a sort of coalescing of energies that act as the stimuli for associational work that leads to the improvements suggested by good EBPs and processes (Figure 12.5).

The behaviors of providers and patients are the best indicators of whether an intertwined culture of innovation and care exists in the organization. There are five behavioral indicators that suggest the context of innovation and care are successfully operating within the system:

1. The ability to openly and frankly probe and question in an effort to challenge for clarity and creativity in a way that leads to a deeper look into existing decisions, processes, and actions subject to the potential for improvement and positive change.
2. The capacity to network collaterally within and across the system with a wide variety of people with diverse capacities and skills, which helps provide access to dynamic thinking and stimulates openness and availability (equity) between providers, resulting in increased value from their relationships and interactions.

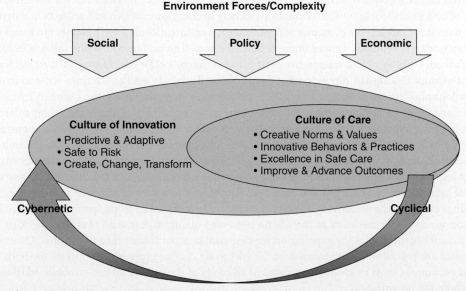

Figure 12.5: Environmental Forces: Coalescing of energies

3. Availability and awareness of the changing external environment and the ability of leaders and clinicians to predict and adapt internal dynamics and practices to reflect these changes and to assure that clinical and care responses are relevant, contemporary, and demonstrate the best in care.

4. Sustaining and advancing experimental awareness that no practice is permanent and that evidence-based design and practice demands a level of mobility, portability, and personal behavior that embraces the journey rather than the event. This demonstrates the role of the provider to appropriately change practice as soon as the evidence demands. This more fluid and flexible characterization of the professional's role is a requisite for the essential capacity to adapt as a way of ensuring that clinical practice is current, relevant, and continuously effective.

5. There must be a willingness to act on evidence. Identifying areas of concern and opportunities to improve are often quite simple to do, more than the courage to do something about those identified issues. Leaders must be willing to take rational risks and challenge long-held assumptions for the good of the healthcare system.

Building a culture of innovation in health care often seems paradoxical. We focus on reliability and consistency, yet there is an ever-present need to continue to assure that our practices are complementary to current evidence, changing environmental circumstances, and new innovations. Nonetheless, the importance of being skilled in dynamic competence rather than an either-or (operations or innovation) cannot be overstated—it is a requirement.

Advancing organizational culture requires time and knowledge. Oftentimes, leaders may believe that creating initiatives and billboards and buttons will drive new behaviors. Nothing could be further from the truth. Advancing or changing a culture requires knowledge of the critical elements and impacts of cultural attributes (Schein, 2004). There are numerous descriptions of organizational culture that have been studied for many years. The combination of Schein and Hatch's work provides a fairly clear framework to understand the levels of complexity. Understanding the levels of complexity provides critical information about the challenges and requirements to effect change in an organization. Schein's model identified assumptions, values, and artifacts as the three fundamental layers of an organization. Hatch advanced Schein's work with the addition of symbols (1993). The identity of an organizational culture is formed by the underlying assumptions about people, activities, and expectations. This is the deepest layer of an organization and often difficult to discern. Values form the middle layer of organizational culture. Artifacts are considered the superficial layer of an organization such as posters, slogans, directives, and other types of shared information. Symbols, introduced by Hatch, added the interpretive aspect of culture and focus on the relationships linking assumptions, values, and artifacts in a dynamic rather than static model. The dynamics of organizational culture include a forth element to assess organizational culture, symbols. This addition permits the model to accommodate the influences of both Schein's theory and symbolic-interpretive perspectives (Hatch, 1993). The reformulated model focuses on relationships linking assumptions, values, symbols, and artifacts with a shift from static to dynamic conceptions of culture by looking at interactions between key elements rather than elements themselves.

As one seeks to advance change or innovation in an organization, the levels of organizational culture and the dynamic relationship among the elements must be considered. Further, alignment of the elements is critical for change to advance. Long-term, lasting change requires firm grounding in organizational culture assumptions. When change or new ideas and expectations are introduced at the artifact level, without agreement on values and assumptions, it is difficult for the change to be sustained. Consider the numerous checklists that have been introduced to assure compliance with standards and reporting criteria. If the underlying assumptions are not directly linked to safe patient care, there is less attention given to the checklists as there is no perceived quality threat. And thus, the checklist (artifact) becomes ineffective as the expectation for cost-containment is identified as the goal. Quality and economics are perceived to be inconsistent. To effectively change processes, the values for both quality and economics must be clearly articulated at all levels of the culture and in symbolic relationships throughout the organization.

Culture is more about context than content. The context for innovation and EBP has in it clear requisites and characteristics that affect strategy, tactics, and clinical decisions and actions (Heskett, 2012). The interplay between innovation and patient care demonstrates a seamless and fluid network of interactions, intersections, and relationships. This exemplifies the network's capacity to engage it stakeholders in the essential activities of change and in advancing and continuously improving service and quality (Anderson & Ackerman-Anderson, 2010). Evidence-based processes represent and demonstrate the character and capacity of a culture of innovation where the ability to adapt and change clinical practices based on the constant generation of evidence is simply an organizational way of life.

IMPACT AND CHANGE: INNOVATION AND EVIDENCE AT WORK

All innovation must end up at some time creating a product or generating an impact. The innovation dynamic and processes associated with it have no purpose or value if there is not a change, a product, or outcome. Impact, outcome, or change is a necessary terminal point of the process and, at the same time, the point at which the cyclical, cybernetic dynamic of innovation and evidence cycles back upon itself and initiates the cyclic processes at their point of inception. At the end of this process, the impact stage is reached where a combination of evidence and the determination of the metrics and measures prove efficacy and effectiveness (Hoggarth & Comfort, 2010). At the point of impact, the evidence-based process enters into the "evaluation zone" where plan, performance, and outcome meet to show the essential character of their interaction and relationship and the convergence of factors that influence value.

Metrics and measures related to impact and value should have been constructed in the earlier stages of the evidentiary process so they might act as both enumerators and potential predictors of desired outcome. Of course, the outcome must result in some specific change that represents improvement, enhancement, or an effective change in course. Ultimately, of course, the result must be articulated in some measure of difference as seen in Box 12.1.

It is here also where the potential for innovation accelerates. At the point of evaluation, the innovative organization looks carefully at the trajectory and processes associated with evidence-driven activities and determines the challenges, opportunities, insights, and capacity to predict change, alter or adjust processes and practices, shift the trajectory, and incorporate new knowledge and technology (Maddock, Uriarte, & Brown, 2011). Here, they integrate the insight from these factors in a way that contributes to the design and modeling of innovative approaches within the cybernetic process of innovation and evidence.

Box 12.1	Examples of Innovation and Evidence at Work

◆ New knowledge, learning, skills, practices (Note: new knowledge may reflect processes or products that do not positively advance change and are now abandoned)
◆ Standards affecting episodes, persons, populations
◆ Changes in policy, protocol, procedure
◆ Changes in the capacity of providers, patients, populations, communities
◆ Changes in patient, provider, community behaviors
◆ Changes in the organization, systems, community (resources, structures, support systems)
◆ Changes in capacity, utility, use
◆ Changes in quality, service, continuity, integrity, viability

Assessment and evaluation at the point of impact also lead to reflection and evaluation of both the core of innovation and evidence and the effectiveness of the evidentiary dynamic and its associated processes. The effectiveness and seamlessness of the interface from knowledge creation, practice expertise, clinical values, and care culture to outcome and impact is as important an element of the evaluation as are the clinical dynamics and provider practices. How the gaps were identified, analyzed, accommodated, and addressed and how response to them led to a more seamless interface between the evidentiary stages are important to creating a more seamless evidentiary dynamic (Ouden, 2012). The implications for innovation here are exemplified by the degree in intensity of creative approaches that enhanced or advanced evidentiary dynamics and associated processes and validated the utility of the culture of innovation (Figure 12.6).

Evaluation of the environment of innovation (culture) is as important as the embedded components of evaluation in EBP. The key is to observe how the leadership and organizational environment facilitated the creation of a context resulting in openness, responsiveness, timeliness, process-seamlessness, timeliness of response, predictive/adaptive capacity, and the value of essential changes (Goldstein, Hazy, & Lichtenstein, 2010). Leadership and management capacity and skills are also ripe territory for the evaluation of effectiveness of evidence-based processes and practices and the human interaction and dynamics that facilitate and advance them. How open, available, and accessible data and information are demonstrates in the most visible way the culture and action of innovation at work. The point-of-service capacity to react, deliberate, act, and change also clearly demonstrates the dynamic impact of the culture of innovation. This innovation engine provides the energy within which the dynamics and processes of EBP are generated and supported in a way that assures their relevance and usefulness (Howie, 2011).

The culture of innovation provides the contextual framework that feeds and facilitates all of the structural, organizational, and human infrastructure and capacities that support EBP as a way of doing business in any endeavor. The complementarity between innovation and evidence is the same as that between context and content—one providing the frame, the other providing the processes. This interdependence defines the essentially interdependent relationship between innovation and evidence, necessitating a fundamental correlation between each of these dynamics in a way that is generative, supportive, and advances the human experience. Commitment to evidence suggests a corollary commitment to the innovation that both supports and enables it. It is the enduring work of leadership to advance the integrity of this partnership between innovation and evidence in a way that enables to provide value, sustain quality, and advance the human enterprise in the delivery of effective patient care.

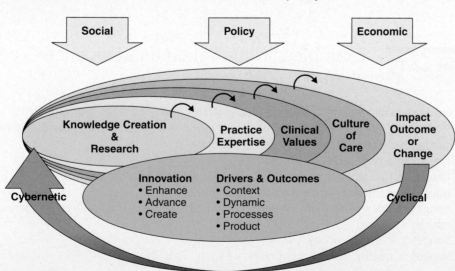

Figure 12.6: Environmental Forces: Implications for Innovation

EBP FAST FACTS

◆ Innovation does least well in organizations that are rigidly controlled and policy dominated, with a narrow locus of control and an overpowering/overwhelming management authority structure.

◆ Innovation is not successfully driven from the top of any system; it is generated from the center of the system and enabled by the institutional infrastructures to move in a way that allows the innovation to grow, adapt, and succeed.

◆ Metrics and measures related to impact and value should have been constructed in the earlier stages of the evidentiary process so they might act as both enumerators and potential predictors of desired outcome.

◆ All innovation must create a product or generate an impact; the innovation dynamic and processes associated with it have no purpose or value if there is not a change, a product, or outcome.

References

Aiken, L. H., Clarke, S. P., Sloane, D., Lake, E. T., & Cheney, T. (2008). Effects of hospital care environment on patient mortality and nurse outcomes. *Journal of Nursing Administration, 38*(5), 223–229.

Anderson, D., & Ackerman-Anderson, L. S. (2010). *Beyond change management : How to achieve breakthrough results through conscious change leadership.* San Francisco: Pfeiffer.

Anderson, D. L. (2012). *Cases and exercises in organization development & change.* Thousand Oaks, CA: SAGE.

Andrews, M. M., & Boyle, J. S. (2012). *Transcultural concepts in nursing care.* Philadelphia, Wolters Kluwer Health/ Lippincott Williams & Wilkins.

Baggs, J. G., Ryan, S. A., Phelps, C. E., Richeson, J. F., & Johnson, J. E. (1992). The association between interdisciplinary collaboration and patient outcomes in medical intensive care. *Heart & Lung, 21*, 18–24.

Blegen, M., Goode, C. J., Spetz, J., Vaughn, T., & Park, S. H. (2011). Nurse staffing effects on patient outcomes: Safety-net and non-safety-net hospitals. *Medical Care, 49*(4), 406–414.

Braithwaite, J., Hyde, P., & Pope, C. (2010). *Culture and climate in health care organizations.* Houndmills, Basingstoke, Hampshire; New York: Palgrave.

Brown, S. J. (2009). *Evidence-based nursing: The research-practice connection.* Sudbury, MA: Jones and Bartlett Publishers.

Brown, V. A., Harris, J. A., & Russell, J. Y. (2010). *Tackling wicked problems: Through the transdisciplinary imagination.* London: Earthscan.

Brynteson, R. (2013). *Innovation at work: 55 activities to spark your team's creativity.* New York: American Management Association.

Burman, M. E., Robinson, B., & Hart, A. M. (2013). Linking evidence-based nursing practice and practice-centered care through patient preferences. *Nursing Administration Quarterly, 37*(3), 231–241.

Burns, L. R. (2012). *The business of healthcare innovation.* Cambridge, UK: Cambridge University Press.

Cross, B. L. (2013). *Lean innovation : Understanding what's next in today's economy.* Boca Raton: CRC Press.

Curlee, W., & Gordon, R. L. (2011). *Complexity theory and project management.* Hoboken, NJ: Wiley.

Dayer-Berenson, L. (2011). *Cultural competencies for nurses: Impact on health and illness.* Sudbury, MA: Jones and Bartlett Publishers.

Dodgson, M., Gann, D., & Salter, A. (2005). *Think, play, do: Technology, innovation, and organization.* New York: Oxford University Press.

Endsley, S. C. (2010). *Putting healthcare innovation into practice.* Chichester, West Sussex, UK: Wiley-Blackwell.

Erickson, J. I., Ditomassi, M., & Adams, J. M. (2012). Attending registered nurse: An innovative role to manage between spaces. *Nursing Economics, 30*(5), 282–287.

Giger, J. N. (2012). *Transcultural nursing: Assessment & interventions.* St. Louis, MO: Elsevier/Mosby.

Goldstein, J., Hazy, J. K., & Lichtenstein, B. B. (2010). *Complexity and the nexus of leadership: Leveraging nonlinear science to create ecologies of innovation.* New York: Palgrave Macmillan.

Gray, M., Coates, J., & Hetherington, T. (2013). *Environmental social work.* Milton Park, Abingdon, Oxon; New York, NY: Routledge.

Grebel, T. (2011). *Innovation and health: Theory, methodology and applications.* Northampton, MA: Edward Elgar Pub.

Hast, A. S., DiGioia, A. M., Thompson, D., & Wolf, G. (2013). Utilizing complexity science to drive practice change through patient- and family-centered care. *Journal of Nursing Administration, 43*(1), 44–49.

Hatch, M. J. (1993). The dynamics of organizational culture. *Academy of Management Review, 18*(4), 657.

Heilbron, J. L. (2003). *The Oxford companion to the history of modern science.* New York: Oxford University Press.

Henneman, E. A., Kleppel, R., & Hinchey, K. T. (2013). Development of a checklist for documenting team and collaborative behaviors during multidisciplinary bedside rounds. *Journal of Nursing Administration, 43*(5), 280–285.

Heskett, J. L. (2012). *The culture cycle: How to shape the unseen force that transforms performance.* Upper Saddle River, NJ: FT Press.

Ho, K. (2012). *Technology enabled knowledge translation for eHealth: Principles and practice.* New York, NY: Springer.

Hoggarth, L., & Comfort, H. (2010). *A practical guide to outcome evaluation.* Philadelphia: Jessica Kingsley Publishers.

Hook, J. M., Pearlstein, J., Samarth, A., & Cusack, C. (2008). *Using barcode medication administration to improve quality and safety: Findings from the AHRQ Health IT Portfolio.* Agency for Healthcare Research and Quality. Retrieved from http://healthit.ahrq.gov/sites/default/files/docs/page/09-0023-EF_bcma_0.pdf

Hovmand, P., & Gillespie, D. (2010). Implementation of evidence-based practice and organizational performance. *The Journal of Behavioral Health Service & Research, 37*(1), 79–84.

Howie, P. J. (2011). *Evolution of revolutions: How we create, shape, and react to change.* Amherst, NY: Prometheus Books.

Institute of Medicine. (2001). *Crossing the quality chasm: A new health system for the 21st century.* Washington, DC: National Academy Press.

Institute of Medicine. (2011). *The future of nursing: Leading change, advancing health.* Washington, DC: National Academies Press.

Kinney, E. D. (2011). Comparative effectiveness research under the Patient Protection and Affordable Care Act: Can new bottles accommodate old wine? *American Journal of Law & Medicine, 37*(4), 522–566.

Kohn, L. T., Corrigan, M., & Donaldson, M. S. for the Committee on Quality Health Care in America. Institute of Medicine. (2000). *To err is human: Building a safer health system.* Washington, DC: National Academy Press.

Kolbasovsky, A., Zeitlin, J., & Gillespie, W. (2012). Impact of point-of-care case management on readmissions and costs. *The American Journal of Managed Care, 18*(8), e300–e306.

Koppel, R., Wetterneck, T., Telles, J. L., & Karsh, B. (2008). Workaround to barcode medication administration systems: Their occurrences, causes, and threats to patient safety. *Journal of the American Medical Informatics Association, 15*, 408–423.

Kuratko, D. F., Hornsby, J. S., & Goldsby, M. G. (2012). *Innovation acceleration: Transforming organizational thinking.* Boston: Pearson.

Lalley, C. (2013). Work-arounds: A matter of perception. *Nurse Leader, 11*(2), 36–40.

Leonard-Barton, D. (2011). *Managing knowledge assets, creativity and innovation.* Hackensack, NJ: World Scientific.

Lorenz, J. M., Beyea, S. C., & Slattery, M. J. (2009). *Evidence-based practice: A guide for nurses.* Marblehead, MA: HCPro.

MacGregor, S. P., & Carleton, T. (2012). *Sustaining innovation: Collaboration models for a complex world.* New York, NY: Springer.

Maddock, G. M., Uriarte, L. C., & Brown, P. B. (2011). *Brand new: Solving the innovation paradox—How great brands invent and launch new products, services, and business models.* Hoboken, NJ: Wiley.

Makic, M. B., Rauen, C. A., & VonRueden, K. T. (2013). Questioning common nursing practices: What does the evidence show? *American Nurse Today, 8*(3), 10–13.

Malloch, K. (2010). Innovation leadership: New perspectives for new work. *Nursing Clinics of North America, 45*(1).

Malloch, K., & Porter-O'Grady, T. (2009). *Introduction to evidence-based practice in nursing and healthcare.* Boston, MA: Jones & Bartlett.

Malloch, K., & Porter-O'Grady, T. (2010). *The quantum leader: Applications for the new world of work.* Boston, MA: Jones & Bartlett.

Marshall, E. S. (2011). *Transformational leadership in nursing: From expert clinician to influential leader.* New York, NY: Springer Publishing Company.

Mattimore, B. W. (2012). *Idea stormers: How to lead and inspire creative breakthroughs.* San Francisco: Jossey-Bass.

Mauk, K. L. (2010). *Gerontological nursing: Competencies for care.* Boston: Jones and Bartlett Publishers.

McCarthy, J. A. (2011). *Beyond genius, innovation & luck: The "rocket science" of building high-performance corporations.* Los Altos, CA: 4th Edition Publishing.

Melnyk, B., & Fineout-Overholt, E. (2012). *Evidence-based practice and nursing and healthcare. A guide to best practice* (2nd ed.). Philadelphia: Wolters Kluwer/Lippincott Williams & Wilkins.

Merrill, J. A., Yoon, S., Larson, E., Honig, J., & Reame, N. (2013). Using social network analysis to examine collaborative relationships among PhD and DNP students and faculty in a research-intensive university school of nursing. *Nursing Outlook, 61*(2), 109–116.

Needleman, J., Buerhaus, P., Pankratz, V. S., Leibson, C. L., Stevens, S. R., & Harris, M. (2011). Nurse staffing and inpatient hospital mortality. *New England Journal of Medicine, 364*(11), 1037–1045.

Ouden, E. D. (2012). *Innovation design: Creating value for people, organizations and society.* London; New York: Springer.

Payne, M. (2011). *Humanistic social work: Core principles in practice.* Chicago, IL: Lyceum Books.

Porter-O'Grady, T., & Malloch, K. (2010). *Quantum leadership: Advancing innovation, transforming healthcare.* Boston: Jones & Bartlett.

Raup, C. M., & Spegman, A. M. (2013). Interprofessional collaboration promotes collaboration. *American Nurse Today, 8*(3), 43–46.

Ridenour, J. (2010). Evidence-based regulation: Emerging knowledge management to inform policy. In K. Malloch & T. Porter O'Grady (Eds.), *Introduction to evidenced-based practice in nursing and healthcare* (pp. 275–299). Boston: Jones & Bartlett.

Rundquist, J. M. & Givens, P. L. (2013). Quantifying the benefits of staff participation in shared governance. *American Nurse Today, 8*(3), 38–42.

Salas, E,, Sims, D. E., & Burke, C. S. (2005). Is there a "big five" in teamwork. *Small Group Research, 36*(5), 555–559.

Schein, E. H. (2004). *Organizational culture and leadership.* San Francisco, CA: Wiley & Sons.

Schultz, A. A. (2009). *Evidence-based practice.* Philadelphia, PA: Saunders.

Sharts-Hopko, N. C. (2013). Tackling complex problems, building evidence for practice, and educating doctoral nursing students to manage the tension. *Nursing Outlook, 61*(2), 102–108.

Smith, M. D. and Institute of Medicine Committee on the Learning Health Care System in America. (2012). *Best care at lower cost: The path to continuously learning health care in America.* Washington, DC: National Academies Press.

Stanhope, M., & Lancaster, J. (2010). *Foundations of nursing in the community: Community-oriented practice.* St. Louis, MO: Mosby/Elsevier.

Starr, P. (2011). *Remedy and reaction: The peculiar american struggle over health care reform.* Hartford, CT: Yale University Press.

Straus, S. E., Tetroe, J., & Graham, I. D. (2013). *Knowledge translation in health care: Moving from evidence to practice.* Chichester, West Sussex: John Wiley & Sons.

Tait, A., & Richardson, K. A. (2010). *Complexity and knowledge management: Understanding the role of knowledge in the management of social networks.* Charlotte, NC: Information Age Pub.

Tocknell, M. D. (2013). Risk and reward in collaborative care. *HealthLeaders, April,* 22–24.

Topol, E. J. (2012). *The creative destruction of medicine: How the digital revolution will create better health care.* New York, NY: Basic Books.

Chapter 13

Models to Guide Implementation and Sustainability of Evidence-Based Practice

Deborah Dang, Bernadette Mazurek Melnyk, Ellen Fineout-Overholt, Donna Ciliska, Alba DiCenso, Laura Cullen, Maria Cvach, June H. Larrabee, Jo Rycroft-Malone, Alyce A. Schultz, Cheryl B. Stetler, and Kathleen R. Stevens

> Change is inevitable...adapting to change is unavoidable, it's how you do it that sets you together or apart.
>
> —William Ngwako Maphoto

- Home visitation to low-income pregnant women misprevents major depressive episodes (Tandon, Leis, Mendelson, Perry, & Kemp, 2013).
- Patient-directed music can reduce anxiety and sedative exposure in critically ill patients who are mechanically ventilated (Chlan et al., 2013).
- A school-based healthy lifestyle intervention program (i.e., COPE [Creating Opportunities for Personal Empowerment] Healthy Lifestyles TEEN [Thinking, Emotions, Exercise and Nutrition]) that includes cognitive behavioral skills building can prevent overweight/obesity, improve social skills and academic performance, and lesson depression in severely depressed adolescents (Melnyk et al., 2013).

The clinical interventions described above are but a few of many interventions that have been evaluated and shown to have a positive impact on patient outcomes and often on cost savings for the healthcare system. However, are healthcare providers aware of these studies? How do they learn about them? How can healthcare providers keep up to date with new knowledge that relates to their practice? Once they acquire new knowledge, how do healthcare providers change their own practices and influence others to change practice behaviors within their organizations? Are evaluations conducted to determine whether evidence-based changes in clinical practice result in beneficial outcomes? All of these questions are important to the effective implementation of evidence-based findings in clinical practice (Box 13.1).

Healthcare providers are highly motivated to be evidence-based practitioners. However, there are many individual and organizational obstacles. At the individual level, clinicians frequently (a) have inadequate skills in searching for and critically appraising research studies (Parahoo, 2000), (b) lack confidence to implement change (Parahoo), and (c) have misperceptions that evidence-based practice (EBP) takes too much time (Melnyk, Fineout-Overholt, Gallagher-Ford, & Kaplan, 2012).

However, organizational factors often create the most significant barriers to EBP (Parahoo; Retsas, 2000). Lack of interest, motivation, leadership, vision, strategy, and direction among managers for EBP poses a significant organizational barrier. Findings from a survey of a random sample of nurses across the United States also identified their nurse leaders and managers as a major barrier to EBP (Melnyk et al., 2012). This is especially true for the nursing profession because a change in practice, especially if it involves purchasing new equipment or changing a policy or procedure, requires administrative support (Parahoo; Retsas). For example, in the case of pressure sore prevention, nurses have the decision-making autonomy to ensure position changes. However, other interventions, such as the purchase of high-specification foam mattresses, require approval of the organization.

Changing clinical practice is complex and challenging. As a result, many models have been developed to systematically guide the implementation of EBP. This chapter begins by describing the components of evidence-based clinical decision making. The chapter then goes on to describe models that are designed to assist clinicians in changing practices based on evidence in their organizations.

> ### Box 13.1   Definition of Evidence-Based Practice
>
> Evidence-based practice is the integration of best research evidence with clinical expertise (including internal evidence) and patient values to facilitate clinical decision making (Sackett et al., 2000).
> Evidence-based practice includes the following steps (Melnyk & Fineout-Overholt, 2011):
>
> 0. Cultivate a spirit of inquiry.
> 1. Ask the burning clinical question in PICOT format.
> 2. Search for and collect the most relevant best evidence.
> 3. Critically appraise the evidence (i.e., rapid critical appraisal, evaluation, and synthesis).
> 4. Integrate the best evidence with one's clinical expertise and patient preferences and values in making a practice decision or change.
> 5. Evaluate outcomes of the practice decision or change based on evidence.
> 6. Disseminate the outcomes of the EBP decision or change.

EVOLUTION FROM RESEARCH UTILIZATION TO EVIDENCE-BASED CLINICAL DECISION MAKING

In the past, nurses and other healthcare providers used the term *research utilization (RU)* to mean the use of research knowledge in clinical practice. EBP is broader than RU because the clinician is encouraged to consider a number of dimensions in clinical decision making, one of which is evidence. Along with the integration of the best research evidence, evidence-based practitioners are encouraged to consider **internal evidence** (e.g., the patient's clinical status and circumstances, and evidence generated internally from outcomes management or quality improvement (QI) and EBP projects), the patient's preferences and actions, healthcare resources, and clinical expertise when making clinical decisions (DiCenso, Ciliska, & Guyatt, 2004; Melnyk & Fineout-Overholt, 2011; Figure 13.1).

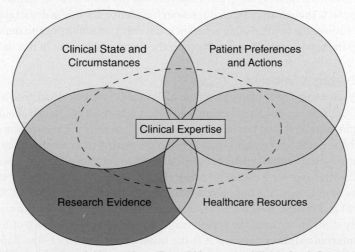

Figure 13.1: Evidence-based decision making. (From DiCenso, A., Ciliska, D., & Guyatt, G. [Eds.] [2004]. *Evidence-based nursing: A guide to clinical practice.* St. Louis, MO: Elsevier.)

Implementation of the Clinical Decision-Making Model

To illustrate how this clinical decision-making model can be implemented, consider the following examples.

Patient Preferences, Actions, Clinical State, Setting, and Circumstances

For many years, public health nurses have been visiting at-risk postpartum mothers in their homes to provide education and support. The nurses have the clinical expertise; the funding is available to the health department to support this nursing intervention; and the evidence shows that it has produced positive outcomes in terms of preventing postpartum depression (Dennis & Dowswell, 2013). However, when the community health nurse calls some clients to arrange a home visit, the clients are reluctant to agree and sometimes refuse to be visited. *Patient preferences and actions* will be the dominant elements in this decision regarding a home visit. Optimally, patient values and preferences are based on careful consideration of information that provides an accurate assessment of the patient's condition and possible treatments as well as the likely benefits, costs, and risks. In this way, clients can make informed decisions based on the best current knowledge. Patient preferences play a large role in cancer treatments where patients, having heard and understood the benefit of a chemotherapy treatment, choose not to have it because of its detrimental effects on quality of life in terms of hair loss and general malaise.

In addition to patient preferences, clinicians need to consider the *patient's clinical state, setting, and circumstances*. For example, patients who live in remote areas may not have access to the same diagnostic tests or interventions as those who live near a tertiary care medical center. Also, the effectiveness of some interventions may vary, depending on the patient's stage of illness or symptoms. Furthermore, outcomes from patients on a specific unit (i.e., internal evidence) might also be integrated into evidence-based decisions.

Availability of Healthcare Resources

Another component of clinical decision making is the availability of *healthcare resources*. Sometimes, even the best evidence cannot be used because the intervention is too costly. Now return to the home visiting example where the local health department would like to replace some of the community health nurses with paraprofessionals (lay home visitors) in hope of delivering similar education and support and achieving comparable outcomes at a lower cost. The nurse manager conducts a literature search and finds an article by Olds and colleagues (2002), which concludes that paraprofessionals had greater effects on mothers than nurse visits, while public health nurses achieved more significant and important effects on child outcomes than paraprofessionals; the differences did not warrant development of a paraprofessional visiting program. Though armed with this research evidence, the health department no longer has the resources to continue the home visiting program using only community health nurses, and it begins to hire and train paraprofessionals. Resources become the dominant element in this decision.

High-Quality Research Evidence

It is the clinician's responsibility to identify current, high-quality *research evidence* to inform his or her clinical decisions. Consider an in-hospital example in which nurses are concerned about the high rate of central venous catheter-related blood stream infections. They currently use transparent dressings on the catheter sites, and one nurse, who recently transferred to this setting from another institution, notes that there seemed to be far fewer central venous catheter-related blood stream infections where she previously worked when gauze dressings were used. This nurse offers to search the literature for studies that compare the two types of dressings. She finds a systematic review by Webster, Gillies, O' Riordan, Sherriff, and Rickard (2011) and reviews it with the clinical instructor on the unit. Together, they conclude that it is a high-quality study in terms of the review methods, and although the risk of bias in individual studies is high (**internal validity**), they feel it is the best available evidence. The population and setting of the included studies are sufficiently similar to theirs that they can apply the results in their unit (**external validity**). From the study's findings, the clinicians conclude that gauze dressings on central venous catheter sites may result in fewer catheter-related blood stream infections. The nurses talk to their administrator about changing to gauze dressings. Their administrator agrees but encourages them to evaluate whether the new type of dressing actually results in a reduction in catheter related infections by recording the number of infections for two months before and after switching to gauze dressings. Gathering internal evidence on the unit with their own patients will provide further evidence to support their change in practice.

Clinical Expertise

Evidence-based decision making is influenced by the practitioner's experience and skills. Clinician skills include the expertise that develops from multiple observations of patients and how they react to certain interventions. *Clinical expertise* is essential for avoiding the mechanical application of care maps, decision rules, and guidelines. Consider an example in which healthcare providers who work in a psychiatric outpatient facility are wondering whether they are providing the best possible care to their patients with schizophrenia. One of these providers offers to search the literature and finds a recent systematic review reporting that social skills training supported employment programs and that cognitive behavior therapy improved some outcomes in patients with schizophrenia (Wykes, Steel, Everitt, & Tarrier, 2008). In considering these interventions, the healthcare providers believed that they had the expertise to conduct social skills training as well as access to employment programs to which they could refer their clients. However, they also believed that they did not have the skills to provide cognitive behavior therapy. As a result, the healthcare providers decided to investigate avenues for learning this skill, then presented a proposal to the clinic director that summarized the research evidence and outlined a plan for their continuing education and program development.

In the clinical decision-making model, clinical expertise is the mechanism that provides for the integration of the other model components. For example, the practitioner's clinical expertise will influence the following:

- Quality of the initial assessment of the client's clinical state and circumstances
- Problem formulation
- Decision about whether the best evidence and availability of healthcare resources substantiate a new approach
- Exploration of patient preferences
- Delivery of the clinical intervention
- Evaluation of the outcome for that particular patient

Integrating Best Evidence With Clinical Expertise

The following scenario exemplifies integrating the best available scientific evidence with clinical expertise. The local school board is concerned about the string of suicides and additional attempts at self-harm in the high schools in the last year. It asks the school nurses and counselors to implement a program for students who have attempted suicide or are otherwise engaging in self-harm. The teachers and school board are very supportive of the program, the school nurses and counselors have the skills to implement this program and resources are sufficient to mount the program. However, the nurses and counselors search the literature and find a high-quality systematic review that shows evidence that these sorts of programs are not effective (Crawford, Thomas, Khan, & Kulinskaya, 2007). The school nurses and counselors recommend that the self-harm program not be offered but that instead, the school board participates in offering and evaluating a "healthy school" approach, which includes an ongoing curriculum in self-esteem enhancement, conflict resolution, and positive relationship building.

The factors in each EBP model will vary in their extent of influence in clinical decision making, depending on the decision to be made. In the past, EBP has been criticized for its "cookbook approach" to patient care. Some believe that it focuses solely on research evidence and, in so doing, ignores patient preferences. Figure 13.1 shows that research evidence is only one factor in the evidence-based decision-making process and is always considered within the context of the other factors. Depending on the decision, the primary determining factor will vary. One of the advantages of this model is that healthcare providers have not traditionally considered research evidence in their decision-making process, and this model reminds them that such evidence should be one of the factors they consider.

MODELS TO CHANGE PRACTICE IN AN ORGANIZATION

There is increasing recognition that efforts to change practice should be guided by conceptual models or frameworks (Graham, Tetroe, & KT Theories Research Group, 2007). Early in the EBP movement, healthcare scientists, including many nurse scientists, developed models to organize our thinking about EBP and understand how various aspects of EBP work together to improve care and outcomes. These models guide the design and implementation of approaches intended to strengthen evidence-based decision making and help clinicians implement an evidence-based change in practice. Graham and colleagues conducted a literature review of the many models that exist and identified commonalities in terms of their steps or phases. These include the following:

- Identify a problem that needs addressing.
- Identify stakeholders or change agents who will help make the change in practice happen.
- Identify a practice change shown to be effective through high-quality research that is designed to address the problem.
- Identify and, if possible, address the potential barriers to the practice change.
- Use effective strategies to disseminate information about the practice change to those implementing it.
- Implement the practice change.
- Evaluate the impact of the practice change on structure, process, and outcome measures.
- Identify activities that will help sustain the change in practice.

According to a thematic analysis of theoretical models (Mitchell, Fisher, Hastings, Silverman, & Wallen, 2010), major EBP models can be grouped into three categories:

1. EBP, RU, and Knowledge Transformation Processes;
2. Strategic/Organizational Change Theory to Promote Uptake and Adoption of New Knowledge; and
3. Knowledge Exchange and Synthesis for Application and Inquiry. A thematic analysis of theoretical models for translational science in nursing: Mapping the field.

Each model brings forth strengths and can be selectively applied for a wide array of purposes, including evidence identification, implementation and integration, and educating current and future workforces. The following eight models were created to facilitate integration of EBP for change improvement:

1. The Stetler Model of Evidence-Based Practice
2. The Iowa Model of Evidence-Based Practice to promote quality care
3. The Model for Evidence-Based Practice Change
4. The Advancing Research and Clinical practice through close Collaboration (ARCC) model for implementation and sustainability of EBP
5. The Promoting Action on Research Implementation in Health Services (PARIHS) framework
6. The Clinical Scholar model
7. The Johns Hopkins Nursing Evidence-Based Practice model
8. The ACE Star Model of Knowledge Transformation

The Stetler Model of Evidence-Based Practice

The original Stetler/Marram model for RU was published in 1976 to fill a void regarding the realistic application of research findings to practice (Stetler & Marram, 1976). The original model has undergone three revisions to strengthen its underpinnings through (a) the use of research on knowledge utilization,

(b) the integration of emerging concepts of EBP, and (c) clarifying and highlighting critical concepts (Stetler, 1994a, 2001a, 2001b). Critical thinking and use of research findings remain the core of the model. However, as introduced in 1994, the model long recognized the value of information beyond research and, in 2001, explicitly introduced additional sources of both *external* and *internal* evidence (described later in the definitions section) that could influence an ultimate "use" decision (Stetler, 1994a, 2001b). Through work on an organizational model of EBP at Baystate Medical Center, with the Stetler model as its underpinning, the 2001 version became integrally related to the concept of evidence-based nursing practice (i.e., practice that stresses "the use of research findings and, as appropriate, QI data, other operational and evaluation data, the consensus of recognized experts and affirmed experience to substantiate practice" [Stetler et al., 1998, p. 49]).

Overview of the Stetler Model

The Stetler model (Figure 13.2A) outlines a series of steps to assess and use research findings to facilitate safe and effective evidence-based nursing practice. Over the years of its evolution, the model has grown in complexity in order to provide more guidance around critical utilization concepts as well as details and options involved in applying research to practice in the real world. In 2009, more modifications were made to the narrative in both pages of the model to better clarify the role of supplemental evidence and to highlight implementation tools (Stetler, 2010).

    The Stetler model has long been known as a practitioner-oriented model because of its focus on critical thinking and use of findings by the individual practitioner (Kim, 1999; Stetler & Marram, 1976). The 2001 version provided clarification that this guided problem-solving process also applies to groups of practitioners engaged in RU/EBP. Yet, the model maintains the bottom-line assumption that even prepackaged, research-based recommendations are applied at the skilled practitioner level to individual patients, staff members, or other targets of use.

Definitions of Terms in the Stetler Model

The term *evidence* first appeared in the model in 1976 and, at that stage, referred only to research findings. However, in 1994, Stetler broadened the concept of "substantiating evidence" to include additional sources of information because research indicates that "experiential and theoretical information are more likely to be combined with research information than they are to be ignored" (Stetler, 1994a, p. 17). By 2001, the concept of evidence had become a key element of the model (see Figure 13.2; Stetler, 2001b). The following definitions underpin the multifaceted meaning of evidence within the current version (Stetler, 2001a, 2001b; Stetler, Brunell, et al., 1998):

◆ Evidence, within the context of health care, is defined as information or facts that are systematically obtained (i.e., obtained in a manner that is replicable, observable, credible, verifiable, or basically supportable; Stetler, 2002).
◆ Evidence, within the context of health care, can come from different sources and can vary in the degree to which it is systematically obtained and, thus, the degree to which it is perceived as basically *credible* or supportable for safe and effective use.

Different sources of evidence can be categorized as external and internal. **External evidence** comes primarily from research, but where research findings are lacking, the consensus opinion/experience of widely recognized experts and credible program evaluations in the literature are considered supportable evidence and will often be used to supplement research-based recommendations. **Internal evidence** comes primarily from systematically but locally obtained facts or information. It includes data from local performance, planning, quality, outcome, and evaluation activity as well as data collected through use of RU/EBP models to assess current practice and measure progress. In addition, internal evidence includes the consensus opinion and experience of local groups as well as experiential information from individual professionals—*if affirmed*. Although an individual's isolated, unsystematic experience and related opinion are not considered to be credible evidence, those experiential observations or ways of thinking that have been reflected on, externalized, or exposed to explorations of truth and

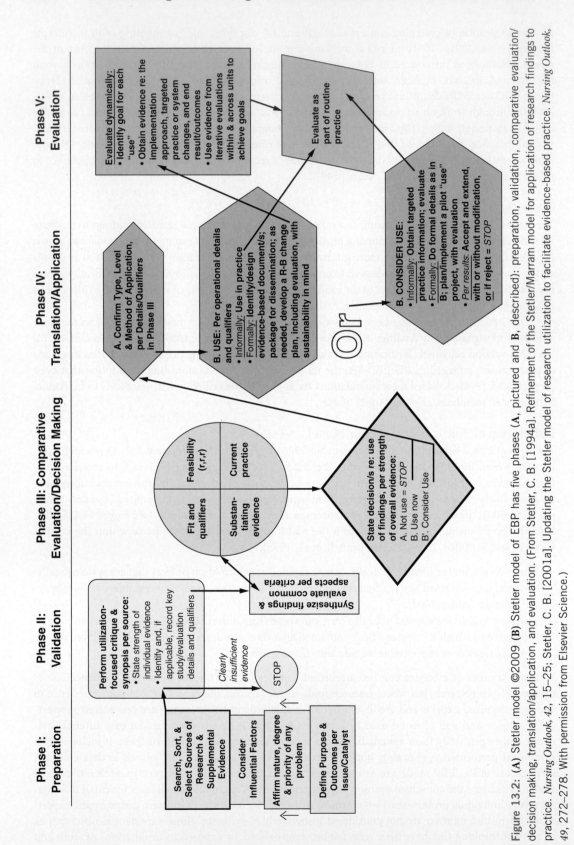

Figure 13.2: **(A)** Stetler model ©2009 **(B)** Stetler model of EBP has five phases (**A**, pictured and **B**, described): preparation, validation, comparative evaluation/ decision making, translation/application, and evaluation. (From Stetler, C. B. [1994a]. Refinement of the Stetler/Marram model for application of research findings to practice. *Nursing Outlook, 42,* 15–25; Stetler, C. B. [2001a]. Updating the Stetler model of research utilization to facilitate evidence-based practice. *Nursing Outlook, 49,* 272–278. With permission from Elsevier Science.)

Phase I: Preparation	Phase II: Validation	Phase III: Comparative Evaluation/Decision Making	Phase IV: Translation/Application	Phase V: Evaluation
Purpose, Context, & Sources of Evidence:	Credibility of Evidence & Potential for/Detailed Qualifiers of Application:	Synthesis & Decisions/Recommendations per Criteria of Applicability:	Operational Definition of Use/Actions for Change:	Alternative Evaluations:
• **Potential Issues/Catalysts** = *a problem, including unexplained variations; less-than-best practice; routine update of knowledge; validation/routine revision of procedures, etc; or innovative program goal*	• **Critique & synopsize essential components, operational details, and other qualifying factors, per source** ° *See instructions for use of utilization-focused review tables,* with evaluative criteria, to facilitate this task; fill in the tables for group decision making or potential future synthesis*	• ****Synthesize the cumulative findings:** ° *Logically organize & display the similarities and differences across multiple findings, per common aspects or sub-elements of the topic under review*	• **Types** = *cognitive/conceptual, symbolic &/or instrumental*	• **Evaluation per type, method, level: e.g., consider conceptual use at individual level&&**
• **Affirm/clarify perceived problem/s, with internal evidence re: current practice** *[baseline]*	• Critique ***systematic reviews and guidelines**	° *Evaluate degree of substantiation of each aspect/sub-element; reference any qualifying conditions for application*	• **Methods** = *informal or formal; direct or indirect*	• **Consider cost-benefit of change + various evaluation efforts**
• **Consider other influential internal and external factors, e.g., timelines**	• ***Rate the level & quality of each individual evidence source per a "table of evidence"**	• **Evaluate degree & nature of other criteria: **feasibility (r,r,r = risk, resources, readiness); pragmatic fit,** including potential qualifying factors to application, & nature of ****current practice,** including the urgency/risk of current issues/needs	• **Levels** = *individual, group or department/organization*	• **Use RU-as-a-process to enhance credibility of evaluation data**
• **Affirm and focus on high priority issues**	• **Differentiate statistical and clinical significance**	• **Make a decision whether/what to use:** ° *Can be a personal practitioner-level decision or a recommendation to others*	• **Direct instrumental use:** *change individual behavior (e.g., via assessment tool or Rx intervention options); or change policy, procedure, protocol, algorithm, program, etc.*	• **For both dynamic & pilot evaluations, include:** ° ***formative, regarding actual implementation & goal progress*
• **Decide if need to form a team, involve formal stakeholders, &/or assign project lead/facilitator**	• **Eliminate non-credible sources**	° *Judge strength of decision; indicate if primarily "research-based" (R-B) or, per hi use of supplemental info, "E-B"; note level of strength of recommendation/s per related* table; note any qualifying factors that may influence individualized variations*	• **Cognitive use:** *validate current practice; change personal way of thinking; increase awareness; better understand or appreciate condition/s or experience/s*	° *summative, regarding identified end goal and end-point outcomes*
• **Define desired, measurable outcome/s**	• **End the process if there is clearly insufficient, credible external evidence that meets your need**	• **If decision = "Not use" research findings:** ° *May conduct own research or delay use till additional research done by others*	• **Symbolic use:** *develop position paper or proposal for change; or persuade others regarding a way of thinking*	
• **Seek out systematic reviews/guidelines first**		° *If still decide to act now, e.g., on evidence of consensus or another basis for practice, consider need for rigorous planned change and evaluation.*	• **CAUTION: Assess whether translation/product or use goes beyond actual findings/evidence:** ° *Research evidence may or may not provide various details for a complete policy, procedure, etc.; indicate this fact to users, and note differential levels of evidence therein*	**NOTE:** Model applies to all forms of practice, i.e., educational, clinical, managerial, or other; **to use effectively read 2001 & 1994 model papers.**
• **Determine need for an explicit type of research evidence, if relevant**		• **If decision = "Use/Consider Use," can mean a recommendation for or against a specific practice**	• **Formal dissemination & change/implementation strategies should be planned per relevant research and local barriers:** ° *Passive education is usually not effective as an isolated strategy. Use Dx analysis** & an ***implementation framework to develop a plan. Consider multiple strategies; e.g., opinion leaders, interactive education, reminders & audits.*	****Stetler et al, 2006 re: dx analysis**
• **Select research sources with conceptual fit**			° *Focus on context§ to enhance sustainability of organizational-related change*	*****E.g.: Rogers' re: implications of attributes of a change; Rycroft-Malone et al. &PARIHS (2002) & Green & Krueter's PRECEDE (1992) models re: implementation**
	*Stetler, Morsi, Rucki, et al. *Appl Nurs Res* 1998; 11(4):195–206 for noted tables, reviews, & synthesis process		• **Consider need for appropriate, reasoned variation**	**§Stetler, 2003 on context**
			• **WITH B, where made a decision to use in the setting:** ° *With formal use, may need a dynamic evaluation to effectively implement & continuously improve/refine use of best available evidence across units & time*	**&&Stetler & Caramanica, 2007 on outcomes**
			• **WITH B', where made a decision to consider use & thus obtain additional, pragmatic information before a final decision** ° *With formal consideration, do a pilot project* ° *With a pilot project, must assess if need IRB review, per relevant institutional criteria*	

Figure 13.2: *(Continued)*

verification from various sources of data—and thus *affirmed*—are considered valid evidence in the model (Rycroft-Malone et al., 2002; Rycroft-Malone & Stetler, 2004; Stetler, 2001b; Stetler, Brunell, et al., 1998).

   It is also important to note, as Haynes (2002) did, the need to consider "evidence of patients' circumstances and wishes" (p. 3). Patient wishes are commonly included in EBP definitions, usually labeled as patient preferences, and at the individual level can be considered internal evidence (Goode & Piedalue, 1999; Haynes, Sackett, Gray, Cook, & Guyatt, 1996).

Using the Stetler Model

The basic "how to" of EBP using the Stetler model is divided into the following five progressive categories or phases of activity. Figure 13.2B and related publications provide specific guidance and rationale for each of these steps (Stetler, 1994a, 2001b; Stetler & Caramanica, 2007; Stetler, Morsi, et al., 1998).

1. *Preparation*: Getting started by defining and affirming a priority need, reviewing the context in which use would occur, organizing the work if more than an individual practitioner is involved, and systematically initiating a search for relevant evidence, especially research.
2. *Validation*: Assessing a body of evidence by systematically critiquing each study and other relevant documents (e.g., a systematic review or guideline), with a *utilization* focus in mind, then choosing and summarizing the collected evidence that relates to the identified need.
3. *Comparative evaluation/decision making*: Making decisions about use after synthesizing the body of summarized evidence by applying a set of utilization criteria, then deciding whether and, if so, what to use in light of the identified need.
4. *Translation/application*: Converting findings into the type of change to be made/recommended, planning application as needed for formal use, putting the plan into action by using operational details of how to use the acceptable findings, and then enhancing adoption and actual implementation with an evidence-based change plan.
5. *Evaluation*: Evaluating the plan in terms of the degree to which it was implemented and whether the goals for using the evidence were met.

Despite the appearance that the systematic utilization of evidence is a linear, clear-cut process, it is more fluid. Figure 13.2B has serrated lines between the phases to indicate this fluidity and the need to occasionally revisit decisions (e.g., the relevance of specific studies and fit of various findings). Despite the model's complex appearance, its steps and concepts can be integrated into a professional's routine way of thinking about RU and EBP in general. This in turn influences how one routinely reads research and applies related findings (Stetler, 1994b; Stetler, Bautista, Vernale-Hannon, & Foster, 1995).

Critical Assumptions and Model Concepts

Key underlying assumptions that generate this model's critical thinking and practitioner orientation must be considered (Stetler, 1994a, 2001b). For example, the model assumes that both formal and informal use of research findings—with supplemental use of other evidence—can occur in the practice setting. Formal, organization-initiated and -sanctioned RU/EBP activity is most frequently discussed in the nursing literature. Often, this activity results in new policies, procedures, protocols, programs, and standards. After formal documents are disseminated, individuals are expected to use these translated and packaged findings. However, as Geyman suggests, EBP "requires the integration, patient by patient, of clinical expertise and judgment with the best available relevant external evidence" (1998, pp. 46–47). This may require reasoned variation (Stetler, 2010) in the context of a patient's circumstances, status, and preferences. Additionally, the practitioner's contextual and personal factors influence the process. Finally, research and evaluative data provide probabilistic information rather than absolutes about each person for whom the evidence is believed to "fit." In light of these assumptions, use of the model requires an RU/EBP competent individual.

   Individual, RU/EBP-competent practitioners (i.e., those who are skilled in the process of research/evidence utilization) can also informally use the model's critical thinking process in their routine practice and interactions with others (Cronenwett, 1994; Stetler, 1994a, 1994b). These practitioners may use evidence to substantiate or improve a current practice, change their way of thinking about an issue or routine, expand their repertoire of assessment or intervention strategies, or change a colleague's way of thinking about a treatment plan or issue (Stetler & Caramanica, 2007). Again, the user must possess a certain level of knowledge and skills specifically related to the use of research and other forms of evidence (Stetler, 2001b). Such knowledge and skills for the safe, appropriate, and effective use of findings include, for example, knowledge regarding research/evidence and its utilization—such as use of tables of evidence and a set of applicability criteria to determine the desirability and feasibility of using guidelines or a credible study, plus knowledge of the substantive area under consideration (Stetler).

Advanced-level practitioners (e.g., clinicians with master's and doctorate degrees) are most likely to fulfill such expectations and are also more likely to routinely integrate research findings into their practices (Cronenwett, 1994; Stetler, 1994a, 1994b). Advanced-level clinicians are able to do so because of their critical thinking skills and advanced knowledge of their specialty areas— knowledge that provides them with a *body of evidence* with which to comparatively evaluate any study under consideration for application in their practice. With sufficient education and skills preparation, baccalaureate-prepared providers—in collaboration with advanced-level clinicians— can and should participate in the identification of issues, development of formal EBPs, and facilitation of related use.

Another of the model's underlying assumptions is that research findings and other credible evidence, such as consensus guidelines, may be used in multiple ways. Practitioners use evidence directly in observable ways to change how they behave or provide care through assessments, clinical procedures, and behavioral interventions. They also use evidence indirectly or conceptually, which is not as easy to observe but is very important to EBP. This can involve using evidence to change how one thinks about a patient or an issue. It also can involve adding evidence to one's body of knowledge, merging it with other information, and using it in the future (Stetler, 1994a). Finally, research findings and related evidence can be used symbolically (i.e., strategically) to influence the thinking and behavior of others. A key to safe use in such multiple forms, however, is that competent users will understand the strength of evidence underlying targeted uses, as well as the status of applicability criteria.

To thoroughly understand the Stetler model, it is most useful to read the 1994 paper—in particular when interested in use of research and related evidence for individual decision making—*and* the 2001 paper, in particular when interested in the safe and effective use of research and related evidence for collective, formal decision making and related policies and practice documents.

The Iowa Model of Evidence-Based Practice to Promote Quality Care

The *Iowa Model of Evidence-Based Practice to Promote Quality Care* (Titler et al., 2001) provides guidance for nurses and other clinicians in making decisions about clinical and administrative practices that affect patient outcomes. The Iowa model (Figure 13.3) outlines a pragmatic multiphase change process with feedback loops. The original model has been revised and updated (Titler et al., 1994, 2001; Watson, Bulechek, & McCloskey, 1987). The model is currently being reviewed and may be updated soon. The model is based on the problem-solving steps in the scientific process and is widely recognized for its applicability and ease of use by multidisciplinary healthcare teams.

Overview of and Using the Iowa Model

Identify "Triggers." The Iowa model begins by encouraging clinicians to identify practice questions or "triggers" either through identification of a clinical problem or from new knowledge. Important triggers often come from questioning current practice. Problem-focused triggers will often have existing data that highlight an opportunity for improvement. Knowledge-focused triggers come from disseminated scientific knowledge (e.g., national guidelines, new research) leading practitioners to question current practice standards. Knowledge-focused triggers are more likely to create top-down change and require more planning for implementation (B. Rakel, personal correspondence May 21, 2013).

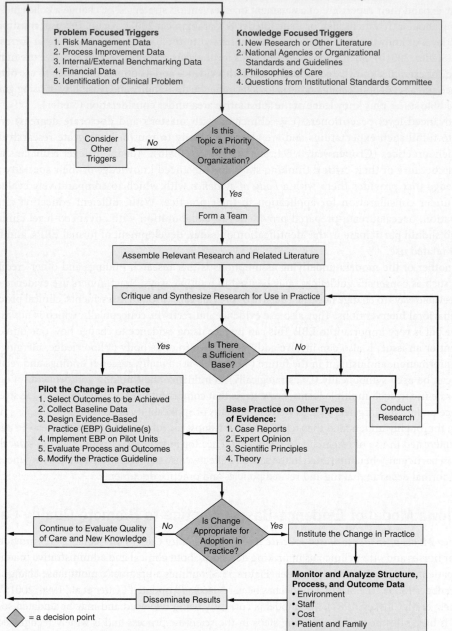

Figure 13.3: The Iowa model of evidence-based practice to promote quality care. (Used with permission from Marita G. Titler, PhD, RN, FAAN, University of Iowa Hospitals and Clinics, © 1998. For permission to use or reproduce the model, please contact the University of Iowa Hospitals and Clinics at (319) 384. 9098.)

Clinical Applications. Nurses identify important and clinically relevant practice questions that can be addressed through the EBP process. A number of clinically important topics have been addressed using the Iowa model, including verification of nasogastric tube placement (Farrington, Lang, Cullen, & Stewart, 2009), hypothermia management (Block, Lilienthal, Cullen, & White, 2012), newborn hyperbilirubinemia (Nelson, Doering, Anderson, & Kelly, 2012), oral mucositis (Farrington, Cullen, &

Dawson, 2013), newborn skin-to-skin contact (Haxton, Doering, Gingras, & Kelly, 2012), fragility fracture (Myrick, 2011), and depression screening (Yackel, McKennan, & Fox-Deise, 2010).

Operational topics and programs have also been addressed using the Iowa model (Chung, Davis, Moughrabi, & Gawlinski, 2011; Krom, Batten, & Bautista, 2010; Mark, Latimer, & Hardy, 2010; Popovich, Boyd, Dachenhaus, & Kusler, 2012; Schulte, Bejciy-Spring, & Niese, 2012). Important issues have been addressed using the Iowa model well ahead of regulatory standards or changes in reimbursement (e.g., pain, falls, suicide risk, urinary catheter use) by supporting EBP projects on important clinical topics identified by clinicians. Administrators and nurses in leadership positions can support clinicians' use of the EBP process by creating a culture of inquiry, clinician ownership, and a system supporting evidence-based care delivery (Cullen, Hanrahan, Tucker, Rempel, & Jordan, 2012; Everett & Sitterding, 2011; Gerrish et al., 2012; Gifford, Davies, Edwards, Griffin, & Lybanon, 2007; Gifford et al., 2013; Hauck, Winsett, & Kuric, 2013; Kelly et al., 2011; Saint et al., 2010).

Organizational Priorities. Not every clinical question can be addressed through the EBP process. Identification of issues that are a priority for the organization will facilitate garnering the support needed to complete an EBP project. Higher priority may be given to topics that address high-volume, high-risk, or high-cost procedures, those that are closely aligned with the institution's strategic plan, or those that are driven by other institutional or market forces (e.g., changing reimbursement). Considering how a topic fits within the organizational priorities can aid in obtaining support from senior leadership and other disciplines as well as in obtaining the resources necessary to carry out the practice change. Discussions determining if the clinical issue is an organizational priority create early opportunities to connect with stakeholders. If the trigger is not an organizational priority, practitioners may want to consider a different focus, different project outcomes, or other triggers for improving practice that better fit organizational needs. This and similar feedback loops within the model highlight the nonlinearity of the work and support continuing efforts for improving quality care through the EBP process.

Forming a Team. Once there is commitment to addressing the topic, a team is formed to develop, implement, and evaluate the practice change. The team is composed of stakeholders that may include staff nurse(s), unit managers, advanced practice nurses (APNs), interdisciplinary colleagues, and organizational leaders. Team membership requires several considerations to maximize the use of team members' skills and organizational linkages.

During a recent project addressing oral mucositis using the Iowa model, team membership was designed to capture key linkages clinically and within the governance structure (Farrington et al., 2013). The team included members from pediatric and adult ambulatory and inpatient settings representing staff nurses, nurse managers, and APNs. Committee members also provided active linkages within the governance structure through their membership on or links to nursing quality, hospital dentistry, dietary, hematology–oncology, radiation oncology, oral pathology, patient education, staff education, the products committee, nursing policy committee, and the nursing management council (Figure 13.4) (Cullen et al., 2012). The team used these linkages to support communication, coordination, and reporting about the initiative. This coordination and collaboration promotes delivery of evidence-based health care (Ida, Adelaide, & Stefania, 2012).

Initially, the team selects, reviews, critiques, and synthesizes available research evidence. Collaboration with nursing librarians can be particularly helpful in optimizing yields from online bibliographic databases and other library resources (Deberg, Adams, & Cullen, 2012; Flynn & McGuinness, 2011; Krom et al., 2010). Librarians' expert knowledge and skills in the functionality of online resources, when matched with clinicians' expertise, will result in yields with the best specificity to address the project trigger. If high-quality research evidence is not available or sufficient for determining practice, the team may recommend using lower levels of evidence (Harmon et al., 2013; Sen et al., 2013) or conduct research to improve the evidence available for practice and operational decisions (Lopes & Galvao, 2010; Staggers & Blaz, 2013; Tucker, Bieber, Attlesey-Pries, Olson, & Dierkhising, 2012). When the evidence is sufficient or lower levels of evidence are used, a practice change is piloted. The team tries the practice change to determine the feasibility and effectiveness of the EBP change in clinical care.

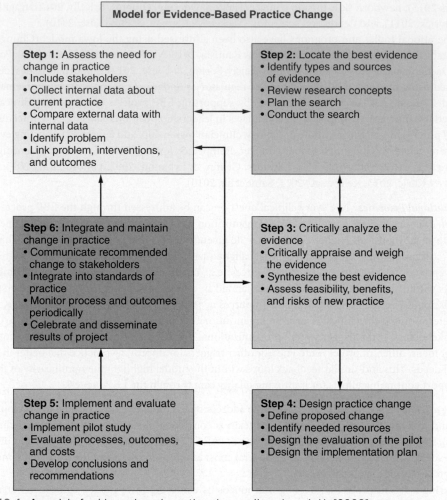

Figure 13.4: A model of evidence-based practice change. (Larrabee, J. H. [2009]. *Nurse to nurse: Practice.* New York: McGraw-Hill. Used with permission.)

Piloting a Practice Change. Piloting is an essential step in the process. Outcomes achieved in a controlled environment, when a researcher is testing a study protocol in a homogenous group of patients, may be different than those found when the EBP is used by multiple caregivers in a natural clinical setting without the tight controls of a research study. Thus, trialing the EBP change is essential for identifying issues before instituting a house-wide rollout.

Piloting involves multiple steps when planning for both implementation and evaluation. The research evidence will provide direction for selecting process and outcome indicators to use for baseline data measurement, although significant simplification of research measures is needed when evaluating QI indicators for EBP. Pilot evaluation is not replication research (i.e., replicating the results of another study) and must be narrowed to key indicators needed to provide direction for clinical decision making. Designing a draft practice guideline or protocol can take many forms, including development of an evidence-based policy, procedure, care map, algorithm, or other document outlining the practice and decision points for clinician users. Implementation during the pilot requires planning and selection of effective implementation strategies (Cullen & Adams, 2012; Titler, 2008; Titler, Wilson, Resnick, & Shever, 2013; van Achterberg, Schoonhoven, & Grol, 2008). Evaluation of the process and outcome indicators is completed before and after implementation of the practice change. A comparison of pre-pilot and post-pilot data will determine the success of the pilot, effectiveness of the evidence-based protocol, and need for modification of either the implementation process or the practice protocol.

Evaluating the Pilot. Following the pilot, a determination is made regarding appropriateness of adoption in the pilot and beyond. A decision regarding adoption or modification of the practice is based on the evaluative data from the pilot. If the practice change is not appropriate for adoption and rollout, quality or performance improvement monitoring is needed to ensure high-quality patient care. Additional steps for clinicians include watching for new knowledge, collaborating with researchers in the area, or conducting research to guide practice decisions. If the pilot results in positive outcomes, rollout and integration of the practice are facilitated through leadership support, education, and continuous monitoring of outcomes (Cheema et al., 2011; Mayer et al., 2011; McMullan et al., 2013).

Evaluating Practice Changes and Dissemination of Results. EBP changes need ongoing evaluation with information incorporated into quality or performance improvement programs to promote integration of the practice into daily care. Monitoring and reporting trends of structure, process, and outcomes indicators with actionable feedback to clinicians can promote sustained integration of the practice change (Hysong, Best, & Pugh, 2006; Ivers et al., 2012; Mayer et al., 2011).

Dissemination of results is important for professional learning. Sharing project reports within and outside of the organization through presentations and publications supports growth of an EBP culture in the organization, expands nursing knowledge, and encourages EBP changes in other organizations as well. Project reports can be used to learn the EBP process, to learn of practice updates, or to generate additional practice questions or triggers. Dissemination of project results is a key step in the cycle promoting adoption of EBPs within the healthcare system (Hauck et al., 2013; STTI, 2008).

The Iowa model guides clinicians through the EBP process. The model includes several feedback loops, reflecting analysis, evaluation, and modification based on evaluative data of both process and outcome indicators. These are critical to individualizing the evidence to the practice setting and promoting adoption within the varying healthcare systems and settings within which nurses work. The feedback loops highlight the messy and nonlinear nature of EBP and support teams moving forward. The Iowa model was designed to support evidence-based healthcare delivery by interdisciplinary teams (Block et al., 2012; Ida et al., 2012; McMullan et al., 2013) by following a basic problem-solving approach using the scientific process, simplifying the process, and being highly application oriented. The large number of nurses and organizations using the Iowa model attests to its usefulness in practice. In fact, over 2,500 requests have been received to use the Iowa model (unpublished data).

Model for Evidence-Based Practice Change

Overview of the Model for Evidence-Based Practice Change

This model is a revised version of the model by Rosswurm and Larrabee (1999). The revised steps and schematic (Figure 13.4) were prompted by Larrabee's experience with teaching and leading nurses in the application of the original model since 1999 at West Virginia University Hospitals and prior experience with teaching and leading nurses in RU and QI (Larrabee, 2004).

The title of the revised model was changed to clarify that it was designed for guiding multiple practice change projects because the author thought the original title, "Model for Change to Evidence-Based Practice," could infer a one-time philosophical decision to pursue EBP. In its application, the actions of the original Step 3, synthesize the best evidence, required a disproportionately longer time to conduct than the other steps. To distribute the actions in Step 3 across two steps and to retain six steps in the model, the original Step 2 was added to Step 1 and the original Step 3 was divided into two: Step 2, "locate the best evidence," and Step 3, "critically analyze the evidence" (Larrabee, 2009, p. 23). The revised model also integrates principles of QI, use of team work tools, and evidence-based translation strategies to promote adoption of a new practice. The handbook (Larrabee) describing the revised model includes a number of forms and examples of their use that may be helpful to nurses applying the model. Progression through the six steps is illustrated by a fabricated EBP project focused on improving outcomes for patients with chronic heart failure.

Step 1: Assess the Need for Change in Practice

Key actions consist of identifying a practice problem or opportunity for improvement; creating an EBP team of stakeholders to address the practice problem; collecting internal data about that practice; collecting external data for benchmarking with the internal data; and refining the practice problem statement by linking the problem with possible interventions and desired outcomes or by developing a PICOT (population-intervention-comparison-outcome-time frame) question.

Often, recognition of a practice problem prompts an EBP project. Practice problems can be identified by members of a clinical unit's RU team or solicited from practicing nurses. Other times, an existing EBP team with the goal of conducting at least one EBP project per year will need to consider what patient outcomes most need improvement. Structured brainstorming and multivoting are teamwork tools that may be helpful during this process. Developing creative avenues for problem identification that increase active involvement from the nurses who will be participating with the implementation stage, such as placing an idea box on the unit for nurses, is crucial for establishing group ownership for the change project.

Once the EBP team has selected a practice problem as the focus of a project, team members should collect internal and external data relevant to that practice problem to confirm that there is an opportunity for improvement. It is important to justify the focus of the EBP project because such projects are resource intensive. Statistical process control tools that may be useful during this activity include histograms and Pareto charts. The EBP team members must prepare a practice problem statement or PICOT question to clarify for themselves and others what the project focus is and to use the statement or question to guide their work during Step 2.

Step 2: Locate the Best Evidence

Key actions are identifying the types and sources of evidence; planning the search for evidence; and conducting the search for the best evidence. Types of evidence include clinical practice guidelines, systematic reviews, single studies, critical appraisal topics, and expert committee reports. Sources of evidence include electronic bibliographic databases, websites, journals, and books. The search for evidence should be planned as a rigorous systematic review, which includes formulating the research question to guide the search, deciding on the search strategy, selecting the inclusion and exclusion criteria, and planning the synthesis. While planning, EBP team members can add rigor to the systematic review by selecting forms for critically appraising evidence sources, for organizing data from the evidence sources in a table of evidence, and identifying key points to use when synthesizing the evidence during Step 3. Critical appraisal forms or checklists are available in journal articles (Rosswurm & Larrabee, 1999) and online, including some that are for systematic reviews and specific research designs (Scottish Intercollegiate Guidelines Network, 2007).The handbook includes examples of forms and completed examples of their use (Larrabee, 2009).

Step 3: Critically Analyze the Evidence

Key actions are critically appraising and judging the strength of the evidence; synthesizing the evidence; and assessing the feasibility, benefits, and risks of implementing the new practice. Critical appraisal of the evidence is conducted using the forms selected during Step 2. Likewise, the forms selected during Step 2 are used to display information about the data sources in an evidence table that is then used to prepare the synthesis worksheet. After synthesizing the evidence, the EBP team members judge whether the body of evidence is of sufficient quantity and strength to support a practice change. If so, EBP team members consider whether or not benefits and risks of the new practice are acceptable and whether the new practice is feasible in their workplace.

Step 4: Design Practice Change

Key actions include defining the proposed practice change; identifying needed resources; designing the evaluation of the pilot; and designing the implementation plan. The description of the new practice may be in the form of a protocol, policy, procedure, care map, or guideline and should be supported by the body of evidence synthesized in Step 3. Needed resources will be specific for the new practice and may include personnel, materials, equipment, or forms. Even if the new practice is specific to just one unit, its use should be pilot tested to evaluate it for any necessary adaptation before making it a standard of care. Therefore, EBP team members need to design the implementation plan and the evaluation plan, considering translation strategies that promote adoption of a new practice. Some strategies include use of change champions, opinion leaders, educational sessions, educational materials, reminder systems, and audit and feedback. After designing the evaluation plan, EBP team members collect baseline data on the process and outcome indicators for which they will collect post-pilot data during Step 5.

Step 5: Implement and Evaluate Change in Practice

Key actions include implementing the pilot study; evaluating process, outcomes, and costs; and developing conclusions and recommendations. The EBP team members follow the implementation plan designed during Step 4, obtaining verbal feedback from those expected to use the new practice and from the change champions who are promoting the use of the new practice. That feedback will be used to make minor adjustments in the implementation plan, if necessary. After the pilot phase concludes, the EBP team members collect and analyze the post-pilot data, comparing with the baseline data. Team members use those data together with the verbal feedback to decide if they should adapt, adopt, or reject the new practice. Few teams reach this stage and decide to reject the new practice. More commonly, the new practice needs to be slightly adapted for a better fit with the organization. Once team members make this decision, they prepare conclusions and recommendations to share with administrative leaders during Step 6.

Step 6: Integrate and Maintain Change in Practice

Key actions include sharing recommendations about the new practice with stakeholders; incorporating the new practice into the standards of care; monitoring the process and outcome indicators; and celebrating and disseminating results of the project. Team members provide information about the project and their recommendations to all stakeholders, including administrative leaders who must approve making the new practice a standard of care.

Once that approval is given, the EBP team members can arrange to provide inservice education to all providers expected to use the new practice. It is important to include all stages of the process in the inservice education, such as problem identification and the strength of the evidence, as teams that emphasize only the practice change have higher rates of noncompliance during the implementation phase. They should also make plans for ongoing monitoring of the process and outcome indicators. The frequency of this monitoring can be based on judging how well the indicators are being met. The data from ongoing monitoring can be used to identify the need for further refinements in the new practice or the need for a new EBP project. The handbook (Larrabee, 2009) provides a timeline template for preparing an annual calendar with multiple EBP projects, including ongoing monitoring of completed projects. Finally, EBP team members should consider disseminating information about their project outside the organization through presentation at professional conferences and publication.

The Evidence-Based Advancing Research and Clinical Practice Through Close Collaboration (ARCC©) Model: A Model for System-Wide Implementation and Sustainability of Evidence-Based Practice

The purpose of the ARCC© model is to provide healthcare institutions and clinical settings with an organized conceptual framework that can guide system-wide implementation and sustainability of EBP to achieve quality outcomes. Since evidence-based clinicians are essential in cultivating an entire system culture that implements EBP as standard of care, the ARCC© model encompasses key strategies for individual and organizational change to and sustainability of best practice.

Overview of the ARCC© Model

The original version of the ARCC© model was conceptualized by Bernadette Melnyk in 1999 as part of a strategic planning initiative to unify research and clinical practice in order to advance EBP within an academic medical center for the ultimate purpose of improving healthcare quality and patient outcomes (Melnyk & Fineout-Overholt, 2002). Shortly following conceptualization of the ARCC© model, Dr. Fineout-Overholt surveyed advanced practice and point-of-care nurses in the medical center about the barriers and facilitators of EBP. The results of this survey along with control theory (Carver & Sheier, 1982, 1998) and cognitive behavioral theory (CBT; Beck, Rush, Shaw, & Emery, 1979) guided the formulation of key constructs in the current ARCC© model. An important facilitator of EBP identified by nurses who completed the survey was a mentor, which eventually became the central mechanism for implementing and sustaining EBP in the ARCC© model. For more than a decade, Melnyk and Fineout-Overholt have further developed the ARCC© model through empirical testing of key relationships in the model and their extensive work with healthcare institutions across the nation and globe to advance and sustain EBP.

The Conceptual Framework Guiding the ARCC© Model

Control theory (Carver & Scheier, 1982, 1998) contends that a discrepancy between a standard or goal (e.g., system-wide implementation of EBP) and a current state (e.g., the extent to which an organization is implementing EBP) should motivate behaviors in individuals to reach the goal. However, many barriers exist in healthcare organizations that inhibit clinicians from implementing EBP, including (a) inadequate EBP knowledge and skills, (b) lack of administrative support, (c) lack of an EBP mentor, (d) lack of belief that EBP improves patient care and outcomes, (e) perceived lack of authority to change patient care procedures, and (f) nurse leader/manager resistance (Hutchinson & Johnston, 2006; Melnyk, 2007; Melnyk et al., 2012; Melnyk & Fineout-Overholt, 2011). In the ARCC© model, EBP mentors (i.e., healthcare providers who have in-depth knowledge and skills in EBP as well as individual and organizational change strategies along with mentorship skills) are developed and placed within the healthcare system as a key strategy to remove barriers commonly encountered by practicing clinicians when implementing EBP (Figure 13.5). As barriers diminish, clinicians enhance their implementation of EBP to improve patient outcomes.

In the ARCC© model, CBT is used to guide behavioral change in individual clinicians toward EBP. CBT stresses the importance of individual, social, and environmental factors that influence cognition, learning, emotions, and behavior (Beck et al., 1979; Lam, 2005). The basic foundation of CBT is that an individual's behaviors and emotions are, in large part, determined by the way he or she thinks or his or her beliefs (i.e., the thinking–feeling–behaving triangle; Melnyk & Moldenhauer, 2006). Based on CBT, a tenet of the ARCC© model contends that when clinicians' beliefs about the value of EBP and their ability to implement it are strengthened through strategies such as education and skills building, there will be greater implementation of evidence-based care. In the ARCC© model, EBP mentors work with point-of-care clinicians to strengthen their beliefs about the value of EBP and their ability to implement it through evidence-based decisions.

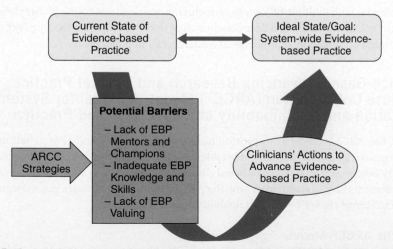

Figure 13.5: Control theory as a conceptual guide for the ARCC model© (Melnyk & Fineout-Overholt, 2005).

....
By changing your thinking, you change your beliefs.
—Author Unknown
....

Central Constructs Within and Evidence to Support the ARCC© Model

Organizational Assessment of Readiness. The first step in the ARCC© model is an organizational assessment of culture and readiness for system-wide implementation of EBP (Figure 13.6). The culture and environment of an organization can foster EBP or stymie it. If sufficient resources are not allocated to support the work of EBP, progress in advancing EBP throughout the organization will be slow. Leaders, administrators, and point-of-care providers alike must adopt the EBP paradigm for system-wide implementation to be achieved and sustained. Assessment of organizational culture can be determined with the use of the Organizational Culture and Readiness Scale for System-Wide Integration of Evidence-Based Practice (OCRSIEP) (Fineout-Overholt & Melnyk, 2006). With the use of this 26-item Likert scale, a description of organizational characteristics, including strengths and opportunities for fostering EBP within a healthcare system, is identified. Examples of items on the OCRSIEP include the following:

(a) To what extent is EBP clearly described as central to the mission and philosophy of your institution?
(b) To what extent do you believe that EBP is practiced in your organization?
(c) To what extent is the nursing staff with whom you work committed to EBP?

In the ARCC© model, higher organizational culture is expected to increase EBP beliefs and implementation, which influences healthcare outcomes. The OCRSIEP scale has established face and content validity, with internal consistency reliabilities consistently greater than 0.85 across many populations (see Appendix K for a sample of the OCRSIEP scale).

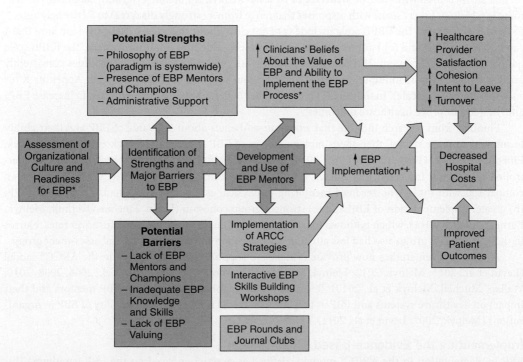

*Scale Developed
+ Based on the EBP paradigm and using the EBP process

Figure 13.6: Melnyk and Fineout-Overholt's ARCC model© (Melnyk & Fineout-Overholt, 2005).

EBP Mentors. Once key strengths and opportunities for fostering EBP within the organization are identified with the OCRSIEP scale, a cadre of EBP mentors is developed within the healthcare system. EBP mentors are healthcare providers, typically APNs, transdisciplinary clinicians, or baccalaureate-prepared nurses where health systems do not have APNs who work directly with point-of-care staff to implement EBP. These mentors assist in (a) shifting from a traditional practice paradigm to an EBP paradigm, (b) conducting EBP implementation (EBPI) projects, and (c) generating and integrating practice-based data to improve healthcare quality as well as patient and/or system outcomes. EBP mentors also have knowledge and skills in individual behavior and organizational change strategies to facilitate changes in clinician behavior and spark sustainable changes in organizational culture, which require specific intervention strategies, time, and persistence.

Key components of the EBP mentor role as defined in the ARCC© model include (a) ongoing assessment of an organization's capacity to sustain an EBP culture; (b) building EBP knowledge and skills by conducting interactive group workshops and one-on-one mentoring; (c) stimulating, facilitating, and educating nursing staff toward a culture of EBP, with a focus on overcoming barriers to best practice; (d) role modeling EBP; (e) conducting ARCC© EBP enhancing strategies, such as EBP rounds, journal clubs, webpages, newsletters, and fellowship programs; (f) working with staff to generate internal evidence (i.e., practice-generated) through outcomes management and EBPI projects; (g) facilitating staff involvement in research to generate external evidence; (h) using evidence to foster best practice; and (i) collaborating with interdisciplinary professionals to advance and sustain EBP. These mentors also have excellent strategic planning, implementation, and outcomes evaluation skills so that they can monitor the impact of their role and overcome barriers in moving the system to a culture of best practice (Melnyk, 2007). Mentorship with direct care staff on clinical units by ARCC EBP mentors© is important in strengthening clinicians' beliefs about the value of EBP and their ability to implement it (Melnyk & Fineout-Overholt, 2002, 2011).

EBP Beliefs Scale. In the ARCC© model, beliefs about the value of EBP and a clinician's ability to implement it are measured with the EBP Beliefs (EBPB) scale (Melnyk & Fineout-Overholt, 2002). This instrument is a 16-item Likert scale, with responses that range from 1 (strongly disagree) to 5 (strongly agree). Examples of items on the EBPB scale include (a) I am clear about the steps in EBP, (b) I am sure that I can implement EBP, and (c) I am sure that evidence-based guidelines can improve care. The EBPB scale has established face, content, and construct validity, with internal consistency reliabilities consistently greater than 0.85 across multiple studies (Melnyk, Fineout-Overholt, & Mays, 2008; see Appendix K for a sample copy of the scale). In the ARCC© model, higher beliefs about EBP are expected to increase EBPI and, thereby, improve healthcare outcomes.

Findings from research indicate that when nurses' beliefs about the value of EBP and their ability to implement it are strong, then their implementation of EBP is greater (Melnyk et al., 2004; Melnyk, Fineout-Overholt, Giggleman, & Cruz, 2010). Additionally, findings from a recent randomized controlled pilot study indicated that nurses who received mentoring from an ARCC© EBP mentor, in comparison with those who received mentoring in physical assessment skills, had (a) stronger EBPB, (b) greater implementation of EBP, and (c) stronger group cohesion (Levin, Fineout-Overholt, Melnyk, Barnes, & Vetter, 2011), which is known to be a predictor of nurse satisfaction and turnover rates. Nurses in the ARCC© EBP group also had less attrition/turnover than nurses in the physical assessment group.

A total of seven studies now provide evidence to support the relationships in the ARCC© model (Levin et al., 2011; Melnyk, 2012; Melnyk & Fineout-Overholt, 2002; Melnyk et al., 2004, 2008, 2010; Wallan, Mitchell, Melnyk et al., 2010). Research is also ongoing on the role of EBP mentors and their impact on healthcare systems and EBP as they are likely to be the key to sustainability of EBP in organizations (Melnyk, 2007; Levin et al., 2011).

Implementing the Evidence-Based ARCC© Model
EBP implementation in the ARCC© model is defined as practicing based on the EBP paradigm. This paradigm uses the EBP process to improve outcomes. The process begins with asking clinical questions and incorporates research evidence and practice-based evidence in point-of-care decision making.

However, simply engaging the process is not sufficient. The results of the first three steps of the process (i.e., establishing valid and reliable research evidence) must be coupled with (a) the expertise of the clinician to gather practice-based evidence (i.e., data from practice initiatives such as QI; gather, interpret, and act on patient data; and effectively use healthcare resources and (b) what the patient and family value and prefer (see Figure 13.4). This amalgamation leads to innovative decision making at the point of care with quality outcomes. While research evidence, practice evidence, and patient/client data as interpreted through expertise and patient preferences must always be present, a context of caring allows each patient–provider encounter to be individualized (see Chapter 1, Figure 1.2). Within an organization and ecosystem or environment that fosters an EBP culture, this paradigm can thrive at the patient–provider level as well as across the organization, resulting in transformed health care.

The ARCC© model is implemented in hospitals and healthcare systems through a 12-month program to prepare a cadre of EBP mentors who work directly with point-of-care clinicians to implement and sustain EBP throughout the entire system or institution. A series of six workshops that consist of 8 days of educational and skills building sessions are conducted over the 12-month ARCC program©, which is focused on implementing the seven-step EBP process and necessary strategies for building an EBP culture and environment. Content of the ARCC© workshops includes (a) EBP skills building, (b) creating a vision to motivate a change to EBP, (c) transdisciplinary team building and effective communication, (d) mentorship to advance EBP, (e) strategies to build an EBP culture, (f) QI processes, (g) data management and outcomes monitoring/evaluation, and (h) theories and principles of individual behavior change and organizational change.

Before the first workshop, a baseline assessment is conducted in order to assess the clinicians' EBP beliefs, EBP implementation, organizational culture and readiness for EBP, job satisfaction, and group cohesion. Data on patient problems identified for improvement by the clinicians in the ARCC program© are also collected and analyzed. Each team who attends the series of workshops implements an EBP implementation project during the course of the ARCC program©, which is focused on improving quality and reliability (i.e., safety) of care as well as patient outcomes.

Recent implementation of the ARCC© model at Washington Hospital Healthcare System, a 355-bed community hospital system in the Western region of the United States revealed the following findings: (a) Early ambulation in the intensive care unit resulted in a reduction in ventilator days from 11.6 days to 8.9 days and no ventilator associated pneumonias; (b) Pressure ulcer rates were reduced from 6.07% to 0.62% on a medical surgical unit; (c) Education of congestive heart failure patients led to a 14.7% reduction in hospital readmissions, and (d) 75% of parents perceived the overall quality of care as excellent after implementation of an evidence-based family centered care program compared with 22.2% preimplementation (Melnyk et al., 2012).

EBP implementation in the ARCC© model is measured with the EBPI scale (Melnyk & Fineout-Overholt, 2002). Clinicians respond to each of the 18 Likert scale items on the EBPI by answering how often in the last 8 weeks they have performed certain EBP initiatives, such as (a) generated a PICOT question about my practice, (b) used evidence to change my clinical practice, (c) evaluated the outcomes of a practice change, and (d) shared the outcome data collected with colleagues. The EBPI has established face, content, and construct validity as well as internal consistency reliabilities greater than 0.85 across multiple studies (Melnyk et al., 2008; see Appendix K for a sample copy of the scale). In the ARCC© model, it is contended that greater EBPI is associated with higher nurse satisfaction, which will eventually lead to fewer turnover rates and healthcare expenditures.

Several healthcare systems and hospitals throughout the United States and globe have now implemented the ARCC model in their efforts to build and sustain an EBP culture and ecosystem in their organizations. As a part of building this culture, groups of nurses and other transdisciplinary healthcare providers have attended a week-long EBP mentorship immersion program, conducted by the authors of the ARCC© model. These programs have prepared more than 400 nurses and transdisciplinary clinicians across the nation and globe as ARCC EBP mentors©. Some of the individuals who have attended these immersion programs have negotiated roles as EBP mentors within their healthcare organizations. The EBP mentorship program is now available as an onsite workshop or through an online program offered by the Center for Transdisciplinary EBP at The Ohio State University College of Nursing (see http://www.nursing.osu.edu/sections/ctep/).

The final step in the ARCC© model is for EBP mentors and other clinicians who practice according to the EBP paradigm to have an impact on provider, patient, and system outcomes. EBP mentors and those they influence focus on achieving the best outcomes of care, thereby making a difference in patients' lives and the success of the organization.

Using and Evaluating the Evidence-Based ARCC© Model

Because valid and reliable instruments are available to measure key constructs in the ARCC© model, barriers and facilitators to EBP along with clinicians' beliefs about and actual implementation of EBP can be readily assessed and identified by organizations. There are also well-established workshops and online offerings available that develop EBP mentors who can work closely with point-of-care staff to strengthen their beliefs about and implementation of EBP (see www.nursing.osu.edu/sections/ctep/). The availability of tools to measure an organization's EBP culture and readiness for EBP as well as clinicians' EBPB and implementation also allow an organization to monitor its progress in the system-wide implementation and sustainability of EBP.

Promoting Action on Research Implementation in Health Services Framework

Overview of the PARIHS Framework

Getting evidence into practice is complex, multifaceted, and dynamic. The Promoting Action on Research Implementation in Health Services (PARIHS) framework was developed in an attempt to reflect these complexities, representing the interdependence and interplay of the many factors that appear to play a role in the successful implementation (SI) of evidence in practice. Previous research exploring why research evidence is not routinely used in practice has tended to focus at the level of individual practitioners and on barriers to utilization (e.g., Hunt, 1991; McSherry, Artley, & Holloran, 2006; Parahoo, 1999). While individual factors are important, getting evidence into practice requires more than a focus on addressing individual influencing factors. The PARIHS framework, which provides a conceptual map, is premised on the notion that the implementation of research-based practice depends on the ability to achieve significant and planned behavior change involving individuals, teams, and organizations. SI is represented as a function (f) of the nature and type of evidence (e), the qualities of the context (c) in which the evidence is being introduced, and the way the process is facilitated (f), whereby SI = f(E,C,F). The three elements (i.e., evidence, context, and facilitation) are each positioned on a high-to-low continuum, where in each implementation effort the aim is to move toward *high* in order to optimize the chances of success.

Development and Refinement

The PARIHS framework has developed over time (Kitson, Harvey, & McCormack, 1998; Rycroft-Malone et al., 2002; Rycroft-Malone, Harvey, et al., 2004). It was originally conceived inductively from an analysis of practice development, QI, and research project work (Kitson et al., 1998). Theoretical and retrospective analysis of four studies led to the proposal that the most SI seems to occur when evidence is scientifically robust; matches professional consensus and patients' preferences (high evidence); when the context is receptive to change with sympathetic cultures, strong leadership, and appropriate monitoring and feedback systems (high context); and when there is appropriate facilitation of change with input from skilled external and internal facilitators (high facilitation).

Since the framework's conception and publication, it has undergone research and development work. Most notably this has included a concept analysis of each of the dimensions (Harvey et al. 2002; McCormack et al., 2002; Rycroft-Malone, Seers, et al., 2004) and a research study to assess content validity (Rycroft-Malone, Harvey, et al., 2004). This enabled some conceptual clarity to be gained about the framework's constituent elements and verification of its content validity. As a result of this work, the framework has been refined over time with the addition, for example, of subelements (Table 13.1). The next phase of work, currently underway, is tool development (Kitson et al., 2008).

Table 13.1 PARIHS Elements and Subelements

Elements	Subelements	
Evidence	**Low**	**High**
Research	• Poorly conceived, designed, and/or executed research • Seen as the only type of evidence • Not valued as evidence • Seen as certain	• Well-conceived, designed, and executed research, appropriate to the research question • Seen as one part of a decision • Valued as evidence • Lack of certainty acknowledged • Social construction acknowledged • Judged as relevant • Importance weighted • Conclusions drawn
Clinical experience	• Anecdote, with no critical reflection and judgment • Lack of consensus within similar groups • Not valued as evidence • Seen as the only type of evidence	• Clinical experience and expertise reflected upon, tested by individuals and groups • Consensus within similar groups • Valued as evidence • Seen as one part of the decision • Judged as relevant • Importance weighted • Conclusions drawn
Patient experience	• Not valued as evidence • Patients not involved • Seen as the only type of evidence	• Valued as evidence • Multiple biographies used • Partnerships with healthcare professionals • Seen as one part of a decision • Judged as relevant • Importance weighted • Conclusions drawn
Local data/ information	• Not valued as evidence • Lack of systematic methods for collection and analysis • Not reflected upon • No conclusions drawn	• Valued as evidence • Collected and analyzed systematically and rigorously • Evaluated and reflected upon • Conclusions drawn
Context	**Low**	**High**

Culture	• Unclear values and beliefs
	
	• Low regard for individuals
	• Task-driven organization
	• Lack of consistency
	
	• Resources not allocated
	• Not integrated with strategic goals
		• Able to define culture(s) in terms of prevailing values/beliefs
		• Values individual staff and clients
		• Promotes learning organization
		• Consistency of individual's role/experience to value:
		  • Relationship with others
		  • Teamwork
		  • Power and authority
		  • Rewards/recognition
		• Resources—human, financial, equipment—allocated
		• Initiative fits with strategic goals and is a key practice/patient issue

Elements	Subelements	
Leadership	• Traditional, command, and control leadership • Lack of role clarity • Lack of teamwork • Poor organizational structures • Autocratic decision-making processes • Didactic approaches to learning/teaching/managing	• Transformational leadership • Role clarity • Effective teamwork • Effective organizational structures • Democratic inclusive decision-making processes • Enabling/empowering approach to teaching/learning/managing

Evaluation	• Absence of any form of feedback
	• Narrow use of performance information sources
	• Evaluations rely on single rather than multiple methods
		• Feedback on:
		  • Individual
		  • Team
		  • System
		  • Performance
		• Use of multiple sources of information on performance
		• Use of multiple methods:
		  • Clinical
		  • Performance
		  • Economic
		  • Experience
		  • Evaluations

Facilitation	**Low Inappropriate Facilitation**	**High Appropriate Facilitation**
Purpose Role *Doing for others:*	Task • Episodic contact • Practical/technical help • Didactic, traditional approach to teaching • External agents • Low intensity—extensive coverage	Holistic
Enabling others:		
	• Sustained partnership • Developmental	
	• Adult learning approach to teaching	
	• Internal/external agents • High intensity—limited coverage	
Skills and attributes	*Task/doing for others* • Project management skills • Technical skills • Marketing skills • Subject/technical/clinical credibility	*Holistic/enabling others* • Co-counseling • Critical reflection • Giving meaning • Flexibility of role • Realness/authenticity

PARIHS Elements

Evidence. Evidence is conceived in a broad sense within the framework including propositional and nonpropositional knowledge from four different types of evidence (1) research, (2) clinical experience, (3) patients and caregivers' experience, and (4) local context information (see Rycroft-Malone, Seers, et al., 2004 for a detailed discussion). For evidence to be located toward high, certain criteria have to be met, including that research evidence (qualitative and quantitative) is well conceived and conducted and that there is consensus about it and that clinical experience has been made explicit and verified through critical reflection, critique, and debate. Patient experience is high when patients (and/or significant others) are part of the decision-making process and when patient narratives are seen as a valid source of evidence. Finally, local information/data could be considered as part of the evidence base if it has been systematically collected, evaluated, and considered. Clearly, this conceptualization indicates the need for an interaction between the scientific and experiential, which requires a dialectical process, that is, a resolution of disagreement through rational and logical discussion.

Context. Context refers to the environment or setting in which the proposed change is to be implemented (see McCormack et al., 2002, for a detailed discussion). Within PARIHS, the contextual factors that promote SI fall under three broad subelements: culture, leadership, and evaluation, which operate in a dynamic, multileveled way. It is proposed that organizations that have cultures that could be described as learning organizations are those that are more conducive to change (high). Such cultures contain features such as decentralized decision making, a focus on relationships between managers and workers, and management styles that are facilitative. Leaders have a key role to play in creating such cultures. Transformational leaders, as opposed to those who command and control, have the ability to challenge individuals and teams in an enabling, inspiring way (high). Finally, contexts with evaluative mechanisms that collect multiple sources of evidence of performance at individual, team, and system levels comprise the third element of a high context.

Facilitation. Facilitation refers to the process of enabling or making easier the implementation of evidence into practice (see Harvey et al., 2002 for a detailed discussion). Facilitation is achieved by an individual carrying out a specific role—a facilitator—with the appropriate skills and knowledge to help individuals, teams, and/or organizations apply evidence in practice. With PARIHS, the purpose of facilitation can vary from being task-orientated, which requires technical and practical support, to enabling, which requires more of a developmental, process-orientated approach. The skills and attributes required to fulfill the role are likely to depend on the situation, individuals, and contexts involved. Therefore, skilled facilitators are those who can adjust their roles and styles to the different stages of an implementation project and the needs of those with whom they are working.

Using the Framework

As each of the elements and subelements are on a continuum of high to low, it is suggested that implementation activities and processes be aimed at moving each of them toward high to increase the chances of success. As such, the framework provides a map of the elements that might require attention and a set of questions that could be asked at the outset of any implementation activity (see Kitson et al., 2008, for examples). This could provide a diagnosis of the current state or readiness to change and provide some indication of what needs to be done to move forward (e.g., Brown & McCormack, 2005). Additionally, PARIHS has the potential to be used as an evaluative tool or checklist, which could be used during or following the completion of an implementation project to assess progress or outcome (e.g., Ellis, Howard, Larson, & Robertson, 2005; Sharp, Pineros, Hsu, Starks, & Sales, 2004). Furthermore, others have used the framework to model and predict the factors involved in RU (Wallin, Estabrooks, Midodzi, & Cummings, 2006).

Future Work

There is a small but growing body of evidence from research and practice that shows that the PARIHS framework has conceptual integrity, face, and concept validity. However, there are still a number of issues that require exploration and further work. These include gaining a clearer understanding of how the elements interact during implementation and how and whether some elements are more important than others. Additionally, there are measurement challenges concerning the development of both diagnostic and evaluative tools. The next phase of work is in collaboration with a wider community of researchers, practitioners, and other stakeholders.

The Clinical Scholar Model©

Overview of the Clinical Scholar Model©

The Clinical Scholar Model© was developed and implemented to promote the spirit of inquiry, educate direct care providers, and guide a mentorship program for EBP and the conduct of research at the point of care. The words of Dr. Janelle Krueger planted the seeds for the model when she encouraged the conduct and use of research as a staff nurse function and promoted the notion that clinical staff are truly in a position to be able to link research and practice. The philosophy and process used in the Conduct and Utilization of Research in Nursing project, based on diffusion of innovation theory, formed the early thinking for the model (Horsley, Crane, Crabtree, & Wood, 1983; Rogers, 2003). The concepts presented in the clinical scholarship resource paper published by Sigma Theta Tau International provided the overarching principles (Clinical Scholarship Task Force, 1999). The innovative ideas cultivated through the curiosity of clinical nurses and the visionary and creative leadership of a nurse researcher combined to flesh out the Clinical Scholar Model©. The model affords a framework for the Clinical Scholar Program©, building the capacity and skills for conducting new research and using evidence at the point of care, thus providing a sustainable solution for changing patterns of thinking, promoting evidence-based care, and improving patient outcomes. The Clinical Scholar Program began as an interactive, outcomes oriented educational program for nurses but has evolved into an interdisciplinary educational program for direct care providers.

....

In dwelling upon the vital importance of sound observation, it must never be lost sight of what observation is for. It is not for the sake of piling up miscellaneous information or curious facts, but for the sake of saving life and increasing health and comfort.
—Florence Nightingale

....

Goals of the Model and Program

There are four central goals of the Clinical Scholar Model© and its accompanying educational program:

1. Challenge current practices within direct care.
2. Clinical providers need to be able to speak and understand the research language, making day-to-day dialog featuring discussion of new research findings a common occurrence.
3. Critique and synthesis of current research as the core of evidence.
4. Clinical scholars should serve as mentors to other staff and to teams who question their practices and seek to improve clinical outcomes.

The structure provided by these goals is important in providing a sense of direction for those whose purpose is creating a center of excellence for patient care.

Components of the Model and Program

The Clinical Scholar Model/Program© is based on clear definitions for research and EBP. The conduct of research is defined as the generation of new, generalizable knowledge using scientific inquiry. Research is conducted when the evidence is not strong enough to support a practice change, without potentially creating risk or harm to the recipient of that practice change. EBP is defined as an interdisciplinary approach to healthcare practice that bases decisions and practice strategies to improve patient outcomes on (1) the best available evidence that includes research as the core, national benchmark and QI data and reliable forms of internal evidence; (2) incorporation of clinical expertise; (3) consideration of patient values; and (4) taking into account the feasibility of implementation and adoption, the potential risk or harm to the recipient, and the human and material costs.

The Clinical Scholar Model© is based on the principles of scholarship described in the Clinical Scholarship resource paper published by Sigma Theta Tau International (Clinical Scholarship Task Force, 1999). Although the purpose of the paper was not to describe or define clinical scholarship in terms of research or EBP, the concepts of the clinical scholar provide a sustainable approach to improving patient outcomes: observe and reflect, analyze and critique, synthesize, apply and evaluate, and disseminate. Each component of the model is further defined within the content of the Clinical Scholar Program (see Figure 13.7A).

Clinical Scholar Program Workshops. The Clinical Scholar Program© realizes the Clinical Scholar Model© and is currently utilized in several acute care facilities across the country (Brewer et al., 2009; Honess et al., 2009; Mulvenon et al., 2009; Schultz, 2008), is the basis for EBP and research in northern Thailand (Schultz, 2011), and is the framework for at least two nursing EBP collaboratives (Schultz, 2012; Sussong et al., 2009; Weeks et al., 2009). The program is composed of equal parts of educating, processing, and mentoring in a series of six to eight all-day workshops. The primary goals of the workshops are to (a) challenge the current clinical practices through observation and the spirit of inquiry; (b) speak and understand research language; (c) critique, synthesize, implement, evaluate, and disseminate evidence; and (d) educate direct care providers to serve as mentors to other direct care staff. The ultimate goals are to improve the quality of care provided to patients, to measure the impact of EBP outcomes, and to base administrative and clinical decisions on the best available evidence.

Development and sustainability of an evidence-based culture of excellence requires both an infrastructure where change and innovation are supported and valued by management and staff and a critical mass of direct care providers (i.e., the capacity) who can conduct research, critically synthesize the science, integrate the research findings with internal and other external evidence, and provide leadership to practice change. The infrastructure and capacity must be embedded in a culture where interdisciplinary collaboration is fostered, policies and procedures are based on evidence, and there is a systematic approach to the evaluation of care (Stetler, 2003). Participants selected to attend the Clinical Scholar Programs© are curious, critical thinkers who have either had a research course or are currently enrolled in a research course and are supported by their clinical supervisors to attend and carry out evidence-based projects or research studies.

The workshops begin with promoting the spirit of inquiry through **observation and reflection.** The participants learn to write clear, concise researchable questions, paying particular attention to defining the desired outcomes and the significance of the practice issue to healthcare providers, families, and patients. A librarian teaches the participants how to perform efficient and structured searches on multiple literature databases. Once scientific studies that address the clinical issues are obtained, the participants are taught how to critique the studies and identify the salient outcomes that answer their clinical questions. Evaluation of evidence is a very rigorous process, not unlike the research process; however, the emphasis is clearly on applying the evidence in practice. Using an evaluation table to delineate the **analysis and critique** of each type of research design, the principles of synthesis are taught. During these workshops, published guidelines and systematic reviews are also evaluated for their level of evidence and quality of the science. **Synthesis** is the crux of EBP and the Clinical Scholar Model© (Schultz, 2011; Schultz et al., 2013). It is not a summary of the relevant articles but rather a process of critical thinking built on several principles of synthesis (Box 13.2). There may be several synthesis tables, depending on how the outcomes and/or the interventions are defined. The strength of the evidence is based on levels of research designs, the quality of the studies, the consistency of the relevant findings, the number of studies measuring an independent or dependent variable, and the available internal evidence. Recommendations for practice changes are based on the strength of the evidence and utilized in the development of evidence-based guidelines, policies, procedures, or protocols. APNs and physicians can utilize

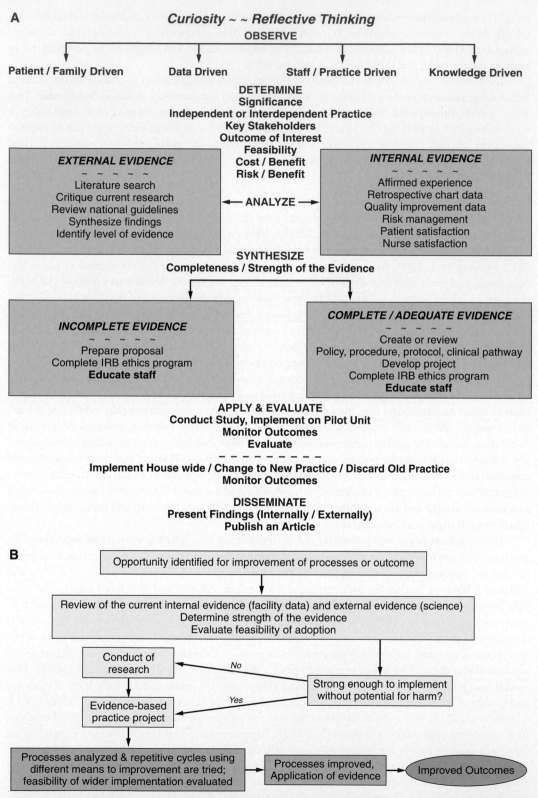

Figure 13.7: (A) The Clinical Scholar Model, as further defined within the content of the Clinical Scholar Program. (Used with permission. © Alyce A. Schultz & Associates, LLC [2008].) (B) Interrelationship between research, EBP, and quality. (From Schultz et al., 2005; used with permission.). Courtesy Alyce A. Schultz RN, PhD, FAAN, Bozeman, Montana.

Box 13.2 Principles of Synthesis

◆ Decide which studies to include/exclude
◆ Arrange studies based on the same or very similar interventions and/or same/similar outcomes measured in the same way
◆ Thoughtfully analyze inconsistencies across studies
◆ Establish consensus on major conclusions for each selected outcome variable
◆ Establish consensus on conclusions drawn from each study
◆ Establish consensus on clinical implications of findings
◆ Determine the strength of the findings for pertinent outcomes
◆ Combine findings into a useful format, with recommendations for implementation in practice if applicable, based on strength of the evidence

the synthesized evidence as they develop care plans for their individual patients. Other healthcare providers often have to work through an organizational change process as the new guidelines, policies, or procedures are **applied** to a small sampling of patients and the outcomes are carefully monitored and **evaluated.** Careful adherence to the steps in the new guidelines or procedures or fidelity of the intervention must also be monitored. If the outcomes for the pilot work are positive, the new guidelines, policies, or procedures are adopted for a broader patient population with outcome measurement continued until the new practices are routinized into daily patterns and positive outcomes are established for the larger group (Schultz, 2007). Finally, the work is **disseminated**, not only to a local audience, but also to a wider audience of direct care providers through poster or podium presentations and publications and through mass media to the general public.

> To be considered true clinical scholars, nurses must identify and describe their work, making it conscious, so that it can be shared with researchers, colleagues, other health care providers and, perhaps most important, the public.
> —Clinical Scholarship Task Force, 1999

Clinical Scholars

Clinical scholars are described as individuals with a high degree of curiosity who possess advanced critical thinking skills and constantly seek new knowledge through continuous learning opportunities. They reflect on this knowledge and seek and use a wide variety of resources in implementing new evidence in practice. They never stop asking "Why?" While most clinical scholars are also highly experienced, experience alone does not assure clinical expertise. Clinical scholarship is not the same as clinical proficiency where performing a task routinely in a highly efficient manner is deemed proficient. Rather, it requires always questioning whether there is a more efficient and effective way to provide care and whether or not a particular procedure or task needs to be performed at all (Clinical Scholarship Task Force, 1999). These characteristics of clinical scholars are very similar to the characteristics of the innovators and early adopters as described by Rogers (2003). The Clinical Scholar Model© is inductive using the innovative ideas generated in direct care and driven by the goal of building a community or cadre of scholars who will serve as mentors to other direct care providers in the critique, synthesis, implementation, and evaluation of internal evidence (e.g., QI, risk management, and benchmarking data) and external evidence (i.e., empirical studies).

Clinical scholar mentors are change agents who promote clinical scholarship through the spirit of inquiry and a willingness to challenge and change traditional practice patterns, mentoring other staff in fostering a culture shift. Practicing as a clinical scholar does not require that one always conducts research, but it does require using an intellectual process that is steeped in curiosity and that continually challenges traditional clinical practice through observation, analysis, synthesis of the evidence, application and evaluation, and dissemination (see Figure 13.7; Schultz et al., 2005). The Clinical Scholar

Model© supports the view that if research and other forms of evidence are to be used in practice, both must be understood and valued by direct care providers.

Sustaining the Clinical Scholar Environment

Evaluation of the model is both iterative and cumulative. The research studies and EBP projects developed during the Clinical Scholar Program© must be continually evaluated for achieving their desired outcomes. The environment in which the work is centered must be evaluated for a sustainable change to a culture of inquiry and a breeding ground for innovation.

EBP may initially be encouraged through the application of knowledge to a single intervention or project but, over time, as more staff are educated regarding the critique, synthesis, application, and evaluation of evidence, the culture and the delivery of care will slowly change to the routine use of evidence—both formally and informally—through inquisitive, reflective, critical thinking. Every healthcare provider becomes responsible and accountable for providing care based on the best available evidence; not to do so is unethical. The institutionalization of evidence use in practice requires creative, critical thinkers and the support and flexibility of management to implement and evaluate change.

Through its focus on the development of new clinical scholars who can act as EBP mentors to their colleagues in the future, the Clinical Scholar Model© is self-sustaining. The Clinical Scholar workshops provide a nurturing, rich environment for direct care providers to create and grow extended networks of professional contacts and colleagues to draw upon for future mentoring. The intensity and fast pace of the Clinical Scholar Program© supports a relatively speedy initial adoption of evidence-based care. As the new clinical scholars begin to serve as mentors to new groups, the model is reinforced and the culture of excellence expands.

In today's environment of limited healthcare budgets, financial support for programs such as the Clinical Scholar Program© can be limited. Financial investment in the program is essential with consideration of the financial implications of any project as an important step in evaluating the probability of adoption of the practice. Evaluating the monetary costs of projects and interventions and including financial outcomes data whenever possible are essential to providing evidence of benefit in this area. Linking the spirit of inquiry to the QI program assures sustainability and financial feasibility (see Figure 13.7B). When the program remains focused on determining what works, for whom, in what situations, with what resources, and with what measurable outcomes, administrative leaders and clinicians alike can find value in and support for the program with the improvement in care that is so central to institutional missions.

The Johns Hopkins Nursing Evidence-Based Practice Model

The Johns Hopkins Nursing Evidence-Based Practice (JHNEBP) model helps bedside nurses translate evidence to clinical, administrative, and educational nursing practice. In 2002, the organizational leadership at The Johns Hopkins Hospital (JHH) recognized a gap in the standard for nursing practice of implementing research results. To accelerate the transfer of new knowledge into practice, nursing leadership set a strategic goal to build a culture of nursing practice based on evidence. The tenets of EBP support this goal because (a) nursing is both a science and profession, (b) nursing practice should be based on the best available evidence, (c) a hierarchy of evidence exists, (d) research findings should be translated to practice, and (e) nursing values efficiency and effectiveness (Newhouse, 2007). The desired outcomes were to enhance nurse autonomy, leadership, and engagement with interdisciplinary colleagues.

A team of JHH nurses and faculty from Johns Hopkins University School of Nursing formed a task force to evaluate published EBP models and tools for application by practicing nurses within the clinical setting. A key objective was to select a model that would demystify the EBP process for bedside nurses and embed EBP into nursing practice. For this reason, it was important that bedside nurses were involved in evaluating and piloting the model and process to be used at JHH.

Nurses' evaluation and feedback from the evaluation of published models was clear—nurses wanted a mentored linear process, with accompanying tools to guide them through each step of the EBP process. Based on this feedback, the JHNEBP model and process were carefully constructed and piloted with a caregiving unit. During the pilot, the team offered EBP educational working seminars in multiple formats, assessed with participants what worked in the pilot as well as the processes that were most challenging. The details of the implementation are reported elsewhere (Dearholt, White, Newhouse, Pugh, & Poe, 2008; Newhouse, Dearholt, Poe, Pugh, & White, 2007). The resulting JHNEBP model includes a conceptual model, a process, and tools to guide nurses through the critical steps of the process.

The model was then implemented organizationally through standardized education and integration of EBP competencies into job performance expectations. An EBP fellowship was funded by Nursing Administration and external funding obtained to test the model in interprofessional teams. The EBP process was subsequently incorporated into undergraduate and graduate research courses at the Johns Hopkins University School of Nursing.

Overview of the Johns Hopkins Nursing Evidence-Based Practice Model
In the JHNEBP model, EBP is

> *a problem-solving approach to clinical decision-making within a health care organization that integrates the best available scientific evidence with the best available experiential (patient and practitioner) evidence, considers internal and external influences on practice, and encourages critical thinking in the judicious application of such evidence to care of the individual patient, patient population, or system.* (Dearholt & Dang, 2012, pp. 4–5)

Consistent with the definition, the conceptual model (Figure 13.8) includes a core of research and non-research evidence within the triad of professional nursing practice (practice, education, and research). Evidence-based nursing practice is influenced by internal organizational (e.g., culture, resources) factors and external factors (e.g., accreditation, licensure). Internal and external factors can enhance or limit implementation of recommendations, conduct of the process, or the existence of EBP itself within organizations.

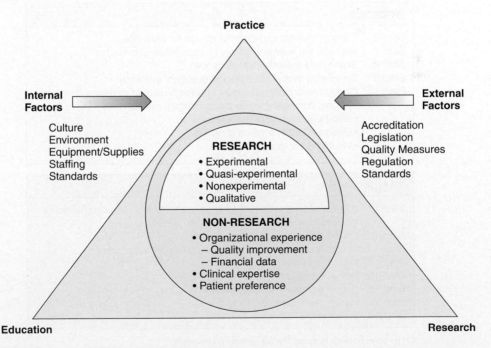

© The John Hopkins Hospital/The John Hopkins University

Figure 13.8: Johns Hopkins nursing evidence-based practice conceptual model. (From Dearholt, S. L., & Dang, D. [2012]. *Johns Hopkins nursing evidence-based practice model and guidelines* (2nd ed.). Indianapolis, IN: Sigma Theta Tau International. Used with permission.)

The Johns Hopkins Nursing EBP model is implemented using the PET process (Figure 13.9) which consists of three phases: *Practice question, Evidence,* and *Translation.* Within these phases, there are 18 prescriptive steps. Although the process appears linear, it may be iterative as the process evolves. For example, teams may discover other sources of the evidence through their review or hand searching which requires refinement of the search strategy or PICO, which moves them back to the prior step(s).

During the practice question stage, a question is refined in answerable terms, a leader is designated, and an interprofessional team is formed. Next, in the evidence phase, a search for evidence is conducted and evidence is screened for inclusion criteria, abstracted, appraised using a rating scale, and then summarized. The evidence phase ends with three distinct activities (1) evidence synthesis; (2) recommendations developed by the team based on the level, quality, and quantity of evidence; (3) selection of one of four path ways to translation based on the overall strength of the evidence. There are four pathways for translating evidence into practice:

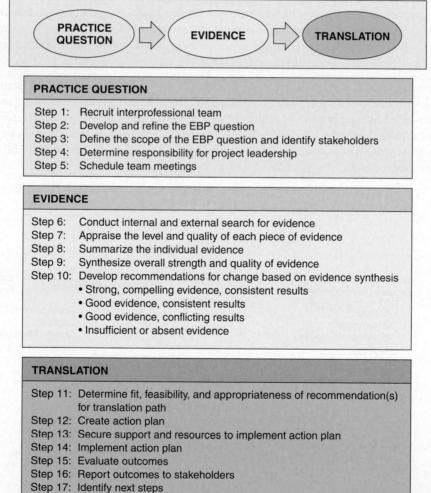

©The John Hopkins Hospital/The John Hopkins University

Figure 13.9: Johns Hopkins nursing process for evidence-based practice (From Dearholt, S. L., & Dang, D. [2012].) *Johns Hopkins nursing evidence-based practice model and guidelines* (2nd ed.). Indianapolis, IN: Sigma Theta Tau International.

1. Strong, compelling evidence and consistent results, a prerequisite for a practice change
2. Good and consistent evidence, an indication for considering a pilot of the practice change or need for further investigation
3. Good but conflicting evidence, requires further investigation for new evidence or a research study
4. Little or no evidence, requires further investigation for new evidence, a research study, or discontinuation of the project.

Finally, in the translation stage, a plan is constructed for implementation of appropriate and feasible recommendations. Implementation, evaluation, and dissemination follow. The translation plan is incorporated into the organization's QI framework to communicate effective (and ineffective) changes and engage the organization in adopting those changes.

Eight tools support critical steps in the process: (1) Question Development, (2) Evidence Level and Quality Guide, (3) Research Evidence Appraisal, (4) Nonresearch Evidence Appraisal, (5) Individual Evidence Summary, (6) Synthesis of Evidence Guide, (7) Synthesis and Recommendations, and (8) Project Management. These tools were developed with input from bedside nurses and include key questions that prompt nurses in the process. The tools were constructed to have high utility with checkbox formats, definitions, and guidelines for use on each form.

After multiple projects using different rating scales, it was clear that many publicly available scales were intended for research evidence based on randomized controlled trials and did not include an approach to evaluate nonresearch sources of evidence. Because the questions proposed by nurses today need an answer tomorrow, the sources of evidence are often found in nonresearch evidence such as integrated reviews, QI data, or expert opinion. Because nursing problems occur in natural settings, they often do not lend themselves to randomized control trials. A rating scale was developed to assess the level and quality of nonresearch evidence to enable nurses to better communicate the strength and quality of evidence on which decisions are made.

The JHNEBP model is applied to clinical, administrative, and educational nursing in any setting where nursing is practiced; and academic settings at schools of nursing at the undergraduate, graduate level. It also has been used for state-level initiatives to review evidence (Newhouse, 2008).

A book is available with the tools to guide teams through the JHNEBP process (Dearholt & Dang, 2012). A teaching guide also is available for faculty that includes strategies for learning activities to boost EBP student competencies at each level (White, Shaefer, & Mark, 2012). The model and tools can be used by bedside nurses to answer important practice questions using the best available evidence to inform decisions.

ACE Star Model of Knowledge Transformation

Development of the ACE Star Model was prompted through the work of the Academic Center for Evidence-Based Practice (ACE) at the University of Texas Health Science Center San Antonio during the early phases of the EBP movement in the United States. Uniquely, the ACE Star Model focuses heavily on the relative utility of several *forms* of knowledge in clinical decision making (Stevens, 2004). From the definition of EBP as *integration of best research evidence with clinical expertise and patient preferences* (Sackett, Straus, Richardson, Rosenberg, & Haynes, 2000, p. ii), it is clear that EBP combines research evidence with clinical expertise and includes individualization of care through incorporation of patient preferences and the circumstances of the setting.

Overview of the ACE Star Model of Knowledge Transformation

Challenges in moving research into practice emerge from a number of sources. The ACE Star Model explains how to overcome the challenges of (1) the volume of research evidence, (2) the misfit between form and use of knowledge, and (3) integration of expertise and patient preference into best practice. Literature and professional knowledge sources contain a variety of knowledge forms, many of which are not useful for direct practice application. For example, results from a single experiment are not suitable to guide best practices because research results from single studies are often not in harmony. One study demonstrates the effectiveness of an intervention while the next may show no difference. Likewise, the sheer volume of research on a topic presents a challenge for real time application. At the same time, many *forms* of knowledge are not suited to direct clinical application. The research report is a form of knowledge that, while valuable, is not well suited for directly informing practice. Nor does a single research report account for gaps in knowledge or consideration of patient preferences.

The Star Model explains how specific forms of knowledge, such as the systematic review and clinical practice the guideline, are solutions for moving research into practice. It is a model for understanding the cycles, nature, and characteristics of knowledge that are utilized in various phases of EBP. The simple, parsimonious Star Model depicts the relationships between various stages of knowledge transformation, from newly discovered knowledge through to best practice and outcomes. It illustrates various *forms* of knowledge in evolutionary sequence, as research evidence is combined with other knowledge and integrated into practice to produce intended outcomes. The Star Model places nursing's previous scientific work within the context of EBP and mainstreams nursing into the formal network of EBP.

Figure 13.10 shows the Star Model configured as a simple 5-point star, illustrating five major stages of knowledge transformation. The Star Model defines the following forms of knowledge: (1) Point 1—Discovery, representing primary research studies; (2) Point 2—Evidence Summary, which is the synthesis of all available knowledge compiled into a single harmonious statement, such as a systematic review; (3) Point 3—Translation into action, often referred to as evidence-based clinical practice guidelines, combining the evidential base and expertise to extend recommendations; (4) Point 4—Integration into practice is evidence-in-action, in which practice is aligned to reflect best evidence; and (5) Point 5—Evaluation, which is an inclusive view of the impact that the EBP has on patient health outcomes, satisfaction, efficacy and efficiency of care, and health policy. QI of healthcare processes and outcomes is the goal of knowledge transformation.

Terms and Premises in the Star Model

A number of basic terms and premises underlie the logic of the Star Model. **Knowledge transformation** is the conversion of research findings from primary research results through a series of stages and forms, to **make an** impact on health outcomes by way of evidence-based action. Underlying premises of knowledge transformation are described in Box13.3.

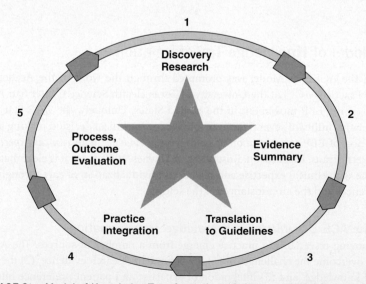

Figure 13.10: ACE Star Model of Knowledge Transformation. (© Stevens, 2004. Reprinted with expressed permission.)

> ## Box 13.3 Premises of the ACE Star Model
>
> 1. Knowledge transformation is necessary before research results are usable in clinical decision making.
> 2. Knowledge derives from a variety of sources. In health care, sources of knowledge include research evidence, experience, authority, trial and error, and theoretical principles.
> 3. The most stable and generalizable knowledge is discovered through systematic processes that control bias, namely, the research process.
> 4. Evidence can be classified into a hierarchy of strength of evidence. Relative strength of evidence is largely dependent on the rigor of the scientific design that produced the evidence. The value of rigor is that it strengthens cause-and-effect relationships.
> 5. Knowledge exists in a variety of forms. As research evidence is converted through systematic steps, knowledge from other sources (expertise, patient preference) is added, creating yet another form of knowledge.
> 6. The form ("package") in which knowledge exists can be referenced to its use; in the case of EBP, the ultimate use is application in healthcare delivery, services, and policy.
> 7. The form of knowledge determines its usability in clinical decision making. For example, research results from a primary investigation are less useful to decision making than an evidence-based clinical practice guideline.
> 8. Knowledge is transformed through the following processes: (a) Summarization into a single statement about the state of the science; (b) Translation of the state of the science into clinical recommendations, with addition of clinical expertise and application of theoretical principles; (c) Integration of recommendations through organizational and individual actions, tailoring care to patient preferences; and (d) Evaluation of impact of actions on targeted actions, care, health outcomes, economic outcomes, and policy.

Source: Stevens, K. *ACE Star Model.* Retrieved from http://www.acestar.uthscsa.edu/acestar-model.asp

Recent recommendations have pointed to systematic reviews (Point 2) and clinical practice guidelines (Point 3) as essential forms of knowledge for knowing what works in clinical practice (IOM, 2008, 2011a, 2011b). These two forms of knowledge were identified as the keystone to understanding whether a clinical intervention works. Both must be developed rigorously, to scientific standards, and in efficient ways (IOM, 2008). Evidence-based clinical practice guidelines have the potential to reduce illogical variations in practice by encouraging use of clinically effective practices.

The Star Model simplifies research evidence for application to clinical decision making. Rather than having practitioners submersed in the volume of research reports, it is better to summarize all that is known on the topic. Likewise, rather than requiring frontline providers to master the technical expertise needed in scientific critique, their point-of-care decisions are better supported by evidence-based recommendations.

Uses of the ACE Star Model

Integrating EBP Competencies. The Star Model has been widely adopted into clinical settings and educational settings as nurses strategize to employ EBP. The ACE Star Model, competencies, and ACE Evidence-Based Practice Readiness Inventory (ACE-ERI) have been adopted into clinical practice settings as nurses strategize to employ EBP. These resources have also been incorporated into educational settings as programs are revised to include EBP skills. The Star Model also provides an anchor for the new sciences of improvement and implementation. As an overarching model, it provides quick insight into archiving best practices. Because it drives to the core of EBP, the *nature of knowledge*, the Star Model is an excellent organizer for more prescriptive detailed EBP models.

As the Institute of Medicine (IOM) urged each profession to develop the details and strategies for integrating EBP competencies into education (National Research Council, 2003), the Star Model was used to develop national consensus on EBP competencies. With a focus on employing EBP, nurses established national consensus on competencies for EBP in nursing in 2004 and extended these in 2009 (Stevens, 2009). The ACE Star Model served as the framework for identifying specific competencies needed to employ EBP in a clinical role. Through multiple iterations, expert panels generated, validated, and endorsed competency statements to guide education programs at the basic (associate and under-graduate), intermediate (masters), and doctoral (advanced) levels in nursing. Between 10 and 32 specific competencies are identified for each of four levels of nursing education. Details were published in *Essential Competencies for EBP in Nursing* (Stevens, 2009). These competencies address fundamental skills of knowledge management, accountability for scientific basis of nursing practice, organizational and policy change, and development of scientific underpinnings for EBP (Stevens, 2009).

From these competencies, a measurement approach was developed. The instrument, called the ACE EBP Readiness Inventory (ACE-ERI) quantifies the individual's confidence in performing EBP competencies. The ACE-ERI exhibits strong **psychometric properties** (reliability, validity, and sensitivity) and is widely used in clinical and education settings to measure nurses' readiness for employing EBP and assessing the impact of professional development programs (Stevens, Puga, & Low, 2012). Available as an online survey, the ACE-ERI reports on an individual's confidence in their abililty (self-efficacy) in their EBP competency.

Organizing and Interpreting Evidence for Clinical Application. As new knowledge resources are developed, the Star Model can be used to organize and interpret relevance to clinical application. For example, systematic reviews from the Cochrane Library can be organized on to Point 2, indicating that the next step is to locate evidence-based clinical practice guidelines. The National Guideline Clearinghouse is an excellent source of knowledge forms on Point 3 of the Star Model. Ideas for integration of EBP into practice (Point 4) can be accessed from the Agency for Healthcare Research and Quality Health Care Innovations Exchange (see http://www.innovations.ahrq.gov/). Finally, Point 5 quality indicators can be found on the National Quality Measures Clearinghouse (see http://www.qualitymeasures.ahrq.gov/).

Research on the Science of EBP. The Star Model also guides research on the *science of EBP*. Point 4 of the Star Model provides a reference for the new fields of improvement and implementation science. Once knowledge is available in sound clinical practice guidelines, the task of actually changing practice is faced. These new scientific fields focus on the study of improvement strategies to increase our understanding of factors that facilitate or hinder integration and implementation of EBP. The aim of improvement science is to determine which improvement strategies work as we strive to assure EBP through safe and effective care; a key feature is that these fields primarily focus on the healthcare delivery system and microsystem (ISRN, 2013). Implementation science is important to EBP improvement in that it asseses ways to link evidence into practice; it adds to our understanding of the effectiveness of strategies to "adopt and integrate evidence-based health interventions and change practice patterns within specific settings" (NIH, 2013).

CONCLUSIONS

Recognizing the challenges inherent in changing practice at an individual or organizational level, numerous models have been created. Common to these models is the recognition of the need for a systematic approach to practice change. Many of the models include common steps such as identification of change agents (e.g., APNs) to lead organizational change; identifying problems' engaging stakeholders to assist with the practice change; comprehensive searching of the literature to find high-quality evidence to inform the practice change; attention to potential organizational barriers to practice change; using effective strategies to disseminate information about the practice change to those implementing it; and evaluating the impact of the practice change.

More research is needed to confirm the advantages of using particular models and how these models could work in tandem. Those who use the models described in this chapter or other models should document their experiences in order to better understand the model's usefulness in facilitating EBP and to provide information to others who might use the model in the future (Graham et al., 2007).

Once the EBP change is implemented, sustainability of the change can be a challenge. Davies et al. (2006) collected data from 37 organizations that had implemented nursing best practice guidelines and found that after 3 years, 59% of the organizations were sustaining implementation of these guidelines. Most of those organizations also expanded their use by implementing the guidelines in more units or agencies, engaging more partners, encouraging multidisciplinary involvement, and integrating the guidelines with other QI initiatives. Top facilitators for sustaining and expanding the use of guidelines were leadership champions, management support, ongoing staff education, integration of the guidelines into policies and procedures, staff buy-in and ownership, synergy with partners, and multidisciplinary involvement. Sustained practice change involves those at the front line as well as at the executive levels. An important element to ensure sustainability is an organizational culture supportive of EBP. Changing nursing practice to be more evidence-informed is a dynamic, long-term, and iterative process.

EBP FAST FACTS

- ◆ Models can guide clinicians and healthcare systems in the implementation and sustainability of EBP.
- ◆ The original Stetler model for RU was published in 1976 to help fill a void regarding the realistic application of research findings into clinical practice; it has five phases, including (1) preparation, (2) validation, (3) comparative evaluation/decision making, (4) translation/application, and (5) evaluation.
- ◆ The Iowa Model of Evidence-Based Practice to Promote Quality Care describes a multiphase change process with feedback loops that provides guidance in making decisions about clinical and administrative practices that affect patient outcomes.
- ◆ The Model for Evidence-Based Practice Change guides clinicians through six steps, including (1) assess the need for change in practice, (2) locate the best evidence, (3) critically analyze the evidence, (4) plan the practice change, (5) implement and evaluate change in practice, and (6) integrate and maintain change in practice.
- ◆ The Advancing Research and Clinical practice through close Collaboration (ARCC©) Model is an evidence-based system-wide implementation and sustainability model for EBP, which uses ARCC© EBP mentors as a key strategy in facilitating evidence-based care with clinicians and creating a culture and environment that supports EBP.
- ◆ The Promoting Action on Research Implementation in Health Services (PARIHS) framework emphasizes that EBP implementation activities and processes should be targeted toward moving the three main elements of evidence, context, and facilitation on a continuum from low to high in order to increase chances of success.
- ◆ The Clinical Scholar Model© was developed and implemented to promote the spirit of inquiry, educate direct care providers, and guide a mentorship program for EBP and the conduct of research at the point of care.
- ◆ The Johns Hopkins Nursing Evidence-Based Practice model facilitates bedside nurses in translating evidence to clinical, administrative, and educational nursing practice.

◆ The ACE Star model explains how to overcome the challenges of (1) the volume of research evidence; (2) the misfit between form and use of knowledge; and (3) integration of expertise and patient preference into best practice.

References

Beck, A., Rush, A., Shaw, B., & Emery, G. (1979). *Cognitive therapy of depression*. New York, NY: The Guilford Press.

Block, J., Lilienthal, M., Cullen, L., White, A., 2012. Evidence-based thermoregulation for adult trauma patients. *Critical Care Nursing Quarterly, 35*(1):50-63. doi: 10.1097/CNQ.0b013e31823d3e9b

Brewer, B. B., Brewer, M. A., & Schultz, A. A. (2009). A collaborative approach to building the capacity for research and evidence-based practice in community hospitals. *Nursing Clinics of North America, 44*(1), 11–25.

Brown, D., & McCormack, B. (2005). Developing postoperative pain management: Utilising the Promoting Action on Research Implementation in Health Services (PARIHS) framework. *Worldviews on Evidence-Based Nursing, 3*(2), 131–141.

Carver, C. S., & Scheier, M. F. (1982). Control theory: A useful conceptual framework for personality-social, clinical, and health psychology. *Psychological Bulletin, 92*, 111–135.

Carver C. S., & Scheier, M. F. (1998). *On the self-regulation of behavior*. Cambridge, UK: Cambridge University Press.

Cheema, A. A., Scott, A. M., Shambaugh, K. J., Shaffer-Hartman, J. N., Dechert, R. E., Hieber, S. M., & Niedner, M. F. (2011). Rebound in ventilator-associated pneumonia rates during a prevention checklist washout period. *BMJ Quality & Safety, 20*(9), 811–817. doi: 10.1136/bmjqs.2011.051243

Chlan, L. L., Weinert, C. R., Heiderscheit, A., Tracy, M. F., Skaar, D. J., Guttormson, J. L., & Savick, K. (2013). Effects of patient-directed music intervention on anxiety and sedative exposure in critically ill patients receiving mechanical ventilator support: A randomized clinical trial. *JAMA, 309*(22), 2335–2344.

Chung, K., Davis, I., Moughrabi, S., & Gawlinski, A. (2011). Use of an evidence-based shift report tool to improve nurses' communication. *MEDSURG Nursing, 20*(5), 255–260, 268.

Clinical Scholarship Task Force. (1999). *Clinical scholarship resource paper*. Retrieved June 3, 2008, from http://www.nursingsociety.org/aboutus/Documents/clinical_scholarship_paper.pdf

Crawford, M. J., Thomas, O., Khan, N., & Kulinskaya, E. (2007). Psychosocial interventions following self-harm: Systematic review of their efficacy in preventing suicide. *British Journal of Psychiatry, 190*, 11–17.

Cronenwett, C. (1994). Using research in the care of patients. In G. LoBiondo-Wood & J. Haber (Eds.), *Nursing research: Methods, critical appraisal, and utilization* (pp. 89–90). St. Louis, MO: Mosby.

Cullen, L., & Adams, S. L. (2012). Planning for implementation of evidence-based practice. *The Journal of Nursing Administration, 42*(4), 222–230. doi: 10.1097/NNA.0b013e31824ccd0a

Cullen, L., Hanrahan, K., Tucker, S., Rempel, G., & Jordan, K. (2012). *Evidence-Based Practice Building Blocks: Comprehensive Strategies, Tools and Tips*. Iowa City, IA: Nursing Research and Evidence-Based Practice Office, Department of Nursing Services and Patient Care, University of Iowa Hospitals and Clinics.

Cullen, L., Smelser, J., Wagner, M., & Adams, S. (2012). Evidence into practice: using research findings to create practice. *Journal of Perianesthesia Nursing, 27*(5), 343–351.

Davies, B., Edwards, N., Ploeg, J., Virani, T., Skelly, J., & Dobbins, M. (2006). *Determinants of the sustained use of research evidence in nursing: Final report*. Ottawa, ON, Canada: Canadian Health Services Research Foundation & Canadian Institutes for Health Research.

Dearholt, S., White, K., Newhouse, R. P., Pugh, L., & Poe, S. (2008). Educational strategies to develop evidence-based practice mentors. *Journal for Nurses in Staff Development, 24*(2), 53–59.

Dearholt, S. L., & Dang, D. (2012). *Johns Hopkins nursing evidence-based practice model and guidelines* (2nd ed.). Indianapolis, IN: Sigma Theta Tau International.

Deberg, J., Adams, S., & Cullen, L. (2012). Evidence into practice: Basic steps for planning your evidence search. *Journal of Perianesthesia Nursing, 27*(1), 37–41. doi: 10.1016/j.jopan.2011.11.001

Dennis, C. L., & Dowswell, T. (2013). Psychosocial and psychological interventions for preventing postpartum depression. *The Cochrane Database of Systematic Reviews, 2*, CD001134

DiCenso, A., Ciliska, D., & Guyatt, G. (2004). Introduction to evidence-based nursing. In A. DiCenso, D. Ciliska, & G. Guyatt (Eds.), *Evidence-based nursing: A guide to clinical practice* (pp. 3–19). St Louis, MO: Elsevier.

Ellis, I., Howard, P., Larson, A., & Robertson, J. (2005). From workshop to work practice: An exploration of context and facilitation in the development of evidence-based practice. *Worldviews on Evidence-Based Nursing, 2*(2), 84–93.

Everett, L. Q., & Sitterding, M. C. (2011). Transformational leadership required to design and sustain evidence-based practice: A system exemplar. *Western Journal of Nursing Research, 33*(3), 398–426. doi: 10.1177/0193945910383056

Farrington, M., Cullen, L., & Dawson, C. (2010). Assessment of oral mucositis in adult and pediatric oncology patients: an evidence-based approach. *ORL-Head and Neck Nursing, 28*(3), 8–15.

Farrington, M., Cullen, L., Dawson, C. (2013). Evidence-based oral care for oral mucositis, *ORL-Head and Neck Nursing, 31*(3), 6–15.

Farrington, M., Lang, S., Cullen, L., & Stewart, S. (2009). Nasogastric tube placement in pediatric and neonatal patients. *Pediatric Nursing, 35*(1), 17–24.

Fineout-Overholt, E., & Melnyk, B. M. (2006). *Organizational culture and readiness scale for system-wide integration of evidence-based practice.* Gilbert, AZ: ARCC, LLC.

Flynn, M. G., & McGuinness, C. (2011). Hospital clinicians' information behaviour and attitudes towards the 'Clinical Informationist': An Irish survey. *Health Information and Libraries Journal, 28*(1), 23–32. doi: 10.1111/j.1471-1842.2010.00917.x

Geyman, J. (1998). Evidence-based medicine in primary care: An overview. *Journal of the American Board of Family Practice, 11*, 46–56.

Gerrish, K., Nolan, M., McDonnell, A., Tod, A., Kirshbaum, M., & Guillaume, L. (2012). Factors influencing advanced practice nurses' ability to promote evidence-based practice among frontline nurses. *Worldviews on Evidence-Based Nursing, 9*(1), 30–39. doi: 10.1111/j.1741-6787.2011.00230.x

Gifford, W. A., Davies, B. L., Graham, I. D., Tourangeau, A., Woodend, A. K., & Lefebre, N. (2013). Developing leadership capacity for guideline use: A pilot cluster randomized control trial. *Worldviews on Evidence-Based Nursing, 10*(1), 51–65. doi: 10.1111/j.1741-6787.2012.00254.x

Gifford, W., Davies, B., Edwards, N., Griffin, P., & Lybanon, V. (2007). Managerial leadership for nurses' use of research evidence: An integrative review of the literature. *Worldviews on Evidence-Based Nursing, 4*(3), 126–145.

Goode, C., & Piedalue, F. (1999). Evidence-based clinical practice. *Journal of Nursing Administration, 29*, 15–21.

Graham, I. D., Tetroe, J., & KT Theories Research Group. (2007). Some theoretical underpinnings of knowledge translation. *Academic Emergency Medicine, 14*(11), 936–941.

Harmon, K. G., Drezner, J. A., Gammons, M., Guskiewicz, K. M., Halstead, M., Herring, S. A., … Roberts, W. O. (2013). American Medical Society for Sports Medicine position statement: Concussion in sport. *British Journal of Sports Medicine, 47*(1), 15–26. doi: 10.1136/bjsports-2012-091941

Harvey, G., Loftus-Hills, A., Rycroft-Malone, J., Titchen, A., Kitson, A., McCormack, B., & Seers, K. (2002). Getting evidence into practice: The role and function of facilitation. *Journal of Advanced Nursing, 37*(6), 577–588.

Hauck, S., Winsett, R. P., & Kuric, J. (2013). Leadership facilitation strategies to establish evidence-based practice in an acute care hospital. *Journal of Advanced Nursing, 69*(3), 664–674. doi: 10.1111/j.1365-2648.2012.06053.x

Haxton, D., Doering, J., Gingras, L., & Kelly, L. (2012). Implementing skin-to-skin contact at birth using the Iowa Model: Applying evidence to practice. *Nursing for Women's Health, 16*(3), 220–229; quiz 230. doi: 10.1111/j.1751-486X.2012.01733.x

Haynes, R. (2002). What kind of evidence is it that evidence-based medicine advocates want health care providers and consumers to pay attention to? *BMC Health Services Research, 2*, 3.

Haynes, R., Sackett, D., Gray, J., Cook, D., & Guyatt, G. (1996). EBM notebook: Transferring evidence from research into practice: 1. The role of clinical care research evidence in clinical decisions. *Evidence Based Medicine, 1*, 196–198.

Horsley, J. A., Crane, J., Crabtree, M. K., & Wood, D. J. (1983). *Using research to improve nursing practice: A guide.* Orlando, FL: Green & Stratton.

Honess, C., Gallant, P., & Keane, K. (2009). The Clinical Scholar Model: Evidence-based practice at the bedside. *Nursing Clinics of North America, 44*(1), 116–130.

Hunt, J. (1991). Barriers to research utilisation. *Journal of Advanced Nursing, 23*(3), 423–425.

Hutchinson, A. M., & Johnston, L. (2006). Beyond the barriers scale: Commonly reported barriers to research use. *The Journal of Nursing Administration, 36*(4), 189–199.

Hysong, S. J., Best, R. G., & Pugh, J. A. (2006). Audit and feedback and clinical practice guideline adherence: Making feedback actionable. *Implementation Science, 28*(1), 1–9.

Ida, R. C., Adelaide, P. M., & Stefania, B. (2012). Supportive care in cancer unit at the National Cancer Institute of Milan: A new integrated model of medicine in oncology. *Current Opinion in Oncology, 24*(4), 391–396. doi: 10.1097/CCO.0b013e328352eabc

Improvement Science Research Network (ISRN). (2013). *What is improvement science?* Retrieved from http://www.isrn.net/about/improvement_science.asp

Institute of Medicine (IOM). (2008). *Knowing what works: A Roadmap for the nation*, J. Eden, B. Wheatley, B. L. McNeil, & H. Sox (Eds.). Washington, DC: National Academies Press.

Institute of Medicine. (2011a). *Clinical guidelines we can trust* [Committee on Standards for Developing Trustworthy Clinical Practice Guidelines]. Washington, DC: National Academies Press.

Institute of Medicine. (2011b). *Finding what works in health care: Standards for systematic reviews* [Committee on Standards for Systematic Reviews of Comparative Effective Research; Board on Health Care Services]. Washington, DC: National Academies Press.

Ivers, N., Jamtvedt, G., Flottorp, S., Young, J. M., Odgaard-Jensen, J., French, S. D., … Oxman, A. D. (2012). Audit and feedback: Effects on professional practice and healthcare outcomes. *Cochrane Database of Systematic Reviews, 6*, CD000259. doi: 10.1002/14651858.CD000259.pub3

Kelly, K. P., Guzzetta, C. E., Mueller-Burke, D., Nelson, K., Duval, J., Hinds, P. S., & Robinson, N. (2011). Advancing evidence-based nursing practice in a children's hospital using competitive awards. *Western Journal of Nursing Research, 33*(3), 306–332. doi: 10.1177/0193945910379586

Kim, S. (1999). *Models of theory-practice linkage in nursing.* Paper presented at the International Nursing Research Conference: Research to Practice, University of Alberta, Edmonton, Canada.

Kitson, A., Harvey, G., & McCormack, B. (1998). Enabling the implementation of evidence based practice: A conceptual framework. *Quality in Health Care, 7*(3), 149–158.

Kitson, A., Rycroft-Malone, J., Harvey, G., McCormack, B., Seers, K., & Titchen, A. (2008). Evaluating the successful implementation of evidence into practice using the PARIHS framework: Theoretical and practical challenges. *Implementation Science, 3*(1), 1–12.

Krom, Z. R., Batten, J., & Bautista, C. (2010). A unique collaborative nursing evidence-based practice initiative using the Iowa Model: A clinical nurse specialist, a health science librarian, and a staff nurse's success story. *Clinical Nurse Specialist, 24*(2), 54–59. doi: 10.1097/NUR.0b013e3181cf5537

Lam, D. (2005). A brief overview of CBT techniques. In S. Freeman & A. Freeman (Eds.), *Cognitive behavior therapy in nursing practice* (pp. 29–47). New York: Springer Publishing Company.

Larrabee, J. H. (2004). Advancing quality improvement through using the best evidence to change practice. *Journal of Nursing Care Quality, 19*(1), 10–13.

Larrabee, J. H. (2009). *Nurse to nurse: Evidence-based practice.* New York: McGraw-Hill.

Levin, R. F., Fineout-Overholt, E., Melnyk, B. M., Barnes, M., & Vetter, M. J. (2011). Fostering evidence-based practice to improve nurse and cost outcomes in a community health setting: A pilot test of the advancing research and clinical practice through close collaboration model. *Nursing Administration Quarterly, 35*(1), 21–33.

Lopes, C. M., & Galvao, C. M. (2010). Surgical positioning: Evidence for nursing care. *Revista Latino-Americana De Enfermagem, 18*(2), 287–294.

Mark, D. D., Latimer, R. W., & Hardy, M. D. (2010). "Stars" aligned for evidence-based practice: A Triservice initiative in the Pacific. *Nursing Research, 59*(1 Suppl), S48–S57. doi: 10.1097/01.NNR.0000313506.22722.53

Mayer, J., Mooney, B., Gundlapalli, A., Harbarth, S., Stoddard, G. J., Rubin, M. A., … Samore, M. H. (2011). Dissemination and sustainability of a hospital-wide hand hygiene program emphasizing positive reinforcement. *Infection Control and Hospital Epidemiology, 32*(1), 59–66. doi: 10.1086/657666

McCormack, B., Kitson, A., Harvey, G., Rycroft-Malone, J., Titchen, A., & Seers, K. (2002). Getting evidence into practice: The meaning of 'context.' *Journal of Advanced Nursing, 38*(1), 94–104.

McMullan, C., Propper, G., Schuhmacher, C., Sokoloff, L., Harris, D., Murphy, P., & Greene, W. H. (2013). A multidisciplinary approach to reduce central line-associated bloodstream infections. *Joint Commission Journal on Quality and Patient Safety, 39*(2), 61–69.

McSherry, R., Artley, A., & Holloran, J. (2006). Research awareness: An important factor for evidence based practice. *Worldviews on Evidence-Based Nursing, 3*(3), 103–115.

Melnyk, B., & Fineout-Overholt, E. (2005). *ARCC Advancing Research and Clinical practice through close Collaboration.* Gilbert, AZ: ARCC Publishing.

Melnyk, B. M. (2007). The evidence-based practice mentor: A promising strategy for implementing and sustaining EBP in healthcare systems. *Worldviews on Evidence-Based Nursing, 4*(3), 123–125.

Melnyk, B. M. (2012). Achieving a high-reliability organization through implementation of the ARCC model for systemwide sustainability of evidence-based practice. *Nursing Administration Quarterly, 36*(2), 127–135.

Melnyk, B. M., & Fineout-Overholt, E. (2002). Putting research into practice. *Reflections on Nursing Leadership, 28*(2), 22–25.

Melnyk, B. M., Fineout-Overholt, E., Feinstein, N., Li, H. S., Small, L., Wilcox, L., & Kraus, R. (2004). Nurses' perceived knowledge, beliefs, skills, and needs regarding evidence-based practice: Implications for accelerating the paradigm shift. *Worldviews on Evidence-Based Nursing, 1*(3), 185–193.

Melnyk, B. M., Fineout-Overholt, E., Gallagher-Ford, L., & Kaplan, L. (2012). The state of evidence-based practice in US nurses: Critical implications for nurse leaders and educators. *Journal of Nursing Administration, 42*(9), 410–417.

Melnyk, B. M., Fineout-Overholt, E., Gallagher-Ford, L., & Stillwell, S. B. (2011). Evidence-based practice, step by step: Sustaining evidence-based practice through organizational policies and an innovative model. *American Journal of Nursing, 111*(9), 57–60.

Melnyk, B. M., Fineout-Overholt, E., Giggleman, M., & Cruz, R. (2010). Correlates among cognitive beliefs, EBP implementation, organizational culture, cohesion and job satisfaction in evidence-based practice mentors from a community hospital system. *Nursing Outlook, 58*(6), 301–308.

Melnyk, B. M., Fineout-Overholt, E., & Mays, M. (2008). The evidence-based practice beliefs and implementation scales: Psychometric properties of two new instruments. *Worldviews on Evidence-Based Nursing, 5*(4), 208–216.

Melnyk, B. M., Jacobson, D., Kelly, S., Belyea, M., Shaibi, G., Small, L., … Marsiglia, F. F. (2013). Promoting healthy lifestyles in high school adolescents. *American Journal of Preventive Medicine, 45*(4), 407–415.

Melnyk, B. M., & Moldenhauer, Z. (2006). *The KySS guide to child and adolescent mental health screening, early intervention and health promotion.* Cherry Hill, NJ: NAPNAP.

Mitchell, S. A., Fisher, C. A., Hastings, C. E., Silverman, L. B., & Wallen, G. R. (2010). A thematic analysis of theoretical models for translational science in nursing: Mapping the field. *Nursing Outlook, 58*(6), 287–300.

Mulvenon, C., & Brewer, M. K. (2009). From the bedside to the boardroom: Resuscitating the use of nursing research. *Nursing Clinics of North America, 44*(1), 145–152.

Myrick, K. M. (2011). Improving follow-up after fragility fractures: An evidence-based initiative. *Orthopaedic Nursing, 30*(3), 174–179; quiz 180-171. doi: 10.1097/NOR.0b013e318219ac9f

National Institutes of Health (NIH). (2013). *Dissemination and implementation research in health.* PAR 10-038. Retrieved from http://grants.nih.gov/grants/guide/pa-files/PAR-10-038.html

National Research Council. *Health professions education: A bridge to quality.* Washington, DC: The National Academies Press, 2003.

Nelson, L., Doering, J. J., Anderson, M., & Kelly, L. (2012). Outcome of clinical nurse specialist-led hyperbilirubinemia screening of late preterm newborns. *Clinical Nurse Specialist, 26*(3), 164–168. doi: 10.1097/NUR.0b013e3182506ad6

Newhouse, R. P. (2007). Creating infrastructure supportive of evidence-based nursing practice: Leadership strategies. *Worldviews on Evidence-Based Nursing, 4*(1), 21–29.

Newhouse, R. P. (2008). Evidence driving quality initiatives: The Maryland hospital association collaborative on nurse retention. *Journal of Nursing Administration, 38*(6), 268–271.

Newhouse, R. P., Dearholt, S., Poe, S., Pugh, L. C., & White, K. (2007). Organizational change strategies for evidence-based practice. *Journal of Nursing Administration, 37*(12), 552–557.

Olds, D. L., Robinson, J., O'Brien, R., Luckey, D. W., Pettitt, L. M., Henderson, C. R., Jr., … Talmi, A. (2002). Home visiting by paraprofessionals and by nurses: A randomized, controlled trial. *Pediatrics, 110*(3), 486–496.

Parahoo, K. (1999). A comparison of pre-project 2000 and project 2000 nurses' perceptions of their research training, research needs and their use of research in clinical areas. *Journal of Advanced Nursing, 29*, 237–245.

Parahoo, K. (2000). Barriers to, and facilitators of, research utilization among nurses in Northern Ireland. *Journal of Advanced Nursing, 31*, 89–98.

Popovich, M. A., Boyd, C., Dachenhaus, T., & Kusler, D. (2012). Improving stable patient flow through the emergency department by utilizing evidence-based practice: One hospital's journey. *Journal of Emergency Nursing, 38*(5), 474–478. doi: 10.1016/j.jen.2011.03.006

Retsas, A. (2000). Barriers to using research evidence in nursing practice. *Journal of Advanced Nursing, 31*, 599–606.

Rogers, E. M. (2003). *Diffusion of innovations* (5th ed.). New York: The Free Press.

Rosswurm, M. A., & Larrabee, J. (1999). A model for change to evidence-based practice. *Image: Journal of Nursing Scholarship, 31*(4), 317–322.

Rycroft-Malone, J., Harvey, G., Seers, K., Kitson, A., McCormack, B., & Titchen, A. (2004). An exploration of the factors that influence the implementation of evidence into practice. *Journal of Clinical Nursing, 13*, 913–924.

Rycroft-Malone, J., Kitson, A., Harvey, G., McCormack, B., Seers, K., Titchen, A., & Estabrooks, C. (2002). Ingredients for change: Revisiting a conceptual framework. *Quality & Safety in Health Care, 11*, 174–180.

Rycroft-Malone, J., Seers, K., Titchen, A., Harvey, G., Kitson, A., & McCormack, B. (2004). What counts as evidence in evidence-based practice. *Journal of Advanced Nursing, 47*(1), 81–90.

Rycroft-Malone, J., & Stetler, C. (2004). Commentary on evidence, research, knowledge: A call for conceptual clarity. *Worldviews in Evidence-Based Nursing, 1*(2), 98f.

Sackett, D. L., Straus, S. E., Richardson, W. S., Rosenberg, W. M. C., & Haynes, R. B. (2000). *Evidence-based medicine: How to practice and teach EBM.* London: Churchill Livingstone.

Saint, S., Kowalski, C. P., Banaszak-Holl, J., Forman, J., Damschroder, L., & Krein, S. L. (2010). The importance of leadership in preventing healthcare-associated infection: Results of a multisite qualitative study. *Infection Control and Hospital Epidemiology, 31*(9), 901–907. doi: 10.1086/655459

Schultz, A. A. (2008). The Clinical Scholar Program: Creating a culture of excellence. *RNL, Reflections on Nursing Leadership*, June. Retrieved from http://www.nursingsociety.org/pub/rnl/pages/vol34_2_schultz.aspx

Schultz, A. A. (Guest Editor). (2009). Evidence-based practice. *Nursing Clinics of North America, 44*(1), xv–xvii.

Schultz, A. A. (Guest Editor), Honess, C., Gallant, P., Kent, G., Lancaster, K., Sepples, S., et al. (2005). Advancing evidence into practice: Clinical scholars at the bedside [Electronic version]. *Excellence in Nursing Knowledge.*

Scottish Intercollegiate Guidelines Network. (2007). *Critical appraisal: Notes and checklists.* Retrieved July 3, 2007, from http://www.sign.ac.uk/methodology/checklists.html

Schulte, S. J., Bejciy-Spring, S., & Niese, J. (2012). Evidence in action rounds: Collaborating with nursing to improve care. *Journal of Hospital Librarianship, 12*(3), 199–207.

Schultz, A. A. (2007). Implementation: A team effort. *Nursing Management*, 38(6), 12, 14.

Schultz, A. A. (Guest Editor). (2009). Evidence-based practice. *Nursing Clinics of North America, 44*(1), xv—xvii.

Schultz, A. A. (2011). *Practical Strategies for EBP and Clinical Research Collaboration*. Minot, ND: Minot State University, Presentation.

Schultz, A. A. (2011). *The Clinical Scholar Program: A Fulbright Collaboration in Northern Thailand*. 41st Biennial Convention, Grapevine, TX: Sigma Theta Tau International, November 2nd. Presentation.

Schultz, A. A. (2012) Basics of Synthesis. *Planning Evidence-based Practice and Research Projects*. Minot, ND: Trinity Health Care System. Presentation.

Schultz, A. A. & Brewer, B. B. (2013). Synthesis, not summary: The core of evidence-based decision-making for the direct care nurse. Unpublished manuscript.

Sharp, N., Pineros, S. L., Hsu, C., Starks, H., & Sales, A. (2004). A qualitative study to identify barriers and facilitators to the implementation of pilot intervention in the Veterans Health Administration Northwest Network. *Worldviews on Evidence-Based Nursing, 1*(4), 129–139.

Sen, S., Kranzler, H. R., Didwania, A. K., Schwartz, A. C., Amarnath, S., Kolars, J. C., & Guille, C. (2013). Effects of the 2011 duty hour reforms on interns and their patients: A prospective longitudinal cohort study. *Journal of the American Medical Association, 173*(8), 657–662. doi: 10.1001/jamainternmed.2013.351

Staggers, N., & Blaz, J. W. (2013). Research on nursing handoffs for medical and surgical settings: An integrative review. *Journal of Advanced Nursing, 69*(2), 247–262. doi: 10.1111/j.1365-2648.2012.06087.x

Stetler, C. B. (1994a). Refinement of the Stetler/Marram model for application of research findings to practice. *Nursing Outlook, 42*, 15–25.

Stetler, C. B. (1994b). Using research to improve patient care. In G. LoBiondo-Wood & J. Haber (Eds.), *Nursing research: Methods, critical appraisal, and utilization* (pp. 1–2). St. Louis, MO: Mosby.

Stetler, C. B. (2001a). *Evidence-based practice and the use of research: A synopsis of basic strategies and concepts to improve care*. Washington, DC: Nova Foundation.

Stetler, C. B. (2001b). Updating the Stetler model of research utilization to facilitate evidence-based practice. *Nursing Outlook, 49*, 272–278.

Stetler, C. B. (2002). *Evidence-based practice: A fad or the future of professional practice?* Paper presented at the Fourth Annual Evidence Based Practice Conference: Creating Momentum! Improving Care! Ann Arbor, MI.

Stetler, C. B. (2003). Role of the organization in translating research into evidence-based practice. *Outcomes Management, 7*, 97–103.

Stetler, C. B. (2010). Stetler model. In J. Rycroft-Malone & T. Bucknall (Eds.), *Evidence-based practice series. Models and frameworks to implementing evidence-based practice: Linking evidence to action*. Oxford: Blackwell Publishing Limited.

Stetler, C. B., Bautista, C., Vernale-Hannon, C., & Foster, J. (1995). Enhancing research utilization by clinical nurse specialists. *Nursing Clinics of North America, 30*, 457–473.

Stetler, C. B., Brunell, M., Giuliano, K., Morsi, D., Prince, L., & Newell-Stokes, G. (1998). Evidence based practice and the role of nursing leadership. *Journal of Nursing Administration, 8*, 45–53.

Stetler, C. B., & Caramanica, L. (2007). Evaluation of an evidence-based practice initiative: Outcomes, strengths and limitations of a retrospective, conceptually-based approach. *Worldviews on Evidence-Based Nursing, 4*(4), 187–199.

Stetler, C. B., & Marram, G. (1976). Evaluating research findings for applicability in practice. *Nursing Outlook, 24*, 559–563.

Stetler, C., Morsi, D., Rucki, S., Broughton, S., Corrigan, B., Fitzgerald, J., … Sheridan, E. A. (1998). Utilization-focused integrative reviews in a nursing service. *Applied Nursing Research, 11*(4), 195–206.

Stevens, K. R. (2004). *ACE Star Model of EBP: Knowledge transformation*. Academic Center for Evidence-based Practice. The University of Texas Health Science Center at San Antonio. Retrieved from www.acestar.uthscsa.edu

Stevens, K. R. (2009). *Essential evidence-based practice competencies in nursing* (2nd ed.). San Antonio, TX: Academic Center for Evidence-Based Practice (ACE) of University of Texas Health Science Center.

Stevens, K. R., Puga, F,, & Low, V. (2012). *The ACE-ERI: An instrument to measure EBP readiness in student and clinical populations*. Retrieved from http://www.acestar.uthscsa.edu/institute/su12/documents/ace/8%20The%20ACE-ERI%20%20Instrument%20to%20Benchmark.pdf

STTI. (2008). Sigma Theta Tau International position statement on evidence-based practice February 2007 summary. *Worldviews on Evidence-Based Nursing, 5*(2), 57–59. doi: 10.1111/j.1741-6787.2008.00118.x

Sussong, A. E., Cullen, S., Theriault, P., Stetson, A., Higgins, B., et al. (2009). Renewing the spirit of nursing: Embracing evidence-based practice in a rural state. *Nursing Clinics of North America, 44*(1), 32–42.

Tandon, S. D., Leis, J. A., Mendelson, T., Perry, D. F., & Kemp, K. (2013). Six-month outcomes from a randomized controlled trial to prevent perinatal depression in low-income home visiting clients. *Maternal Child Health Journal*, June 22 [Epub ahead of print].

Titler, M. G., Wilson, D. S., Resnick, B., & Shever, L. L. (2013). Dissemination and implementation: INQRI's potential impact. *Medical Care, 51*(4 Suppl 2), S41–S46. doi: 10.1097/MLR.0b013e3182802fb5

Titler, M. G. (2008). The evidence for evidence-based practice implementation. In R. G. Hughes (Ed.), *Patient safety and quality: An evidence-based handbook for nurses* (pp. 1–49). [AHRQ Publication No. 08-0043] Rockville, MD: Agency for Healthcare Research and Quality..

Titler, M. G., Klieber, C., Steelman, V., Goode, C., Rakel, B., Barry-Walker, J., ... Buckwalter, K. (1994). Infusing research into practice to promote quality care. *Nursing Research, 43*(5), 307–313.

Titler, M. G., Klieber, C., Steelman, V., Rakel, B. A., Budreau, G., Everett, L. Q., ... Goode, C. J. (2001). The Iowa model of evidence-based practice to promote quality care. *Critical Care Nursing Clinics of North America, 13*(4), 497–509.

Tucker, S. J., Bieber, P. L., Attlesey-Pries, J. M., Olson, M. E., & Dierkhising, R. A. (2012). Outcomes and challenges in implementing hourly rounds to reduce falls in orthopedic units. *Worldviews on Evidence-Based Nursing, 9*(1), 18-29. doi: 10.1111/j.1741-6787.2011.00227.x

van Achterberg, T., Schoonhoven, L., & Grol, R. (2008). Nursing implementation science: How evidence-based nursing requires evidence-based implementation. *Journal of Nursing Scholarship, 40*(4), 302–310.

Wallen, G. R., Mitchell, S. A., melnyk, B., Fineout-Overholt, E., Miller-Davis, C., Yates, J., and Hastings, C. (2010). Implementing evidence-based practice: effectiveness of a structured multifaceted mentorship programme. *Journal of Advanced Nursing 66*(12): 2761–2771.

Wallin, L., Estabrooks, C. A., Midodzi, W. K., & Cummings, G. G. (2006). Development and validation of a derived measure of research utilization by nurses. *Nursing Research, 55*(3), 149–160.

Watson, C. A., Bulechek, G. M., & McCloskey, J. C. (1987). QAMUR: a quality assurance model using research. *Journal of Nursing Quality Assurance, 2*(1), 21-27.

WATSON, C. A., BULECHEK, G. M., & McCLOSKEY,J. C. (1987). QAMUR: A quality assurance model using research. Journal of Nursing Quality Assurance, 2(1), 21-27.

Webster, J.1., Gillies, D., O'Riordan, E., Sherriff, K.L., & Rickard, C.M. (2011). Gauze and tape and transparent polyurethane dressings for central venous catheters. *The Cochrane Database of Systematic Reviews, 11*, CD003827. doi: 10.1002/14651858.CD003827.pub2.

Weeks, S. M., Marshall, J., & Burns, P. (2009). Development of an evidence-based practice & research collaborative among urban hospitals. *Nursing Clinics of North America, 44*(1), 26–31.

White, K. W., Shaefer, S. J. M., & Mark, H. D. (2012). *Instructors' guide for Johns Hopkins nursing evidence-based practice model and guidelines.* Indianapolis, IN: Sigma Theta Tau International.

Wykes, T., Steel, C., Everitt, B., & Tarrier, N. (2008). Cognitive behavior therapy for schizophrenia: Effect sizes, clinical models, and methodological rigor. *Schizophrenia Bulletin, 34*(3), 523–537.

Yackel, E. E., McKennan, M. S., & Fox-Deise, A. (2010). A nurse-facilitated depression screening program in an Army primary care clinic: An evidence-based project. *Nursing Research, 59*(1 Suppl), S58-65. doi: 10.1097/NNR.0b013e3181c3cab6

Chapter 14

Creating a Vision and Motivating a Change to Evidence-Based Practice in Individuals, Teams, and Organizations

Bernadette Mazurek Melnyk and Ellen Fineout-Overholt

Shoot for the moon because even if you miss, you will land amongst the stars.

—Les Brown

In today's rapidly changing healthcare environment in which health professionals are often confronted with short staffing, cost reductions, and heavy patient loads, the implementation of a change to evidence-based practice (EBP) can be a daunting or "character-building" endeavor. Individual, team, and organizational changes are often a complex and lengthy process. However, there are general principles at the individual, team, and organizational levels that will expedite the process of change when an exciting vision is created and a thoughtful and well thought out strategic plan is carefully executed.

Most organizational change theories are conceptual rather than evidence-based, which limits the science base to guide decisions about implementation strategies (Prochaska, Prochaska, & Levesque, 2001). In addition, many organizational change initiatives fail because leaders and teams (a) lose sight of their vision, (b) get steeped in barriers that are challenging to overcome, and (c) forget the stages of change that are a normal part of the process, which can lead to abandoning the change initiative.

This chapter discusses critical principles and steps for implementing change in individuals, teams, and organizations, with an emphasis on four unique nonhealthcare models of organizational change that are useful in guiding successful change efforts in healthcare institutions. Strategies to enhance team functioning as well as the cooperation of individuals with various personality styles are highlighted. The major intent is to stimulate innovative "out-of-the-box" or nontraditional thinking in motivating a change to best practice within individuals, teams, and organizations.

Although it is imperative to consider the structure, culture, ecosystem or environment, and strategy for change within a system, it is also critical that the leaders and individual(s) implementing the change have a clear vision, belief in that vision, and persistence to overcome the many difficult or character-building experiences along the journey to bringing that project to fruition.

ESSENTIAL ELEMENTS FOR SUCCESSFUL ORGANIZATIONAL CHANGE

Among the important elements that must be present for change to be accomplished successfully are vision, belief, strategic planning, action, persistence, and patience.

First Element: Vision and Goals

The first essential element for implementing change, whether it is at the **macro** (i.e., large scale) or **micro** (i.e., small scale) level, is a crystal clear, exciting vision or dream of what is to be accomplished. A clear vision of the desired outcome is needed in order to unify stakeholders (MacPhee, 2007) and outline a plan for implementing success strategies. In numerous biographies of highly successful people, a recurrent theme is that those individuals had big dreams and a clear vision of the projects that they wanted to accomplish in their lives. Although it is important to have a well-planned process for execution, without vision the dream is unlikely to come to fruition.

For example, Dr. Robert Jarvik, the man who designed the world's first artificial heart, was rejected at least three times by every medical school in the United States. However, he also had a large dream that was not going to be denied. He was finally accepted into the University of Utah School of Medicine in 1972, and a decade later, he achieved a medical breakthrough that has gone down in history. Dr. Jarvik had none of the conventional assets (e.g., superior grades, a high score on the medical entrance exam), but he possessed important intangibles (e.g., a big dream, passion, and persistence to achieve his dream).

Dr. William DeVries, the chief surgeon who inserted the first artificial heart in a human patient, commented about how he had the vision of performing this procedure for years. Dr. DeVries repeatedly rehearsed that procedure in his mind in terms of what and how he was going to accomplish it so that when the opportunity finally presented itself, he was ready to perform.

Walt Disney visualized a dream of an amusement park where families could spend quality time together long before that dream became a reality. Walt Disney's strong visualization prompted him to take action and persist in his efforts, despite many character-building experiences. Most individuals do not realize that Walt Disney was bankrupt when he traveled across the country, showing his drawing of a mouse to bankers, investors, and friends. He faced countless rejections and tremendous mockery for his ideas for years before his dream started to become a reality. However, Disney stayed focused on his dream and thought about it on a daily basis. This intense daily focus on his dream facilitated a cognitive plan of a series of events that led him to act on that dream. Walt Disney believed that once you dream or visualize what it is that you want to accomplish, the things you need to accomplish it will be attracted to you, especially if you think about *how you can do it* instead of *why you will not be able to accomplish it*. Walt Disney died before Disney World was completed and, in the opening park ceremony, a reporter commented to his brother that it was too bad that Walt never had the opportunity to see the wonderful idea come to fruition. His brother, however, commented emphatically that the reporter was incorrect and, in fact, that Walt had seen his dream for many years.

Mark Spitz dreamed of becoming an Olympic gold medalist for many years. He prepared himself by swimming many hours a day looking at a black line on the bottom of the pool. As he swam and looked at the black line, he kept the vision of standing on the Olympic platform and receiving an Olympic gold medal. It was that dream that kept him persisting through many character-building days of grinding practice.

If you knew it were impossible to fail, what would be the vision that you have for a change to EBP in your organization? Both within yourself and in your organization, how you think is everything. It is important to *think success* at the outset of any new individual or organizational initiative and to keep your vision larger than the fears of and obstacles associated with implementation.

....

What will you do in the next 3–5 years if you know you cannot fail?
—Bernadette Mazurek Melnyk

....

Establishing an exciting shared vision with the team of individuals who will lead organizational change to EBP is important for buy-in and success of the project. Top-down dictates without involvement of a team is often a formula for failure. However, when a team of leaders and individuals share a common vision for which everyone has had the opportunity for input, there is greater ownership and investment by the team members to facilitate organizational change.

Once the vision for change to EBP in your organization is established, it is imperative to create written goals with designated time frames for how that vision will be accomplished. Individuals with written goals are usually more successful in attaining them than those without written goals. For example, findings from a classic Harvard Business School study indicated that 83% of the population did not have clearly defined goals; 14% had goals that were not written; and 3% had written goals. The study also found that the 3% of individuals with written goals were earning 10 times that of the individuals who did not have written goals (McCormack, 1986).

Second Element: Belief

Belief in one's ability to accomplish the vision is a key element for behavior change and success. Too often, individuals have excellent ideas, but they lack the belief and confidence necessary to successfully spearhead and achieve their initiatives. Thus, many wonderful initiatives do not come to fruition.

A change to EBP in individuals requires a change in their behaviors, which is not easy. Individuals typically do not change behavior because they are provided with information or didactic education. Most individuals change because a crisis happens (e.g., a sibling who did not take his antihypertensive medication as prescribed or engage in regular physical activity dies young of a myocardial infection) or their emotions are raised. Further, behavior change in clinicians requires education plus repeated skills building activities (Melnyk et al., 2012). In their educational programs, clinicians are usually taught models to assist patients with behavior change (e.g., smoking cessation, healthy eating). However, those same models are rarely taken into consideration when working with clinicians on behavior change.

Cognitive theory is a useful framework to guide individual behavioral change toward EBP as it contends that an individual's behaviors and emotions are, in large part, determined by the way he or she thinks or his or her beliefs (i.e., the thinking–feeling–behaving triangle; Beck, Rush, Shaw, & Emery, 1979; Lam, 2005; Melnyk & Jensen, 2013). Findings from research have supported that cognitive beliefs affect emotions and behaviors, including the ability to successfully function or attain goals (Carver & Scheier, 1998; Melnyk et al., 2006, 2013). For example, if an individual does not believe or have confidence in the ability to achieve an important goal, he or she is likely to feel emotionally discouraged and not take any action toward accomplishing that goal. Findings from studies have also supported that when clinicians' beliefs about the value of EBP and their ability to implement it are high, they have greater implementation of evidence-based care than when their beliefs are low (Melnyk et al., 2004; Melnyk, Fineout-Overholt, Giggleman, & Cruz, 2010).

....

Anything that the mind can conceive and believe, it can achieve.
—John Heywood

....

Third Element: A Well-Formulated Strategic Plan

Once an initiative is conceptualized and goals are established with deadline dates, the next essential element required for successful change is a well-defined and written strategic plan. Many initiatives fail because individuals and teams do not carefully outline implementation strategies for each established goal. As part of the strategic planning process, it is important to accomplish a SCOT (**S**trengths, **C**hallenges, **O**pportunities, and **T**hreats) analysis. This analysis will

- Assess and identify the current **S**trengths in the system that will facilitate the success of a new project.
- Assess and identify the **C**hallenges in the system that may hinder the initiative.
- Outline the **O**pportunities for success.
- Delineate the **T**hreats or barriers to the project's completion, with strategies to overcome them.

Other Key Elements: Action, Persistence, and Patience

Other elements for the success of any organizational change project are action, persistence, and patience. All too often, projects are terminated early because of the lack of persistence and patience and faulty execution, especially when challenges are encountered or the results of action are not yet seen.

An analogy to this scenario may be seen in an Asian tree, the giant bamboo. The tree has a particularly hard seed. The seed is so difficult to grow that it must be watered and fertilized every day for 5 years before any portion of it breaks the soil. At the end of the fifth year of watering, the tree shows itself. Once the plant breaks the surface, it is capable of growing as fast as 4 feet a day to a height of 90 feet in less than a month. The question that is often asked is: Did the tree grow 90 feet in under a month or did it grow to its height over the 5 years? Of course, the answer is that it took 5 years to grow. It is critical to stay persistent until your dream and outcomes are realized.

....

Nurse your dreams and protect them through the bad times and tough times to the sunshine and light which always comes.
—Woodrow Wilson

....

Thomas Edison tried 9,000 different ways to invent a new type of storage battery before he found the right combination. His associate used to laugh at him, saying that he had failed 9,000 times. However, Edison kept his dream in front of him and persisted, commenting that at least he found 9,000 ways that it would not work. What would have happened if Edison had stopped his efforts to invent a storage battery on his 8,999th attempt?

The bottom line is that, no matter how outstanding a strategic plan is conceptualized and written, an exciting vision, belief in that vision, action, persistence, and patience are key elements for success in accomplishing any new initiative.

FOUR MODELS OF ORGANIZATIONAL CHANGE

Chapter 13 outlined several models that have been used to stimulate EBP in the health professions. However, four organizational change models are presented here because they take different elements and strategies into consideration. These models were selected because they are based either on hundreds of interviews and real-life experiences by highly qualified change experts who have worked to facilitate change in business organizations for a number of years (Duck, 2002; Kotter & Cohen, 2012; Rogers, 2003), or they are based on a behavior change model that has been empirically supported for a number of years as effective in producing behavior change in high-risk patient populations (e.g., smokers, people who engage in risky sexual behavior). The principles of these models add unique perspectives and could easily be applied to healthcare organizations interested in motivating a change to EBP. Empirical testing of these models could move forward the field of organizational change in healthcare organizations.

The Change Curve Model

Duck's (2002) Change Curve model emphasizes basic assumptions for change in an organization (Box 14.1). In addition, it emphasizes the stages of organizational change with potential areas for failure.

Stage I: Stagnation
The first stage of organizational change in the Change Curve model is *stagnation*. The causes of stagnation are typically a lack of effective leadership, failed initiatives, and too few resources. The emotional climate in the stage of stagnation is one in which individuals feel comfortable, there is no sense of threat, depression occurs, and/or hyperactivity exists and individuals become stressed and exhausted. Stagnation ends when action is finally taken.

Stage II: Preparation
The second stage of the Change Curve model is *preparation*. In this stage, the emotional climate of the organization is one of anxiety, hopefulness, and/or reduced productivity. Buy-in from individuals is essential at this stage in which people must ask themselves what they are willing to do. The opportunity that exists at this stage is getting people excited about the vision. The danger at this stage of change is the length of preparation: the project may fail if it is too short or too long.

> **Box 14.1** Basic Assumptions for Change in an Organization
>
> ◆ Changing an organization is a highly emotional process.
> ◆ Group change requires individual change.
> ◆ No fundamental change takes place without strong leadership.
> ◆ The leader must be willing to change before others are expected to change.
> ◆ The larger and more drastic the change, the more difficult the change.
> ◆ The greater the number of individuals involved, the tougher the change will be to effect.
>
> From Duck, J. D. (2002). *The change monster. The human forces that fuel or foil corporate transformation and change.* New York: Crown Business.

Stage III: Implementation

The third stage of the Change Curve model is *implementation*. In this stage, it is essential to assess individuals' readiness for the change as well as to increase their confidence in their ability to help make the change happen.

In the implementation stage, Duck (2002) emphasizes that individuals must see "what is in it for them" if they are going to commit to making a change. In addition, she asserts that when emotion is attached to the reason, individuals are more likely to change.

Stage IV: Determination

The fourth stage of the Change Curve model is *determination*. If results are not being experienced by now, individuals begin to experience fatigue change. The opportunity in this stage of organizational change is to create small successes along the way to change. The danger is that this is the stage in which the initiative has the highest chance of failure.

Stage V: Fruition

The fifth and final stage in the Change Curve model is *fruition*. In this stage, the efforts are coming to fruition, and positive outcomes can be seen. The opportunity in this stage is to celebrate and reward individuals for their efforts as well as to seek new ways to change and grow. This stage is in danger when individuals revert back to a level of complacency and begin to stagnate again.

....

I have learned that success is to be measured not so much by the position that one has reached in life as by the obstacles which one has overcome while trying to succeed.
—Booker T. Washington

....

Kotter and Cohen's Model of Change

Based on evidence gathered during interviews from more than 100 organizations in the process of large-scale change, Kotter and Cohen (2012) proposed that the key to organizational change lies in helping people to feel differently (i.e., appealing to their emotions). They assert that individuals change their behavior less when they are given facts or analyses that change their thinking than when they are shown truths that influence their feelings. In other words, there is a seeing, feeling, and changing pattern if

Table 14.1 **Eight Steps for Successful Change**

Action	New Behavior
Step 1: Increase urgency	"Let's go" "We need to change"
Step 2: Build the guiding team	A group forms to guide the change and work together
Step 3: Get the vision right	The team develops the right vision and strategy for the change effort
Step 4: Communicate for "buy-in"	People begin to see and accept the change as worthwhile
Step 5: Empower action and remove barriers	People begin to change and behave differently
Step 6: Create short-term wins	Momentum builds Fewer people resist the change
Step 7: Don't let up	The vision is fulfilled
Step 8: Make change stick	New and winning behavior continues

Source: From Kotter, J. P., & Cohen, D. S. (2012). *The heart of change: Real-life stories of how people change their organizations*. Boston, MA: Harvard Business School Press.

successful behavioral change is going to occur. In their book *The Heart of Change* (2012), Kotter and Cohen outline eight steps for successful change in an organization (Table 14.1).

Step 1: Urgency
According to Kotter and Cohen, the first step in changing an organization is creating a *sense of urgency*. This is especially important when individuals in an organization have been in a rut or a period of complacency for some time.

Step 2: Team Selection
The second step is carefully selecting a strong team of individuals who can guide change. Members of the team should possess the needed knowledge, skills, respect, and trust with other individuals in the organization as well as a commitment to the project. They should also show enthusiasm for the project as enthusiasm, like stress, is contagious to others in the environment. In some prior studies that have implemented interventions to facilitate a change to EBP, **opinion leaders** (e.g., individuals who have the ability to influence others) and EBP champions have been a critical element in a change to EBP. It is important to remember that informal leaders (i.e., those individuals without a formal title who have a positive influence over others) can often be as or more effective than formal titled leaders. Therefore, look for informal leaders within the environment to place on the team.

Step 3: Vision and Strategy
In step 3, the team guiding the project creates a clear vision with realistic implementation strategies for accomplishing that vision. In this step, it is important that the strategies are implemented in a reasonable timeframe because implementation that is too slow may lead to the initiative's failure.

Step 4: Communicating the Vision
Step 4 of Kotter and Cohen's organizational change model emphasizes the importance of communicating the vision and strategies with "heartfelt messages" that appeal to people's emotions. For example,

instead of telling individuals that EBP results in better patient outcomes, stories of real-life examples where EBP really made a difference need to be shared with them. For instance, some examples might be that thousands of low-birth-weight infants were saved from dying as a result of a systematic review of randomized controlled trials, which indicated that dexamethasone injections to women in premature labor enhanced lung surfactant production in the fetus; or, mortality rates in intensive care units (ICUs) dropped as a result of a change in endotracheal suctioning procedures. Repetition is also key so that everyone is clear on the strategies that need to be implemented.

Step 5: Empowerment

In step 5, individuals need to be empowered to change their behaviors. Barriers that inhibit successful change (e.g., inadequate resources or skills) should be removed. If not, individuals will become frustrated and change will be undermined.

Step 6: Interim Successes

Step 6 in Kotter and Cohen's model consists of establishing short-term successes. If individuals do not experience some degree of early success in their attempts to change, they will soon become frustrated and the initiative will falter.

Step 7: Ongoing Persistence

In step 7, continued persistence is essential in order to make the vision a reality. Organizational change efforts often fail because individuals try to accomplish too much in a short time or they give up too early, especially when the going gets tough.

Step 8: Nourishment

In step 8, it is important to nourish the new culture to make the change last, even if the leadership team experiences transitions. This nourishment is essential if the new culture and behaviors are to be sustained.

In summary, evidence from Kotter and Cohen's work with organizations to change the behavior of professionals have indicated that change agents must communicate their vision and make their points in ways that are compelling and emotionally engaging. It is this type of communication that enables individuals to identify a problem or the solution to a problem, prompts them to experience different feelings (e.g., passion, urgency, hope), and changes behavior (i.e., they see, feel, and change).

Rogers's Diffusion of Innovations

Concepts in Everett M. Rogers's (2003) theory of diffusion of innovations can be very useful when rolling out an organizational change to EBP. In this theory, a bell-shaped curve is used to describe the rate of adoption of new innovations by individuals (Figure 14.1).

Innovators comprise 2.5% of the innovation curve in Everett's theory. They are out-of-the-box thinkers and readily recognize innovative opportunities. Next are the early adopters or opinion leaders, who comprise 13.5% of the curve. These are individuals who are highly influential in organizations and encourage others to adopt innovations. The next group of individuals, comprising approximately 34% of the innovation curve, is the early majority. This group of individuals follows the lead of the early adopters in implementing the innovation. The late majority also comprises 34% of the innovation curve. This group of individuals spends additional time watching how the innovation is progressing and are more cautious in its adoption. Finally, the last 16% of individuals are the laggards, or the individuals who are fairly steeped in tradition and have much difficulty with change. They eventually adopt the new innovation, but not until it becomes the standard practice. According to the theory, there needs to be a critical mass of 15% to 20% of innovators, early adopters, and early majority before innovative change really begins to take hold (Rogers, 2003).

If leaders who are embarking on an innovative change to EBP do not expect this pattern of diffusion, they can easily be frustrated and relinquish the initiative too prematurely. According to the theory, it is important to target the early adopters in the change effort as they are instrumental in helping to

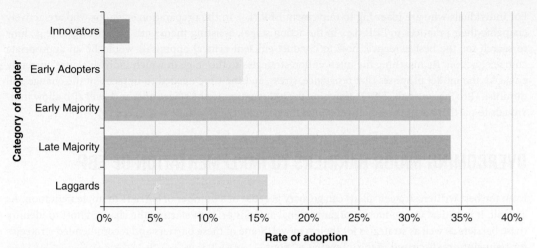

Figure 14.1: How individuals adopt innovation: Innovators to Laggards. Data from Roger's Diffusion of Innovation Theory, 1995.

facilitate a change to EBP in the organization. Many change efforts fail because focus and energy are placed on the late majority as well as on laggards who are much slower to adopt change, instead of targeting the individuals who welcome and/or are receptive to it.

The Transtheoretical Model of Health Behavior Change

For the past two decades, the transtheoretical model of health behavior change (Prochaska & Velicer, 1997) with its five stages (i.e., precontemplation, contemplation, preparation, action, and maintenance) has been empirically supported as being useful in precipitating and explaining behavior change in patients.

In the stage of precontemplation, the individual is not intending to take action in the next 6 months. In contemplation, the individual is intending to take action in the next 6 months. In preparation, the individual plans to take action in the next 30 days. The stage of action is when overt changes were made less than 6 months ago. Finally, the stage of maintenance is when overt changes were made more than 6 months ago (Prochaska et al., 2001).

Research indicates that approximately 40% of individuals in a specific population (e.g., smokers) are in the precontemplation stage, 40% are in the contemplative stage, and 20% are in the preparation phase (e.g., Laforge, Velicer, Richmond, & Owen, 1999).

In applying these statistics, if only approximately 20% of the staff in an organization are preparing (preparation stage) to take action in implementing EBP, it will be challenging for the initiative to succeed because many of these individuals will likely view a change to EBP as imposed and become resistant to the idea (Prochaska et al., 2001).

The transtheoretical model is now beginning to be applied in the field of organizational change (Prochaska et al., 2001). The extension of this model to healthcare providers when a change to EBP is desired could continue to extend the theory's pragmatic efficacy. For example, when attempting to stimulate a change to EBP in individuals who are in the precontemplative and contemplative stages, the focus should be on making a connection with them and assisting them to progress to the next stage of readiness (e.g., from precontemplative to contemplative), rather than working with them on actual behavior change strategies.

Strategies to assist individuals to move from the precontemplative or contemplative stages to a stage of readiness to change might include

◆ Strengthening their beliefs that EBP results in the best patient outcomes and highest quality of care
◆ Supporting their self-efficacy or confidence (i.e., they can indeed make the shift to EBP)

For individuals who are planning to implement EBP (i.e., in the preparation stage) or who are actively changing their practices to EBP (i.e., in the action stage), assisting them with EBP strategies (e.g., how to search for the best evidence, how to conduct efficient critical appraisal) would be an appropriate course of action. By matching the intervention strategies to the stage in which individuals are currently engaged, the model proposes that resistance, stress, and the time needed to implement the change will diminish (Prochaska et al., 2001). Matching the intervention to the stages of change will also allow individuals to participate in the initiative, even if they are not ready to take action.

OVERCOMING MAJOR BARRIERS TO IMPLEMENTATION OF EBP

Even the best written strategic plans can go awry because of a number of barriers to implementation. As a result, it is critical to conduct an organizational analysis prior to starting the change effort to identify these barriers as well as strategies for their removal. Some of these barriers and recommended strategies for removing are discussed in the following sections.

Dealing with Skepticism and Misperceptions About EBP

Any time a change is introduced in a system, there will be some degree of skepticism about it. Individuals tend to be skeptical about a change if they do not clearly understand the reason for it, if they are fearful about it, or if they have misperceptions about why the change is needed. The best strategy for overcoming this barrier to change in implementation of EBP is to allow individuals to express their skepticism, fears, and anxieties about the change as well as to clarify any misperceptions that they may have about EBP (e.g., that it takes too much time). Educating clinicians about EBP in a way that appeals to their emotions and enhances their beliefs about their ability to implement it will enhance the change process.

Knowing Individual Personality Styles and How Best to Motivate Individuals

Any time that change is introduced in a system, it is important to be sensitive to the personality styles of individuals. Knowing the four major personality styles will assist in the change effort by facilitating strategies to work successfully with each of them.

Rohm and Carey (1997), seasoned psychologists who have written books on the different personality styles, use a DISC model (see descriptions in the following sections) for working with individuals who possess different personality styles. Although a particular style tends to predominate, individuals often are in combinations of two or more styles.

D Personality Styles: Drivers

Individuals with **D** personality styles like to take charge of projects and are highly task oriented. They are dreamers, dominant, driving, and determined. An excellent strategy for working with individuals who have this type of personality style is to create excitement by giving them opportunities to lead the way by spearheading specific tasks or initiatives.

I Personality Styles: Inspired

Individuals who possess predominantly **I** personalities are typically people who are socially oriented and like to have fun. They are inspirational, influencing, impressive, and interactive. As such, they usually get excited about a new initiative by being shown that it can be a fun and exciting process.

S Personality Styles: Supportive and Steady

Individuals with predominantly *S* personalities are typically reserved and like to be led. They tend to be supportive, steady, submissive, and shy. The best strategy for working with individuals who have this personality style is to lead the way, telling them that they will be important in helping the project to succeed but that they themselves do not need to spearhead the effort.

C Personality Styles: Contemplators

Individuals with predominantly *C* personality styles are very analytical and detail oriented. They tend to be competent, cautious, careful, and contemplative. At one extreme, they can experience "analysis by paralysis," to a point at which initiatives never get launched. These individuals, although they mean well, may prolong the planning stage of a new initiative so long that others lose enthusiasm for embarking on the change process. The best way to deal with these individuals is to show them all of the details of the specific action plan that will be used to accomplish the change to EBP. Also, consider giving them a leadership role in ensuring that process is being followed and tracking outcomes.

Formulating a Well-Written Strategic Plan with Set Goals

Again, it is essential to have a written strategic plan with clearly established goals for a change to EBP to occur. Lack of a detailed plan is a major barrier to implementing a change to EBP within a system. The goals established should be SMART (i.e., *S*pecific, *M*easurable, *A*ttainable, *R*elevant, and *T*ime bound; Torres & Fairbanks, 1996). The established goals should also be high enough to facilitate growth in individuals and the organization but not so high that people will get easily frustrated by their inability to reach them.

Communicating the Vision and Strategic Plan

Communication is key to any successful organizational change plan. Individuals in the system need to be very clear about the vision and their role in the strategic planning efforts. Repetition and visual reminders of the vision and plan are important for the project's success. Involving individuals in creating the vision and plan will facilitate their buy-in and commitment to the project. Top-down directives typically do not sustain.

> **Change is stressful enough even when people are well prepared for its demands.**
> **Action imposed on people who are not adequately prepared can become intolerable.**
> **—Prochaska et al., 2001, p. 258**

Interprofessional Teamwork

Interprofessional team building and teamwork are essential for successful organizational change to EBP. Research supports that the successful implementation of new best practices is a multilevel process involving healthcare delivery teams and their effectiveness, not just individual clinicians, with the strongest link being team knowledge and skills to make the desired improvements (Lukas, Mohr, & Meterko, 2009). Research has shown that interprofessional teams demonstrate higher quality of patient care and better outcomes than individual professions functioning in silos (IOM, 2013).

It is important to understand that the team-building process is dynamic and that it requires creativity and flexibility. In addition, knowing the typical stages of team development (i.e., forming, storming, norming, and performing) will promote successful development of the team and prevent the early termination of a project due to typical team struggles, especially in the storming phase (Table 14.2).

Table 14.2 Stages of Team Development with Associated Characteristics

Forming	Anxiety, excitement, testing, dependence, exploration, and trust
Storming	Resistance to different approaches; attitude changes; competitiveness and defensiveness; tension and disunity
Norming	Satisfaction increases; trust and respect develops; feedback is provided to others; responsibilities are shared; decisions are made
Performing	Level of interaction is high; performance increases; team members are comfortable with one another; there is optimism and confidence

Source: Egolf, D. B., & Chester, S. L. (2013). *Forming, storming, norming & performing. Successful communication in groups and teams* (3rd ed.). Bloomington, IN: iUniverse.

Organizational Context, Including Resources and Administrative Support

Organizational context (i.e., the environment or ecosystem), including resources and administrative support, has been linked to the diffusion of EBPs throughout an organization (Rycroft-Malone et al., 2004). When leaders visibly express support for change or innovation, the change is more likely to occur (Lukas et al., 2009). In addition, effective leaders adopt innovation early and view change as an opportunity to learn, adapt, and improve (Rogers, 2003).

Assessment of resources in the organization and the level of readiness for system-wide change is an important step in the change process (e.g., web access and data bases for searching, assistance from a librarian, EBP mentors, educational and skills building programs, shared governance model that encourages clinicians to routinely question their practices) (Ogiehor-Enoma, Taqueban & Anosike, 2010). Although a large number of resources are not necessary to begin a change to EBP, there is no doubt that having ample resources as well as support and EBP role modeling from leaders and managers will expedite the process. Findings from a recent study revealed that nurses named leaders and managers as the one thing that prevented them from implementing EBP. Therefore, it is critical that leaders and managers be targeted in change efforts as their role modeling and support is necessary if point-of-care clinicians are going to consistently engage in evidence-based care.

Systems can begin to introduce small initiatives to implement a change to EBP, such as conducting journal clubs or EBP rounds. It is important to remember that small changes can have substantial impact (MacPhee, 2007).

....

What is the smallest change that you can make based on evidence that will have the largest impact?
—Bernadette Mazurek Melnyk

....

Placing PICOT boxes and EBP posters visibly in clinical settings can spark a spirit of inquiry in clinicians to consistently be asking themselves what the evidence is behind the care practices that are being implemented with their patients. These have been used successfully as part of the Advancing Research and Clinical Practice through Close Collaboration (ARCC) model; Melnyk & Fineout-Overholt, 2002 [see Chapter 13]). Effective teams also can be instrumental for sparking a change to EBP when there is a weak organizational context (Lukas et al., 2009).

In EBP rounds, the staff generate an important practice question. Then, they are assisted with searching for and critically appraising the evidence, followed by a presentation to other staff, where findings and implications for practice are discussed.

In systems that lack administrative support for a change to EBP, it is challenging but not impossible to ignite change. Assisting administrators to understand how a change to EBP can improve the quality and cost-effectiveness of patient care and appealing to their emotions with concrete examples of how a lack of evidence-based care resulted in adverse outcomes can help facilitate their support. Sharing of important documents that herald EBP as the standard for quality care and health professional education (e.g., Greiner & Knebel, 2003; Institute of Medicine, 2001) will support the position of implementing a change to EBP in the organization.

Overcoming Resistance

Resistance in an organization is frequently the result of poorly planned implementation and is the major reason that organizational change initiatives often fail (Prochaska et al., 2001). Individuals who display resistance to change are often not clear about the benefits of change and/or they have fears and anxiety about their role in implementing change or how it will impact them.

When confronted with individuals who are resisting a change to EBP, it is essential to facilitate conversations that will help them express their thoughts, hesitations, fears and misperceptions. Listening to these individuals' perspectives on change with respect and acceptance is essential to overcoming resistance (Corey & Corey, 2002; Prochaska et al., 2001). Once concerns and fears are expressed, strategies to overcome them can be implemented.

Organizational Culture and Mentorship: Key Elements for Sustaining Organizational Change

It is one thing to begin implementation of EBP in a healthcare organization, but a whole other entity to sustain the momentum. Organizational culture is the attitudes, beliefs, experiences, and values of the organization. It is defined as "the specific collection of values and norms that are shared by people and groups in an organization that control the way they interact with each other and with stakeholders outside the organization" (Hill & Jones, 2001). In order to sustain EBP, adoption of the EBP paradigm by a critical mass of administrators and managers, leaders, and individual clinicians is essential. This paradigm should be reflected in the vision, mission, and goals of an organization as well as in its standards of practice, clinical ladder promotion systems, and new employee orientations.

The paradigm shift to an EBP culture does not happen overnight; it typically takes years as well as consistent and persistent effort to build and sustain. Unfortunately, many leaders give up prematurely when they are not seeing the outcomes of their efforts materialize in the time frame that they believe they should occur. Therefore, having a mechanism for support and regular recognition within the organization for individuals who are facilitating this shift to an EBP paradigm is important.

EBP mentors are another key ingredient for the sustainability of EBP as first described in the ARCC model by Melnyk and Fineout-Overholt (2002; see Chapter 13 for a full description of ARCC). These healthcare professionals typically have (a) a master's degree; (b) in-depth knowledge and skills in EBP; and (c) knowledge and skills in individual, team, and organizational change strategies. EBP mentors work directly with point-of-care staff on shifting from a traditional paradigm to an EBP paradigm, which includes (a) assisting clinicians in gaining EBP knowledge and skills, (b) conducting EBP implementation projects, (c) integrating practice-generated data to improve healthcare quality as well as patient and/or system outcomes, and (d) measuring outcomes of EBP implementation (Melnyk, 2007). Findings from a study in the Visiting Nurse Service indicated that nurses who received mentorship from an ARCC EBP mentor, compared with those who received instruction in physical assessment (i.e., the attention control group), had higher EBP beliefs, greater EBP implementation, and less attrition/turnover. In addition, there was no significant difference between the ARCC and attention control groups on the outcome variable of nurses' productivity, indicating that nurse involvement in learning about how to integrate EBP into their daily practice along with implementing an EBP project during work time did not affect the number of home visits made by the nurses (Levin, Fineout-Overholt, Melnyk, Barnes, & Vetter, 2011). In other studies, mentors or EBP facilitators have been noted as critical for advancing EBP (Dogherty, Harrison, Graham, Vandyk, & Keeping-Burke, 2013; Melnyk & Fineout-Overholt, 2002). For further evidence on the outcomes of mentoring and additional information on the specific role of the EBP mentor, see Chapter 17.

Preventing Fatigue

The barrier of fatigue typically presents itself when the implementation phase of a project is exceedingly long. An excellent strategy for preventing and/or decreasing fatigue in a system is to create small successes along the course of the change project and to recognize (reward) individuals for their efforts. Recognition and appreciation are very important in demonstrating the value of individuals' efforts and sustaining enthusiasm along the course of a project.

The road to implementing a change to EBP will be challenging but extremely rewarding. Essential elements for success include a clear shared vision, strong leadership, and a well-defined written strategic plan as well as knowledge and skills regarding the process of organizational change, team building, and working with individuals who possess different personality styles. Lastly, an ability to persist through the multiple challenges that will be confronted along the course of an organization's change will be essential for success.

....
Never, never, never, never, never, never, never quit!
—Winston Churchill
....

EBP FAST FACTS

◆ The first step in creating a change to EBP is to create an exciting team vision of what is to be accomplished and belief that it can be accomplished.
◆ A well-formulated strategic plan is necessary with strategies to overcome potential barriers.
◆ Vision without execution in the form of action will not result in the desired outcomes.
◆ Knowing the stages of change and what to expect in each will enhance the chances of success.
◆ An organizational culture and environment in addition to EBP mentors are necessary to sustain the change to EBP.
◆ Persistence through the character-builders is necessary for success, so do not give up!

References

Beck, A., Rush, A., Shaw, B., & Emery, G. (1979). *Cognitive therapy of depression*. New York: The Guilford Press.
Carver, S., & Scheier, M. F. (1998). *On the self-regulation of behavior*. Cambridge, England: Cambridge University Press.
Corey, M. S., & Corey, G. (2002). *Groups: Process and practice* (6th ed.). Pacific Grove, CA: Brooks/Cole.
Dogherty, E., Harrison, M. B., Graham, I. D., Vandyk, A. D., & Keeping-Burke, L. (2013). Turning knowledge into action at the point-of-care: The collective experience of nurses facilitating the implementation of evidence-based practice. *Worldviews on Evidence-based Nursing, 10*(3), 129–139.

Duck, J. D. (2002). *The change monster: The human forces that fuel or foil corporate transformation and change*. New York: Crown Business.

Greiner, A., & Knebel, E. (2003). *Health professions education: A bridge to quality*. Washington, DC: National Academy Press.

Hill, C. W. L., & Jones, G. R. (2001). *Strategic management*. New York: Houghton Mifflin.

Institute of Medicine. (2001). *Crossing the quality chasm: A new health system for the 21st century*. Washington, DC: National Academy Press.

Institute of Medicine (IOM). (2013). *Interprofessional education for collaboration: Learning how to improve health from interprofessional models across the continuum of education to practice: Workshop summary*. Washington, DC: The National Academies Press.

Kotter, J. P., & Cohen, D. S. (2012). *The heart of change: Real-life stories of how people change their organizations*. Boston, MA: Harvard Business School Press.

LaForge, R. G., Velicer, W. F., Richmond, R. L., & Owen, N. (1999). Stage distributions for five health behaviors in the USA and Australia. *Preventive Medicine, 28*, 61–74.

Lam, D. (2005). A brief overview of CBT techniques. In S. Freeman & A. Freeman (Eds.), *Cognitive behavior therapy in nursing practice* (pp. 29–47). New York: Springer Publishing Company.

Levin, R. F., Fineout-Overholt, E., Melnyk, B. M., Barnes, M., & Vetter, M. J. (2011). Fostering evidence-based practice to improve nurse and cost outcomes in a community health setting: A pilot test of the advancing research and clinical practice through close collaboration model. *Nursing Administration Quarterly, 35*(1), 21–33.

Lukas, C. V., Mohr, D. C., & Meterko, M. (2009). Team effectiveness and organizational context in the implementation of a clinical innovation. *Quality Management in Health Care, 18*(1), 25–39.

MacPhee, M. (2007). Strategies and tools for managing change. *Journal of Nursing Administration, 37*(9), 405–413.

McCormack, M. H. (1986). *What they don't teach you at Harvard Business School: Notes from a street smart executive*. New York: Bantam.

Melnyk, B. M. (2007). The evidence-based practice mentor: A promising strategy for implementing and sustaining EBP in healthcare systems [Editorial]. *Worldviews on Evidence-Based Nursing, 4*(3), 123–125.

Melnyk, B. M., & Fineout-Overholt, E. (2002). Putting research into practice, Rochester ARCC. *Reflections on Nursing Leadership, 28*(2), 22–25.

Melnyk, B. M., Fineout-Overholt, E., Feinstein, N. F., Li, H., Small, L., Wilcox, L., & Kraus, R. (2004). Nurses' perceived knowledge, beliefs, skills, and needs regarding evidence-based practice: Implications for accelerating the paradigm shift. *Worldviews on Evidence-Based Nursing, 1*(3), 185–193.

Melnyk, B. M., Fineout-Overholt, E., Giggleman, M., & Cruz, R. (2010). Correlates among cognitive beliefs, EBP implementation, organizational culture, cohesion and job satisfaction in evidence-based practice mentors from a community hospital system. *Nursing Outlook, 58*(6), 301–308.

Melnyk, B. M., Grossman, D. C., Chou, R., Mabry-Hernandez, I., Nicholson, W., Dewitt, T. G., … US Preventive Services Task Force. (2012). USPSTF perspective on evidence-based preventive recommendations for children. *Pediatrics, 130*(2), e399–e407.

Melnyk, B. M., Jacobson, D., Kelly, S., Belyea, M., Shaibi, G., Small, L., … Marsiglia, F. F. (2013). Promoting healthy lifestyles in high school adolescents: A randomized controlled trial. *American Journal of Preventive Medicine, 45*(4), 408–416.

Melnyk, B. M., & Jensen, P. (2013). A practical *guide to child and adolescent mental health screening, early intervention and health promotion* (2nd ed.). New York: National Association of Pediatric Nurse Practitioners.

Melnyk, B. M., Small, L., Morrison-Beedy, D., Strasser, A., Spath, L., Kreipe, R., … Van Blankenstein, S. (2006). Mental health correlates of healthy lifestyle attitudes, beliefs, choices & behaviors in overweight teens. *Journal of Pediatric Health Care, 20*(6), 401–406.

Ogiehor-Enoma, G., Taqueban, L., & Anosike, A. (2010). 6 steps for transforming organizational culture. *Evidence-Based Nursing, 41*(5), 14–17.

Prochaska, J. M., Prochaska, J. O., & Levesque, D. A. (2001). A transtheoretical approach to changing organizations. *Administration and Policy in Mental Health, 28*(4), 247–261.

Prochaska, J. O., & Velicer, W. F. (1997). The transtheoretical model of health behavior change. *American Journal of Health Promotion, 12*(1), 38–48.

Roger, E. (1995). *Diffusion of Innovations* (4th ed.). New York, NY: The Free Press.

Rogers, E. M. (2003). *Diffusion of innovations* (5th ed.). New York: Free Press.

Rohm, R. A., & Carey, E. C. (1997). *Who do you think you are … anyway? How your personality style acts … reacts … and interacts with others*. Atlanta, GA: Personality Insights.

Rycroft-Malone, J., Harvey, G., Seers, K., Kitson, A., McCormack, B., & Titchen, A. (2004). An exploration of the factors that influence the implementation of evidence into practice. *Journal of Clinical Nursing, 13*, 913–924.

Torres, C., & Fairbanks, D. (1996). *Teambuilding: The ASTD trainer's sourcebook*. New York: McGraw-Hill.

Chapter 15

Teaching Evidence-Based Practice in Academic Settings

Ellen Fineout-Overholt, Susan B. Stillwell, Kathleen M. Williamson, John F. Cox III, and Brett W. Robbins

The meaning of 'knowing' has shifted from being able to remember and repeat information to being able to find and use it.

—National Research Council, 2007

Evidence-based practice (EBP) is an imperative in health care and continues to rapidly replace the traditional paradigm of authority in healthcare decision making (Porter-O'Grady & Malloch, 2012). Although making this transition for learners, students, or practitioners can sometimes be challenging, accrediting bodies, healthcare professionals, policy makers, and payers have determined that EBP is essential to providing effective patient care (American Association of Colleges of Nursing [AACN], 2008, American Nurses Credentialing Center, 2014; Centers for Medicare & Medicaid Services, 2014; Joint Commission, 2013). Early in the 21st century, the Institute of Medicine (IOM) set forth a vision that all healthcare professionals would be educated to practice patient-centered care as members of an interdisciplinary team, who, utilizing quality improvement approaches and **informatics,** would base their decision making on valid, reliable evidence (Greiner & Knebel, 2003; IOM, 1999, 2001, 2002). The core competencies for healthcare education to meet the needs of the healthcare system in this century were identified as

- ◆ **Provide patient-centered care**
- ◆ **Work in interdisciplinary teams**
- ◆ **Employ EBP**
- ◆ **Apply quality improvement**
- ◆ **Utilize informatics (Greiner & Knebel, p. 46)**

The Health Professions Educational Summit recommended that everyone involved in education address these competencies from an oversight perspective, in essence from leadership downward. Professional organizations and accrediting bodies have used these competencies as standards for criteria that define successful curricula for academic programs (AACN, 2006, 2008; Association of American Medical Colleges, 2007). Accordingly, to meet the expectations of today's healthcare organizations, clinicians need knowledge, skills, and language that enables them to look past the traditional focus of the conduct of research to the use of this important resource in practice (Ciliska, 2005). Twenty-first-century practitioners are expected to bring the best and latest evidence to bear on their decision making with patients. As such, the primary role of 21st century health professions faculty is to teach learners about how to think like evidence-based clinicians, using language that incorporates into daily practice the appraisal and application of research and practice-based data (i.e., data generated from clinical practice). These faculty will assist learners to shift their primary focus from clinical tasks to a life-long approach of mastery of knowledge and skills for improving outcomes for patients, providers, and systems. Evidence synthesis skills will be valued and required for learners to be up-to-date on current treatments and care modalities. Learners lay the foundation to practicing based on evidence as they embrace inquiry and an in-depth way of thinking and doing in the classroom and associated clinical practica that incorporates valid scientific and theoretical evidence; their own expertise and practice-based data; and their patients' choices, concerns, and values when making clinical decisions to achieve best outcomes (i.e., EBP). This chapter provides a framework designed to assist faculty reflect on how they can integrate EBP into exist-ing curricula. Each aspect of the framework is discussed with suggestions for actualizing the framework in readers' educational organizations.

A CONCEPTUAL FRAMEWORK FOR EVIDENCE-BASED EDUCATORS

To facilitate meeting learners' needs for understanding daily decision making based on the EBP para-digm, educators in academic settings need a framework that can assist them in strategically crafting their approach to achieve evidence-based educational outcomes. The first recommendation is to begin with the end in mind. Consider the program outcomes you desire in your graduates as well as the identified milestones along the way. How do your organization culture, faculty colleagues, and your own teach-ing approach help you to achieve these important results? It is important to understand the educational institution's culture and evaluate whether or not there are sufficient supports for integrating EBP into curricula. For example, do educators have sufficient financial resources to build a foundation of knowl-edge and skills that they can share as they integrate EBP into their courses and other endeavors?

Building a Culture and Support of EBP

Simply having knowledge and/or skills in EBP does not necessarily ensure their use; however, research-ers have repeatedly demonstrated that those with knowledge and *beliefs* in EBP were more likely to share their knowledge with their colleagues (Melnyk et al., 2004; Melnyk, Fineout-Overholt, Giggleman, & Cruz, 2010; Wallen et al., 2010). Building beliefs is therefore imperative for evidence-based educators. Part of building beliefs is diffusely integrating the EBP paradigm and principles across curricula, both in clinical or in academic settings. This in-depth thinking lays the foundation for integration of EBP in daily decisions. Without the EBP paradigm and process along with diffuse integration, there may be a perceived "disconnect" by learners between the paradigm and process and their practice. Learners may view EBP as academic and unrelated to clinical skills they are learning. Furthermore, the EBP paradigm and process must be valued by faculty. For example, faculty must make no distinction regarding the rigor of the courses in which EBP principles and concepts are foundationally taught and other courses with more clinical content. In some cases, faculty may have agreed to an unwritten commitment that students will not fail foundational EBP courses. This sends the message to other faculty and to students that these courses and their content are "less than" clinical courses, such as medical/surgical courses. Rather, EBP principles and concepts must be the foundation of *every* course in the curriculum. Once foundational principles are learned, each course reinforces evidence-based decision making, including use of lan-guage, the EBP process, and evaluation of outcomes. Clinical skills are learned within the context of the EBP paradigm, which focuses on achieving an outcome versus simply mastering a skill.

More broadly, for learners to grasp the need for integrating EBP principles, their relevance must be evi-dent and the culture must be imbued with EBP. The product of our educational endeavors must be learners who have fully engaged the paradigm shift and foster a culture and mindset underpinned by EBP principles. Furthermore, educators need to be mentored to set their own evaluation goals and be encouraged to take time to self-reflect on the extent to which they are meeting them. As an initial step, it is helpful to consider how the organization as a whole embraces integration of EBP across its decision making and curricula. The process for curricula-wide integration is graphically represented in Figure 15.1, the EBP model for educators entitled, Advancing Research and Clinical Practice through Close Collaboration in Education (ARCC-E) (Fineout-Overholt & Melnyk, 2011). This model will provide the structure for the following chapter sections.

....

Without change there is no innovation, creativity, or incentive for improvement. Those who initiate change will have a better opportunity to manage the change that is inevitable.
—William Pollard

....

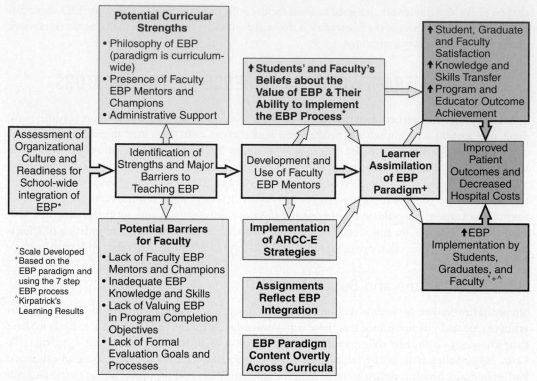

Figure 15.1: Advancing Research, Education and Clinical Practice through Close Collaboration & Education (ARCC-E) copyright Fineout-Overholt & Melnyk, 2011.

ASSESSMENT OF ORGANIZATIONAL CULTURE

The first step in establishing a successful program for teaching EBP, be it large or small, is to assess the organization and its capacity for moving toward school-wide integration of EBP into its curriculum and culture. This includes, among other concerns, the institutional support, resources allotted, and the commitment and engagement in EBP by the educators and learners. Palaima (2010) discovered that organizational factors influenced learners' roles in the organization as well as their use of EBP. Furthermore, learners who practice EBP positively influence the organizational culture. These findings emphasize the importance of conducting an organization assessment prior to any intervention. The assessment questions in this chapter are drawn from EBP scales that were developed to assist in assessment of organizations' efforts to embrace EBP as the foundation of their educational efforts (Fineout-Overholt & Melnyk, 2005; Fineout-Overholt & Melnyk, 2010a, 2010b, 2011; Melnyk & Fineout-Overholt, 2003a, 2003b, see Appendix K). The Organizational Culture and Readiness for School-Wide Integration of EBP (OCRSIEP-E) (Fineout-Overholt & Melnyk, 2011) was specifically developed to provide the initial assessment of this important paradigm shift in education. OCRSIEP-E has been used reliably across multiple educational settings with reliability coefficients of >.80. The sections that follow discuss what is necessary for an educational organization to demonstrate a culture of EBP.

Institutional Support for Evidence-Based Practice

For school-wide integration of EBP, it is essential for EBP language and intent to be present in the philosophy and mission of the organization. For example, the words evidence, synthesis, outcomes, and dissemination should be considered where appropriate. In addition, there are some underlying questions to help determine the extent to which EBP is a basic tenet of an organization (Box 15.1). If the philosophy

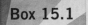

Box 15.1   Questions for Evaluating the Environmental Readiness for Teaching Evidence-Based Practice Successfully

1. Does the philosophy and mission of my institution support EBP?
2. What is the personal commitment to EBP and practice excellence among educators and administration?
3. Are there educators who have EBP knowledge and skills?
4. Do all educators have basic computer skills?
5. Do all students and educators have ready access to quality computers (e.g., that will support Internet access)?
6. Do educators have skills in using databases to find relevant evidence?
7. Are there librarians who have EBP knowledge and skills and who can be involved in teaching EBP?

Adapted from Fineout-Overholt, OCRSIEP-E Scale, 2011.

or culture is less than supportive of EBP (i.e., fully integrated into all curricula and culture), primary efforts may need to focus on demonstrating to the organization the effectiveness of EBP through the success of small initiatives by the committed champions of EBP (e.g., demonstration that courses are taught from an EBP paradigm, including small changes such as changing simple language of assignments to include EBP language [change "what is the rationale" to "what is the evidence"]).

The goals and objectives of an educational organization need to be congruent with a mission to produce evidence-based practitioners. Evaluation of the role of varied goals and competing agendas needs to be conducted to assist faculty with integration of EBP concepts fully across the curricula. The first step toward building an evidence-based curriculum is to obtain buy-in and support from all levels of administration. From this support will flow other necessary resources for a successful EBP program, such as committed, qualified personnel; continuing education; evidence databases; and computers. Another evaluation of buy-in is assessment of the resources available that are or could be dedicated to EBP. Asking further important questions can assist in evaluating the support for EBP that can assist you in getting started (Box 15.2).

Commitment of Educators and Administrators

Demonstrated commitment to the EBP paradigm and process among educators and administrators that results in practice excellence is imperative for EBP to be fully integrated across academic curricula. One way to ascertain whether educators are committed to EBP is to observe their educational practices (e.g., observe whether they teach based on evidence or on tradition [i.e., "we have always done it that way"]; observe how they integrate current scientific and practice-based evidence into their teaching). Other facets of evaluating this commitment may involve what educators read, how they seek to enhance their database-searching skills, their receptivity to discussing supporting evidence for decision making, their willingness to discuss EBP, and their involvement in EBP initiatives. Because commitment is not a tangible outcome, this can be a challenging requirement to demonstrate; however, it is no less important that the latest technological resources, such as computers and databases. According to change theorists (Duck, 2002), it may be wise advice to invite those who are the biggest resisters to assist you in advancing the change, as this may facilitate movement toward a unified commitment among faculty to foster learning through the EBP paradigm. Purposefully engaging those who are not committed to EBP may be what it takes for them to join in the journey toward integration of EBP into the curriculum.

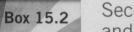

Box 15.2 Secondary Questions: Does the Philosophy and Mission of My Institution Support Evidence-Based Practice?

1. How is EBP taught in my organization, throughout all mediums (e.g., inservices, formal classroom offerings, one-on-one mentoring)?
2. Is it a goal of the institution or practice to promote EBP?
3. If so, how is this mission "lived out" in the atmosphere/curriculum of the institution or practice?
4. Are there champions for EBP at my institution? If so, how would I describe them (having responsibility and authority)?
5. What kind of physical resources are available to practitioners, educators, and students to support reaching EBP goals?
6. What incentives are in place for practitioners and educators to incorporate EBP into practice, curriculum, and courses for which they are responsible?
7. What are the EBP assignments throughout the educational objectives or curriculum that evaluate the integration of EBP concepts?

Adapted from Fineout-Overholt, OCRSIEP-E Scale, 2011.

Unfortunately, lack of commitment to EBP by educators or administrators is not easily remedied. However, persistent exposure of administrators, faculty, and learners to the benefits of EBP and how it improves outcomes in education and practice will hopefully reap the naysayers involvement in building the foundation needed to move EBP forward in academic organizations.

Qualities of Evidence-Based Educators and Learners

Champions for EBP are committed to excellent patient care, whether they are an educator or learner. These individuals continually strive for excellence and want to understand their students' or patients' problems thoroughly and apply the current best evidence appropriately to all aspects of work—they are evidence based. Box 15.3 lists the essential qualities that characterize evidence-based educators and learners. Desiring excellence in patient care is foundational. To foster clinicians who seek after relevant information to address patient issues strive for the highest quality of care requires those who teach EBP to be committed to excellence in education.

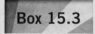

Box 15.3 Qualities for Evidence-Based Practice Teachers and Learners

Commitment to:
1. Excellent patient care
2. Excellent clinical skills
3. Excellent clinical judgment
4. Diligence
5. Perspective

Excellent Clinical Skills. Excellent clinical skills in patient interviewing and physical examination are needed for clinicians to accurately understand the clinical problem, the patient's unique situation and values, and the evidence-based management options related to the identified problem. In addition, excellent communication skills are essential so that practitioners and teachers of EBP can clearly explain to patients and learners the risks and benefits of the available options and evidence-based recommendations.

Excellent Clinical Judgment. Excellent clinical judgment is of paramount importance because it is the skill that enables practitioners to weigh the risks and benefits targeted by the available research evidence in light of the patient's values and preferences. Time and experience are essential elements to developing clinical judgment. Teachers will be expected to have highly developed clinical judgment, whereas early learners will grow in this quality.

Diligence. Diligence is another desirable teacher and learner quality. Teachers and learners of EBP must be consistently willing to work hard, to search the ever-expanding array of available healthcare information resources to find the best evidence for a given clinical question, and to return to the clinical scenario and apply the evidence appropriately. Diligence is needed to communicate and hone the other essential skills of interviewing, physical examination, clinical reasoning, and judgment.

Perspective. Perspective rounds out the essential characteristics for an EBP teaching/learning culture. Perspective allows for incorporating newly appraised evidence appropriately into a greater body of healthcare knowledge and accepted practice, with a particular focus on integration with student/patient preference. Gaining perspective comes from the extensive study required to become proficient in the practice of healthcare and requires tolerance of uncertainty. If a teacher or learner has an "all-or-nothing" attitude, evidence is usually categorized as either good or bad, and this is seldom beneficial to the student or patient. Most of the evidence that exists today is in the in-between category, neither perfectly valid nor worthy of rejection. The more mature perspective of educators will cultivate openness to uncertainty that will benefit learners.

Teacher efforts to cultivate desirable learner qualities must be tailored to the learner's proficiency in the steps of the EBP process. For example, learners without much experience asking questions about their patients should be encouraged to start asking questions, then coached to refine those questions into more searchable, answerable questions. In the process, learners will start to see the benefit of walking through the stages of the EBP process and that careful formulation of the question leads to a more fruitful search for information. Only after learners have developed some proficiency in asking the searchable, answerable question does it make sense to focus teaching efforts on improving searching efficiency.

In the early stages, learners typically are excited about finding out information relevant to their patients in clinical practicums. These early learners may use textbooks to answer most of their questions. This is appropriate because many questions of early learners are background questions (i.e., those questions that ask for general information about a clinical issue). As learners gain knowledge and experience in asking pertinent questions about their patients' care, questions shift from background questions answered by a textbook to foreground questions that require more up-to-date information to answer them. Chapter 2 has an excellent discussion of foreground and background questions. Determining which type of question the learner is asking has implications for how the teacher directs the learning.

For various reasons, early learners may often neglect to report the source of their information for their clinical decision. It is necessary for teachers of EBP to prompt learners explicitly to provide their rationale for their choice of information resources used in clinical decision making. Furthermore, teachers who are at this early stage need to query their learners consistently about which resources they used to find their information and their opinion of the validity of the information they found, as well as the ease of use—or lack thereof—of the resource. Such discussion is useful for all involved because those resources that are updated regularly; are easy to search; and provide clear, evidence-based recommendations are likely to emerge as the favorites.

This discussion sets the stage for the expectation that learners will critically appraise primary articles from the literature when they progress to the point that they are using the research evidence for the purpose of answering their own questions versus performing an academic exercise. This is a shift from traditional education where learners simply received information passively. In EBP, learners must actively formulate clinical questions, search out evidence to answer them, determine the validity of the evidence, and decide how to use it in practice (Fineout-Overholt & Johnston, 2007).

SHIFT IN EDUCATIONAL PARADIGM: FROM TRADITIONAL TO EVIDENCE-BASED PRACTICE

Traditional research education focuses on preparing research generators (i.e., learning to design studies and generate hypotheses) or critiquing research for strengths and weaknesses. EBP education focuses on preparing the learner to be an **evidence user**. The learner is taught to think of issues in the clinical area in a systematic fashion and to formulate questions around the issues in a searchable, answerable way. Teaching learners to find evidence quickly that can answer their clinical questions and critically appraise it, not only for strengths and weaknesses (validity) but also for applicability to the given patient situation, is integral to EBP education. This decision cannot be made solely on the scientific evidence itself but must include consideration of the patient's values and preferences, as well as the clinician's expertise, which incorporates internal evidence. If the scientific evidence is useful to the practitioner, the next step in learning is to understand how to apply the evidence and evaluate the outcomes of the intervention. Assisting learners to understand how the EBP process flows is essential to success in teaching EBP concepts. There are many models for implementing EBP, all of which could be discussed here (see Chapter 11 for more information). However, the EBP paradigm and the ACE Star Model were selected to demonstrate the ease of learning when approached from the perspective of the EBP process.

The Evidence-Based Practice Paradigm

To understand the EBP paradigm, faculty must understand what is considered evidence. In this book, evidence has been described as internal evidence (i.e., practice-generated evidence) and external evidence (i.e., research). When using evidence (i.e., external and internal) for decision making along with patient preferences and clinician expertise, faculty and students must realize that a new responsibility comes with this broadened EBP scope: life-long problem solving that integrates (a) a systematic search for, critical appraisal, and synthesis of the most relevant and best research (i.e., external evidence) to answer a clinical question; (b) clinicians expertise, which includes abilities to interpret information generated from practice (i.e., internal evidence), from patient assessment, and from the evaluation and subsequent careful use of resources available to improved outcomes; and (c) the values and preferences of patients (see Chapter 1, Figure 1.2).

In the EBP paradigm, how the three EBP components will meld together when making a clinical decision is dependent on each patient–clinician interaction. Students practicing from this paradigm have a better sense of why they are learning about Foley catheter insertion or turning every 2 hours. The variability of the weight of each component is directly related to the characteristics of the clinician–patient clinical encounter. Clinical expertise involves how clinicians integrate knowledge of research and what they know about their work and population, as well as what they know about their patients' preferences. The best clinical decisions come when all of these are present and contributing factors in the decision-making process. Patient preferences are not uninformed preferences. When patients are not informed, clinicians have the responsibility to provide needed information in a manner that the patient can appreciate. Once informed, patients determine how they choose to proceed with the decision. For example, evidence from research might support the efficacy of one naturopathic supplement over another in treating gastrointestinal irritation. However, if the patient is likely to experience financial hardship from the preferred supplement because it is so expensive and will likely refuse to take it, and if there is another supplement with similar efficacy, the clinician has a responsibility to discuss these options with the patient. The patient can then decide which supplement works best for him or her. In this case, patient preference will outweigh the evidence from research and perhaps from clinical expertise and the healthcare provider and the patient will choose an alternative supplement with similar efficacy and tolerable financial burden that will achieve the outcome of resolving the gastrointestinal irritation. This is an important foundational paradigm for students and faculty to understand and practice for the EBP process and models of EBP to make sense. Otherwise, these processes and models simply become following steps. The bottom line for educators is to help students grasp why they are learning and what outcome they are striving to achieve. This clarity helps students put their energies into learning to improve outcomes versus studying to pass a test or procedural check-off.

Knowledge of Evidence-Based Practice

When engaging ideas about how to teach EBP to health professions students, a colleague once remarked, "We cannot teach what we do not know" (Dave Hrabe, personal communication 2005). An evidence-based academic organization needs to have educators who have considerable comfort with EBP knowledge and skills. Knowledge of the EBP paradigm and use of the EBP processes is the first human resource to evaluate. For example, do educators construct their educational learning experiences based on the EBP paradigm framework? Do they know how to construct a searchable, answerable clinical question? Can they distinguish clinical from research questions? Can they communicate how to search for relevant evidence? Do they know how to critically appraise (i.e., rapidly critically appraise, evaluate and synthesize) all levels of evidence? Can they apply the evidence to a clinical situation? Can they efficiently guide learners in evaluating outcomes? After it has been determined how much educators are prepared to teach about EBP, the challenge becomes gaining the information needed to close the gaps in knowledge and skills.

A caveat is warranted here in that sometimes faculty may exhibit a high commitment to teaching EBP but may not be able to discern the gaps in their knowledge. In a survey of nurse practitioner faculty, Melnyk, Fineout-Overholt, Feinstein, Sadler, and Green-Hernandez (2008) found that of the sample of 79 graduate educators, 97% indicated they taught EBP in their curricula; however, the top-cited teaching strategy was supporting clinical practice with a single study. The EBP paradigm focuses on what we know (i.e., a body of evidence) versus basing practices on a single study. These findings allude to faculty's commitment to teaching EBP and identify gaps in their knowledge of the EBP paradigm and what teaching EBP requires (Melnyk et al., 2008). Furthermore, Stichler et al. (2011) found that faculty's traditional research knowledge did not necessarily translate to support of EBP, thus faculty knowledge of EBP must be assessed and educational sessions on how to teach EBP may be warranted.

Gaining Knowledge

There are numerous mechanisms available to assist educators in gaining EBP knowledge and skills. There are workshops around the country that present basic and advanced EBP concepts, as well as online tutorials that can be accessed easily at one's convenience to learn about EBP (see Boxes 16.1 and 16.2 for sample listings).

Of course, there are many articles about the basic knowledge of EBP, including the widely used EBP Step-by-Step Series in the *American Journal of Nursing* by Fineout-Overholt and Colleagues (2010–2012), the *Users' Guides to Evidence-Based Practice* (http://www.cche.net/usersguides/main.asp), the *Tips for Teaching EBP* series (e.g., Kennedy et al., 2008; McGinn et al., 2008; Prasad, Jaeschke, Wyer, Keitz, Guyatt, & Evidence-Based Medicine Teaching Tips Working Group, 2008; Richardson, Wilson, Keitz, Weyer, & EBM Teaching Scripts Working Group, 2008; Williams & Hoffman, 2008), and the *Worldviews on Evidence-Based Nursing* journal's most recent recurring column *Tactics for Teaching EBP*, along with the prior *Teaching EBP* column (e.g., Fineout-Overholt & Johnston, 2005; Johnston & Fineout-Overholt, 2005; Kent & Fineout-Overholt, 2007; O'Mathuna, Fineout-Overholt, & Kent, 2008). After determining the level of EBP knowledge of the key people in your institution, consider whether the workloads of those individuals can accommodate a new endeavor. Administrative involvement is essential to this preliminary evaluation step. Organization support, resources, and time have been identified as barriers to teaching EBP (Stichler et al., 2011). Without administrative support of an endeavor to initiate EBP, success will be difficult to achieve (Fineout-Overholt & Melnyk, 2005; Melnyk, Fineout-Overholt, Gallagher-Ford, & Kaplan, 2012).

Informatics and Computer Literacy among Educators

Determining the basic informatics and computer literacy of educators is an important step in building the foundation for teaching EBP. Without educators who are knowledgeable in informatics, including adequate computer skills and the ability to use databases to find relevant evidence, teaching EBP will be challenging. While technology to enhance teaching EBP is important, before any technology can be considered basic skills in informatics must be assessed.

When determining the fiscal resources for teaching EBP, funding for computers is an essential budget item. Foundationally, updated, fast computers with Internet access are a must for educators and learners who will be learning about EBP. Administrators will need to commit to onsite computer access for all students, clinicians, and educators as well as remote access to data bases (e.g., from home). In addition, a commitment by administrators is essential to ensure that all learners and teachers are computer literate at a basic level.

Availability of Medical Librarians

A medical/health science librarian who is knowledgeable about EBP is an invaluable resource on the EBP teaching team. It is imperative that these librarians be involved in the plan to initiate EBP. They can provide perspective and expertise in searching databases as well as facilitate aspects of information literacy needed by students and faculty who strive to successfully teach and learn about EBP. Medical librarians are indispensable to the EBP process and are excellent resources for helping both learners and teachers accomplish the goal of informatics and computer literacy. Often librarians can offer classes on computer basics and database searching techniques, among other helpful topics.

 Online tutorials about basic computer function (e.g., **http://tech.tln.lib.mi.us/tutor/**) are also helpful resources.

> "Tell me and I will forget.
> Show me and I will remember.
> Involve me and I will understand.
> Step back and I will act."
>
> *Old Chinese Proverb*

ARCC-E STRATEGIES FOR TEACHING/ENHANCING EBP IN ACADEMIC SETTINGS

Once the organizational culture and context is evaluated, it is important to introduce the best strategies to enhance the ability for educators to teach EBP as well as integrate it across the curricula. These strategies include securing the necessary human, fiscal, and technological resources. Human resources can include EBP champions and evidence-based librarians who have knowledge of EBP and time to accomplish the goal. Fiscal resources include committed funds for ongoing development of the teaching program to educate the educators and for purchasing the best technology available for enhancing the program and easing the workload of faculty. Technological resources are vast and always changing. Considering how to best use them to enhance EBP is an imperative.

According to a systematic review conducted by Coomarasamy and Khan (2004), knowledge, skills, attitude, and behavior were improved with the clinical integration of EBP; however, stand-alone EBP courses only improved knowledge. Thus, EBP must be incorporated across all settings in healthcare education, to parallel learners' daily experiences (e.g., ambulatory care and inpatient experiences, direct patient care, patient rounds, change-of-shift meetings, and unit-to-unit report when a patient is being transferred).

Teaching EBP should not be restricted to one instructor or to a stand-alone course (e.g., academic or clinical course). Rather, it should be woven into the fabric of academic programs' overall curricula in such a fashion that it becomes part of the culture. Learners need to see EBP used and have the opportunity to learn in every setting to which they are exposed. This ever-present implementation and learning of EBP concepts serves to model for the learners that EBP is not only an academic exercise but also is actively used in clinical practice.

Human Resources

Multilevel support for integration of EBP into curricula is imperative. Administrators, educators, librarians, and learners are key stakeholders in this initiative. Administrators, for the purposes of this chapter, are defined as anyone who provides fiscal and managerial support to an EBP program (e.g., university presidents, vice presidents for academic affairs, academic deans, residency directors, department chairs, chief financial officers, chief executive officers). Administrators must include designated fiscal resources for EBP in their strategic plans and prospective budgets (e.g., for ongoing education, technology, evidence databases, librarian involvement, and recognition of experts' time in training and compensation). Strategic planning must reflect the integration of EBP. Actualization of cultural expectations for integration of EBP should be present in the annual performance appraisal criteria as well as promotion and tenure guidelines. Careful consideration of a proposal outlining the integration of EBP throughout the curricula and the potential benefits and costs will assist in obtaining support from administration.

Involve the Librarian Early

In preparing for integration of EBP across the curriculum, early involvement of the librarian is crucial. It is an evidence-based medical/health sciences librarian's job to be proficient in knowing where and how to get information. Librarians' knowledge of databases, informatics resources, and information retrieval is integral to successful EBP teaching programs. Librarians can assist educators in developing database and Internet searching skills as a means of finding relevant evidence to answer clinical questions. In addition, librarians can set up direct search mechanisms in which the faculty or students pose their PICOT question electronically, the librarian then scours the databases for the answer and sends at minimum the citations and abstracts for the body of evidence to the inquirer. If the articles are available full text, the librarian is responsible for sending them along to the clinician. This approach to evidence retrieval can save enormous amounts of time and use some of the many talents of medical/health sciences librarians well.

Develop and Cultivate EBP Champions

Educators support teaching EBP by being knowledgeable and skilled in EBP and able to meaningfully articulate the concepts to the students. A preliminary investment is required to ensure that educators teaching EBP have the necessary expertise for meaningful and successful delivery and role modeling of EBP concepts. For example, assigning faculty to teach a fundamental critical appraisal methods course when their primary focus is generating evidence and they are novices at using evidence in practice is likely to be frustrating to the faculty member and students. Helping the faculty to become more proficient in understanding the EBP paradigm and how it blends with their research paradigm can facilitate their transition from frustration to being a champion of EBP. Despite faculty having a positive attitude about EBP, they may not rate their EBP knowledge and skills positively (Stichler et al., 2011) Educators need to be familiar with the concepts of EBP to be able to assist students in determining whether observed practice is built on solid evidence or solely on tradition. Educators role modeling EBP concepts (e.g., addressing a student question at the time it is asked with a search of the literature and a discussion of findings and outcomes) can assist learners to integrate EBP concepts into their own practice paradigms.

Additional champions required for successful communication of EBP concepts are the learners themselves. There are always different levels of learners. Those who quickly absorb the concepts of EBP can become champions who assist other learners in integrating EBP principles into their practices. Integration of EBP concepts into one's practice is essential for learners to both see and do. Without learner champions, educating other learners will be less successful. Often in venues such as journal clubs, the learners are the ones who create an environment that encourages the less-than-enthusiastic learner to join in the process. Using ideas such as learning EBP can be analogous to making a quilt may help learners to see the EBP process as wholly integrated. Educators, clinical preceptors, and other learners using EBP concepts are the "patches" in the quilt. When learners see EBP concepts integrated by these patches, there is implied agreement among faculty that integration of EBP is a valued tenet for education. Furthermore, the EBP paradigm and process take on perspective and purpose, much as patches put together make a pattern that can be seen only in the completed quilt. Without faculty and learner champions, broad valuing of the EBP paradigm and process, and implementation of EBP into educational practices (Fineout-Overholt & Melnyk et al., 2010a, 2010b), school-wide integration of EBP is unlikely.

Technological Resources

Technical resources are an imperative for educators as they develop curricula using multiple instructional technologies to provide varied learning opportunities for students to improve their information literacy skills required to engage the 21st-century workplace (Stephens-Lee, Lu, & Wilson, 2013). Furthermore, these skills are required to effectively and efficiently access resources to answer clinical questions (Melnyk et al., 2012; Pravikoff, Pierce, & Tanner, 2005; Schutt & Hightower, 2009). According to the AACN, technology affords an increased collaboration among faculties in teaching, practice, and research. In addition, technology in education may enhance the professional ability to educate clinicians for practice, prepare future healthcare educators, and advance professional science (AACN, 2000, 2008).

The Summit on Health Professions Education (Greiner & Knebel, 2003) identified the use of informatics as one of the core competencies for the 21st-century health education. Through the use of informatics, medical errors can be avoided as students learn in a safe environment from experiences enhanced by technology such as simulation, thereby, making mistakes without the harm to the patient (IOM, 1999, 2001). In the IOM report, *Educating Health Professionals to Use Informatics* (2002), informatics is described as an enabler that may enhance patient-centered care and safety, making possible EBP, continuous improvement in quality of care, and support for interdisciplinary teams. When teaching organizations assume a leadership role in enhancing learning with technology, clinical organizations also benefit (IOM, 2001). To bring these transformative, foundational goals to fruition, organizations such as the American Medical Informatics Association (AMIA, 2013) offers virtual courses to help healthcare professionals gain knowledge and skill above their clinical education to ensure proper guidance and use of technology in health care.

Information technology (IT) provides students and faculty access to evidence-based resources that are necessary for learning about evidenced-based care (Technology Informatics Guiding Education Reform [TIGER], 2007). Through IT support students can collect practice-based evidence (e.g., quality improvement data), combined with external evidence (i.e., research) to make evidence-based decisions at the bedside in their clinical practica (Hinton-Walker, 2010; TIGER Summit Report, 2007). Curricula require an infusion of innovation, including technology, to sustainably reform nursing curricula that will prepare healthcare providers of the future (National League of Nursing [NLN], 2008). All educational programs for all levels of healthcare providers should design evidence-based curricula that are flexible, responsive to students' needs, collaborative, and technology savvy (NLN).

Opportunities abound to infuse technology into the curriculum. Although students use technologies in their everyday lives, they can sometimes revert backward when in the educational milieu, preferring a less technical approach to education. Therefore, many instructional technologies should be included in curriculum planning and delivery, including (a) simulation technology; (b) mobile devices; (c) Internet-accessed social networking sites, such as Facebook, Twitter, and Second Life; (d) course management systems, such as Blackboard™ and Moodle™ that provide distance learning through web-enhanced and online courses; (e) audio and video conferencing through Internet-based programs such as WebEx, Adobe® Acrobat® Connect™ Pro, Zoom™ and Skype™; and (f) clinical decision support systems (CDSSs), such as SimChart, Cerner and PowerChart®.

Simulation, mobile devices, electronic health records (EHRs), and the Internet to access social networking sites via the World Wide Web are expected to be the most used and important technologies in healthcare and healthcare education. These products have the potential of enabling students to access data and information for point-of-care decision making and support healthcare practitioners with work flow, continuing education, collaboration, and access to EBP resources. Innovative technologies are being developed and applied daily to enhance patient care delivery and provider productivity.

Implementing a curriculum that integrates EBP through incorporating technology provides faculty creative avenues for innovation and offers multiple opportunities to increase students' information literacy skills (Schutt & Hightower, 2009). Bloom's taxonomy and Society of College, National and University Seven Pillars of Information Literacy can be helpful to developing students' information literacy skills (Springer, 2010) Educational agencies are on the cutting edge of developing collaborative learning communities with active use of technology to move toward knowledge development, dissemination, and implementation of EBPs (Hinton-Walker, 2010; TIGER, 2009). In addition, technologies need to be people-centered, affordable, useable, universal, useful, and standards-based (TIGER). Healthcare educators have the opportunity to be creatively innovative as they integrate EBP and technology into curricula to give students the ability to practice in real-world settings through simulation, document care, and access to EBP resources.

With technology changing the landscape of education, there is concern over copyright and ensuring protection of intellectual property. For the purposes of this chapter, the U.S. copyright law indicates that a work may be used for the purpose of critique, scholarship, and for teaching, among other uses, which may be considered fair use (U.S. Copyright Law, section #107; see http://www.copyright.gov/title17/92chap1.html#107).

 Additional copyright information can be found at **http://www4.law.cornell.edu/uscode/17/.** Information about the Teach Act, including a checklist for use, can be found in the Teach Act Toolkit at **http://copyright.uncc.edu/copyright/TEACH**

One way of dealing with the copyright issue, which can sometimes be difficult and time consuming, is to use as teaching tools only links to full-text study reports. This places the responsibility on learners to obtain information straight from the source. The disadvantage to this practice is that there are many good teaching tools that are not provided as full text. Despite the challenges that come with electronic information, resources such as the Internet, electronic journals, and other computer databases are essential to a successful EBP teaching program.

There are many strategies that can assist in teaching EBP in academic settings. The key to all of them is to keep it simple. Focusing on the EBP paradigm and how it is being lived/exemplified in course documents and teaching will facilitate this simplicity. A common language and the steps of the EBP process are areas of course curricula that are readily incorporated into existing courses without a tremendous upheaval.

Curricular Resources

Introduce EBP Language into Every Course

The goal of integrating EBP into the curriculum is to do so without getting overwhelmed. A good place to begin is to review course syllabi and related course documents for the opportunity to use language that reflects EBP. For example, something as simple as changing the word "rationale" to "evidence" or "improve client care" to "improve client outcomes" can facilitate learning and shifting of paradigms for learners. These small steps reflect the EBP paradigm, and students and faculty will begin to speak the language.

Another simple step that can be taken is to review the current learning activities and course assignments and reframe them to reflect EBP. For example, in an undergraduate nursing program learning activities could be reviewed and altered, such as adding EBP-related criteria for the assignments. An example of changing evaluation methods is requiring students to develop aesthetic projects that represented their first nursing experience. Peer review of these projects can be important for both the learner and the evaluator. Often learners are asked to integrate EBP but are given a *Critique Form*—an old approach. Simply retitling it to *Appraisal Form* guides learners to reframe the activity and look for the value or worth of the project to clinical practice. This parallels critical appraisal of evidence, which is step 3 of the EBP process. In addition, questions such as "How did this project (either yours or your peers) help you understand the evidence-based practice process?" can be added to the appraisal form used by students to reflect on the EBP process. In this almost effortless way, existing assignments may become framed within the EBP paradigm, making doable the integration of EBP into courses.

Consider the best place to introduce the theoretical underpinnings of EBP and additional courses in which it can be integrated throughout the curriculum. An imperative approach for making EBP real for students is relevance—it must be important enough to them to integrate into their learning. Particularly, since new healthcare professional students may not have sufficient clinical reference points to make examples clear, using current exemplars of how they make decisions, such as purchasing iPods, automobiles, or flight tickets can make the connection.

Use the steps in the EBP process for problem solving across all courses. It is important for faculty to use the EBP process across courses as the chosen process for problem solving. When there are EBP abstainers (i.e., those who choose not to embrace and use the EBP process), students can get a mixed message about the importance of this paradigm for their learning and clinical decision making. When this occurs, it becomes something like, "that's the way that professor wants to do it, but I like this professor's approach that is not so challenging—let's do it this way." Fully embracing the EBP process as the problem-solving approach for the school will require that the resources listed above be present, and it will help ensure that students do not consider evidence-based decision making a course-specific rhetoric; rather, they will use the principles to make daily decisions with and for their patients.

Ask Clinical Questions

First, faculty must keep in mind that step 0 of the EBP process is fostering a spirit of inquiry. Once that step is achieved, students can focus on step 1, formulating clinical questions. Faculty may need to practice this skill before they feel confident teaching students; however, it is easily mastered with practice (see Chapter 2). Creative use of interactive instructional methods can assist students in learning how to frame their inquiry, particularly use of terminology for the formulating the question. The language of the PICOT question does not indicate a direction for the desired outcome (e.g., increased glucose, decreased falls). For example, a PICOT question would be framed as How does yoga compared to simple stretching *affect* back pain? However, the research question uses different language, based on the theoretical approach of the investigator and the expected effectiveness of the intervention or issue (e.g., Do(es) specific interventions have an *increase/decrease effect* on an outcome ?). Some examples could include Do fall prevention programs *decrease* falls? How do fall prevention programs *reduce* falls?

Search for Evidence

Step 2 of the EBP process begins with a well-formulated clinical question. Searching for the evidence involves competency with informatics, as has been discussed. Addressing searching from an EBP perspective will help eliminate some of the reported barriers to finding answers to the clinical question (Ebell, 2009; Ely, Osheroff, Chambliss, Ebell, & Rosenbaum, 2005; Green & Ruff, 2005; Melnyk et al., 2012).

Strategies to teach how to search for the evidence include formal classes on searching electronic databases, online searching PubMed tutorial (Winters & Echeverri, 2012) as well as workshops (Ilic, Tepper & Misso, 2012), and role modeling by faculty. Librarians, whether from academic or clinical settings, are essential for consistency in introducing students to library resources, including access to available electronic databases. In the Internet-mediated classroom, faculty have the opportunity to role-model searching techniques that may be challenging to students, such as using controlled vocabulary, Boolean connectors, and limits (see Chapter 3 for more information). In the clinical setting, student and preceptor can collaborate on clinical questions and searching the databases (Winteres & Echeverri, 2012).

Laptops in the classroom can serve as learning tools for the immediate retrieval of evidence to answer questions generated by case studies. Role modeling proper searching techniques helps learners understand their importance. Requiring search histories as part of written papers (e.g., students capture their search using screenshots that are pasted into their papers; how to http://graphicssoft.about.com/cs/general/ht/winscreenshot.htm) demonstrates the quality of students' searching skills. When a student engages a librarian or faculty with this information, it can reinforce successful skill building through evaluative feedback as well as provide an opportunity for peer review and learner self-assessment of efficiency with searching (McDowell & Ma, 2007; Stillwell, Fineout-Overholt, et al., 2010).

Critically Appraise

Step 3 of the EBP process is critical appraisal. There are a variety of teaching strategies that have been reported in the literature to teach this concept, including journal clubs and letter writing (Edwards, White, Gray, & Fischbacher, 2001; Fineout-Overholt, Melnyk, Stillwell, & Williamson, 2010a, 2010b, 2010c; Laaksonen, Hannele, von Schantz, Ylönen, & Soini, 2013). Laaksonen and colleagues found that over 90% of clinicians found journal clubs satisfactory learning opportunities. Over 75% of students found their skills in EBP to increase overall with a journal club. An example of journal clubs to enhance critical appraisal skills may include a small group structure in which the participants present the appraisal of a preselected paper to their peers. Advanced learners may choose to compose a letter to the article author that outlines the appraisal and subsequent conclusion about usefulness to practice. In a mixed-methods study, Ilic, Hart, Fiddes, Misso, and Villanueva (2013) found that teaching EBP with the blended-learning approach compared to the traditional lecture-type approach significantly improved the confidence students reported in their critical appraisal skills. Bath-Hextall, Wharrad, and Leonardi-Bee (2011) reported that reusable learning objectives supported student learning in appraisal of meta-analyses.

For some educators, the challenge in teaching critical appraisal to students is delineating EBP and research (Fineout-Overholt, 2013). Though there may be an intellectual assent that undergraduate nursing programs need to move away from the traditionally emphasized critiques of research and the development of a research proposal or conducting research, there is still a focus on heavy research methods; however, faculty are increasingly reporting redesigning the traditional research course to an EBP approach (Melnyk et al., 2012). Simple interventions for integration of EBP, such as restructuring research courses into incremental experiential learning opportunities lay the foundation for evidence-based decision making that clinical educators can use to set up occasions for discovery in clinical courses. In these same courses, clinical educators can use levels of evidence as the framework to discussing the appropriate research design to answer a clinical questions as well as critical appraisal of evidence. To fully integrate the concepts of EBP into the curriculum requires that faculty be educated about critical appraisal, participate in curriculum revisions to incorporate this important step in the EBP process, and demonstrate buy-in by actively using critical appraisal in their teaching, no matter what course they teach.

An example of curriculum integration that incorporates critical appraisal into various courses could begin with redesigning an undergraduate nursing research course by reframing course objectives and learning activities to specifically address critical appraisal concepts and principles. A focus on use of research in clinical decision making would be imperative. It is important for faculty to understand the relationship between research and EBP. EBP is the paradigm of care—decisions made at any level must be made with this approach; however, foundational to using this approach, clinicians must understand what methods lead to valid and reliable research. For faculty to teach critical appraisal effectively, they must refocus to producing evidence users not evidence generators. The how-tos of research are not the imperative; however, what makes good research is imperative. This redesign should include the language of research and critical appraisal. All research designs must be included in the discussion of available evidence. Furthermore, for EBP to be a lived experience, there must be an active engagement of EBP initiatives at the educational institution.

As a joint effort among faculty who teach traditional research courses, the group charged with integration of EBP into the curriculum (i.e., recognized champions of EBP), and an EBP expert sanctioned by the curriculum committee to lead the integration of EBP in the curriculum can strategically plan how to best begin the integration of EBP into each course. Sample objectives and learning activities from a redesigned course that shifted the requirements from producing a research proposal to using concepts and principles of EBP can be found in Box 15.4.

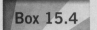

Box 15.4 Sample Course Objectives and Learning Assignments

Course Objective	Example Assignment
Formulate searchable, answerable questions from clinical issues	Generate PICOT questions for written assignment
Examine clinical questions in relation to levels of evidence	Groups share and give feedback on PICOT questions
Find the best evidence to answer the clinical question through searching existing healthcare databases and other sources of evidence	Search two types of questions and post search strategies/results Groups share and give feedback to peers Paper on search for the evidence to a clinical question
Critically appraise best evidence (i.e., evaluating research methodologies for validity, reliability, and applicability) to answer selected clinical questions	Conduct a rapid critical appraisal of a quantitative study Groups share and give feedback to peers Paper on appraisal of the evidence
Discuss strategies for implementing evidence into daily practice	Paper on proposed change in practice

Make Evidence-Based Clinical Decisions

In step 4 of the EBP process, along with evidence, patient values and preferences play an integral part in clinical decision making. Faculty assessment of where learners are taught about the importance of understanding the role of patient preferences is critical. Learning activities focused on heightening students awareness of the importance of patient preferences can be intentionally designed around students' day-to-day experiences with patient-centered care. For example, a learning activity with beginning students can include clinical experiences in which students are obtaining patient histories. This experience can provide a rich forum for discussing patients' preferences, desires, and values about their health and their expectations of health care and how those preferences are being integrated into the care received. For more advanced learners, discussion of strategies to actively include the role of patient preferences in care interventions would be appropriate.

Lectures, Group Learning, Journal Clubs, and More. Methods used to teach EBP should emphasize active participation by the learners as much as possible. Examples of potential strategies include lectures, discussion groups, small- and large-group presentations, journal clubs, elective rotations, grand rounds, unit rounds, and change-of-shift discussions for practica. Teachers are best to act in the facilitator role while learners take front stage in working through the concepts, much like the flipped classroom described by Bergmann and Sams (2012).

Presentations Integrated with Clinical Practicum. A good way to begin any type of educational presentation on EBP is to provide a short synopsis on the definition and EBP process with examples. When teaching EBP in a classroom setting, using an interactive teaching style is preferred (e.g., Socratic questioning and group work), because the students can get lost in the content if not engaging the material. If you want to engage the flipped classroom approach, you would prepare 10-minute interactive videos that provide the essential content, post them online, and spend class time exploring the concepts of EBP and how they relate to clinical care. However you choose to conduct your class, choose methods to facilitate student engagement.

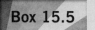

	Hierarchy of Teaching and Learning Activities
Box 15.5	

Level 1	Interactive and clinically integrated activities
Level 2(a)	Interactive but classroom-based activities
Level 2(b)	Didactic but clinically integrated activities
Level 3	Didactic classroom or stand-alone teaching

Clinically integrated teaching-learning activities are superior to classroom teaching alone to improve knowledge, attitude, and behavior. However, classroom teaching that incorporates activities (e.g., case studies, group work, role-play, hands-on learning) can increase educational effectiveness. Clinical teaching can include didactic information by the teacher who directly applies the content to patient situations. Using interactive teaching strategies at a clinical site can make learning more effective. Didactic teaching without interactive teaching strategies is less effective and leads to rote memory. A proposed hierarchy of teaching and learning activities related to educational effectiveness has been suggested by Khan and Coomarasamy (2006) (see Box 15.5).

Small-Group Seminars. Research evidence supports that seminars targeting specific EBP skills can increase those skills to a moderate degree, at least in the short term (Novak & McIntyre, 2010; Shuval et al., 2007; West & McDonald, 2008; Yew & Reid, 2008). If you are in doubt about what sort of topic would be of interest for small-group work, ask for suggestions from the participants. Suggestions can be offered either before the group work seminar so that predigested or preappraised examples can be used or at the time of the seminar in more of an "on-the-fly" setup. These more spontaneous sessions tend to be risky, because if the example is too difficult, the learners quickly can become lost and disheartened, potentially viewing EBP as a tedious and difficult process. A skillful teacher can build confidence in the learner by crafting or framing the issue in such a way that easily guides the learner to a clinical question that can be formulated rather easily, then to an available answer that can be found from a relatively simple search, and then to the evidence that can be easily critically appraised. This is an initial engagement step, and each group work seminar could build in difficulty and ambiguity of the EBP process. Beginning this way will enable the group to feel that the process is not only learnable but also useful and doable, because they have participated in it and accomplished many of the steps themselves.

When moving toward seminars more focused in EBP skills, remember to orient your group of learners to how the skill you are teaching fits into the greater context of the EBP process. For example, if you are teaching a seminar on how to search the healthcare literature, it is important to stress that searching is simply a tool to be used to find the most relevant, valid research evidence and not the only—or even the most important—skill that needs to be learned in the EBP process. Whetting their appetites about the focus of the search and prompting them on to the next steps of critical appraisal and application of evidence to the clinical problem can help learners to realize the broader scope of the EBP process rather than focus on an isolated skill.

Another practical suggestion when establishing small, focused group seminars on EBP concepts is to provide time and means of hands-on practice. For example, when teaching a session on composing and formatting answerable, searchable questions, ask the participants to individually think of clinical questions from their own experience. Provide ample time for them to share their questions with the group then determine whether they are foreground or background questions (see Chapter 2 for more information on formulating clinical questions). If the question was foreground, the group would decide what type of question it was (e.g., treatment, diagnosis, harm, meaning) and construct it in the PICOT format. Then the group would access computers to search for relevant scientific evidence to answer their questions.

Alternatively, the leader could present a case to the group members, asking them to write down questions they generate during the presentation. Then the leader asks each member of the group to share the questions phrased in the PICOT format with their group. This sort of individual practice and skill building as a group is quite powerful as a teaching and learning method. All participants are working actively, not passively, to learn the concepts, and their peers in the group provide immediate feedback and "reality testing" for each individual.

Whether the learning is in a seminar or classroom, learning searching skills led by a medical librarian knowledgeable in EBP should include hands-on practice in searching for evidence to answer their own questions. This combines the principle of relevance to the learner with the evidence-based method of skill-building workshops and thereby fosters more active participation and learning.

For teaching critical appraisal skills, it is useful to work with three small groups, each group focusing on a specific appraisal criterion. (Chapters 4–7 have more information on critical appraisal of evidence.) For example, one small group would report back to the larger group on the results of the study. Another group would discuss the validity of the study results, and the third group would discuss applicability of the study findings to the given patient scenario. This process assists the learners to view the critical appraisal process as a coherent whole.

Incorporating small-group work in a classroom setting adds more opportunity for learners to discuss EBP content in a less threatening atmosphere. Small groups can be a successful forum to formulate PICOT questions from a provided clinical scenario, critically appraise studies, and report back to the class.

Journal Clubs. Another option for teaching EBP is the journal club. Consider that a journal club is not a gathering of faculty or students to passively discuss topics. Rather, a journal club is an active group discussion in which all people involved participate. When establishing a journal club in an academic setting, to optimize attendance it is important to begin by being explicit about the purpose, who should participate, the timing, and the format. The participants can be those interested in learning and teaching EBP or students in a course. Although the leader of the group can rotate among the members, an educator-mentor who is knowledgeable in EBP is essential to validate the journal club's importance and to provide mentoring when the group needs her or his expertise to ask facilitating questions about each step of the EBP process.

The timing of a journal club should be amenable to participants' schedules. Scheduling journal clubs over the lunch hour may work well for some; others can attend those held in the early evening. Whatever the time, food and camaraderie are great incentives to increase attendance. Box 15.6 contains the essential elements of a journal club, which were supported in systematic review of how to run an effective journal club (Deenadayalan, Grimmer-Somers, Prior, & Kumar, 2008).

Journal Club Teaching Formats: Grazing or Hunting. In journal clubs, determining which teaching format will work best for your participants is crucial. Consider first whether a "grazing" format or a "hunting"

Box 15.6   Characteristics of a Successful Journal Club

Regular and anticipated meetings
Mandatory attendance
Clarity of purpose
Appropriate times to meet
Incentives for meeting
A leader to choose articles and lead the discussion
Having articles circulated before the meeting
Internet use for dissemination and storing data
Applying established critical appraisal criteria
Providing a summary of the club's findings

format would best meet learners' needs. Grazing formats have been the most common to this point and typically begin with a group of individuals, such as faculty wanting to learn more about EBP or students post-conference, dividing the relevant journals in their field among themselves. Each individual is then responsible for perusing—or grazing on—one to three journals for recent publications of interest to the group. At the small-group meeting, members of the group take their turns in presenting the information they have found to the rest of the group members.

Unless it is a required component during clinical experiences for students, the grazing process has its inherent inefficiencies. First, in this format, the number of journals reviewed tends to be a function of the number of individuals in the group. Thus, the group is likely to leave several journals unreviewed and, therefore, miss evidence. Second, the group effect is further complicated by members' abilities to make it to the meetings. Third, there are many citations in given journals that are of poor quality. Wading through several journals looking for quality research evidence can be quite tedious. Fourth, the time required by the group members to accomplish the given goal tends to be quite high. Due to these inefficiencies of grazing, many members may relegate the small-group meeting to just another thing on their already full to-do lists.

Despite the inherent inefficiencies, grazing is still an essential activity in keeping up with the latest information. Fortunately, there are now secondary publications that do the grazing, cutting down the time it takes to find quality research evidence. The editorial boards of these resources systematically survey the existing literature. Any relevant studies that meet certain methodologic criteria are abstracted in a quickly readable format. Examples of sources for predigested or preappraised evidence are the *Evidence-Based Nursing Journal*, *Worldviews on Evidence-Based Nursing*, *American College of Physicians Journal Club*, *Clinical Evidence*, *InfoPoems*, and *American Academy of Pediatrics Grand Rounds*. Thus, grazing is very helpful in keeping current, especially when grazing in these greener pastures.

An alternative to grazing is a hunting format. This format begins with a clinical issue and the question of interest to the individual or group. A question is posed from a concern about a clinical issue. The question is then converted into a PICOT question, one that is answerable and searchable. A literature search to find relevant research evidence is performed. Finally, any relevant studies are brought back to the group to critically appraise and discuss application to clinical decision making.

The hunting format has two distinct advantages. First, it is by definition relevant to the group because its own members posed the original question, rather than relying on whatever happened to be published since the last meeting. Second, it includes the question and search components of the EBP process, which are left out of the grazing format. The hunting format can easily be adapted for use in formal coursework. Simply assign group members the task of presenting the results of their question, search, and critical appraisal at the various meetings on a rotating basis.

It is important to make a distinct link between the applicable clinical scenario; the searchable, answerable search question; the search findings; and the subsequent critical appraisal and application of research evidence to allow the group to see the process as a coherent whole. Otherwise, because so much time is spent in learning critical appraisal, learners can quickly equate EBP with only critical appraisal instead of seeing it as a comprehensive process.

TEACHERS AS EBP MENTORS/STUDENTS AS EBP MENTORS

The final champion for successfully teaching EBP is the EBP mentor, sometimes called a coach, information broker, or confidant (see Chapter 17). This individual's job is to provide one-on-one mentoring of educators, providing them with on-site assistance in problem solving about a how to teach EBP. Mentoring has been a long-standing tradition in academia. It is important that these efforts are supported by administration, purposeful and focused to maximize success. Faculty who believe in EBP and desire to teach students to be evidence-based clinicians may find that competing priorities within an academic environment must be overcome in order for them to provide the amount of guidance they would like to their fellow educators. An EBP mentor's primary focus in the academic setting is on improving the student's and faculty's understanding and integration of EBP in practice and educational paradigms. This is often accomplished through providing the right information at the right time that can assist the student to provide the best possible care to the patient and the faculty to provide the best evidence-based education to the student. These mentorships need to be formal, paid positions with time dedicated for teaching EBP. Through mentored relationships, students and faculty have the opportunity to reflect on how well they are achieving their learning goals and advancing EBP.

EVALUATING SUCCESS IN TEACHING EVIDENCE-BASED PRACTICE

Evaluation of outcomes based on evidence is an essential step in the EBP process and in teaching EBP. Effective outcome evaluation of EBP teaching programs is as imperative as their existence. Evaluation involves an assessment of (a) learners, (b) educators/preceptors, (c) curricula, and (d) the program (Fineout-Overholt, 2013). Most instruments used to evaluate educational programs measure the self-efficacy about EBP skills, knowledge, behaviors, outcome expectation, and attitudes of the learners (Bernhardsson & Larsson, 2013; Chang & Crowe, 2011; Hart et al., 2008; Ireland et al., 2009; Shaneyfelt et al., 2006; Sherriff, Wallis, & Chaboyer, 2007; Varnell, Haas, Duke, & Hudson, 2008; Wallin, Bostrom, & Gustavsson, 2012). Shaneyfelt and colleagues conducted a systematic review evaluating EBP in education and found that a number of instruments were used to evaluate some dimension of EBP and could be used to evaluate individuals as well as educational programs. These studies did not measure the outcome of the impact EBP has on patient outcomes. A protocol for standardizing the reporting EBP educational interventions and teaching is currently being proposed (Phillips et al., 2013).

Evaluation of Learner Assimilation of EBP

The outcome of ARCC-E strategies is learner assimilation of the EBP paradigm. This means that learners' clinical decisions inherently include external evidence, internal evidence, their expertise, and patient preferences. The role of the health professions educator is to transfer the EBP paradigm to new healthcare providers as the basis of their practice. This ensures that the mantle of professional health professions will be thoughtfully handed down to clinicians who will uphold their profession with the honor, pride, commitment, dedication, and determination of their predecessors.

Learner Evaluation
Evaluating learners' integration of EBP concepts into their thinking, problem solving, and practice is not an easy task. However, several mechanisms are discussed that can assist in determining how well learners have integrated EBP concepts into their practices.

Classroom Learning. Depending on the educational delivery program (e.g., formal classroom, online, seminars), there are many options for evaluating the specific levels of the cognitive domain related to EBP concepts. Formal testing or specific EBP assignments can assist the learners to identify areas in the process that need remedial work. However, synthesis is a higher cognitive level, and synthesis papers or presentations seem to be a common option that educators use to determine the learner's ability to comprehend, synthesize, and apply EBP concepts and principles in formal educational settings and can be assigned as a group, individual or combined assignment (Box 15.7).

Student perception is another valuable evaluation strategy. Box 15.8 contains an exemplar of how these evaluations can provide important feedback on the value of a course to those taking it.

Clinical Experiences. Traditionally, clinical experiences in nursing programs used care plans, care maps, and logs to evaluate clinical knowledge and application. Other evaluation methods include the objective structure clinical examination (OSCE) and other simulated evaluations, such as a case study. The Fresno Test for evidence-based medicine (Ramos, Schafer, & Tracz, 2003) offers another objective evaluation method for determining how well clinicians assimilate EBP into their daily decisions. Another

Box 15.7 Description of a Combined Group and Individual Synthesis Assignment

Learning Outcome: Find the best evidence to answer a clinical question through the search of existing healthcare databases and other sources of valid and reliable evidence: The purpose of this assignment is for students to enhance their skills in evidence synthesis and communication of best practice to the professional nursing community.

Groups will be assigned a clinical scenario from which a PICOT question can be formulated that has a known body of evidence. **Each person in the group must have a specific part of the presentation to be responsible for, complete their part of the appraisal, create the slides and present the information during the presentation (see criteria below).** Group evaluation will be a part of this process.

Required Criteria for Creative PowerPoint Presentation

◆ Clinical issue, background and significance; statistics that demonstrate there is a significant issue required
◆ PICOT question in PICOT format (appropriate template)
◆ Search strategy with resultant cohort of studies found, screenshots of search required
◆ Appraisal of evidence: evaluation and synthesis tables required (evaluation table may be as handout, but synthesis is required in the presentation)
◆ Applicability for practice & recommendations for evidence-based decision making
◆ APA for citations and reference slide

*Each student is responsible for writing up a three-page paper that reflects this project, using the criteria above. Screenshots of the group search will be included as a figure in the paper and will be in the appendix along with any other tables or figures students choose to use. The culminating paragraphs will be the conclusion from the evidence and recommendations for clinical practice change that is based on the evidence.

Adapted from Core EBP Course, East Texas Baptist University, Fall 2012.

Box 15.8 On Change…An Exemplar for Using Student Evaluation to Demonstrate Effective Teaching

Context: Beginning paradigm shift within the college; however, traditional focus of research course was introduction of the conduct of nursing research, including concepts, issues, processes, and methods without explicit attention to EBP.
Course: The course structure (e.g., course syllabus) remained unchanged; however, the faculty taught it with a "spirit" of inquiry. The course was launched with a simple question: "What are you curious about?" The language of research and EBP was modeled. Course content and assignments were modified. Nursing research core content was taught in the context of EBP concepts, principles, and practices. The course evaluation was simply a question: "What changes have you made?"

(continued)

Invitation: A substantial body of education and nursing literature supports the importance of reflective practice; that is, taking time to "take stock" and integrate experiences from practice, peer interactions, and educational endeavors. I tapped into this powerful learning tool to assess the students' perception of their journey to a better understanding of self and their professional nursing role related to nursing research and EBP. I began the undergraduate research course (i.e., NUR362) with a reflection on change, citing the following 1872 Nightingale quote, to create an early anticipatory set for an end of course Discussion Board forum designed to capture student self-evaluation of change during their course journey and provide qualitative impact/outcome evaluation data. As the course reached its conclusion, students were invited to engage in thoughtful self-reflection and post a response to the following question: What personal and/or professional change(s)/progress have you made over the duration of NUR362?

....

"For us who Nurse, our Nursing is a thing, which, unless in it we are making progress every year, every month, every week, take my word for it, we are going back."
—Nightingale (1872)

....

Captured Reflections: A PowerPoint presentation was created using selected quotes by each student, capturing the nature and power of the students' learning and change journey. This became a "surprise" presentation for the students during the last class session, and served to reinforce the student's shared perceptions, experiences, and pride related to their achievements and learning across all learning domains.

Impact/Outcomes: The student quotes speak for themselves in providing insight into the impact and outcomes of their course experience. Change in knowledge, skills, and attitudes were reflected in responses that captured:

- "I have been able to understand how important research will be in my future career."
- "I have a stronger knowledge of how research will play a part in the daily things I will be doing."
- "The idea of…actually being able to look for the answers to my questions instead of just wondering…really piqued my interest."
- "I feel more confident in tackling the sometimes overwhelming research journals or articles."
- "When I first began this class, I was thinking to myself how boring this class was going to be….I have come to realize that research is essential for the nursing profession to further itself and to provide the best care we can."

Submitted by Karen Saewert, PhD, RN, CPHQ, CNE
Clinical Associate Professor & Director, E³: Evaluation & Educational Excellence
Arizona State University College of Nursing & Health Innovation

Ulrich, B. T. (1992). Change. In *Leadership and management according to Florence Nightingale* (pp. 10–13). Norwalk, CT: Appleton & Lang.

evaluative method, depending on the level of student, is to have the learner find and critically appraise the scientific evidence to support a chosen intervention, then describe in an EBP application paper how this evidence influenced decision making, taking into consideration the clinical team's expertise and the patient's preferences and values.

In addition, checklist to assist in evaluation of students' clinical skills can be helpful. Table 15.1 contains an EBP skills inventory that may be used to assess learners' self-perceived strengths and weaknesses regarding the essential skills of EBP. Informal assessment has demonstrated that learners as well as teachers have gained valuable perspective from this self-assessment. Using this type of questionnaire, EBP teachers can discover learners' comfort with learning to be an evidence-based practitioner. In addition, teachers can discern the importance they attach to improving their EBP skills.

Making learning relevant is one of the most important strategies for developing learners' enthusiasm for and skill in practicing EBP. The examples, assignments, and concepts used in teaching must be based on real patients. In addition, applying the results of the process to learners' current or future practice helps to cement the concepts for them. In the academic setting, if students are given assignments that are not relevant to practice, all but the most highly motivated EBP students will perceive it as busy work and lose enthusiasm.

An effective reflection tool is the **educational prescription** (EP). Though it was originally described by Sackett, Haynes, Guyatt, and Tugwell (1991) to teach people how to "do" critical appraisal, it is easily applicable to clinical practica. The educator writes an EP for an early learner when a learner does not know the answer to a question that is pertinent to the evaluation or management of his or her patient. Given that the hope is that learners eventually start to identify their own knowledge deficits and write their own EPs, this tool can become an evaluation method for clinical post-conference. Furthermore, learners can prepare EPs as a self-assessment of learning the EBP process and journal these prescriptions, reflecting on what they need to learn, how they plan to learn the information, and on what they have learned. Box 15.9 contains an example of the elements of an EP and emphasizes the qualities that are desirable in learners and teachers. Asking learners to report how the evidence they find will alter the management of their patients teaches them perspective. Fundamental to the successful use of EPs is educators' willingness to admit they do not know everything, write their own EPs, and present them to

Table 15.1 **Evidence-Based Practice Skills Inventory**

To help your preceptor improve your skills in EBP, please indicate your experience by checking the appropriate box

	No Experience	Some Experience	Much Experience
Asking answerable questions about my patients	☐	☐	☐
Performing efficient searches for evidence that answers my clinical questions	☐	☐	☐
Selecting the best evidence from what is found in the search	☐	☐	☐
Critically appraising the evidence	☐	☐	☐
Applying the evidence to my practice			

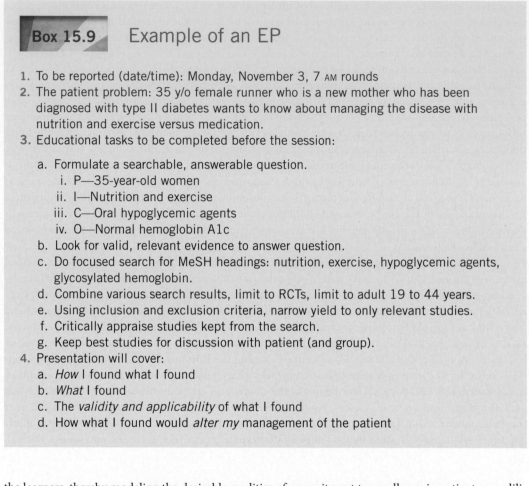

Box 15.9   Example of an EP

1. To be reported (date/time): Monday, November 3, 7 AM rounds
2. The patient problem: 35 y/o female runner who is a new mother who has been diagnosed with type II diabetes wants to know about managing the disease with nutrition and exercise versus medication.
3. Educational tasks to be completed before the session:

   a. Formulate a searchable, answerable question.
      i. P—35-year-old women
      ii. I—Nutrition and exercise
      iii. C—Oral hypoglycemic agents
      iv. O—Normal hemoglobin A1c
   b. Look for valid, relevant evidence to answer question.
   c. Do focused search for MeSH headings: nutrition, exercise, hypoglycemic agents, glycosylated hemoglobin.
   d. Combine various search results, limit to RCTs, limit to adult 19 to 44 years.
   e. Using inclusion and exclusion criteria, narrow yield to only relevant studies.
   f. Critically appraise studies kept from the search.
   g. Keep best studies for discussion with patient (and group).
4. Presentation will cover:
   a. *How* I found what I found
   b. *What* I found
   c. The *validity and applicability* of what I found
   d. How what I found would *alter my* management of the patient

the learners, thereby modeling the desirable qualities of commitment to excellence in patient care, diligence, and perspective. More can be learned about EPs from the toolbox on the website for the Centre for Evidence-Based Medicine (**http://www.cebm.utoronto.ca/practise/formulate/eduprescript.htm**).

> **What is experienced and seen in the clinical area is what will likely predict future behavior.**
> **—Bob Berenson**

Educator and Preceptor Evaluation

Preparing educators and preceptors for teaching EBP to learners is imperative. It is known that learners emulate what they see modeled in their preceptors and educators. Berenson (2002) made that point very clear when he articulated, in a discussion about healthcare professionals' education, that even if the benefits of EBP are clearly presented in a didactic venue, what is experienced and seen in the clinical area is what will likely predict future behavior.

Whether the educational program is nursing, physical therapy, or medicine, or the level of education is baccalaureate, graduate, or postgraduate, educators/preceptors should make clear the course objectives and expectations of the learning about EBP. Knowledge of EBP should be evident in the educators'/preceptors' clinical discussions with learners and should be central to the teaching–learning process. An example of a great opportunity for demonstrating operation of the EBP process is preceptors asking advance practice nurses questions about why a particular treatment option was chosen or a care trajectory was decided. For instance, during the clinical experience of a student at a large southeast university, the healthcare team was discussing the appropriateness of the common practice of prescribing multiple tests for those who test negative for *Clostridium difficile*. One of the preceptors indicated that current evidence supports single assay testing and that routine use of multiple testing increases the likelihood that a false-positive test would occur (Bobo, Dubberke, & Kollef, 2011). Further discussion focused on the cost savings, avoidance of inappropriate treatment, and patient comfort by implementing current evidence. Another clinician in the group discussed how difficult it was for clinicians to accept the variation from traditional practice. A discussion ensued, reflecting on the use of science, expertise, and patient concerns and choices together to make the best clinical decision. The role of uncertainty in clinical practice and the benefits of clinical inquiry were also discussed. Subsequently, the student was asked to design a project that would apply EBP principles to this clinical situation and evaluate the plan, including measurement of practice outcomes. This kind of preceptor interaction to foster application of EBP principles in the clinical area is invaluable to the learner. Gerrish et al. (2011) found that advanced practice nurses who were committed to facilitating EBP in the clinical setting used a knowledge broker approach. These nurses facilitated EBP in clinical nurses through role modeling, teaching, clinical problem solving, and facilitating change. These principles and roles used are also the ones by which they would be evaluated. Evaluation forms can be constructed that delineate these principles that students and preceptors complete to indicate the extent to which they perceive the principles were present in the learning experience.

An additional measure to evaluate educator/preceptor teaching is peer review. Course syllabi, teaching materials, lesson plans, or case studies, as well as peer observation of the educator/preceptor in the clinical or classroom setting can be one source of evaluation data to assess teaching effectiveness. Student evaluations of teaching can also assist the educator/preceptor to reflect on aspects of teaching that are helpful or can be improved to foster student learning. Establishing a peer review rubric assists with consistency of evaluation. There are many online sources of such rubrics. For example, Google results for *peer review rubric* elicited more than a dozen readily available peer review rubrics, ranging from paper rubrics to team work rubrics.

Curricula Evaluation

The design of the curriculum guides the content and activities that are implemented in a health professions educational program. Competence as an outcome must be clearly linked with the expected learner outcomes. EBP as the foundation of a curriculum should be sequenced logically allowing for incremental learning of the depth and breadth of all essential content. One way to determine this is to develop a grid or matrix that identifies EBP program outcomes and course objectives reflecting Bloom's taxonomy (http://www.nwlink.com/~donclark/hrd/bloom.html). The EBP content, the learning activities that relate to the objectives, and the evaluative methods that measure the learner outcomes can be entered into the matrix to determine internal consistency and vertical organization. The curricular design should mirror the institution's mission and philosophy statements, which should actively reflect EBP. Specific courses can be reviewed to determine the internal consistency of course objectives, content, learning activities, and evaluative methods and their placement in the curriculum and how they reflect EBP knowledge, skills, and attitudes. In informal workshop or seminar formats, it is equally important to evaluate the objectives, content, learning activities, and outcomes to foster successful learning about EBP.

Program Evaluation

To evaluate the program, careful consideration of what to evaluate, when to evaluate, and who to evaluate is imperative. Evaluating learners' ongoing absorption of EBP concepts throughout an educational program is integral to knowing the success of the program. However, other outcomes of the overall program that need to be examined include program goal(s) and environmental outcomes. Some of these outcomes may be evaluated on a continual basis (e.g., graduates application of EBP in daily practice) and some may be a one-time assessment (e.g., number of attendees from different locations to measure scope of attendance).

Continual monitoring of the environment and outcomes (goals) is necessary for either teaching or implementing EBP. Periodically, the educator/preceptor champions of EBP need to determine where they are in reaching the goals of the EBP program. This first requires a commitment to setting measurable program goals that can be monitored on an ongoing basis. Evaluation of the program's foundation (environment) can be obtained by examining the questions raised in the first part of this chapter. If there are insufficient answers (e.g., educators' knowledge of up-to-date EBP concepts is lacking), the program has not been completely successful in that area. Steps then would be taken to address the areas that lack support (e.g., send the educators to an EBP conference or hold an EBP conference on the program site). The learners can provide feedback on the courses and learning experiences at the conclusion of the courses. This input can be analyzed and used to make decisions about the courses.

Program goals should address whether learners can formulate a searchable, answerable clinical question; efficiently find relevant evidence; discern what is best scientific evidence; and apply the best scientific evidence with clinical expertise and patient input to clinical decision making. Part of the Summit on Health Professions Education (Greiner & Knebel, 2003) competency regarding practicing using evidence stated that across and within disciplines, efforts must be focused on the development of a scientific evidence base. The final goal for a teaching program must be for learners to actively evaluate outcomes based on evidence.

In addition, the Summit recommended that funding sources such as the Agency for Healthcare Research and Quality (AHRQ) support ongoing clinical and education research that evaluates care based on the five specified competencies. An example of this type of research could be a study to evaluate educational outcomes for an EBP teaching program across two or more disciplines (e.g., nursing and medicine).

Final Assessment

There is usually some type of cumulative assessment for learners completing a degree program, such as comprehensive exams. However, not every discipline uses this form of outcome evaluation. National licensure and certifying exams may provide outcome evaluation for some disciplines and some levels of education. Whatever form of final assessment a teaching program in EBP employs (e.g., EBP implementation project), it must address the EBP paradigm, particularly application and evaluation. These are the most challenging steps of the EBP process to evaluate. Without evaluating the EBP process in a final evaluation, educators cannot know whether learners are prepared to apply principles they have learned in their daily practices.

Program Effectiveness

The overall EBP program is effective if the learners are successful in integrating EBP concepts into their thinking and practice. Integration of EBP concepts into daily practice can be discerned by periodic follow-up with graduates to ask them about the integration of EBP in their practices. Although self-report has its drawbacks, querying what EBP initiatives learners have been involved in during the past 12 months can assist the educator in obtaining more objective information on how they have applied EBP knowledge to practice.

An example could be that EBP concepts and principles are integrated throughout the health professions major. Evaluation of the impact of EBP integration on students' EBP beliefs and implementation of concepts and principles would be planned and executed before the first introduction to EBP content. Foundational concepts for EBP should be introduced in the first semester while learning about the healthcare professions, with specific learning activities placed in specific courses in that semester. An introduction to the evaluation of research and its use in practice are the focus of the second semester. A foundational course focuses on the underpinnings of EBP paradigm with at least two other courses providing the incremental learning. These courses would replace any traditional research generation course. As students progress in their learning, no further didactic information would be presented; however, building skills in critical appraisal and application of evidence to practice would be emphasized in all clinical settings. Competence in effecting change and improving outcomes through the integration and amalgamation of evidence, clinician expertise, and patient preference would be demonstrated through a culmination capstone project in final semester of their healthcare education.

Tools such as Evidence-based Practice Beliefs (Melnyk & Fineout-Overholt, 2003a), Evidence-Based Practice Implementation for Educators (EPBI-E; Fineout-Overholt & Melnyk et al., 2010a), Evidence-Based Practice Implementation for Students (EBPI-S; Fineout-Overholt & Melnyk et al., 2010b), and the Organizational Culture and Readiness for School-Wide Integration of Evidence-based Practice in Education (OCRSIEP-E; Fineout-Overholt & Melnyk et al., 2011c) are being used to determine the impact of an EBP-integrated curriculum. These tools can be used to compare total beliefs, implementation and organizational culture scores as well as individual belief and implementation statements, which can provide information about the curriculum in terms of strengths and areas to focus EBP learning. A full assessment of the environment is imperative for moving forward.

To know if the change to evidence-based curricula was effective, the transition requires focused evaluation. This could be part of ongoing quality improvement of the EBP integration, during which students' beliefs about EBP and use of EBP principles were measured. Students who had a more traditional approach could be compared with those who used an EBP approach. Evaluating the impact of EBP programs on learners and healthcare providers' performance may involve various approaches, such as tests, papers, EPs, and self-report, to evaluate various outcomes (e.g., knowledge, attitude, and behaviors). In more formal academic settings, to facilitate ease of evaluation, the use of a portfolio may be used to capture the integration of the EBP paradigm.

BARRIERS FOR TEACHING/ENHANCING EBP IN ACADEMIC SETTINGS: LESSONS LEARNED

Reflection offers opportunity to learn from our life journey. Among lessons learned about the structure and content of an EBP integration curriculum, five are noted here: ensure incremental learning, set clear deadlines, carefully assess skill levels, assure education has meaning, and foster learning and growth.

First Lesson: Ensure Incremental Learning

Building knowledge and skills in EBP can be overwhelming. Teaching EBP to undergraduates with no or minimal clinical experience requires offering opportunities to learn the language of EBP, its principles, and the EBP paradigm over time and in small doses. Heavier doses may lead to discontent with learning and may be perceived as competitive versus complementary (i.e., foundational) to learning the clinical tasks associated with health professions. Furthermore, advanced learners students will appreciate the opportunity to incrementally assimilate knowledge and skills into their practice as well.

Second Lesson: Set Clear Deadlines

Deadlines for any product of learning are crucial. Clinicians, both teachers and learners, are very busy in a complex clinical setting. Because there are many distractions, it is important to be explicit about the goals and timeline of any assigned learning experience. Examples of this are a 2-day return on search results for a question generated by both teacher and learner, assigning an EP on a question to be presented the next day on rounds or in report, and breaking up a large project into smaller ones with shorter deadlines (e.g., divide an EBP paper assignment into three stages due 1 month apart: question and search strategy, critical appraisal, and application of evidence). In short, it is important to keep the learning experience on the learner's radar screen within the context of the experience, workshop, seminar, or coursework.

Third Lesson: Carefully Assess Skill Levels

The third lesson learned is that learners begin an educational program with widely varied skills in informatics and EBP. Determining learners' skills prior to starting the teaching program is essential. Because becoming an evidence-based provider is a complex task, much like becoming a licensed practitioner, the program should be broken down into reasonable parts that learners can accomplish. It is important to meet learners where they are and to foster growth in knowledge and skills from that point. Any bar to reflect learner growth should be flexible enough to be angled upward or downward for a specific learner. This avoids the frustration that sets in when learners are overwhelmed with the material or process. Setting realistic expectations for each experience and providing formative feedback along the way in addition to summative information at the end of the experience will encourage learners' growth.

Fourth Lesson: Assure Education Has Meaning

The fourth lesson learned is to make the content, settings, formats, and methods meaningful to learn ers. This shows learners first hand that EBP is applicable and useful to them in their particular practice setting. Use relevant examples and scenarios. This is best accomplished by beginning the process with a question generated by the learner. It is incredibly powerful to learn the EBP process by working through a clinical issue that the learner actually cares about and that the learner can imagine herself or himself using in the future. One teaching–learning experience that can assist students to synthesize the EBP process and make it relevant is developing a shared partnership between academia and clinical agency where students would engage in best practice and improve patient outcomes in real time (Odell & Barta, 2011).

Fifth Lesson: Foster Learning and Growth

The fifth lesson learned is to foster learning and growth in those you teach, with the goal that they, in turn, will share their EBP knowledge with their colleagues. Focusing on getting a particular grade or checking off a required assignment will not produce life-long learners who will improve outcomes. Learners who do not readily understand PICOT questions, patient preferences, effect size, or intention-to-treat will improve their knowledge and comfort with the subject matter if they experience mentored learning. According to Thomas, Saroyan, and Dauphinee (2011), a cognitive apprenticeship approach can provide students with opportunities to learn EBP from clinicians and faculty.

PROPOSAL AND CASE EXEMPLAR FOR TEACHING EVIDENCE-BASED PRACTICE IN ACADEMIC SETTINGS

Degree programs need to integrate EBP so that knowledge and skills are built upon throughout the program. The leveling of EBP courses throughout the program focuses on building an understanding of the EBP paradigm and principles of critical appraisal and theory in the first few semesters while students are gaining expertise in clinical specialty. This sequencing enables learners to incrementally engage the EBP paradigm as they integrate it into their practices. Capstone experience, whether in undergraduate or graduate programs, offers a wonderful opportunity for students to bring to culmination what they have learned in courses across the curriculum. Furthermore, across courses within the curriculum, faculty could integrate building blocks for their capstone project, thus enabling students to avoid the need to complete the entire project in one semester. For example, students could complete a synthesis of a body of evidence to answer a clinical question in their first or second semester (e.g., graduate: exhaustive; undergraduate: guided). As they engage in clinical experiences, they can work with clinicians to build a plan for implementing that evidence and determining outcomes to demonstrate the impact of the evidence. As a culmination of their learning, within their capstone course students can engage evidence implementation and outcome evaluation. Finally, learners can reflect on their projects and their impact on local organizations with whom they partnered and choose a method of dissemination that matches their project. As faculty plan for incremental learning, it would be important for a clinical component to be planned, outlining specific EBP milestones that assist learners with benchmarking where they are in the process and evaluate their progress. Boxes 15.10 and 15.11 contain some suggested educational evaluation methods that help health professions students assimilate EBP concepts as they learn their craft.

Box 15.10 Example of Outcomes Management Project Assignment Criteria

◆ Background and significance of project are clear. (Support that there is insufficient evidence to answer the clinical question.)
◆ Clinically meaningful question is clear. (Use PICOT to identify question components.)
◆ Sources and process for identifying outcomes for project are clear. (The outcomes flow from the question. All possible outcomes are considered and addressed to answer the question.)
◆ Sources and process for collecting data are clear. (How approval was obtained, collection tool, who is collecting data, and from whom or what.)
◆ Data analysis approach assists in answering the clinical question. (Was the right statistical test for the level of data collected?)
◆ Proposed presentation of data is clear. (Graphs are readable on slide/handout. All data are synthesized and presented to audience in written form, slide/handout.)
◆ Implications for practice changes based on the data are clear. (What the data indicate that needs to be different in practice.)
◆ Plan for change is clear. (Specific steps for change.)
◆ Anticipated barriers, facilitators, and challenges to plan are clear.
◆ Outcomes for evaluation of plan are clear and measurable.
◆ Dissemination plan is clear and feasible. (What is going to be done with the information gathered in the project?)
◆ PowerPoint presentation and supporting documents enhance presentation.
◆ Overall argument is compelling and worthy of change in practice.

Box 15.11 Example of Requirements for an Evidence Implementation Project

Purpose

This small-group project (two people per group) has been designed to assist students in searching for the best evidence and appraising it so that scholarly, up-to-date care for patients can be provided.

(continued)

Instructions

1. Identify a clinical question of interest from a patient you have cared for in your clinical experiences. Topics must be preapproved by the course faculty.
2. Briefly describe the background to the problem, its clinical significance, and how you searched for the best evidence to answer your question.
3. Present the best evidence to answer this clinical question.
4. Critically appraise the evidence.
5. Discuss implications for practice and future research.
6. Include a glossary of all research terms used in your paper.
7. All studies appraised must accompany paper submission (paper must be in hard and disk copy).

ACADEMIC TEACHING EBP EXEMPLAR

The University of Rochester Internal Medicine, Pediatrics, and Medicine-Pediatrics offers a variety of teaching–learning methods in both clinical *practicum* and academic *courses* as part of residents' learning experiences (e.g., morning report, journal club, ambulatory conferences, skills blocks, and an EBP elective). During morning report, participants are required to present an EP once every month as they rotate to different patient units. The clinical questions are to be drawn from their practice experiences, with the search, critical appraisal, and application discussed among the group. This 1-hour teaching conference usually consists of two cases being presented and discussed, each for half of an hour. Once per week, an EP is presented and discussed instead of a case. The group in attendance (including a seasoned mentor) gives immediate feedback to the resident.

Journal club meets once per week. During this noon conference, a hunting format is used, and the group is divided into smaller groups, each with the task of analyzing one aspect of a systematic review or study and presenting back to the large group. Skills blocks are specific 2-week rotations set aside for nonclinical, classroom learning of clinical concepts, with a large portion of these sessions being devoted to the teaching of EBP concepts. These skill block minicourses are quite successful in bringing beginners to a common place of facility with EBP. Table 15.2 illustrates a workable skill block minicourse schedule.

For the more advanced learner, an EBP elective is offered. This is a 2-week course that consists of two 2-hour sessions daily. Attendance is limited to 8 to 10 participants for optimizing individual participation. In an introductory session where individual and group goals are set, learning needs are identified. A session on asking an answerable and searchable question; a search tutorial with a medical librarian; and sessions on the critical appraisal and application of articles of therapy, diagnosis, prognosis, overview, and harm using preselected articles follow the introductory session. The remainder of the elective is left open for the group to decide what to present and discuss. Individuals are required to take turns in leading these open sessions, teaching the group something they did not know beforehand. This program is designed to address the three ingredients of optimal adult learning:

1. A pretest that reveals a knowledge deficit
2. A learning phase to fill the knowledge deficit
3. A posttest where the learner presents what she or he has learned

To conclude the elective, group members individually present a project of their choosing, ranging from an appraisal of related single studies to formulating a complete EP.

There are many considerations when planning to integrate EBP into a curriculum. The ARCC-E framework provides guidance into what are the critical elements to foster in learners. Techniques and interventions have been suggested in this chapter. Educators will have ideas of their own for how to

Table 15.2 Example of Workable Skill Block Minicourse Schedule

Session	Topic
1. 3 h	Introduction of principles of EBP (large group)
	Session on asking answerable questions (large group)
	Break into small groups of 8–10 and select project topics
2. 2 h (large group)	Search tutorial by medical librarian
3. 1 h (small groups)	Critically appraise and discuss an article on therapy—preselected article
4. 1 h (small groups)	Critically appraise and discuss an overview (meta-analysis) This overview optimally contains the article on therapy from the previous session
5. 1 h (small groups)	Critically appraise and discuss an article on diagnostic testing—preselected article
6. 1 h (small groups)	Critically appraise and discuss an article on prognosis—preselected article
7. 2 h	Small groups—participants present their project (EP)
	Large group—wrap up and answer any overall questions

address the mandate of evidence-based education. The key is for educators to move, not stand still. Be brave—know that you will not always do things perfectly and you may get results you didn't desire; however, that is an opportunity to put your knowledge to the test and re-plan so that the next time your results are different. Charles Swindoll, a noted theologian, offered the following perspective with which educators and learners alike must embrace integration of EBP into current healthcare professions' curricula:

> **Words can never adequately convey the incredible impact of attitude toward life [integration of EBP]. The longer I live the more convinced I become that life is 10% what happens to us and 90% how we respond to it. I believe the single most significant decision I can make on a day-to-day basis is my choice of attitude. It is more than my past, my education, my bankroll, my successes or failures, fame or pain, what other people think of me or say about me, my circumstances, or my position. Attitude keeps me going or cripples my progress. It alone fuels my fire or assaults my hope. When my attitudes are right, there's no barrier too high, no valley too deep, no dream too extreme, no challenge too great for me.**
> **—Charles S. Swindoll**

EBP FAST FACTS

- ◆ A systematic approach is necessary to teaching EBP in academic settings (e.g., using the ARCC-E framework).
- ◆ Offering plenty of step-by-step learning opportunities facilitates learning EBP incrementally.
- ◆ Assessment, ongoing evaluation, and data-driven improvements are essential elements of teaching EBP in academic settings.

References

American Association of Colleges of Nursing. (2000). Distance technology in nursing education: Assessing a new frontier. AACN white paper. *Journal of Professional Nursing, 16*(2), 116–122.

American Association of Colleges of Nursing. (2006). *The essentials of doctoral education for advanced nursing practice.* Retrieved August 29, 2013, from http://www.aacn.nche.edu/DNP/pdf/Essentials.pdf

American Association of Colleges of Nursing. (2008). *The essentials of baccalaureate education for professional nursing practice.* Retrieved August 29, 2013, from http://www.aacn.nche.edu/education-resources/baccessentials08.pdf

American Medical Informatics Association. (2013). *AMIA 10X10 Programs.* Retrieved December 13, 2013, from http://www.amia.org/education/10x10-courses

American Nurses Credentialing Center. (2014). *ANCC Magnet Recognition Program.* Retrieved September 29, 2013, from http://www.nursecredentialing.org/magnet/

Association of American Medical Colleges. (2007). *Advancing educators and education: Defining the components and evidence of educational scholarship.* Retrieved December 8, 2013, from https://members.aamc.org/eweb/upload/Advancing%20Educators%20and%20Education.pdf

Bath-Hextall, F., Wharrad, H., & Leonardi-Bee, J. (2011). Teaching tools in evidence-based practice: Evaluation of reusable learning objects (RLOs) for earning about meta-analysis. *BMC Medical Education, 11*(18), 2–10.

Berenson, B. (2002). *Crossing the quality chasm: Next steps for health professions education.* Major stakeholders comment on key strategies and action plans. Retrieved May 17, 2003, from http://www.kaisernetwork.org/health_cast/uploaded_files/Transcript_6.18.02_IOM_Major-Stakeholders.pdf

Bergmann, J., & Sams, A. (2012). *Flip your classroom: Reach every student in every class, every day.* Colorado: International Society for Technology in Education (ISTE).

Bernhardsson, S., & Larsson, M. E. (2013). Measuring evidence-based practice in physical therapy: Translation, adaptation, further development, validation, and reliability test of a questionnaire. *Physical Therapy, 93*(6), 819–832.

Bobo, L., Dubberke, E., & Kollef, M. (2011). *Clostridium difficile* in the ICU: The struggle continues. *Chest, 140*(6), 1643–1653.

Centers for Medicare & Medicaid Services. (2014). *Quarterly provider updates.* Retrieved January 1, 2014, from http://www.cms.gov/Regulations-and-Guidance/Regulations-and-Policies/QuarterlyProviderUpdates/index.html

Chang, A., & Crowe, L. (2011). Validation of scales measuring self-efficacy and outcome expectancy in evidence-based practice. *Worldviews on Evidence-Based Nursing, 8*(2), 106–115.

Ciliska, D. (2005). Educating for evidence-based practice. *Journal of Professional Nursing, 21*(6), 345–350.

Coomarasamy, A., & Khan, K. (2004).What is the evidence that postgraduate teaching in evidence-based medicine changes anything? A systematic review. *British Medical Journal, 329*, 1017–1022.

Deenadayalan, Y., Grimmer-Somers, K., Prior, M., & Kumar, S. (2008). How to run an effective journal club: A systematic review. *Journal of Evaluating Clinical Practice, 14*(5), 898–911.

Duck, J. D. (2002). *The change monster: The human forces that fuel or foil corporate transformation and change.* New York: Crown Business.

Ebell, M. H. (2009). How to find answers to clinical questions. *American Family Physician, 79*(4), 293–296.

Edwards, R., White, M., Gray, J., & Fischbacher, C. (2001). Use of a journal club and letter writing exercise to teach critical appraisal to medical undergraduates. *Medical Education, 35*, 691–694.

Ely, J. W., Osheroff, J. A., Chambliss, M. L., Ebell, M. H., & Rosenbaum, M. E. (2005). Answering physicians' clinical questions: Obstacles and potential solutions. *Journal of the American Medical Informatics Association, 12*(2), 217–224.

Fineout-Overholt, E. (2013). Outcome evaluation for programs teaching EBP. In R. F. Levin & H. R. Feldman (Eds.), *Teaching evidence-based practice in nursing* (2nd ed., pp. 205–224). New York: Springer.

Fineout-Overholt, E., & Colleagues. (2010–2012). *EBP Step-by-Step Series.* Retrieved from the American Journal of Nursing Collections: http://journals.lww.com/ajnonline/pages/collectiondetails.aspx?TopicalCollectionId=10

Fineout-Overholt, E., & Johnston, L. (2005). Teaching EBP: A challenge for educators in the 21st century. *Worldviews on Evidence-Based Nursing, 2*(1), 37–39.

Fineout-Overholt, E., & Johnston, L. (2007). Evaluation: An essential step to the EBP process. *Worldviews on Evidence-Based Nursing, 4*(1), 54–59.

Fineout-Overholt, E., & Melnyk, B. (2005). Building a culture of best practice. *Nurse Leader, 3*(6), 26–30.

Fineout-Overholt, E., & Melnyk, B. M. (2011). ARCC Evidence-Based Practice Mentors: The Key to Sustaining Evidence-Based Practice. *In Evidence-based Practice in Nursing and Healthcare: A Guide to Best Practice.* 2nd ed., Philadelphia: Lippincott, Williams & Wilkins (pp. 344–352).

Fineout-Overholt, E., & Melnyk, B. M. (2010a). *Evidence-based practice implementation for educators.* Gilbert, AZ: ARCC Publishing.

Fineout-Overholt, E., & Melnyk, B. M. (2010b). *Evidence-based practice implementation for students.* Gilbert, AZ: ARCC Publishing.

Fineout-Overholt, E., & Melnyk, B. M. (2011). *Organizational culture & readiness for school-wide integration of evidence-based practice*. Marshall, TX: ARCC Publishing.

Fineout-Overholt, E., Melnyk, B. M., Stillwell, S. B., & Williamson, K. M. (2010a). Evidence-based practice step by step: Critical appraisal of the evidence: part I. *American Journal of Nursing, 110*(7), 47–52.

Fineout-Overholt, E., Melnyk, B. M., Stillwell, S.B., & Williamson, K. M. (2010b). Evidence-based practice, step by step: Critical appraisal of the evidence: part II. *American Journal of Nursing, 110*(9), 41–48.

Fineout-Overholt, E., Melnyk, B. M., Stillwell, S. B., & Williamson, K.M. (2010c). Evidence-based practice, step by step: Critical appraisal of the evidence: part III. *American Journal of Nursing, 110*(11), 43–51.

Gerrish, K., McDonnell, A., Nolan, M., Guillaume, L., Kirshbaum, M., & Tod, A. (2011). The role of advanced practice nurses in knowledge brokering as a means of promoting evidence-based practice among clinical nurses. *Journal of Advanced Nursing, 67*(9), 2004–2014.

Green, M. L., & Ruff, T. R. (2005). Why do residents fail to answer their clinical questions? A qualitative study of barriers to practicing evidence-based medicine. *Academic Medicine, 80*(2), 176–182.

Greiner, A., & Knebel, E. (Eds.). (2003). *Health professions education: A bridge to quality*. Washington, DC: National Academy Press.

Hart, P., Eato, L., Buckner, M., Morrow, B., Barrett, D., Fraser, D., … Sharrer, R. L. (2008). Effectiveness of a computer-based educational program on nurses' knowledge, attitude, and skill level related to evidence-based practice. *Worldviews on Evidence-Based Nursing, 5*(2), 75–84.

Hinton-Walker, P. (2010). The TIGER initiative: A call to accept and pass the baton. *Nursing Economics, 28*(5), 352–355.

Ilic, D., Tepper, K., & Misso, M. (2012). Teaching evidence-based medicine literature searching skills to medical students during the clinical years: a randomized controlled trial. *Journal of the Medical Library Association, 100*(3), 190–196.

Institute of Medicine. (1999). *To err is human: Building a safe health system*. Washington, DC: National Academy Press.

Institute of Medicine. (2001). *Crossing the quality chasm: A new health system for the 21st century*. Washington, DC: National Academy Press.

Institute of Medicine. (2002). *Educating health professionals to use informatics*. Washington, DC: National Academy Press.

Ireland, J., Martindale, S., Johnson, N., Adams, D., Eboh, W., & Mowatt, E. (2009). Blended learning in education: Effects on knowledge and attitude. *British Journal of Nursing, 18*(2), 124–130.

Johnston, L., & Fineout-Overholt, E. (2005). Teaching EBP: "Getting from zero to one." Moving from recognizing and admitting uncertainties to asking searchable, answerable questions. *Worldviews on Evidence-Based Nursing, 2*(2), 98–102.

Kennedy, C. C., Jaeschke, R., Keitz, S., Newman, T., Montori, V., & Wyer, P. C. Evidence-Based Medicine Teaching Tips Working Group. (2008). Tips for teachers of evidence-based medicine: Adjusting for prognostic imbalances (confounding variables) in studies on therapy or harm. *Journal of General Internal Medicine, 23*(3), 337–343.

Kent, B., & Fineout-Overholt, E. (2007). Teaching EBP: Clinical practice guidelines: part 1. *Worldviews on Evidence-Based Nursing, 4*(2), 106–111.

Khan, K. S., & Coomarasamy, A. (2006). A hierarchy of effective teaching and learning to acquire competence in evidence-based medicine. *BMC Medical Education, 6*(59). Retrieved January 11, 2014, from http://www.biomedcentral.com/1472-6920/6/59/abstract.

Laaksonen, C., Hannele, P., von Schantz, M., Ylönen, M., & Soini, T. (2013). Journal club as a method for nurses and nursing students' collaborative learning: A descriptive study. *Health Science Journal, 7*(3), 285–292.

McGinn, T., Jervis, R., Wisnivesky, J., Keitz, S., Wyer, P. C., & Evidence-based Medicine Teaching Tips Working Group. (2008). Tips for teachers of evidence-based medicine: Clinical prediction rules (CPRs) and estimating pretest probability. *Journal of General Internal Medicine, 23*(8), 1261–1268.

Melnyk, B., & Fineout-Overholt, E. (2003a). *Evidence-based practice beliefs scale*. Rochester, NY: ARCC Publishing.

Melnyk, B., & Fineout-Overholt, E. (2003b). *Evidence-based practice implementation scale*. Rochester, NY: ARCC Publishing.

Melnyk, B. M., Fineout-Overholt, E., Feinstein, N., Li, H. S., Small, L., Wilcox, L., & Kraus, R. (2004). Nurses' perceived knowledge, beliefs, skills, and needs regarding evidence-based practice: Implications for accelerating the paradigm shift. *Worldviews on Evidence-Based Nursing, 1*(3), 185–193.

Melnyk, B. M., Fineout-Overholt, E., Feinstein, N. F., Sadler, L. S., & Green-Hernandez, C. (2008). Nurse practitioner educators' perceived knowledge, beliefs, and teaching strategies regarding evidence-based practice: Implications for accelerating the integration of evidence-based practice into graduate programs. *Journal of Professional Nursing, 24*(1), 7–13.

Melnyk, B. M., Fineout-Overholt, E., Gallagher-Ford, L., & Kaplan, L. (2012). The state of evidence-based practice in US nurses: Critical implications for nurse leaders and educators. *Journal of Nursing Administration, 42*(9), 410–417.

Melnyk, B. M., Fineout-Overholt, E., Giggleman, M., & Cruz, R. (2010). Correlates among Cognitive Beliefs, EBP Implementation, Organizational Culture, Cohesion and Job Satisfaction in Evidence-based Practice Mentors from a Community Hospital System. *Nursing Outlook, 58*(6), 301–308.

National League for Nursing. (2008). *Position statement: Preparing the next generation of nurses to practice in a technology-rich environment: An informatics agenda*. Retrieved on December 8, 2013, from http://www.nln.org/aboutnln/positionstatements/informatics_052808.pdf

Novak, I., & McIntyre, S. (2010). The effect of education with workplace supports on practitioners' evidence-based practice knowledge and implementation behaviours. *Australian Occupational Therapy Journal, 57*, 386–393.

Odell, E., & Barta, K. (2011). Teaching evidence-based practice: The bachelor of science in nursing essentials at work at the bedside. *Journal of Professional Nursing, 27,* 370–377.

O'Mathuna, D. P., Fineout-Overholt, E., & Kent, B. (2008). How systematic reviews can foster evidence-based clinical decisions: part II. *Worldviews on Evidence-Based Nursing, 5*(2), 102–107.

Palaima, M. (2010). *Evidence based practice: Clinical experiences of recent doctor of physical therapy graduates.* UMI # AAI3430468. (83p). ISBN: 978-112-429-8047047

Phillips, A. C., Lewis, L. K., McEvoy, M. P., Galipeau, J., Glasziou, P., Hammick, M., … Williams, M. (2013). Protocol for development of the guidelines for reporting evidence based practice educational interventions and teaching (GREET) statement. *BMC Medical Education, 13*(9), 2–11.

Porter-O'Grady, T., & Malloch, K. (2012). *Leadership in nursing.* Sudbury, MA: Jones & Barlett.

Prasad, P., Jaeschke, R., Wyer, P., Keitz, S. Guyatt, G., & Evidence-Based Medicine Teaching Tips Working Group. (2008). Tips for teachers of evidence-based medicine: Understanding odds ratios and their relationship to risk ratios. *Journal of General Internal Medicine, 23*(5), 635–640.

Pravikoff, D. S., Pierce, S. T., & Tanner, A. (2005). Evidence-based practice readiness study supported by academy nursing informatics expert panel. *Nursing Outlook, 53*(1), 49–50.

Ramos, K., Schafer, S., & Tracz, S. (2003). Validation of the Fresno test of competence in evidence based medicine. *British Medical Journal, 326,* 319–321.

Richardson, W. S., Wilson, M. C., Keitz, S. A., Weyer, P. C., & EBM Teaching Scripts Working Group. (2008). Tips for teachers of evidence-based medicine: Making sense of diagnostic test results using likelihood ratios. *Journal of General Internal Medicine, 23*(1), 87–92.

Sackett, D. L., Haynes, R. B., Guyatt, G. H., & Tugwell, P. (1991). *Keeping up to date–The educational prescription in clinical epidemiology* (2nd ed.). Boston, MA: Little Brown & Co.

Schutt, M. S., & Hightower, B. (2009). Enhancing RN-to-BSN students' information literacy skills through the use of instructional technology. *Journal of Nursing Education, 48*(2), 101–105.

Shaneyfelt, T., Baum, K. D., Bell, D., Feldstein, D., Houston, T., Kaatz, S., … Green, M. (2006). Instruments for evaluating education in evidence-based practice: A systematic review. *American Medical Association, 296*(9), 1116–1127.

Sherriff, K. L., Wallis, M., & Chaboyer, W. (2007). Nurses' attitudes to and perceptions of knowledge and skills regarding evidence-based practice. *International Journal of Nursing Practice, 13,* 363–369.

Shuval, K., Berkovits, E., Netzer, D., Hekselman, I., Linn, S., Brezis, M., & Reis, S. (2007). Evaluating the impact of an evidence-based medicine educational intervention on primary care doctors' attitudes, knowledge and clinical behaviour: A controlled trial and before and after study. *Journal of Evaluation in Clinical Practice, 13*(4), 581–598.

Stichler, J., Fields, W., Kim, S. C., & Brown, C. (2011). Faculty knowledge, attitudes and perceived barriers to teaching evidence-based nursing. *Journal of Professional Nursing, 27*(2), 92–100.

Springer, H. (2010). Learning and teaching in action. *Health information and Libraries Journal, 27,* 327–331.

Stephens-Lee, C., Lu, D., & Wilson, K. (2013). Preparing students for an electronic workplace. *Online Journal of Nursing Informatics (OJNI), 17*(3). Retrieved from http://ojni.org/issues/?p=2866

Technology Informatics Guiding Education Reform. (2007). *The TIGER initiative: Evidence and informatics transforming nursing: 3-year action steps toward a 10-year vision.* Retrieved January 11, 2014, from http://www.tigersummit.com/uploads/TIGERInitiative_Report2007_Color.pdf

Technology Informatics Guiding Education Reform. (2009). *The TIGER initiative: Collaborating to integrate evidence and informatics into nursing practice and education: An executive summary.* Retrieved January 11, 2014, from http://www.tigersummit.com/uploads/TIGER_Collaborative_Exec_Summary_040509.pdf

The Joint Commission. (2013). *Revised requirements for the hospital accreditation program.* Retrieved January 11, 2014, from http://www.jointcommission.org/assets/1/6/PrepublicationReport_CMS_HAP.pdf

Thomas, A., Saroyan, A., & Dauphinee, W. D. (2011). Evidence-based practice: A review of theoretical assumptions and effectiveness of teaching and assessment interventions in health professions. *Advances in Health Sciences Education: Theory & Practice, 16*(2), 253–276.

Varnell, G., Haas, B., Duke, G., & Hudson, K. (2008). Effect of an educational intervention on attitudes toward and implementation of evidence-based practice. *Worldviews on Evidence-Based Nursing, 5*(4), 172–181.

Wallen, Mitchell, Melnyk, Fineout-Overholt, Miller-Davis, Yates, et al. 2010; Wallen, G. R., Mitchell, S. A., Melnyk, B. M., Fineout-Overholt, E., Miller-Davis, C., Yates, J., & Hastings, C. (2010). Implementing evidence-based practice: Effectiveness of a structured multifaceted mentorship programme. *Journal of Advanced Nursing, 66*(12): 2761–71.

Wallin, L., Bostrom, A., & Gustavsson, J. P. (2012). Capability beliefs regarding evidence-based practice are associated with application of EBP and research use: Validation of a new measure. *Worldviews Evidence-based Nursing, 9*(3), 139–148.

West, C. P., & McDonald, F. S. (2008). Evaluation of a longitudinal medical school evidence-based medicine curriculum: A pilot study. *Journal of General Internal Medicine, 23*(7), 1057–1059.

Williams, B. C., & Hoffman, R. M. (2008). Teaching tips: A new series in JGIM. *Journal of General Internal Medicine, 23*(1), 112–113.

Winters, C. A., & Echeverri, R. (2012). Teaching strategies to support evidence-based practice. *Critical Care Nurse, 32*(3), 49–54.

Yew, K. S., & Reid, A. (2008). Teaching evidence-based medicine skills: An exploratory study of residency graduates' practice habits. *Family Medicine, 40*(1), 24–31.

Chapter 16

Teaching Evidence-Based Practice in Clinical Settings

Karen Balakas and Ellen Fineout-Overholt

In learning you will teach, and
in teaching you will learn.

—Phil Collins

It is critically important for all healthcare providers and leadership to consider how and why evidence-based practice (EBP) is a part of the culture of any organization. For best practice to thrive, the EBP paradigm must be a core value held by leadership and point-of-care providers, not just an edict from the top down. As part of this cultural shift, educators in health care are essential facilitators for EBP to flow to the point of care (Rickbeil & Simones, 2012). Furthermore, many educators are designated EBP mentors whose role is to foster a culture of EBP within an organization (Gawlinski & Becker, 2012).

One method that healthcare educators can employ to shift the thinking of point-of-care clinicians to EBP is to document how others have changed outcomes through the implementation of EBP. There are many examples in the literature of how clinicians have used the EBP process to improve patient outcomes. For example, hourly rounding has been documented as an effective intervention to reduce fall rates in acute care settings (Tucker, Bieber, Attlesey-Pries, Olson, & Dierkhising, 2012). Sedwick, Lance-Smith, Reeder, and Nardi (2012) found that an evidence-based bundle greatly reduced their incidence of ventilator-associated pneumonia. However, EBP change may be seen as temporary, unless all clinicians are aware of the purpose and the process for each evidence-based initiative. In the situation with Tucker and colleagues, an unexpected clinical situation emerged at the time the hourly rounding was being implemented that resulted in a mandate from administration rather than the training that had been planned. Subsequently, the fidelity of the intervention (i.e., how well the intervention was followed as it was described in the research) was quite variable, with nursing staff reporting that they felt a lack of decision making. Real-life examples such as these are very helpful to educators who are working with clinicians who daily experience the competing priorities of "getting the work done" and of ensuring evidence-based care.

Not only is EBP the right thing to do, as it improves healthcare outcomes (Jeffs et al., 2013; Kim et al., 2013; Linton & Prasun, 2013; Lusardi, 2012; Murphy, Wilson, & Newhouse, 2013), but also regulatory and accrediting agencies have indicated that, from a safety standpoint as well as a reimbursement standpoint, organizations that are practicing based on evidence will reap rewards. Patient safety is an imperative. Organizations must know the best initiatives that reliably produce the safest environments. Educators must be able to translate for clinicians the evidence that demonstrates these expected safety outcomes. Every clinician must be aware that lives are lost every year due to preventable errors by clinicians and systems (Institute of Medicine, 2001). The National Patient Safety Goals (The Joint Commission, 2013) clearly indicate that evidence-based initiatives are to be put into place to achieve best outcomes for patients. Furthermore, the Center for Medicare & Medicaid Services (DHHS, 2012) has mandated that preventable, nosocomial infections (e.g., urinary tract infections), and other complications (e.g., pressure ulcers) will no longer be reimbursed and that evidence-based care must be manifest. Such a mandate can foster opportunity to bring the evidence to the clinician that supports why these clinical issues are so important to address. This partnership enables innovative decision making between the patient and the provider that will bring about outcomes that will be best for the patient, impact potential disengagement by the point-of-care provider, and, as a matter of course, comply with the mandate.

Evidence-based care makes sense from a safety perspective and from a best care perspective. Best care cannot be distilled down into safe-only care. There are issues such as cost effectiveness, quality, and satisfaction also that are important to consider. The American Nurses Credentialing Center's (ANCC) Magnet program has become another driver in the EBP movement by setting standards of clinical excellence (Schreiber, 2013). These standards hinge on the EBP paradigm as the underpinning philosophy for health care, from care delivered at the bedside to decisions made in the executive boardroom. Healthcare educators have the privilege of making these standards meaningful to point-of-care clinicians as well as leadership. While this may sound simple, there are challenges to bringing EBP alive in clinical settings.

CHALLENGES IN THE CLINICAL SETTING

EBP has become recognized as a necessary component of quality patient care, prompting many healthcare organizations to invest resources into the creation of a culture that sustains the integration of evidence into direct care decision making. Nurses at the point of care are essential to the implementation of EBP; therefore, it is important to ascertain factors that may hinder its adoption by these care providers. Identification of barriers to achievement of EBP has been studied extensively (Barako, Chege, Wakasiaka, & Omondi, 2012; De Pedro-Gomez et al., 2011; Grant, Janson, Johnson, Idell, & Rutledge, 2012; Rickbeil & Simones, 2012). Among the most cited barriers remain individual nurses' EBP skill level and the time needed to find sufficient research (Dalheim, Harthug, Nilsen, & Nortvedt, 2012; Maaskant, Knops, Ubbink, & Vermeulen, 2013).

Today's nurses are increasingly being challenged by patients and healthcare organizations to demonstrate high-quality and measurable patient care outcomes. However, nurses report that they continue to use experience-based knowledge collected from their own observations and input from colleagues (Dalheim et al., 2012). Thus, since nurses most often practice nursing guided by what they learned in nursing school and their clinical experiences, evaluating how age and educational preparation of the registered nurse (RN) population affects their decision making may offer insights.

According to the 2008 National Sample Survey of Registered Nurses (NSSRN; Health Resources and Services Administration [HRSA]), the median age of the nurse remained steady at 46 years, reflecting no increase since 2004. This change from a rising median age is a reflection of the increasing number of nurses under the age of 30 entering the workforce. Over the past several years there have been rising enrollments in schools of nursing, in particular in bachelor's nursing programs whose student population can be younger than that of other initial nursing education programs. However, it is important to note that over 50% of the nursing workforce is nearing retirement (NNSRN).

Educational preparation is an important factor that needs to be considered when planning strategies to teach EBP. Since the 2008 NSSRN reported that over half of RNs (56.7%) obtained their primary nursing education in an associate degree program, nurses who graduated from these programs, even 5 years ago, may have not had formal education in research or EBP. From 2004 to 2008, the percentage of nurses whose highest initial nursing preparation was a baccalaureate degree increased only from 40.1% to 40.3%, while the number of diploma prepared nurses continued to steadily decline (HRSA, 2008). Although these figures reflect a slight change in initial nursing preparation and therefore foundational knowledge of EBP, there is some evidence to support that today's nursing population will still require education specific to research and EBP in the clinical environment (Winters & Echeverri, 2012).

According to Kim et al. (2013), nurses have difficulty interpreting and applying study findings, and knowledge resulting from scientific research is seldom used in practice. Kelly and colleagues (2011) reported that the majority of nurses did not appreciate the contribution of research for practice. Their study found that the relationship between research findings and patient care outcomes had not been stressed to most practicing nurses. They also noted that by not conducting process and patient outcome evaluations after planned practice changes, the application of research to practice was not emphasized. The possible limited ability of clinical nurses to understand research is of great concern, since nurses are expected to evaluate research to determine which findings produce better outcomes before they apply it. Nurses stated that although they were aware of the importance of research to guide practice, it was often implemented through a top-down hierarchy that eliminates the staff nurse from the process. The result is decreased commitment by staff nurses to adopt EBP or implement research findings (Kelly et al., 2011).

Nurses report that although they believe that practice should be based on all evidence, including research, they rarely consult with healthcare librarians or use nursing research. Nurses often lack the skills and the time needed to locate research information and indicate that they feel much more confident asking colleagues or searching the Internet (e.g., Google Scholar) than using bibliographic databases such as PubMed or CINAHL (Linton & Prasun, 2013; Rickbeil & Simones, 2012). Heavy patient loads and outdated policies and procedures were additional factors that decrease the application of evidence among nurses (Barako et al., 2012). Heaslip, Hewitt-Taylor, and Rowe (2012) found that the organization did not structure the workplace environment itself to foster prioritization of research, thus limiting the ability of the staff to use current best external evidence to inform practice.

Results from the 2008 NSSRN also indicated that although there have been substantial changes in the healthcare delivery system, hospitals still remain the primary setting in which nurses are employed. Stressors related to shortages in the RN workforce and the demands associated with long shifts and increased patient loads are well documented (American Association Colleges of Nursing, 2012; Zinn, Guglielmi, Davis, & Moses, 2012). It is not surprising that a lack of time is frequently cited as one of the major barriers to the implementation of EBP (Barako et al., 2012; Hauck, Winsett, & Kuric, 2012; Heaslip et al., 2012; Linton & Prasun, 2013). Nurses reported that they had little time either during scheduled working hours or during their personal time to engage in activities required for EBP. For many nurses, not only was there no time to search for evidence; there was no time to read or appraise research.

Prior to the current initiative to incorporate EBP into the workplace, staff nurses and other healthcare providers may have had no expectation to question current practice. Adherence to institutional policies and procedures and following physician orders were anticipated nursing behaviors. Nurses incorporated safety into their practice, such as checking medication doses and interactions, but may not have sought information to support or change patient care interventions. Within the current, changing healthcare environment, nurses are being asked to formulate clinical questions and translate research findings to ensure cost-efficient, clinically effective patient care.

Nurses also report that managers do not always support the implementation of EBP and that there is a lack of organizational commitment to engage in research activities (Hauck et al., 2012; Rickbeil & Simones, 2012). These studies support that there may be a discrepancy between a stated goal for EBP implementation and competing organizational priorities. Hospitals focus on achieving and maintaining a balance that considers patient and staff safety, productivity, improved clinical outcomes, hospital financial viability, enhanced patient satisfaction, and increased staff satisfaction. Support from immediate managers and unit educators is critical to facilitate change toward evidence-based care (Hauck et al., 2012; Sandstrom, Borglin, Nilsson, & Willman, 2011; Wilkinson, Nutley, & Davies, 2011).

For bedside clinicians to engage in EBP, they must have the necessary tools; therefore, teaching EBP has become an imperative for healthcare organizations. Since bedside clinicians directly influence patient care outcomes, it is essential for organizational leadership to understand their ability to implement EBP in the real practice environment (for more information, see Chapter 12). This understanding drives the design of educational initiatives to meet point-of-care providers' learning needs. The introduction of EBP education must be carefully planned and executed so that clinicians truly can incorporate EBP into their everyday practice.

According to Melnyk, Fineout-Overholt, Stillwell, and Williamson (2010), the key to teaching nurses and other healthcare providers about EBP is *buy-in*. Perhaps buy-in is not strong enough—perhaps ownership is truly the key to successful integration of EBP into an organizational culture. When teaching point-of-care providers or healthcare administrators about EBP, the first place to start is with what motivates daily care decisions. Often this is the traditional practice paradigm, which embraces the comfort of "we've always done it that way." While most of those reading this chapter would agree that this is not the best paradigm to follow, we also would likely admit that it is reassuring to be able to predict how things are going to be done. However, the difficulty with this paradigm is that tradition does not guarantee predictable outcomes. Rather, the outcomes vary with the clinician and the interpretation of the norm.

Practicing based on the EBP paradigm (see Figure 1.2) enables variation of care processes with some standardization regarding the inclusion of the external evidence (i.e., research), patient preferences, clinical expertise, and internal evidence. This paradigm focuses on patient outcomes which, for all clinicians and administrators, is the unifying factor. When initiating care practices, the outcome is the driver of decisions. Consider teaching all those involved in health care about why they engage in care practices such as inserting an intravenous line, administering a medication, or performing a diagnostic test. Often clinicians may indicate that processes are the goal of care initiatives; however, processes lead to outcomes. The outcomes are bottom-line drivers for fiscal and resource allocation, and other decisions that establish priorities in health care. Some may see EBP as a burden, a challenge, or a disturbance of the status quo; however, without this kind of disruption, transformation of health care will not occur (Ubbink, Guyatt, & Vermeulen, 2013). Educators, particularly as EBP mentors, are the key to this paradigm shift at the bedside.

ORGANIZATIONAL READINESS FOR TEACHING EVIDENCE-BASED PRACTICE

Teaching EBP in clinical settings is not an option, it is a necessity and, therefore, a leadership responsibility. Although the individual staff nurse may lack the skills for EBP, it is the nursing leaders who must establish a culture for EBP (Fitzsimons & Cooper, 2012), which includes providing the resources and leadership needed to transform the culture to one that uses EBP on a daily basis. The American Nurses Credentialing Center's Magnet program has long indicated that transformational leadership is a requirement for an evidence-based organization. Through this leadership, the vision and value for EBP are communicated to clinicians and an appeal for their active involvement is clearly conveyed. Leaders must be innovative and challenge assumptions. They need to partner with point-of-care providers to achieve outcomes. Transformational leaders demonstrate their commitment by setting forth the vision and providing resources necessary to establish an EBP culture (Everett & Sitterding, 2011; Hauck et al., 2012). Although the incorporation of EBP into nursing curricula has occurred in most baccalaureate programs, the culture must be present to support these new nurses to ask the clinical questions and seek the answers. Leaders are challenged to ensure that the organization is structured to provide the supportive environment needed for EBP to flourish. Nurse scientists and advanced practice nurses need to be accessible and responsive to the bedside nurses who provide direct care (Pierce, 2011).

One method for achieving mutual goals is through shared governance. Establishing a councilor structure in an EBP organization includes an EBP or Research/EBP Council to address clinical issues with evidence. This becomes part of an EBP culture. Clinicians begin to rely on this council for tackling the clinical issues that are important to bedside staff and providing guidance for applying the evidence to their organization. A Practice Council can be a partner that takes the evidence compiled and synthesized by the EBP Council and operationalizes plans for putting standards of care and other policies into place across the organization to address the given clinical issue based on evidence. Commitment to shared governance is key to providing a voice for point-of-care providers so that they are able to actively participate in evidence-based initiatives and improve outcomes (Fitzsimons & Cooper, 2012; Ubbink et al., 2013). Having an EBP Council provides an opportunity to have an impact on the spread of evidence-based decision making. When all councils begin to use evidence-based thinking, the EBP process becomes the norm for making decisions in the organization. An Education Council can make sure that programs offered are evidence based and that EBP is an essential component of orientation and continuing education for all clinical staff. A Leadership Council can ensure that essential resources are provided for clinicians to practice based on evidence and educators to facilitate a culture of EBP.

ESSENTIAL RESOURCES FOR TEACHING EVIDENCE-BASED PRACTICE

Assess Available Resources

One of the first steps in establishing an educational program for EBP in the clinical setting is to assess the resources that are available or could be dedicated to EBP. Challenges to the implementation of EBP can occur at the institutional level as well as with individuals. Solomons and Spross (2011) found that competing priorities, difficulty with recruiting and sustaining a workforce, and insufficient funds to purchase database subscriptions were among the top institutional barriers. Leadership in the development of educational strategies is contingent upon the human resources within the healthcare organization. A clinically focused nurse researcher who is dedicated to the vision of EBP can provide guidance and support as a program is developed. Teaching the EBP process and its associated skills requires the ability to pose searchable, answerable questions; assist in searching for relevant evidence; critically appraise and synthesize evidence; apply evidence in the clinical setting; and guide providers in evaluating outcomes based on evidence (Pierce, 2011; Sawin et al., 2010). If an individual with in-depth knowledge of EBP and research is not available within the organization, establishing a partnership with an academic institution can help to facilitate the development of a program (Linton & Prasun, 2013; Schreiber, 2013).

Assess Educators' Knowledge of EBP

The next step is to assess the knowledge level about EBP among educators within the organization to determine whether additional education may be needed. Building a team of EBP educators and mentors is a crucial component of any educational strategy and EBP culture (Aitken et al., 2011; Fitzsimons & Cooper, 2012; Pierce, 2011). Interdisciplinary teams are an essential factor for building an evidence-based framework in the clinical setting (Sibbald, Wathen, Kothari, & Day, 2013). Once the gaps are identified regarding knowledge and skills needed to teach EBP, there are numerous workshops, courses, and online programs that are available throughout the country to assist team members in gaining basic and advanced EBP knowledge and skills. Some of the more established programs are listed in Box 16.1, and online tutorials that can be easily accessed are listed in Box 16.2.

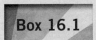

Box 16.1 A Sampling of Available Educational Programs to Learn About Evidence-Based Practice

◆ **McMaster University** offers a 5-day course that is designed to help participants advance their critical appraisal skills, improve their skills in acknowledging and incorporating patient values and preferences in clinical decision making, and learn how to teach EBP using a variety of educational models. (http://ebm.mcmaster.ca/)

◆ **The University of Texas Health Science Center's Academic Center for Evidence-Based Nursing (ACE)** offers a 3-day institute on EBP that is geared toward preparing participants for an increasingly active role in EBP. Knowledge and skills gained through this interdisciplinary conference are directly pertinent to integrating EBP preparation into nursing education programs. Additional learning modules at the basic, intermediate and advanced levels are also available. (http://www.acestar.uthscsa.edu/)

(continued)

◆ **The Johanna Briggs Institute** offers a 6-month workplace, evidence-based, implementation program involving two 5-day intensive training residencies. (http://www.joannabriggs.edu.au/Short%20Courses). In addition, there is an online RAPid critical Appraisal Training Program consisting of seven modules that can be accessed at http://www.joannabriggs.edu.au/RAPcap%20Critical%20Appraisal%20 Training%20Program. In partnership with Sigma Theta Tau International, the Johanna Briggs Institute offers a course titled "Transforming Nursing Practice Through Evidence: The Joanna Briggs Institute Approach" that can be accessed at: http://www.nursingknowledge.org/transforming-nursing-practice-through-evidence -the-joanna-briggs-institute-approach.html

◆ **The Center for Transdisciplinary Evidence-Based Practice at The Ohio State University** offers a 5-day immersion program targeted for clinicians to develop effective strategies to integrate and sustain EBP within their organization as well as change the organizational culture. For academic educators, a 3-day EBP Mentorship Program is designed to prepare faculty to integrate EBP across their nursing curricula. In addition to these initiatives, EBP conferences, workshops, and online programs are offered throughout the year. (http://nursing.osu.edu/sections/ctep/)

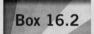

Box 16.2 A Sampling of Available Tutorials on Evidence-Based Practice

◆ *Evidence-Based Medicine: Finding the Best Clinical Literature* from University of Illinois at Chicago (http://www.uic.edu/depts/lib/lhsp/resources/ebm.shtml)
◆ *Centre for Evidence-Based Medicine* from the Mt. Sinai Hospital and University Health Network (Toronto, Ontario, Canada)—this website offers comprehensive and detailed materials on evidence-based practice (http://www.cebm.utoronto.ca/teach/)
◆ *Users' Guides to Evidence-Based Practice* from the Canadian Centre for Health Evidence. These are similar to the series of *JAMA Users' Guides to the Medical Literature*. (http://www.cche.net/text/usersguides/therapy.asp)
◆ Penn State tutorial on EBP for nurses: http://www.libraries.psu.edu/instruction/ ebpt-07/index.htm
◆ Johns Hopkins Nursing Evidence-Based Practice online course can be accessed at http://www.ijhn.jhmi.edu/contEd_3rdLevel_Class.asp?id=EvidBasedHome &numContEdID=4

Assessing Computer Literacy

Determining the basic informatics and computer literacy of educators is necessary in developing the groundwork for teaching EBP in clinical settings. Without educators who are knowledgeable in informatics, including adequate computer skills and the ability to use databases to find relevant evidence, teaching EBP will be challenging. Chapter 3 provides in-depth information for developing effective search strategies for finding relevant evidence in multiple databases to answer clinical questions.

Include Knowledgeable Medical Librarian

Another important issue in the preliminary evaluation of resources is to assure that you have a clinical (i.e., on the unit) or medical librarian on the teaching team who is knowledgeable about EBP. It is imperative that medical librarians be involved in the plan to initiate EBP. It is important to plan early involvement of librarians in preparing an EBP teaching program. If your organization does not have an on-site librarian, it would be important to work toward a partnership with a librarian in a nearby agency or educational institution. As active partners, evidence-based librarians can provide perspective and expertise in search strategy development as well as access to databases and other sources of evidence. In addition, healthcare librarians are experts in informatics and information literacy and can facilitate teaching the skills needed by nurses, physicians, and other healthcare providers who strive to be successful at EBP. Evidence-based librarians foster a culture of EBP within an organization.

An essential resource that facilitates the work of EBP mentors and educators to teach about and sustain EBP implementation is ready access to databases and evidence to support changes in practice. Both PubMed and the Cochrane Library offer free access to search and read abstracts, but clinicians need full-text articles to appraise and apply the evidence. Subscriptions to databases such as CINAHL and online resources such as Nurse or MD Consult can be very helpful for obtaining clinical information. Many hospitals have healthcare libraries and can include vital resources in their holdings that are necessary for clinicians to provide evidence-based care to their population of patients. If a hospital does not have a library, there are online resources that clinicians can join for a fee. DynaMed is an online reference developed for point-of-care clinicians that contains thousands of summaries. This resource is updated daily and monitors the content of more than 500 medical journals and systematic review databases. The literature is critically appraised, integrated into existing content, and synthesized to deliver the best available evidence. Another tool is *Isabel,* a decision-support tool that helps providers expand their differential diagnosis at the point of care providing evidence-based critical information. Another online peer-reviewed resource providing evidence-based reviews is UpToDate, which contains thousands of articles in over 30 categories and provides the user with synthesized recommendations upon which to make treatment decisions. Point-of-care clinicians can also subscribe to the Nursing Reference Center to obtain relevant clinical information. All of these resources can help clinicians model and teach the critical value of EBP to provide improved patient outcomes. Chapter 3 contains more information on sources of evidence.

 Information on DynaMed and a free trial can be found at http://www.ebscohost.com/dynamed/

 Information on UpToDate can be found at http://www.uptodate.com/home

 Information on the Nursing Reference Center can be found at http://ebscohost.com/uploads/thisTopic-dbTopic-1045.pdf

 Information on *Isabel* can be found at http://www.isabelhealthcare.com/home/default

Financial Support

A final crucial element required to teach EBP is financial support. Clinicians need protected time to participate in classes, develop clinical questions, locate evidence, read and appraise the evidence, plan for application of the evidence and implementation of practice changes, and determine evaluation strategies to assess outcomes. This means that administrators and unit-level managers must include time for EBP in their budgets. This time must be reflected as valuable on the schedule as well as the budget. Terms such as "nonproductive time" do not facilitate valuing of EBP among staff, managers, or agency leadership.

A budget that provides for dedicated time to engage in evidence-based project work demonstrates to staff nurses that the education for and implementation of EBP is valued by leadership (Ingersoll, Witzel, Berry, & Qualls, 2010; Ubbink et al., 2013).

EDUCATIONAL STRATEGIES FOR TEACHING EVIDENCE-BASED PRACTICE

Teaching EBP requires a tiered educational approach. It is not enough to just offer classes to bedside clinicians without first engaging direct-line managers in the process. Managers, unit educators, and advanced practice nurses serve as models of change for point-of-care staff. They can foster the implementation of EBP, if they too understand its value, their role in the process, and can see the link between the use of external and internal evidence and improved patient outcomes (Hauck et al., 2012; Linton & Prasun, 2013; Sandstrom et al., 2011). One way to accomplish this undertaking is to first determine the model(s) upon which to base the program. The next step is to schedule one or several meetings to introduce the EBP model(s), discuss the steps of EBP, and present the clinicians' unique role in developing and sustaining EBP on the unit. An example from my work with organizations includes one pediatric hospital's professional practice department's decision to host a luncheon meeting for nurse managers and administrators prior to launching an educational program for staff nurses. This preliminary step proved to be a crucial one, since each nurse manager was needed to identify a staff nurse whose leadership skills might grow from being involved in an EBP program. In another institution, the Nursing Research/EBP Committee developed a strategic plan that specifically addressed establishment of a culture to support EBP. The role of nursing leadership in promotion of an EBP culture was listed among the plan's objectives (Hauck et al., 2012). It is vital to the success of an EBP project that it is fully supported by managers with clearly identified benefits for each unit's population (Balakas, Sparks, Steurer, & Bryant, 2012; Wilkinson et al., 2011). Similar meetings to present EBP to supervisors, case managers, and clinical educators also are needed to sustain adoption of EBP.

Once a team of educators and EBP mentors has been developed, additional intensive efforts can begin to educate bedside caregivers. Numerous EBP educational programs for clinical staff have been documented in the literature (Bromirski, Cody, Coppin, Hewson, & Richardson, 2011; Gawlinski & Becker, 2012; Grant et al., 2012; Kelly et al., 2011; Kim et al., 2013; Lusardi, 2012; Rickbeil & Simones, 2012). The length and depth of each program vary, but the basic content is consistent and includes a comprehensive overview of EBP, a presentation for each step in the process, a discussion of change theory, and often an opportunity to complete a project using what has been taught. Some of the programs are offered in a workshop format that may range from 1 day to 7 days and are presented at one point in time or over several months. Some of these programs include a formal application process and are delivered in a combination of didactic classes, discussion groups, and mentored projects. Classes within these programs provide the clinician with intensive guidance on the development of a PICOT question, building searching skills to locate and retrieve evidence, learning critical appraisal skills, and application of evidence for practice change. Requiring the identification of a clinical question or area of interest prior to participation in a program is very helpful, as it makes it easier for the clinicians to quickly focus on their thinking about evidence-based decision making and applying the steps of EBP. Using clinicians' PICOT questions and providing computers for interactive sessions while teaching searching skills is very effective. If a computer lab is not available, securing laptop computers and encouraging participants to work as partners can help to facilitate learning. Given that most hospitals have clinical guidelines readily available, some programs incorporate critical review and updating of the guidelines as a component of the EBP course. This exercise provides the learner with a relevant example to illustrate one aspect of applying the principles of EBP. These programs serve to not only educate clinical staff but also build a cadre of EBP mentors to lead and promote EBP initiatives within the organization. An outline of potential class topics and exercises is listed in Box 16.3.

Since not all clinicians are able to commit to a mentoring role, classes that introduce the concepts of EBP and highlight its potential for improving patient care outcomes can support continued adoption of EBP. At

Box 16.3	Topical Outline for an Evidence-Based Practice Program

1. Introducing the principles of EBP
2. Incorporating the vision for EBP
3. Understanding the institutional EBP model
4. Developing focused clinical questions
   - Defining the clinical problem
   - Developing PICOT questions
5. Recruiting an interdisciplinary team
6. Searching for relevant external evidence
   - Using search engines and EBP databases
   - Finding clinical guidelines
   - Exploring EBP websites
   - Benchmarking
7. Searching for internal evidence
8. Determining performance improvement indicators
9. Critically analyzing the evidence
   - Research designs
   - Using rapid appraisal forms
   - Understanding the statistics
10. Synthesizing evidence
    - Using an evaluation table
    - Using a synthesis table
11. Translating evidence into practice
    - Implications for practice change
    - Defining and evaluating outcomes
    - Piloting the change
12. Evaluating the outcomes to sustain the change
13. Disseminating the evidence

one institution, following participation in an EBP Mentorship Program, three nurses at an academic hospital partnered with a medical librarian and two academic nurse educators and began offering 2-day workshops for bedside staff to deliver an overview of the EBP process. Staff who participate in the workshops are then eligible to apply for a 26-week EBP fellowship that includes more in-depth classes and individual mentoring to complete a project. Teaching smaller classes can adapt content for relevance to the participant's clinical background and prepare a significant number of caregivers who embrace inquiry and value EBP for best practice.

Self-directed learning has been a part of healthcare education for several decades, and the benefits have been documented in the literature for more than 25 years. Self-directed learning incorporates adult learning principles and encourages participants to take an active role in the learning process. This approach may be helpful for motivated clinicians who are not able to attend face-to-face classes or conferences and wish to learn the principles of EBP. Through self-directed learning, participants have the opportunity to set their own priorities and determine their own timeframe for learning. The Department of Nursing at the University of Iowa Hospitals and Clinics offers an online continuing education course to introduce EBP and present a summary of the current state of the science of EBP (https://www.uihealthcare.org/Nursing/Post.aspx?id=235965).

Additional initiatives can be created within the work environment to provide staff with opportunities for learning EBP outside of more traditional methods. One hospital, intent on creating a supportive culture for EBP, conducted an educational needs assessment and discovered inconsistent use of EBP principles by staff. To stimulate consistent integration of EBP, nursing administration partnered with an academic institution to provide several introductory EBP lectures that were open to all staff. Following this fundamental education, they developed a competitive EBP award program to fully engage staff in the integration of EBP. After an application process and critical review by nurse representatives from administration, education, performance improvement, research, and frontline staff, three teams were awarded $5,000 to conduct their projects. Post-award mentoring and seminars were provided to help participants overcome barriers and complete their projects (Kelly et al., 2011).

Another hospital created a proposal and obtained a grant from a local foundation to develop a 1-day hands-on workshop that focused on achievable, small-scale projects. The workshop discussed the elements of EBP and quality improvement considerations. Small group activities were included to help participants develop project ideas and work with a librarian to complete an initial search for evidence. Nurses could attend individually or in teams, and participants were then mentored for 12 months to complete the projects (Grant et al., 2012).

Within the past several years, EBP Fellowships for staff nurses have been developed to foster professional development and skills in making EBP changes. A collaborative regional fellowship program was created by healthcare professionals from academic institutions and several hospitals in California. The program targets nurse leaders (managers, educators, advanced practice nurses, and directors) to become primary mentors for selected staff nurses. The dyads (groups of two each) complete a clinical practice project in their home institution over a 9-month period. The recent evaluation of the program indicted that it has been successful in reducing the barriers to EBP at both the individual and organizational levels (Kim et al., 2013).

Additional fellowship programs have been created at individual institutions to further support development of EBP and leadership skills. The need for mentoring throughout the process so that outcomes are achieved, documented and evaluated has been recognized as a critical need for the success of EBP programs (Gawlinski & Becker, 2012). The length of these programs varies but each includes mentoring through dissemination as an important component.

The committee structure of the organization provides another venue for teaching EBP. Hospitals traditionally support a committee dedicated to the development and review of policies and procedures that impart guidance for the care frontline staff provide to patients and families. Policies and procedures provide the direction to implement procedures, deliver patient education, and evaluate interventions. Establishing a process that supports the integration of evidence into policies, procedures, and guidelines ensures safety and rigor while embracing EBP (Lusardi, 2012). To accomplish this goal, participants need to learn skills necessary to implement EBP. Evidence can be located, appraised, and then used to further develop or update documents as well as to create an evidence-based process or algorithm to guide the committee's work.

Journal clubs have been used effectively for decades in the clinical setting to assist providers who want to improve the application of research into practice. Traditionally, journal clubs that have been either *topic-based* or *teaching-based* provided a forum for healthcare providers to discuss clinical issues, the current research available on the topic, and the recommended basis for clinical decisions related to treatment options. They have also been used as a teaching/learning strategy to help clinicians learn about EBP and how evidence can be used for clinical decision making. EBP-skills-focused journal clubs teach participants the steps needed for EBP from development of a PICOT question through application of evidence and evaluation of clinical outcomes.

Active participation in a journal club is frequently dependent on some knowledge of the research appraisal process. Providing classes about the critical appraisal of research, including evaluating the validity of research methods, can support bedside clinicians to become involved in unit-based journal clubs. However, participation in such classes may seem daunting for some clinical staff. Also, the additional time commitment for another meeting may compete with other hospital committees and the daily demands of patient care needs. Incorporating a modified journal club format into existing unit committee meetings is an effective teaching strategy to teach appraisal skills and engender interest in the use of research to guide practice. The EBP mentor/teacher can locate an article relevant to the unit's patient population and either post it on the unit's bulletin board or distribute it electronically prior to the meeting. The beginning of the meeting can then be used to role model appraisal of the article and brainstorm with the group potential applications for practice. This strategy has been used successfully in one hospital during unit practice committee meetings to implement bedside reporting, a new tube-feeding protocol, fall-prevention rounds, family presence during resuscitation, the effective use of capnography, and the use of noninvasive technology to assess tissue oxygenation and stroke volume. Committee members have learned the steps of EBP and can clearly articulate why they chose specific practices. As the clinical staff have become educated about EBP, they are able to communicate more effectively with other disciplines and engage more frequently in scholarly discussions (Honey & Baker, 2011).

Teaching EBP in the clinical setting can also be enhanced through partnerships with academic institutions. A collaborative EBP effort encompassing two projects was developed by faculty from two nursing programs and a clinical nurse specialist at one institution. A need for a comprehensive oral hygiene program for adult and pediatric patients in critical care and acute care settings was the focus of 20 nursing students. The second project centered on best practices for sleep apnea patients. Both projects involved frontline nurses along with students in the EBP process as policies were developed and education delivered to hospital committees and staff. Students were able to contribute their expertise in searching the literature and appraising the findings; staff nurses could identify significant problems and knew hospital processes (Rickbeil & Simones, 2012).

As clinicians become skilled in the steps of EBP and complete projects, they will need guidance in learning how to share their work through oral and poster presentations. Some staff will be required to deliver a presentation following the completion of an educational program, while others will want to communicate the results of their endeavors internally and externally. In addition to individual guidance, classes in how to develop presentations can be very helpful. Promotion of attendance and presentations at local, state, and national conferences by the EBP leadership team supports previous teaching efforts and strengthens the clinician's knowledge base. One example from my work with organizations includes nurses from one community and one academic hospital participated in a 12-month EBP Fellowship program that produced 12 completed projects. When a call for abstracts from the state university was issued, the staff nurses were encouraged to submit their projects. EBP mentors helped them write and submit the abstracts and then helped them develop their posters. Hospital administration from both institutions financially supported the nurses' attendance at the regional EBP conference where they expanded their knowledge of EBP and returned with increased enthusiasm and commitment to EBP.

Teaching EBP in a clinical setting requires commitment, diligence, enthusiasm, creativity, and teamwork. It is not accomplished through one program, one committee, or one project. It requires an ability to set goals and then evaluate progress toward the attainment of those goals. Teaching EBP is a continuous process that will result in improved patient care outcomes, professional growth, and an empowered clinical staff. Teaching EBP can be a personally and professionally rewarding experience.

EBP FAST FACTS

- ◆ EBP is essential for optimal patient outcomes and clinical educators must be able to promote and sustain its everyday implementation.
- ◆ Although nurses state they believe practice should be based on research, over 56% of today's nurses have had no education specific to research or EBP.
- ◆ Barriers to EBP implementation remain in the clinical setting, most often reported as the skill level of the individual nurse, lack of time, and lack of managerial support.

- For bedside nurses to engage in EBP, they must have the necessary tools, thus teaching EBP has become an imperative for healthcare organizations.
- Teaching EBP is a leadership responsibility and requires organizational commitment to provide the resources needed to support a cultural change for EBP.
- Following assessment of organizational readiness, financial support, and available resources, a tiered educational approach is needed to engage managers, educators, and point-of-care staff in EBP.

References

Aitken, L. M., Hackwood, B., Crouch, S., Clayton, S., West, N., Carney, D., & Jack, L. (2011). Creating an environment to implement and sustain evidence based practice: A developmental process. *Australian Critical Care: Official Journal of the Confederation of Australian Critical Care Nurses, 24*(4), 244–254. doi:10.1016/j.aucc.2011.01.004

American Association Colleges of Nursing. (2012). *Nursing shortage.* Retrieved from http://www.aacn.nche.edu/media-relations/fact-sheets/nursing-shortage

Balakas, K., Sparks, L., Steurer, L., & Bryant, T. (2012). An outcome of evidence-based practice education: Sustained clinical decision-making among bedside nurses. *Journal of Pediatric Nursing 28*(5), 479–485. doi:10.1016/j.pedn.2012.08.007 (Epub ahead of print).

Barako, T. D., Chege, M., Wakasiaka, S., & Omondi, L. (2012). Factors influencing application of evidence-based practice among nurses. *African Journal of Midwifery and Women's Health, 6*(2), 71–77.

Bromirski, B. H., Cody, J. L., Coppin, K., Hewson, K., & Richardson, B. (2011). Evidence-based practice day: An innovative educational opportunity. *Western Journal of Nursing Research, 33*(3), 333–344.

Dalheim, A., Harthug, S., Nilsen, R. M., & Nortvedt, M. W. (2012). Factors influencing the development of evidence-based practice among nurses: A self-report survey. *BMC Health Services Research, 12*, 367. doi:10.1186/1472-6963-12-367. Retrieved from http://www.biomedcentral.com/1472-6963/12/367

Department of Health and Human Services, Centers for Medicare and Medicaid Services. (2012). *Hospital Acquired Conditions (HAC) in Acute Inpatient Prospective Payment System (IPPS) Hospitals.* Retrieved from http://www.cms.gov/Medicare/Medicare-Fee-for-Service-Payment/HospitalAcqCond/downloads/hacfactsheet.pdf

De Pedro-Gomez, J., Morales-Asencio, J. M., Bennasar-Veny, M., Artigues-Vives, G., Perello-Campaner, C., & Gomez-Picard, P. (2011). Determining factors in evidence-based clinical practice among hospital and primary care nursing staff. *Journal of Advanced Nursing, 68*(2), 452–459. doi:10.1111/j.1365-2648.2011.05733.x

Everett, L. Q., & Sitterding, M. C. (2011). Transformational leadership required to design and sustain evidence-based practice: A system exemplar. *Western Journal of Nursing Research, 33*(3), 398–426. doi:10.1177/0193945910383056

Fitzsimons, E., & Cooper, J. (2012). Embedding a culture of evidence-based practice. *Nursing Management, 19*(7), 14–19.

Gawlinski, A., & Becker, E. (2012). Infusing research into practice. *Journal for Nurses in Staff Development, 28*(2), 69–73. doi:10.1097/NND.0b013e31824b418c

Grant, M., Janson, J., Johnson, S., Idell, C., & Rutledge, D. N. (2012). Evidence-based practice for staff nurses. *The Journal of Continuing Education in Nursing, 43*(3), 117–124. doi:10.3928/00220124-20110901-02

Hauck, S., Winsett, R. P., & Kuric, J. (2012). Leadership facilitation strategies to establish evidence-based practice in an acute care hospital. *Journal of Advanced Nursing, 69*(3), 664–674. doi:10.1111/j.1365-2648.2012.06053.x

Health Resources and Services Administration. (2008). *The registered nurse population: Findings from the 2008 national sample survey of registered nurses*, September 2010. Retrieved from http://bhpr.hrsa.gov/healthworkforce/rnsurveys/rnsurveyfinal.pdf

Heaslip, V., Hewitt-Taylor, J., & Rowe, N. E. (2012). Reflecting on nurses' views on using research in practice. *British Journal of Nursing, 21*(22), 1341–1346.

Honey, C. P., & Baker, J. A. (2011). Exploring the impact of journal clubs: A systematic review. *Nurse Education Today, 31*(8), 825–831. doi: http://dx.doi.org/10.1016/j.nedt.2010.12.020

Ingersoll, G. L., Witzel, P. A., Berry, C., & Qualls, B. (2010). Meeting Magnet® research and evidence-based practice expectations through hospital-based research centers. *Nursing Economics, 28*(4), 226–236. doi:http://search.ebscohost.com/login.aspx?direct=true&db=ccm&AN=2010764399&site=nrc-live

Institute of Medicine. (2001). *Crossing the quality chasm.* Washington, DC: National Academies Press.

Jeffs, L., Sidani, S., Rose, D., Espin, S., Smith, O., Martin, K., … Ferris, E. (2013). Using theory and evidence to drive measurement of patient, nurse and organizational outcomes of professional nursing practice. *International Journal of Nursing Practice, 19*(2), 141–148. doi:10.1111/ijn. 12048

Kelly, K. P., Guzzetta, C. E., Mueller-Burke, D., Nelson, K., DuVal, J., Hinds, P. S., & Robinson, N. (2011). Advancing evidence-based nursing practice in a children's hospital using competitive awards. *Western Journal of Nursing Research, 33*(3), 306–332. doi:10.1177/0193945910379586

Kim, S. C., Brown, C. E., Ecoff, L., Davidson, J. E., Gallo, A. M., Klimpel, K., & Wickline, M. A. (2013). Regional evidence-based practice fellowship program: Impact on evidence-based practice implementation and barriers. *Clinical Nursing Research, 22*(1), 51–69. doi:10.1177/1054773812446063

Linton, M. J., & Prasun, M. A. (2013). Evidence-based practice: Collaboration between education and nursing management. *Journal of Nursing Management, 21*, 5–16. doi:10.1111/j.1365-2834.2012.01440.x

Lusardi, P. (2012). So you want to change practice: Recognizing practice issues and channeling those ideas. *Critical Care Nurse, 32*(2), 55–63. doi:10.4037/ccn2012899

Maaskant, J. M., Knops, A. M., Ubbink, D. T., & Vermeulen, H. (2013). Evidence-based practice: A survey among pediatric nurses and pediatricians. *Journal of Pediatric Nursing, 28*, 150–157. doi:10.1016/j.pedn.2012.05.002

Melnyk, B., Fineout-Overholt, E., Stillwell, S., & Williamson, K. (2010). Transforming healthcare quality through innovations in evidence-based practice. In T. Porter-O'Grady & K. Malloch (Eds.), *The leadership of innovation: Creating the landscape for healthcare transformation* (pp. 167–194). Sudbury, MA: Jones & Bartlett.

Murphy, L. S., Wilson, M. L., & Newhouse, R. P. (2013). Improving care transitions through meaningful use stage 2: Continuity of care document. *Journal of Nursing Administration, 43*(2), 62–65. doi:10.1097/NNA.0b013e31827f2076

Pierce, C. J. (2011). Establishing a methodology for development and dissemination of nursing evidence-based practice to promote quality care. *U.S. Army Medical Department Journal, Oct.–Dec.*, 41–44.

Rickbeil, P., & Simones, J. (2012). Overcoming barriers to implementing evidence-based practice. *Journal for Nurses in Staff Development, 28*(2), 53–56. doi:10.1097/NND.0b013e31824b4141

Sandstrom, B., Borglin, G., Nilsson, R., & Willman, A. (2011). Promoting the implementation of evidence-based practice: A literature review focusing on the role of nursing leadership. *Worldviews on Evidence-Based Nursing, 8*(4), 212–223. doi:10.1111/j.1741-6787.2011.00216.x

Sawin, K. J., Gralton, K. S., Harrison, T. M., Malin, S., Balchunas, M. K., Brock, L. A., … Schiffman, R. F. (2010). Nurse researchers in children's hospitals. *Journal of Pediatric Nursing, 25*(5), 408–417. doi:10.1016/j.pedn.2009.07.005

Schreiber, J. A. (2013). Beyond evidence-based practice: Achieving fundamental changes in research and practice. *Oncology Nursing Forum, 40*(3), 208–210. doi:10.1188/13.ONF.208-210

Sedwick, M. B., Lance-Smith, M., Reeder, S. J., & Nardi, J. (2012). Using evidence-based practice to prevent ventilator-associated pneumonia. *Critical Care Nurse, 32*(4), 41–50. doi:10.4037/ccn2012964

Sibbald, S. L., Wathen, C. N., Kothari, A., & Day, A. M. B. (2013). Knowledge flow and exchange in interdisciplinary primary health care teams (PHCTs): An exploratory study. *Journal of the Medical Library Association, 101*(2), 128–137. doi:10.3163/1536-5050.101.2.008

Solomons, N. M., & Spross, J. A. (2011). Evidence-based practice barriers and facilitators from a continuous quality improvement perspective: An integrative review. *Journal of Nursing Management, 19*(1), 109–120. doi:10.1111/j.1365-2834.2010.01144.x

The Joint Commission. (2013). *Hospital: National Patient Safety Goals*. Retrieved from http://www.jointcommission.org/standards_information/npsgs.aspx

Tucker, S. J., Bieber, P. L., Attlesey-Pries, J. M., Olson, M. E., & Dierkhising, R. A. (2012). Outcomes and challenges in implementing hourly rounds to reduce falls in orthopedic units. *Worldviews on Evidence-Based Nursing, 9*(1), 18–29. doi:10.1111/j.1741-6787.2011.00227.x

Ubbink, D. T., Guyatt, G. H., & Vermeulen, H. (2013). Framework of policy recommendations for implementation of evidence-based practice: A systematic scoping review. *BMJ Open 2013, 3*, e001881. doi:10.1136/bmjopen-2012-001881

Wilkinson, J. E., Nutley, S. M., & Davies, H. T. O. (2011). An exploration of the roles of nurse managers in evidence-based practice implementation. *Worldviews on Evidence-Based Nursing, 8*(4), 236–246. doi:10.1111/j.1741-6787.2011.00225.x

Winters, C. A., & Echeverri, R. (2012). Teaching strategies to support evidence-based practice. *Critical Care Nurse, 32*(3), 49–54. doi:10.4037/ccn2012159

Zinn, J. L., Guglielmi, C. L., Davis, P. P., & Moses, C. (2012). Addressing the nursing shortage: The need for nurse residency programs. *AORN Journal, 96*(6), 652–657. doi:10.1016/j.aorn.2012.09.011

Chapter 17

ARCC Evidence-Based Practice Mentors: The Key to Sustaining Evidence-Based Practice

Ellen Fineout-Overholt and Bernadette Mazurek Melnyk

Mentoring is more an affair of the heart than the head—it is a 2 way relationship that is based on trust. A mentor wins and sustains the mentee's trust through constancy (staying the course), reliability (being there when it counts), integrity (honoring commitments and promises), and walking the talk.

—M. J. Tobin

OVERVIEW OF THE ARCC MODEL AND EVOLUTION OF EVIDENCE-BASED PRACTICE (EBP) MENTORS

A mentor is a trusted coach or teacher, whether in EBP or any other endeavor. Tobin (2004) describes the following roles of a mentor: (a) teacher, (b) sponsor, (c) advisor, (d) agent, (e) role model, (f) coach, and (g) confidante. A mentor typically provides directional guidance, fosters self-confidence, and instills values in the mentee (Wensel, 2006). Unlike having a preceptor who sets specific goals to be met in a limited period of time (Funderburk, 2008), the mentor–mentee relationship usually is enduring and dynamic. One might call it synergistic (Figure 17.1). The relationship changes over time to meet the mentee's and mentor's needs (Bellack & Morjikian, 2005; Wensel, 2006). Characteristics of effective mentors include a minimum of beginning expert knowledge and skills, patience, enthusiasm, a sense of humor, respect, positive attitude, and good communication and listening skills (Fawcett, 2002; Kanaskie, 2006). Characteristics of good mentees include leadership, self-awareness, creative thinking, receptiveness to constructive feedback, good judgment, integrity, and political awareness (Abedin et al., 2012).

This chapter provides a foundational overview of the role and purpose of the ARCC EBP mentor. ARCC EBP mentors have a unique mentor/mentee relationship that is focused on improving patient care along with professional healthcare practice through EBP. Consider that the implementation of EBP is known to improve the quality of care and patient outcomes, which is a major reason why third-party payers are incentivizing organizations to deliver evidence-based care, yet, healthcare systems are having challenges sustaining a culture of EBP. *Sustainability* has become a buzz word in today's world and, in its broadest sense, means an emphasis on cultivating a high quality of life for generations to come by promoting and maintaining security, clean air, and health (Fineout-Overholt, Williamson, Gallagher-Ford, Melnyk, & Stillwell, 2011; Gallagher-Ford, Fineout-Overholt, Melnyk, & Stillwell, 2011; Melnyk, 2007). For EBP to be sustained in healthcare systems, there needs to be a key mechanism inherent in organizations to promote the continued system-wide advancement of evidence-based care once it is initiated. As first proposed in the Advancing Research and Clinical practice through close Collaboration (ARCC) Model (Melnyk & Fineout-Overholt, 2002; Melnyk, Fineout-Overholt, Gallagher-Ford, & Stillwell, 2011), this key mechanism is an **EBP mentor**, typically an advanced practice clinician with in-depth knowledge and skills in EBP as well as individual behavioral and organizational change strategies. An EBP mentor, however, can be any clinician with expert knowledge of EBP and a desire to assist others in advancing excellence through evidence-based care. A facilitator works with individuals, teams, and organizations to prepare, guide, and support them through the evidence implementation process. While a facilitator and an EBP mentor are both focused on evidence implementation and its context and

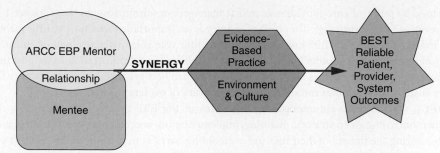

Figure 17.1: Unique relationship between ARCC EBP mentor and mentee.

change in patient outcome, an EBP mentor is also concerned with development of the clinician who is caring for the patient, which leads to sustainable changes in the organizational environment. As with other mentoring relationships, careful consideration of role expectations of both the EBP mentor and those receiving mentorship should include building rapport between mentor/mentee; selecting mechanisms for regular communication in which feedback is shared between mentor/mentee; advocating for a supportive environment in which administrative as well as overall psychosocial support is evident; striving for work/life balance while maximizing career progression options; and fostering social networking (Nick et al., 2012). Both mentor and mentee require clear expectations. The ARCC EBP mentor role should be outlined in the role description as well as performance appraisal criteria. These specialized roles require seminars on how to be an EBP mentor, including how to negotiate and effectively leverage release time for this role.

The ARCC Model is a guide for system-wide implementation and sustainability of EBP in healthcare organizations that focuses on assisting clinicians with EBP knowledge, beliefs, and skills building to consistently implement evidence-based care and the building of EBP cultures to sustain best practices. The model was first conceptualized to provide a framework for advancing EBP within an academic medical center and surrounding community (see Chapter 13). Nurses identified mentorship as an important success strategy to assist point-of-care staff with the implementation of EBP (Melnyk & Fineout-Overholt, 2002, 2010). Thus, the term *EBP mentor* was coined to emphasize the key role of mentorship in promoting and sustaining the use of evidence-based care by point-of-care staff and in building cultures that support EBP (Melnyk, 2007; Melnyk & Fineout-Overholt, 2010).

In the ARCC Model, EBP mentors use findings from an assessment of the readiness and culture of an organization for system-wide implementation of EBP to guide them in developing a strategic plan to enhance clinicians' knowledge and skills in EBP and to foster a culture of best practice. Evidence from research has supported that EBP mentors enhance point-of-care providers' beliefs about the value of EBP and their ability to implement it, which in turn leads to greater EBP implementation (EBPI) (Levin, Fineout-Overholt, Melnyk, Barnes, & Vetter, 2011; Mariano et al., 2011; Melnyk et al., 2004; Wallen et al., 2011). Research further supports that when EBPI is enhanced, group cohesion is strengthened and turnover rates are less (Levin et al., 2011). A key outcome of reduced staff turnover is substantial cost savings for healthcare organizations. For more specific information about the ARCC Model, see Chapter 13.

THE ARCC EBP MENTOR ROLE

EBP mentors first ensure that those they mentor and others with whom they work have a common understanding of the definition of EBP. For these mentors, EBP is defined as a problem-solving approach to clinical practice that integrates the *best evidence* (after systematic appraisal of both internal and external evidence) with a *clinician's expertise* and *patient preferences and values* to make decisions about the type of care that is provided in their setting and which are the most appropriate outcomes to be evaluated to demonstrate sustainable best care. In addition, these mentors ensure that the seven-step EBP process is well understood by point-of-care providers as well as managers or administrators (see Chapter 1 for more on the seven-step EBP process). The spirit of inquiry is an important focus for the EBP mentor. Without this initial element of an EBP culture, the EBP mentor role is less effective and often can be perceived as nothing more than another bureaucratic role established by administration to support their agenda. EBP mentors can serve both as catalysts for change toward best practice and as the stability factors that foster sustainable outcomes through consistent delivery of evidence-based care.

In the ARCC Model, there are important components of the EBP mentor role (Box 17.1) that enable these mentors to engage in strategic planning, implementation, and outcomes evaluation that are focused on monitoring the impact of their role and overcoming barriers in moving the system to a culture of best practice (Melnyk, 2007; Wallen et al., 2011). There is determined purpose in the mentoring of direct care staff on clinical units, in primary care practice, or in public health practice—to strengthen clinicians' beliefs about the value of EBP and their ability to implement it (see Figure 17.1) (Holliman, Resler, Edmunds, & Child Life Council, 2010; Levin et al., 2011; Melnyk & Fineout-Overholt, 2002; Olson Keller, Strohschein, & Schaffer, 2011; Wallen et al., 2011).

Each agency can individualize the role of the EBP mentor. Imperative to the role are the components in Box 17.1 and a focus on reliable best outcomes. Often, health care has been focused on processes, such as measurement of time from door to discharge in the emergency department or sign-in to exit for a primary care practice. EBP mentors are focused on both the outcomes of these processes as well as the processes themselves. These mentors assist with refining processes for the purpose or improving outcomes (Melnyk, Fineout-Overholt, Giggleman, & Cruz, 2010; Roe & Whyte-Marshall, 2011).

As systems strategists, EBP mentors (a) strategically plan, implement, and monitor/evaluate outcomes; (b) evaluate the impact of their role as EBP mentors; and (c) overcome barriers in moving to a culture of best practice (Table 17.1). These mentors play a strategic role in sustaining an EBP culture (Ervin, 2005; Fineout-Overholt, Melnyk, & Schultz, 2005; Levin et al., 2011; Melnyk & Fineout-Overholt, 2002; Melnyk et al., 2010; Morgan, 2012; Wallen et al., 2011). Mentorship makes a difference (Sambunjak, Straus, & Marušic, 2006). Dr. Rona Levin and Dr. Linda Olson-Keller indicated that they had taught clinicians about EBP for many years, but not until the mentor was introduced into their respective groups did the clinicians embrace the use of evidence (Levin et al., 2011; L. Olson-Keller, personal communication, June 9, 2009). The problem was not a knowledge deficit and could not be resolved by teaching alone. What was missing was the mentoring component that moves EBP into the realm of the everyday, the expected norm for professional practice.

Box 17.1   Components of the ARCC EBP Mentor Role

- ◆ Ongoing assessment of an organization's capacity to sustain an EBP culture
- ◆ Building EBP knowledge and skills through conducting interactive group workshops and one-to-one mentoring
- ◆ Stimulating, facilitating, and educating clinicians toward a culture of EBP, with a focus on overcoming barriers to best practice
- ◆ Role modeling EBP
- ◆ Conducting ARCC strategies to enhance the implementation of EBP, such as journal clubs, EBP rounds, web pages, newsletters, and fellowship programs
- ◆ Working with staff to generate internal evidence (i.e., practice-generated) through quality improvement, outcomes management, and EBP implementation projects
- ◆ Facilitating staff involvement in research to generate external evidence
- ◆ Using evidence to foster best practice
- ◆ Collaborating with interdisciplinary professionals to advance and sustain EBP

Table 17.1 Identified Barriers and Facilitators of the EBP Mentor Role

Barriers	Facilitators
• Competing clinical priorities	Continued contact with the mentorship program faculty
• Time	The ability to ask questions
• Allocated resources	The availability of assistance with data analysis
• Existing politics in the organization	Assistance with project development
• Lack of administrative support	A supportive chief nursing officer or director of EBP or nurse researcher
• No accountability for EBP	A network of fellow EBP mentors
	EBP as an expectation of the Joint Commission on the Accreditation of Healthcare Organizations (JCAHO) and Magnet

....

What is experienced and seen in the clinical area is what will likely predict future behavior.
—Bob Berenson

....

EVIDENCE TO SUPPORT THE POSITIVE IMPACT OF MENTORSHIP ON OUTCOMES

There is a growing body of evidence that supports the positive impact that mentors have on individual and system outcomes (Table 17.2) (Melnyk et al., 2010; Roe & Whyte-Marshall, 2011; Varkey et al., 2012). Researchers found that students had a more satisfactory learning experience with mentors (Collins et al., 2011). Students stated, "It is wonderful to have someone who cares for us personally and professionally. It is nice to have a complete stranger who now wants to help me make myself a better clinician" (p. 229). In another study, mentoring was found to influence career success in a group of physicians; however, there were not enough mentors for all students, particularly females (Stamm & Buddeberg-Fischer, 2011).

Table 17.2 Evidence Supported Outcomes of Mentoring

Outcome	Impact
Satisfaction	⇧
Career progression/development	⇧
Self-confidence	⇧
Publications	⇧
Research	⇧
Grants	⇧

Findings of the 2006 systematic review of 42 mainly cross-sectional descriptive studies that evaluated the evidence about the prevalence of mentorship and its impact on career development (Sambunjak et al., 2006) continue to be relevant. This review indicated that less than 50% of medical students and, in some fields, less than 20% of faculty had mentors. Overall, individuals with mentors had significantly higher career satisfaction scores than those without mentors. Eight studies from this systematic review reported the positive influence that mentorship had on personal development and career guidance. Furthermore, 21 studies in the review described the impact of mentoring on research development and productivity. Findings indicated that mentors increased mentees' self-confidence and provided resources and support for their activities. Mentees were more productive in the number of publications and grants than those individuals without mentors. They were also more likely to complete their theses. A lack of mentorship was reported as a barrier to completing scholarly projects and publications. Mentors were viewed as an important motivating factor in pursuing a research career. Overall, the studies from this systematic review indicated that mentorship was perceived to be important for career guidance, personal development, career choice, and productivity. Despite these compelling studies, mentorship programs are not necessarily commonplace in education of health professionals (Harrington, 2011).

> **Mentoring is a brain to pick, an ear to listen, and a push in the right direction.**
> **—John Crosby**

As a result of the benefits of mentoring, The Academy of Medical Surgical Nurses (AMSN) developed a mentoring program entitled Nurses Nurturing Nurses (N3) (Reeves, 2004). Some of the benefits of mentoring for mentors outlined by the Academy included

- development of professional colleagues, self-awareness, and interpersonal relationships;
- professional development;
- stimulation to question practice; and
- improved political skills.

In addition, benefits for those being mentored proposed by the Academy included

- recipient of one-to-one nurturing,
- insight into unwritten rules and politics,
- assistance with career development,
- increased network of contacts, and
- development of self-confidence and problem-solving skills.

The AMSN continues to offer a mentoring program, complete with a mentor guide, mentee guide and site coordinator guide to facilitate smooth program delivery (AMSN, 2013). The IOM (2010) recommended mentorship programs for nurses as part of their recommendations for building leaders to advance health. Finally, in 2011 the American Nurses Association put forward a call to fund five demonstration projects to develop mentoring programs for nurses. These initiatives dovetail with the process that hospitals must embark upon to seek Magnet status from the American Nurses Credentialing Center, which is considered the gold standard for nursing practice, and includes mechanisms for mentoring and professional development of nurses as well as succession planning (e.g., mentoring nurses into leadership roles). In the application process, examples must be provided that speak to mentoring for these purposes (American Nurses Credentialing Center, 2014).

ARCC EBP MENTORS: MAKING A DIFFERENCE?

Ideally, every healthcare organization would have ARCC EBP mentors who could assist staff and others to practice based on evidence to achieve better outcomes. However, some organizations, healthcare educators, and providers continue to practice as they always have—without attention to the evidence, inclusion of the patient's preferences and with no recognition of the role of clinical expertise. Given that EBP mentors are central to implementation of the ARCC Model, an educational intervention was designed as a 5-day EBP Mentorship Program and was held as an immersion program to prepare staff nurses, advanced practice nurses, nurse researchers, and other healthcare providers to serve as leaders and mentors in changing organizational cultures through the promotion, implementation, and sustainability of EBP from administration to the bedside.

The educational intervention program fostered a shift to the EBP paradigm and covered the seven-step EBP process:

1. cultivate a spirit of inquiry,
2. ask the clinically relevant question in PICOT format,
3. search for the best evidence,
4. critically appraise and synthesize the evidence,
5. plan and implement evidence,
6. evaluate the outcomes, and
7. disseminate the outcome.

Additional foci included the implementation of what is known from a body of evidence and development of the EBP mentor role. The EBP mentors returned to their home institutions with a strategic plan for implementing and evaluating at least one EBP project and a description of the EBP mentor role individualized for their agency.

In a postprogram evaluation survey, almost 40% of the 38 EBP mentors from across the United States and the world (Table 17.3) who responded were from the Southwestern United States. More than 40% were from medium-sized community hospitals, with a mean tenure of 6.16 years in their current role and 26.84 years as a nurse. The EBP mentors who responded to the survey were primarily Caucasian (95%) and female (97%). The majority of the respondents' exposure to EBP came from the EBP Mentorship Program (84%), with continuing education coming in as the second source of learning about EBP (52.6%). In addition, less than 20% formally learned about EBP in school.

To help understand the culture in which these EBP mentors worked, they completed the 25-item Organizational Culture & Readiness for System-wide Integration of EBP Scale (OCRSIEP; Fineout-Overholt & Melnyk, 2006). Examples of scale items include (a) To what extent is EBP clearly described in the mission and philosophy of your institution? (b) To what extent do practitioners model EBP? and (c) To what extent are fiscal resources used to support EBP? The range of summed scores was between 25 and 125, with 25 representing *not much EBP organizational support for an EBP culture*; 50 representing *marginal organizational support for an EBP culture*; 75 representing *some organizational support for an EBP culture*; 100 representing *moderate organizational support for an EBP culture*; and 125 representing *full organizational support for an EBP culture*. The EBP mentors' OCRSIEP scores were compared with a similar sample of EBP workshop participants and were found to have a slightly higher mean (83 [SD = 16] and 80 [SD = 18], respectively). The EBP mentors perceived their organizations to fall between some and moderate organizational support for EBP. This is an expected finding in that organizations that already support the formal role of EBP mentor would reasonably provide organizational support for system-wide EBP. While it is encouraging to find that organizations with EBP mentors have moderate support for EBP, these findings indicate that healthcare systems in which these EBP mentors work still have room for growth to establish a sustained culture of EBP.

The EBP mentors' beliefs about EBP were measured by the 16-item EBP Beliefs (EBPB) Scale (Melnyk & Fineout-Overholt, 2003a). Participants responded from 1 (strongly disagree) to 5 (strongly agree) to each of the 5-point Likert scale items. Examples of the items on the EBPB scale include (a) "I believe that EBP results in the best clinical care for patients," (b) "I am clear about the steps of EBP," and (c) "I am sure that I can implement EBP." Scoring consists of reverse scoring two negatively phrased items (i.e., "I believe EBP takes too much time"; "I believe EBP is difficult") and then summing all 16 items, with a total score that ranges between none (16), marginal (32), some (48), moderate (64), and very strong beliefs (80) (Melnyk, Fineout-Overholt, & Mays, 2008). The Cronbach's alpha (i.e., reliability coefficient) for this sample was 0.83. The EBP mentors' mean EBPB scores increased from a less than moderate beliefs at baseline ($X = 61$,

Table 17.3 **Description of EBP Mentors Who Completed the EBP Mentorship Program Evaluation Survey (*n* = 38)**

Home Area	Percent	Description of Institution	Percent	Roles	Percent
Northeast	2.6	Academic Medical Center (affiliated with Nursing School/ Division/Department)	34.2	Staff nurse	2.6
Southeast	7.8	Large Medical Center (>600 beds)	7.9	Charge nurse	0.0
Northwest	13.2	Community or Medium-sized Hospital (>150 beds and <600 beds)	42.1	Nurse manager	5.3
Southwest	39.5	Small or Rural Hospital (<150 beds)	0.0	Advanced practice nurse (clinical nurse specialist or nurse practitioner)	18.4
Midwest	31.6	Urgent Care Clinic, Primary Care or Long Term care	0.0	Clinical educator	23.7
International	5.3	Nursing Education (College of Nursing)	10.5	Academic faculty	15.8
		Other	5.3	EBP mentor	10.5
				Other	23.7

SD = 7.4) to moderate belief after program completion (X = 68, SD = 6.2). In addition, compared to a similar sample of EBP workshop participants, these mentors were found to have a slightly higher EBPB mean score (60 [SD = 6.2] and 68 [SD = 9.5], respectively). Although EBP mentors' beliefs were higher approximately 1 year after completing the EBP Mentorship Program than when they began, their beliefs in EBP remained in the moderately strong category versus moving to the high beliefs category (Figure 17.2).

The final evaluation of the effectiveness of the EBP mentorship program was actual implementation of EBP, which was measured by the 18-item EBPI Scale (Melnyk & Fineout-Overholt, 2003b). EBP

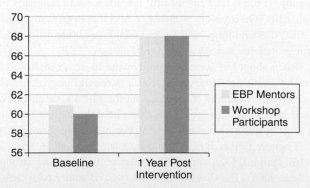

Figure 17.2: EBP beliefs at baseline and 1 year after educational intervention.

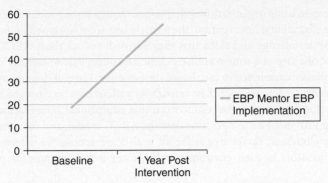

Figure 17.3: EBP mentor EBP implementation at baseline and 1 year after educational intervention.

mentors responded to each of 18 items on the 5-point frequency scale by indicating how often in the past 8 weeks they performed the item. Sample items include (a) used evidence to change my clinical practice, (b) shared an EBP guideline with a colleague, (c) promoted the use of EBP to my colleagues, and (d) shared the outcome data collected with colleagues. Scoring of the instrument consists of summing all 18 items with a range between 0 and 72, with none equal to 0 times within the past 8 weeks; 18 equal to *1 to 3 times* within the past 8 weeks; 36 equal to *4 to 5 times* within the past 8 weeks; 54 equal to *6 to 8 times* within the past 8 weeks; and 72 equals *greater than 8 times* within the past 8 weeks (Melnyk et al., 2008). The reliability coefficient of the EBPI with this sample was 0.95. As a group, the EBP mentors reported a mean implementation score at baseline of 19 (SD = 13.2) (e.g., 1–3 times per week they used evidence, talked about outcomes; see Appendix K for sample scales), which is consistent with other EBP workshop samples at baseline (X = 20 [SD = 15.5]). About 1 year after attending the program, the mentors reported a mean implementation score of 55 (SD = 18.6) (i.e., they used evidence in their practice approximately 6–8 times within the past 8 weeks) (Figure 17.3). In addition to increasing EBP beliefs and implementation, EBP mentors reported other outcomes of the educational intervention (Box 17.2).

While EBP beliefs and implementation increased and were sustained for approximately one year after the 5-day immersion program, EBP mentors identified barriers to the EBP mentor role that challenged the mentor to carry out the role to its fullest degree as well as facilitators to their role (Box 17.2). Many of these barriers have been documented in the literature (Amodeo et al., 2011; Pravikoff et al., 2005). These findings are valuable to organizations that want to move toward an EBP culture and ensure that their clients are provided the best evidence-based care possible.

Findings from this program evaluation with ARCC EBP mentors indicated that they were able to strengthen and sustain their EBP beliefs and increase EBPI for as long as 1 year following attendance

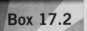 **Box 17.2**   Impact of EBP Mentor Educational Intervention

EBP Mentors reported that they were able to:
◆ Become more influential
◆ Speak more intelligently about evidence
◆ Improve outcomes
◆ Formulate the question and find the evidence
◆ Read research
◆ Lead EBP initiatives (e.g., through gaining promotions that facilitated their influence on organizational change)
◆ Advance their education through returning to school
◆ Provide valued contributions to care
◆ Serve as sought after consultants/resources for EBP

at the workshop, despite some organizational challenges. With a strong focus on education and skills building during the educational intervention, the participants were equipped to implement into clinical practice the EBP knowledge and skills that they learned. Just as these ARCC EBP mentors are making a difference one step at a time with their clinician colleagues, so can any clinician who has a sincere desire to enhance excellence in care based on evidence. Careful documentation of outcomes will assist EBP mentors to demonstrate their impact on patient care, system outcomes, and the care practices of their colleagues. Given the results from this educational intervention designed specifically for developing EBP mentors to operationalize the ARCC model, and the other evidentiary support for mentoring clinicians, the charge is for all healthcare settings to determine how best they can actualize EBP mentors in their environments to foster best outcomes for patients, providers, and systems.

EBP FAST FACTS

◆ EBP Mentors are central to an EBP culture.
◆ Engaging in specific education designed to prepare EBP mentors can demonstrate a return on the investment through improved organizational patient, provider and system outcomes.

References

Abedin, Z., Biskup, E., Silet, K., Garbutt, J., Kroenke, K., Feldman, M. D., … Pincus, H. A. (2012). Deriving competencies for mentors of clinical and translational scholars. *Clinical Translational Science, 5*(3), 273–280. doi:10.1111/j.1752-8062.2011.00366.x

American Medical Surgical Nurses. (2013). *AMSN mentoring program.* Retrieved from http://www.amsn.org/professional-development/mentoring on September 20, 2013.

American Nurses Association. (2011). *Call for proposals for mentoring programs in nursing.* Retrieved September 20, 2013, from http://www.nursingworld.org/DocumentVault/NewsAnnouncements/ANA-Demonstration-Mentoring-Program-Memo.pdf

American Nurses Credentialing Center. (2014). *The magnet application manual.* Silver Spring, MD: Author.

Amodeo, M., Lundgren, L., Cohen, A., Rose, D., Chassler, D., Beltrame, C., & D'Ippolito, M. (2011). Barriers to implementing evidence-based practices in addiction treatment programs: Comparing staff reports on motivational interviewing, adolescent community reinforcement approach, assertive community treatment, and cognitive-behavioral therapy. *Evaluation and Program Planning, 34,* 382–389.

Bellack, J. P., & Morjikian, R. L. (2005). The RWJ Executive Nurse Fellows Program, Part 2: Mentoring for leadership success. *Journal of Nursing Administration, 35*(12), 533–540.

Craik, J., & Rappolt, S. (2006). Enhancing research utilization capacity through multifaceted professional development. *American Journal of Occupational Therapy, 60,* 155–164.

Collins, L., Arenson, C., Jerpbak, C., Kane, P., Dressel, R., & Antony, R., (2011). Transforming chronic illness care education: A longitudinal interprofessional mentorship curriculum. *Journal of Interprofessional Care, 25*(3), 228–230.

Ervin, N. E. (2005). Clinical coaching: A strategy for enhancing evidence-based nursing practice. *CNS, 19*(6), 296–301.

Fawcett, D. (2002). Mentoring: What it is and how to make it work. *AORN Journal, 75*(2), 950–954.

Fineout-Overholt, E., & Melnyk, B. (2006). *Organizational culture & readiness for system-wide integration of evidence-based practice.* Gilbert, AZ: ARCC Publishing.

Fineout-Overholt, E., Melnyk, B. M., & Schultz, A. (2005). Transforming healthcare from the inside out: Advancing evidence-based practice in the 21st century. *Journal of Professional Nursing, 21*(6), 335–344.

Fineout-Overholt, E., Williamson, K. M., Gallagher-Ford, L., Melnyk, B. M., & Stillwell, S. B. (2011). Following the evidence: Planning for sustainable change. *American Journal of Nursing, 111*(1), 54–60.

Funderburk, A. E. (2008). Mentoring: The retention factor in the acute care setting. *Journal for Nurses in Staff Development, 24*(3), E1–E5.

Gallagher-Ford, L., Fineout-Overholt, E., Melnyk, B. M., & Stillwell, S. (2011). Implementing an evidence-based practice change: Beginning the transformation from an idea to reality. *American Journal of Nursing, 111*(3), 54–60.

Greene, M. T., & Puetzer, M. (2002). The value of mentoring: A strategic approach to retention and recruitment. *Journal of Nursing Care Quality, 17*(1), 63–70.

Harrington, S. (2011). Mentoring new nurse practitioners to accelerate their development as primary care providers: A literature review. *Journal of the American Academy of Nurse Practitioners, 23* (4), 168–174.

Holliman, J., Resler, R., Edmunds, T., & Child Life Council. (2010). *The leaders of the pack: Three EBP models used in pediatric settings.* Poster retrieved from http://www.childlife.org/files/EBPPoster2010.pdf

Institute of Medicine (IOM) (2010). *The future of nursing: Leading change, advancing health.* Washington, DC:Institute of Medicine of the National Academies Press.

Kanaskie, M. L. (2006). Mentoring: A staff retention tool. *Critical Care Nursing Quarterly, 29*(2), 248–252.

Levin, R. F., Fineout-Overholt, E., Melnyk, B. M., Barnes, M., & Vetter, M. J. (2011). Fostering evidence-based practice to improve nurse and cost outcomes in a community health setting: A pilot test of the advancing research and clinical practice through close collaboration model. *Nursing Administration Quarterly, 35*(1), 21–33.

Mariano, K., Caley, L., Eschberger, L., Woloszyn, A., Volker, P., Leonard, M., & Tung, Y. (2011). Building evidence-based practice with staff nurses through mentoring. *Journal of Neonatal Nursing, 15*, 81–87.

Melnyk, B. M. (2007). The evidence-based practice mentor: A promising strategy for implementing and sustaining EBP in healthcare systems. *Worldviews on Evidence-Based Nursing, 4*(3), 123–125.

Melnyk, B. M., & Fineout-Overholt, E. (2002). Putting research into practice. *Reflections on Nursing Leadership, 28*(2), 22–25.

Melnyk, B., & Fineout-Overholt, E. (2003a). *Evidence-based practice beliefs scale.* Rochester, NY: ARCC Publishing.

Melnyk, B., & Fineout-Overholt, E. (2003b). *Evidence-based practice implementation scale.* Rochester, NY: ARCC Publishing.

Melnyk, B., & Fineout-Overholt, E. (2010). ARCC (Advancing Research and Clinical practice through close Collaboration): A model for system-wide implementation & sustainability of evidence-based practice. In J. Rycroft-Malone & T. Bucknall (Eds.), *Models and frameworks for implementing evidence-based practice.* Indianapolis, IN: Wiley-Blackwell & Sigma Theta Tau International.

Melnyk, B. M., Fineout-Overholt, E., Feinstein, N., Li, H. S., Small, L., Wilcox, L., & Kraus, R. (2004). Nurses' perceived knowledge, beliefs, skills, and needs regarding evidence-based practice: Implications for accelerating the paradigm shift. *Worldviews on Evidence-Based Nursing, 1*(3), 185–193.

Melnyk, B M., Fineout-Overholt, E., Gallagher-Ford, L., & Stillwell, S. (2011). Evidence-based practice, step by step: Sustaining evidence-based practice through organizational policies and an innovative model. *American Journal of Nursing*, 111(9), 57–60.

Melnyk, B. M., Fineout-Overholt, E., Giggleman, M., & Cruz, R. (2010). Correlates among cognitive beliefs, EBP implementation, organizational culture, cohesion and job satisfaction in evidence-based practice mentors from a community hospital system. *Nursing Outlook, 58*(6), 301–308.

Melnyk, B. M., Fineout-Overholt, E., & Mays, M. (2008). The evidence-based practice beliefs and implementation scales: Psychometric properties of two new instruments. *Worldviews on Evidence-Based Nursing, 5*(4), 208–216.

Morgan, L. (2012). A mentoring model for evidence-based practice in a community hospital. *Journal for Nurses in Staff Development, 28*(5), 233–237.

Nick, J., Delahoyde, T., Del Prato, D., Mitchell, C., Ortiz, J., Ottley, C., … Siktberg, L. (2012). Best practices in academic mentoring: A model for excellence, *Nursing Research and Practice, 2012*, Article ID 937906, 9p. doi:10.1155/2012/937906

Olson Keller, L., Strohschein, S., & Schaffer, M. (2011). Cornerstones of public health nursing. *Public Health Nursing, 28*(3), 249–260.

Pravikoff , D. S., Pierce, S. T., & Tanner, A. (2005). Evidence-based practice readiness study supported by academy nursing informatics expert panel. *Nursing Outlook, 53*, 49–50.

Reeves, K. A. (2004). Nurses nurturing nurses: A mentoring program. *Nurse Leader, 2*(6), 47–54.

Roe, E., & Whyte-Marshall, M. (2011). Mentoring for evidence-based practice: A collaborative approach. *Journal for Nurses in Staff Development, 28*(4), 177–181.

Sambunjak, D., Straus, S. E., & Marušic, A. (2006). Mentoring in academic medicine: A systematic review. *The Journal of the American Medical Association, 296*(9), 1103–1115.

Stamm M & Buddeberg-Fischer B. (2011). The impact of mentoring during postgraduate training on doctors' career success. *Medical Education.* 45(5), 488–96

Tobin, M. J. (2004). Mentoring: Seven roles and some specifics. *American Journal of Respiratory and Critical Care Medicine, 170*, 114–117.

Varkey, P., Jato, A., Williams, A., Mayer, A., Ko, M., Files, J., … Hayes, S. (2012). The positive impact of a facilitated peer mentoring program on academic skills of women faculty. *BMC Medical Education 2012, 12*, 14. Retrieved from http://www.biomedcentral.com/1472-6920/12/14

Wallen, G.R., Mitchell, S.A., Melnyk, B.M., Fineout-Overholt, E., Miller-Davis, C., Yates, J., & Hastings, C. (2010). Implementing evidence-based practice: Effectiveness of a structured multifaceted mentorship programme. *Journal of Advanced Nursing,* 66(12):2761–71.

Wensel, T. M. (2006). Mentor or preceptor: What is the difference? *American Journal Health-System Pharmacy, 63*, 1597.

Zucker, B., Coss, C., Williams, D., Bloodworth, L., Lynn, M., Denker, A., & Gibbs J. D. (2006). Nursing retention in the era of a nursing shortage. *Journal for Nurses in Staff Development, 22*(6), 302–306.

Mercy Heart Failure Pathway

Robin Kretschman, MSA, RN, NEA-BC

Vice President Nursing Excellence
Mercy Health

Introduction

Pathways typically focus on stable, predictable conditions. Mercy pathways go beyond stable conditions to address complex conditions and chronic progressive diseases. The Mercy pathway development process combines evidence-based practice (EBP), electronic functionality, and lean and manufacturing disciplines with collaborative specialty teams that integrate evidence into practice. Between June 2012 and September 2013, 24 pathways were deployed using this strategy.

The work begins with an evaluation of diagnosis-related groupings (DRGs). Pathways chosen for development meet specific criteria: populations with high patient volumes, similar treatment needs, and foreseeable benefits. These are evaluated in conjunction with the cost of care.

The national vital statistics report lists heart disease as the leading cause of death in 2010 (Murphy, Jiaquan, & Kochanek, 2013). Heart failure represents a large segment of this population and was therefore chosen as the pilot for the Mercy pathway strategy.

The challenges facing health care today demand innovations and operational diligence. The per capita amount spent on health care in America is $8,608 (World Bank, 2013). Although we spend more money on health care than other nations, we "die sooner and experience more illness than residents in many other countries" (IOM Committee on Population, Division of Behavioral and Social Sciences and Education, 2013). Healthcare reform is a challenge to develop a more efficient and effective healthcare process.

Strategy for EBP Integration

The electronic health record (EHR) has become so much more than a longitudinal record of patient health information for one or more encounters. It is the basis of healthcare business intelligence, providing the data required for clinical and financial analysis. As the primary vehicle for interdisciplinary communication, decision support, and care planning, the EHR is a key component in the Mercy strategy for EBP integration.

To assure that decision support within the EHR is the current best practice, a team responsible for content development makes up the second major component in this strategy. Master's prepared nurses with specialty and clinical workflow expertise are selected as pathway leads and then equipped with EBP mentor skills and lean training. These coworkers assemble the evidence, define patient outcomes and daily goals, and then partner with physician leads to make evidence-based recommendations. Comprehensive pathways are then built into the EHR.

Audience

The target audience for Mercy heart failure pathways is the 35,000 patients in the Mercy service area with heart failure. Mercy has 5,320 physicians on the medical staff, 1,900 clinic physicians, and over 12,000 nurses. Going forward, pathways will support each of these clinicians.

Setting

The setting for this work is Mercy, the sixth largest Catholic healthcare system in the United States, a complex system that spans four states and the entire healthcare continuum. Mercy is made up of 32 hospitals (4,571 beds) and over 300 outpatient facilities.

The Impetus for Designing This Strategy

The current healthcare environment is the impetus for this change. From a healthcare reform perspective, the Affordable Care Act, Value-Based Purchasing, Readmission Reduction, Healthcare-Associated Conditions reduction, Hospital Compare measures, Accountable Care organizations, Medical Homes, and Meaningful Use have all been designed to challenge health-care organizations and providers to redesign care delivery.

Mercy's own analysis of supply cost trends, the cost of providing care trends, avoidable costs, and projections of shifts in payer mixes clearly articulate a need to create systems that address the key clinical drivers of optimal outcomes.

As a national leader in EHR implementation, physician integration, and adoption of Meaningful Use measures, Mercy was in a perfect position to integrate EBP through technology.

Description of Strategy

Once a patient population is selected for the pathway approach, nurse and physician specialists are identified from across the organization to serve as pathway leads. Nurses participate in an EBP immersion that allows them to hone the skills required to assemble the pathway content.

Competencies for the role include being able to define the clinical questions associated with the population, using PICOT questions to conduct literature searches, critically appraising research, and evaluating and synthesizing the body of evidence.

No longer viewed apart from our work, technology is core to the work in health care. The EHR automates portions of the clinicians' workflow, provides communication channels and information flow, captures discrete data, and generates the legal medical record. Decision support based on the evidence is embedded in the electronic system to direct clinicians to needed interventions.

As the pathway is constructed, the team identifies the appropriate clinical, operational, and financial outcomes associated with each pathway. A data warehouse and real time feeds are then used to provide the most up-to-date pathway measures.

Communication and information flow are crucial to the project's success. In addition to the EHR, an intranet site houses a pathway library and pathway dashboards. The library provides detailed information about each pathway, including the EBP references used to determine physician orders, nursing interventions, daily patient goals, documentation requirements, and tasks associated with the care. Dashboard reporting tracks outcomes and provides a mechanism for Mercy benchmarking.

A key tactic used for pathway development is a 14- to 16-week production cycle. Leveraging lean methodologies and the manufacturing discipline, Mercy has invested in a performance acceleration department dedicated to supporting the pathway leads. Many of the typical barriers associated with implementing EBP are eliminated using this approach. Time is allocated to develop EBP knowledge, skills, and competencies. Time is also allocated to compile the evidence. Nurses' positions in patient care units are backfilled to free them up for the production cycle. Nurses, physicians, librarians, pharmacists, ancillary leaders, administrative assistants, clinical informatics specialists, and information technology specialists are all identified as members of a collaborative team: the right people doing the right work at the right time. The work to be done is mapped out in flow sheets, and all resources are brought to bear to create the most efficient and effective process. Additionally, leaders are incentivized to assure pathway success.

Results

Measures tracked for all pathways include length of stay, readmission rates, direct care variable costs, and compliance/utilization of pathways. Unique critical to process and specialty specific measures are also tracked. For heart failure, this includes hours to first order, hours to a diuretic, severity index, and morality risk.

In the heart failure population, this process has reduced length of stay and cost of care as well as successfully reduced variation in care.

Next Steps

Achieving a standard of care across a large population will enable us to conduct regression studies, determine key clinical drivers, and utilize feedback loops to improve the interventions included on the pathway.

Pathways are only one component of a larger effort to create care paths across the continuum. The principles used to identify evidence and create lean clinical and electronic workflow are being used in emergency departments, care management, ambulatory settings, and in the chronic disease center. An interactive patient portal completes the tools used to coordinate care across the continuum. Metric dashboards provide valuable information. Pathway measures are reviewed by executives, operations teams, and physicians.

As the first organization to leverage pathway functionality for complex conditions and chronic progressive diseases, there are many opportunities to publish. Evidence-based pathways built into the EHR is the strategy Mercy has adopted to meet the challenges of the future.

References

IOM Committee on Population, Division of Behavioral and Social Sciences and Education. (2013). *U.S. health in international perspective: shorter lives, poorer health.* Washington, DC: The National Academies Press.

Murphy, S. L., Jiaquan, X., & Kochanek, K. D. (2013, May 8). *National vital statistic reports, deaths: Final data for 2010.* Retrieved September 20, 2013, from http://www.cdc.gov/nchs/data/nvsr/nvsr61/nvsr61_04.pdf

World Bank. (2013). *Health expenditure per capita.* Retrieved September 20, 2013, from http://data.worldbank.org/indicator/SH.XPD.PCAP/countries?display=map

Step Six: Disseminating Evidence and Evidence-Based Practice Implementation Outcomes

Chapter 18

Disseminating Evidence Through Publications, Presentations, Health Policy Briefs, and the Media

Cecily L. Betz, Kathryn N. Smith, Bernadette Mazurek Melnyk, and R. Terry Olbrysh

The seven-step evidence-based practice (EBP) process is a major emphasis of this book along with implementation of the best evidence to improve clinical practice and patient outcomes. However, new evidence will not achieve its maximum value to practice and better patient outcomes unless it is communicated effectively. While clinicians communicate constantly with patients, peers, and colleagues in their work, many are not familiar with or confident in use of the intricacies, tools, processes, and opportunities to professionally communicate evidence findings.

Despite the many changes driven by communication technology advances, guidelines on best practices for healthcare professionals to disseminate evidence and evidence-based information remain the same. To speak before an audience, present a poster, publish a paper, place a story with the media, or write a health policy brief requires sufficient preparation, planning, and, in most cases, the use of the same communications principles. Excellent preparation reduces performance anxiety, builds confidence, and enhances the success of any communications initiative. The primary goal of disseminating evidence, whatever the channel or tool as described in this chapter, is to facilitate the transfer and adoption of research findings into clinical practice (Majid et al., 2011). For the majority of clinicians in advanced practice and leadership roles, enrollment in some type of instructional program (e.g., a continuing education course, staff development class, or college course) to learn the knowledge and skills to successfully make presentations or publish manuscripts is readily available (Lannon, Gurak, & Daemon, 2012). Moreover, many websites have helpful information for creating and delivering professional oral presentations. However, most learning to obtain advanced professional skills is gained through practical experience, mentoring by experienced colleagues, and modeling the observable behavior and materials demonstrated by leading professionals (Marble, 2009; Tinkham, 2013).

This chapter presents information on the strategies and communications tools that can be used by healthcare professionals to disseminate evidence. Content covered includes podium/oral, panel, roundtable, poster, and small-group presentations, as well as podcasts/vodcasts, hospital-based and professional committees, journal clubs, and community meetings. A discussion follows on professional publishing and dissemination of evidence to influence health policy and enhance care. In addition, suggestions for disseminating evidence through the news media conclude the chapter.

DISSEMINATING EVIDENCE THROUGH PODIUM/ORAL PRESENTATIONS

Conference presentations offer rich and dynamic opportunities to share and learn knowledge and enhance clinical expertise pertaining to EBP, quality improvement, case studies, program evaluation, and research. Whether the presenter has been invited or submitted an abstract that has been accepted, the process for developing the oral presentation is similar (Billings & Kowalski, 2009a).

An effective evidence-based presentation begins with an understanding of audience characteristics and needs, conference characteristics, and topical focus. It would be incorrect to make unwarranted assumptions about the presentation to be given. Each conference will be uniquely different from others. In preparing for a podium or oral presentation, it is important to know the audience composition, the context of the presentation, the desired length and format, and any special considerations (Sawatzky, 2011). Therefore, the first step to developing an effective oral presentation is to conduct a thorough analysis of the expectations and guidelines. This can be accomplished by gathering the necessary information from the conference announcements, speaker handbook, and contact with the conference representative, be it the conference manager or member of the organizing committee.

....

Whether you think you can or think you can't, you're right.
—Henry Ford

....

Analyzing Audiences for Presentations

As you begin preparing the presentation, ask the following substantive questions:

- What is the educational level and practice specialty of the audience?
- What is the audience's current knowledge of the material to be presented?
- Is the content for an audience with limited knowledge of the evidence-based topic?
- Why is the audience interested in the presentation?
- Is the audience expected to use evidence-based approaches in providing clinical care?
- What other information, if any, will the audience be receiving?
- What previous exposure has the audience had to the content of the presentation?
- How might the members of the audience use the information from the presentation to improve their practices, teaching, or other aspects of their work?
- How many people are expected to attend the presentation?

Additional logistical questions to consider include:

- Availability of audiovisual equipment (e.g., LCD projector for PowerPoint presentations)
- Whether the presentation will be transmitted to satellite sites or taped (this will limit podium mobility)
- Capacity to incorporate multimedia into presentation
- Internet access
- Type of microphone available (i.e., podium, lavaliere [personal/clip microphone])
- Length of the presentation
- Format of the presentation (amount of time allocated for questions and answers)
- Expectations regarding handouts
- Specific content to be addressed (Ranse & Hayes, 2009).

Once these questions are answered, development of the presentation can begin. The first step is development of learner objectives. If this is an invited presentation, the objectives may be defined by the organizer. Otherwise, objectives are developed solely by the presenter. The development of the objectives will be further facilitated following the conversation with the conference representative using the analysis format for determining the needs of the audience and conference purpose (Rogoschewsky, 2011). For presenters whose conference abstract was accepted, the objectives are to be closely aligned with it. For presentations to disseminate evidence from a study, the following topical outline is suggested:

1. Introduction to the clinical problem (e.g., depression affects approximately 25% of adults in the United States)
2. The purpose/primary aim of the study (e.g., to determine the short- and long-term effects of cognitive behavior therapy [CBT] on depressive symptoms in young adults)
3. The theoretical framework used to guide the study

4. Hypotheses (e.g., young adults who receive CBT will have less depressive symptoms than young adults who do not receive CBT) or study questions (what are the effects of CBT on depressed adults?)
5. The design (e.g., a randomized controlled trial)
   a. A description of the interventions used if an experimental study is being presented
   b. A description of the sample with inclusion and exclusion criteria (e.g., the sample included 104 depressed adults between the ages of 21 and 30 years; potential subjects were excluded if they had a mental health problem with psychotic features), as well as a concise description of the demographics of the sample
   c. The dependent variables and instruments used to measure the study's outcomes, along with validity and reliability information of each instrument (e.g., the Beck Depression Inventory was used to measure depressive symptoms; construct validity of the Beck Inventory has been supported in prior work, and internal consistency reliability is reported as consistently higher than 0.80)
6. Findings from the study
   a. Approach to statistical analyses (e.g., types of statistical tests used [an independent t-test was used to test the study hypothesis])
   b. Findings (it is best to represent the findings in easy-to-read graphs or tables)
7. Discussion of the findings, along with major strengths and limitations of the study (e.g., substantial attrition rate, difficulties in recruitment)
8. Implications
   a. Implications for future research (e.g., what was learned from this study that can guide future research in the area)
   b. Implications for clinical practice (e.g., how this evidence can be used to improve practice)

Once the outline is developed, major points and the content for each section of the outline can be developed along with the time allocation for each component of the presentation. Many conferences limit research/evidence-based presentations to 20 minutes or less, with it being commonplace for three to four individuals to deliver related talks in the same session. For presentations with short time frames, it is critical to deliver only nuts-and-bolts information. Because many beginning presenters often go beyond the allocated time limit, it is valuable to hold a practice presentation with colleagues before the actual conference to time and critique it.

Other more lengthy presentations will require a more thoughtful approach to the allocation of time to each section. Although the objectives will guide the development of the presentation, the extent to which each section is developed is based on the audience analysis and conference purpose. The interdisciplinary BOPPPS model (**B**ridge, **O**bjectives, **P**retest, **P**articipatory learning, **P**ost-test, and **S**ummary) provides a template for developing a presentation. The BOPPPS model can be accessed at http://hlwiki.slais.ubc.ca/index.php/BOPPPS_Model (HLWIKI International, 2013).

Slides to Enhance the Presentation

When presentation content is completed, slides should be developed to enhance delivery and hold the attention of the audience. A rule of thumb is that a minimal amount of information should be contained on each slide and that the total number of slides presented should not distract from the flow of the presenter' remarks. The tempo for slides is no more than one slide every 30 to 60 seconds (Billings & Kowalski, 2009b). However, it may be that far fewer slides are needed as the presenter uses the slide as a prompt for expanding upon the bullet points presented on the slide. The use of slides is not a substitute for the oral presentation. That is, the speaker's remarks are not restricted to the slide content as this approach would become one-dimensional and stilted.

Another helpful guideline is to create simple slides in terms of the colors, graphics, and fonts used. A dark or medium background (e.g., navy blue or maroon) with light color lettering (e.g., yellow or white) is most readable by viewers, although may not photocopy well if copies are to be distributed. White or pale-colored backgrounds should be avoided. Individuals in the back of a room should be able to read all text. Fonts should be simple, using font size between 24 and 32 points, and san serif font such as Arial. Font and background color should be consistent throughout the slide presentation, and important points should appear in boldface. Excessive use of bolding, italics, and underlining can be distracting for the reader. Underlining can be problematic as it is may be misconstrued as an Internet hyperlink (Sawatzky, 2011). In addition, photographs enhance presentations, hold the audience's attention, and help emphasize major points (see this book's companion website at http://thepoint.lww.com/Melnyk3e for an example of a slide presentation for a 20-minute research report). If multimedia is to be incorporated into the slide presentation, the feasibility of using it will be dependent on the conference technical capacity and costs, as the presenter may be expected to incur the additional costs associated with Internet and electronic linkages. The presenter needs to have absolute confidence that the integration of multimedia into the presentation will not cause technical problems. A dry run or rehearsal of the slide presentation may be available at the conference just prior to the presentation in the speakers' preparation room. Avoid the use of comics and entertaining sound effects to maintain a professional tone. When acronyms are used, they should be defined by the speaker when first referenced, enabling tremendous convenience for presenters (Coumoyer, 2012).

Excellent tutorials on creating PowerPoint™ slides by Epson Presenters Online, where registration is free, and templates and clip art are downloadable at www.presentersonline.com/

Other Types of Evidence-Based Oral Presentations

The following guidelines for presenting evidence from a study also apply to delivering evidence-based implementation projects. The format for presenting *systematic reviews* of evidence should include:

◆ Introduction to the clinical problem
◆ Purpose of the systematic review or the clinical question addressed
◆ Methods (e.g., search strategy)
◆ Results (i.e., presentation and critical appraisal of the evidence)
◆ Implications for future research and practice

It is important to be aware that conference presentation materials can be converted into a manuscript for publication with additional effort. The information communicated at a conference would also be appropriate and timely for an audience targeted by print and/or electronic media (Cleary, Happell, Lau, & Mackey, 2013).

DISSEMINATING EVIDENCE THROUGH PANEL PRESENTATIONS

Panel presentations are an effective strategy to convey divergent perspectives on evidence-based topics. This type of presentation format is especially effective to convene colleagues from various clinical settings to disseminate evidenced-based information. For example, during a panel presentation, clinicians can discuss their various evidenced-based approaches to promoting spiritual support services on their hematology–oncology units. Listening to different views enriches the session for the audience. The style and purpose of panel presentations vary according to the roles of the moderator and panelists. The moderator may serve as the coordinator, meaning that this individual manages the agenda of the panel by first giving background or introductory information and commentary on the subject matter to be discussed. Then, the moderator asks questions of the panel members to elicit their opinions on the topic. Questions from the audience are taken as a means of delving further into particular areas of interest or understanding the panelists' views better.

Another panel model takes a more formalized approach in which members of the panel present prepared remarks, with the moderator serving as a discussion facilitator by offering commentary for panel response and encouraging audience questions. The panel format is dependent on a number of factors, including panelist expertise, public speaking experience, organizational practices, and the moderator's competence in the role. Participation in a panel requires close adherence to the allotment of time given to each panel member in order to assure that each is able to present their material.

Panelist Preparation

Serving as a panelist requires knowing the expectations for participation (e.g., delivering a prepared presentation or sharing expert opinions with the audience). The panel format will dictate the type of preparation necessary for the presentation. Whatever the format, it is necessary to know the context in which the information is to be presented.

First, the prospective panelist must know the theme of and rationale for the panel, as well as session objectives. For example, is the panelist expected to provide a clinically based or theoretically oriented presentation? Coupled with this information, it is important to know the backgrounds of the other panelists, their areas of expertise, and the topics that the other panelists will address, along with their particular biases or perspectives. It is also necessary to know the time frame for the entire panel, including time allotted for audience questions, each panelist's prepared remarks, and the moderator's commentary (Griffin, Buccino, Klein, & Thaler-Carter, 2010).

In addition, the following strategies will ensure success of the panel presentation:

◆ Limit the number of slides to prevent distraction from the topic and to highlight what is said. It is helpful to have a brief conversation with the other panelists and agree on a number of slides and timeframes so that none of the panelists dominate.
◆ Develop a time clock system (e.g., set a timepiece in front of the speaker or have the moderator invoke the time with signage or some other method).
◆ Use an active voice that holds the audience's attention and illustrate content with real-life examples.
◆ Identify the major theme of the presentation, and add three to five major points to support the thrust of the theme.

If a panelist is expected to offer expert opinions in response to questions, the following preparatory steps are needed:

◆ Similar to preparing for presentations, panelists need to gather information on their audience and gear responses to the needs of the group. Consulting with colleagues before the panel presentation is also useful.
◆ Anticipate audience questions; colleagues can be asked to contribute to a potential list of questions for advance preparation.
◆ Paraphrase questions asked from the audience before responding; this allows everyone in the audience to hear the questions and allows the presenter time to organize his or her thoughts.
◆ Treat all questions with the same importance so as not to display a bias or preference for certain individuals in the audience.

During the session, panelists are expected to conduct themselves professionally, with sensitivity to the fact that they are only one of several experts sharing the stage from whom the audience wants to hear new information and practice ideas. Box 18.1 lists suggestions for panelist do's and don'ts.

Moderator Preparation

The moderator's role during a panel presentation is to ensure that the session objectives are met, that the panelist presentations are pulled together in a cohesive fashion, and that all participants fulfill their duties without dominating the presentation. The moderator will begin the session by providing introductory remarks that include an overview of the panel's purpose, a brief biographical introduction, and the evidence-based topic of each panelist. The moderator's role is to ensure the even flow of the panel discussion and questions from the audience. At the conclusion of the panel, the moderator should provide summary statements of the major themes of each evidence-based presentation; therefore, note taking

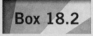

Box 18.1 A Panelist's Do's and Don'ts

DO

◆ Be sensitive to time limitations for both prepared and spontaneous remarks.
◆ Make notations of other speakers' comments for response and essential points for an organized, well-thought-out reply.

DON'T

◆ "Jump" on the remarks of other speakers (i.e., enable them to speak without interruption).
◆ Look at another panelist when responding to his or her comments; rather, speak directly to the audience.
◆ Express political or partisan opinions.

Box 18.2 Responsibilities of the Moderator During a Panel Presentation

◆ Provide a brief introduction of each panelist, emphasizing his or her expertise or experience with the evidence-based topic.
◆ Select audience members who have questions to ask of panelists.
◆ Repeat questions (or have panelists do it) for the audience's benefit.
◆ Remind the audience members or panelists of time constraints if too much time is used.
◆ Redirect the panelists' comments as needed to ensure that one or two panelists do not dominate the session.

during the session will be necessary while being attentive to coordinating questions from the audience and panelist responses. Box 18.2 presents specific responsibilities of the moderator during a panel presentation.

Prior to the panel session, the moderator should contact each panelist to obtain sufficient information about their presentation and area of expertise. An exchange of information about the other panel members should also occur, including contact information so that coordination by panel members can be made before the presentation. Additionally, the moderator can serve as a liaison for exchanging logistic information (e.g., audiovisual needs, room setup, projected number of individuals attending the presentation for distribution of handouts, and confirmation of the meeting time and place). The moderator also needs to ensure that the panel conforms to time constraints and clearly conveys to panelists time remaining in their speaking slots.

DISSEMINATING EVIDENCE THROUGH ROUNDTABLE PRESENTATIONS

Roundtable presentations are a third way to "narrowcast" EBP data. They are an informal way to share information with a small group of people—literally, the number of individuals that fit around a table. Roundtable presentations offer the opportunity not only to share specific information with a group but also to allow the group discussion about experiences and how the content could be used within their practices.

Because the group for a roundtable is generally small—6 to 12 persons—it is appropriate to introduce group members first, which will make them more comfortable to engage in discussion. The use of audiovisual equipment is often not possible in this setting, but printed handouts of slides can be used to identify key points or provide supplemental information. As in the case of a formal lecture, it is important to understand the needs of the audience and their reasons for attending the roundtable (Larkin, Griffith, Pitler, Donahue, & Sbrolla, 2012).

Preparation for a Roundtable Discussion

In planning the presentation, it is important to allow ample time for discussion. Anticipate that one half to one third of the allotted time will be spent in discussion related to the prepared evidence-based material. Advance discussion questions distributed by the presenter help to facilitate dialogue among the participants, should conversation lapse.

Content for a roundtable is prepared in the same way as for a lecture presentation. Delivery of the material will be different, given the small group size and intimate setting in which the roundtable takes place. After introductions, the goals of the evidence-based presentation are stated. Any handouts are distributed and described in terms of their utility and relevance to the EBP topic. The content of the presentation is then delivered. Because the group is small, it is important to scan the group regularly, making eye contact with each person, in order to engage all present. Questions can be answered either during the presentation or at the end. If questions are taken and discussion allowed during the delivery of the content, it is important to watch the time to assure that all content will be covered (Griffin et al., 2010).

At the end of a roundtable session, participants should be thanked for attending, and any final questions that require additional clarification should be answered. The group may wish to exchange business cards or other identification or information so that dialogue among the members may continue. The presenter should offer his or her business card to allow future follow-up and may stay in the vicinity of the roundtable for a period of time after the session to answer individual questions.

DISSEMINATING EVIDENCE THROUGH POSTER PRESENTATIONS

Poster presentations provide an alternative option for presenting evidence-based information to professional audiences, but they are different from those given from a podium in a number of ways. Podium presentations are more formal in both style and format. There are several types of poster presentations: display, easel, and table top (DeSilets, 2010). More recently, laptop poster presentations, wherein the poster is displayed via computer, have been introduced at conferences as more economical, "green," and space saving (Health Care Transition Research Consortium [HCTRC], 2013). The presenter typically provides more information from the podium as contrasted with the poster, wherein only the most essential aspects of information about a study or evidence-based project are given. The podium presenter adheres to a fairly standard format for providing information, with little or no time allowed to take audience questions. The poster presenter also adheres to a defined format for displaying information; however, this type of presentation allows for more interaction between colleagues in the area of clinical interest, enabling the sharing and learning that otherwise would not have been possible with a podium presentation (Billings & Kowalski, 2010).

Typically, the presenter stands near his or her poster during the times designated by conference planners. Standing to the side of the poster will enable participants to read and reflect upon the poster content without feeling intruded upon or intimidated by the presenter's presence (Billings & Kowalski, 2010). When the participant is ready, the poster presenter is available to answer questions or discuss key points. Individuals displaying posters can explore any number of issues that are not possible with podium presentations. For example, colleagues might discuss in greater detail the clinical implications of the evidence presented, such as implementation challenges in a community-based setting compared with those in a tertiary care setting. Poster presentations also enable the dissemination of preliminary research data or evidence reviews (Miracle, 2008). Having business cards available for conference attendees facilitates additional consultation and conveys the message of accessibility.

Podium presentations have time limits of usually 15 to 20 minutes while posters are displayed for longer periods of time, allowing the presenter more time to speak directly with colleagues about his or her work. A poster presentation is less intimidating than a podium presentation because public speaking can be uncomfortable for professionals who are not accustomed to presenting before large numbers of people (Christenbery & Latham, 2013). Displaying information also may be preferable to giving an oral presentation for individuals who process information better in visual rather than verbal format.

The key to developing an effective visual poster is to construct it in a way that captures the attention of the conference participants. It is useful to think about the attractive characteristics of poster presentations seen at various professional conferences (see http://thepoint.lww.com/Melnyk3e for two well-designed posters that were displayed at national/international conferences). Notable aspects of these posters include their design and symmetry, the contrast of colors used, use of key words or phrases to emphasize important content, and use of graphs/figures to present study findings. A poster that is content dense is not an effective poster as the essence of the messaging is obscured, visually unattractive, and difficult to read (Billings & Kowalski, 2010; DeSilets, 2010). Posters that are poorly designed often present content in a disorganized format, contain too much or too little information, use colors that clash, and do not use figures/graphs to display content.

However, the display of graphics and organization of a poster are not enough. Knowing how to present information to colleagues in succinct, scholarly, and precise terms is just as important. Substance and design, when combined effectively in a poster, can serve as an effective vehicle for conveying information to colleagues. The poster becomes a magnet for attracting colleagues, not only to read about one's work but also to provide a comfortable setting for additional discussion with sharing of information that is the cornerstone of collegial discourse (DeSilets, 2010; Miracle, 2008).

If resources are available, it is useful to consult with a graphic design expert when developing a poster. Consulting with an expert certainly makes it easier, but the designer has limitations as well because this individual's area of expertise is limited to graphic design, not the poster content (Sherman, 2010). If consulting with a designer is not an option, then accessing examples of posters from print resources or the Internet or from colleagues is an alternative. Several software programs are available for developing posters, which include Microsoft PowerPoint, Adobe Illustrator, and InDesign (Billings & Kowalski, 2010). When a poster is accepted for presentation at a conference, authors typically receive size guidelines for construction and display of their posters from a conference organizer and/or an association. These guides are critical to the presenter before beginning the poster's design so that time is not lost in preparing a product that does not meet the requirements of the poster session.

The Pragmatics of Constructing a Poster: Getting Started

The first step in developing a poster presentation is to translate ideas and images into graphic form. Sketching out or developing a mock-up of the poster with self-sticking notes or using a computer template may be useful (Hamilton, 2008).

Evidence-Based Poster Presentations

The content of an evidence-based poster presentation is similar to other EBP presentation forms and generally include the following sections:

- **Background/Significance**: Provide background as to the nature or status of the clinical problem (e.g., prevalence data or other statistics demonstrating the growing importance of the problem).
- **Clinical Question**: Specifically identify what clinical problem or question was investigated.

- **Search for Evidence/Accepted Practice**: Identify briefly the methods and sources used to collect evidence (e.g., search strategy for the review of literature, focus groups, and surveys of institutional practices).
- **Presentation and Critical Appraisal of the Evidence**: Provide a succinct summary of the conclusions drawn from evaluating the scope of evidence available.
- **Clinical Practice Implications**: Describe clinical practice implications, based on the process of collecting and evaluating the evidence.

It is also important to obtain and carefully review poster guidelines received, such as the poster size that is standard for the conference (e.g., the typical size is 4 × 6 feet) so that the poster text and graphics are readable from a distance of 4 feet. Keeping the following principles in mind will enhance the readability of the poster:

- Remember that English-speaking participants will read the poster from left to right and from top to bottom.
- Number the order of the poster presentation to assist the reader in information sequencing.
- Vary the font size on the poster according to the type of information being presented, for example, 100 point (pt.) or larger for the poster title (readable from 20 feet), 72 pt. or larger for authors' names and affiliations, 36 to 48 pt. or larger for poster headings and subheadings, and 24 pt. for poster text.
- Use graphics or illustrations in lieu of text when appropriate, such as when reporting findings.
- Keep headings and subheadings brief (fewer than five words).
- Use bulleted phrases or short sentences of seven words or less.
- Use high contrast between lettering and background.
- Use familiar fonts (e.g., Times New Roman, Courier New, and Arial) and the same font style throughout the poster (some recommend a different font for the title).
- Keep in mind that sans serif fonts (without ascenders or descenders) are more readable.
- Avoid using shadowing and underlines; use bold instead for areas of emphasis.
- Use active tense (e.g., "Findings reveal…") and plain language.
- Organize poster in four sections: background information, methodology, findings, and implications; *or*
- Organize poster in three sections: purpose/methods; findings, implications
- Limit the number of references cited on the poster by listing them on the handout or at the end of a corresponding section.
- Limit text blocks to 50 or fewer words.
- Insert institutional branding logo at the top of poster

The presentation of content should follow a logical sequence from beginning to end—the same format used for publishing research papers. The presentation of research content, although dependent on the specifications of the conference, typically includes:

- **Introduction/Background**: The focus of the introduction section is to attract the attention of colleagues about the significance of the project by emphasizing the need, prevalence of the problem, or clinical issue.
- **Objectives(s)**: This section should be brief in that it states the focus of the study.
- **Design/Methods**: Brevity is the key unless there is something of interest about the methods or design that warrants emphasis (e.g., recruiting and training interviewers for culturally diverse populations).
- **Data Analysis**: This section should be concise in terms of listing analyses conducted.
- **Study Findings**: The emphasis in this section is on presenting graphs or tables with limited explanatory text to accompany them.
- **Conclusions:** Brief statements are made regarding the most significant findings as well as the clinical implications for practice.
- **Acknowledgment:** When appropriate, it is important to recognize the names of other colleagues on the project and/or the funding source.

Expectations of Poster Presenters

Poster presenters are expected to stand beside their posters in accordance with the designated display times. It is disappointing for colleagues to walk among posters without the authors or investigators present, as one of the primary purposes for a poster presentation is to facilitate scholarly and clinical dialogue among colleagues. Having PowerPoint handouts of the poster presentation available for distribution is also helpful (Bingham & O'Neal, 2013). The handouts may contain additional information that was not possible to include in the poster display (e.g., more detail on the review of pertinent literature, the theoretical framework, research instruments, and references). Contact information for later correspondence is helpful as well (Billings & Kowalski, 2010; Hamilton, 2008).

Helpful Resources for Constructing Posters

The Internet has many excellent resources to help with constructing posters, and these resources provide practical details (e.g., durable poster materials, display layout and format, logistics of color selection, photos, and graphics). Some sites provide information on using PowerPoint and creating posters for online purposes. These sites are contained in Box 18.3.

Listed below are some fail-safe suggestions to avoid poster presentation mistakes.

◆ Develop a timeline that accommodates unexpected delays in processing over which one has no control (e.g., use of graphic designer, photography).
◆ Back up files as the poster is being developed so that no data are lost through computer malfunctioning or as a result of a virus.
◆ Determine the best method for transporting the poster while traveling because it may have to be carried to the passenger section and stored overhead. Shipping the poster in advance risks not having it arrive for your presentation.

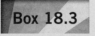

Box 18.3 Helpful Websites for Creating Poster Presentations

1. *Creating Effective Poster Presentations: An Effective Poster*. This website provides succinct information on the construction of posters akin to listing of "helpful hints." Background information is presented on the rationale and benefits for considering poster sessions as an option for professional presentation.
http://www.ncsu.edu/project/posters/NewSite/
2. *Creating Medical Poster Presentations*. This website provides information about poster sessions for medical and scientific presentations using PowerPoint software.
http://www.free-power-point-templates/articles/create-poster-powerpoint-2010/
3. *Designing Effective Posters*. This website provides the most comprehensive and detailed information about poster sessions of any website. Jeff Radel, Department of Occupational Therapy Education, University of Kansas Medical Center, provides detailed information on every aspect of creating a poster, from formatting the poster title to transport and storage. This website is really a must.
http://www.kumc.edu/SAH/OTEd/jradel/Poster_Presentations/PstrStart.html
4. *The University of Medicine and Dentistry of New Jersey Center for Teaching Excellence*. This website contains numerous links to other websites to provide comprehensive information on the development of poster presentations. It is an excellent resource for obtaining information on all aspects of poster presentations.
http://cte.umdnj.edu/career_development/career_posters.cfm

◆ Bring a flash drive or upload the file onto the laptop computer of the poster in case it gets lost, damaged, or destroyed in transit.

◆ Locate the business office at the conference site or nearby copy center if needed prior to leaving, in case the poster needs to be reprinted.

◆ Label the poster to ensure its security if staying at a hotel to prevent loss in transit.

◆ Remember to bring materials (e.g., masking tape, double-sided tape, push pins) to display the poster, although they will often be provided.

◆ Have handouts available for colleagues who want additional information on the literature review, methodology, and references.

◆ Bring sufficient numbers of business cards.

Laptop Poster Presentations

Laptop poster presentations are a new electronic iteration of the hard copy poster. The content of the laptop poster is similar to the hard copy version; however, its appearance and format are similar to a PowerPoint presentation. The laptop poster is composed of a limited number of slides (five to six). The poster presenter engages actively with one or more individuals as he or she provides a brief oral commentary as the slides are shown. The attendees are encouraged to ask questions and make comments as the poster presentation is given (HCTRC, 2013). The laptop poster is an electronic innovation; its widespread application remains to be seen in the years to come.

DISSEMINATING EVIDENCE TO SMALL GROUPS

Evidence-Based Grand Rounds

Grand rounds can serve as a major forum for evidence-based presentations. Departments within tertiary care and academic settings often host grand rounds or forums designed for clinicians to speak directly to their colleagues on topics that are innovative or that call for new approaches to care. Usually, speakers present empirically based answers to clinical practice questions, typically findings from their own or others' studies or policy updates with clinical implications for staff. Grand rounds usually consist of formal oral presentations accompanied by audiovisual slides or video presentations. Generally, a question-and-answer period follows the speaker's presentation.

Just as there are journal club websites (discussed in more detail later in the chapter), grand rounds presentations can be found on Internet websites. Internet-based grand rounds are another setting for experts to share evidence-based information with colleagues on topics of mutual interest. Internet grand rounds topics may be presented or reviewed by several clinical experts, enabling users to e-mail questions that can later be posted on the website. The advantages of Internet usage are the widespread access that is available to users, the ability to combine the perspectives and expertise of many clinical specialists, and the convenience for the users. Additionally, users are not bound by the time constraints of real-time meetings, enabling them to participate at their convenience.

Evidence-Based Clinical Rounds

Evidence-based clinical rounds, smaller in scope than grand rounds, are another effective medium to present evidence to guide clinical practice changes, as well as meaningfully involve clinical staff in the process. Evidence-based clinical rounds have been used very successfully as part of the Advancing Research and Clinical Practice through Close Collaboration (ARCC) model. One or a few clinicians will do the following in preparation for these rounds:

◆ Identify a clinical question (e.g., What is the most effective medication to decrease pain in postsurgical cardiac patients?).

- Conduct a systematic search for the evidence to answer the clinical question.
- Critically appraise the evidence found.
- Recommend guidelines for practice changes based on the evidence.

These clinicians then present the information that they gathered and make recommendations for clinical practice to their colleagues, based on the evidence, in the form of an oral presentation during a more casual session than the more formal, larger grand rounds.

Brief Consultations

The ultimate goal of excellence in clinical care is to integrate evidence into clinical practice as a standard of care for *all* patients under *all* circumstances. This level of practice can only be achieved by fostering the organizational environment to support it. As one expert has stated, "hallway consultations," that occur informally between colleagues in the hallways about patients, are an on-the-ground approach to facilitate discussion about nursing care interventions that are evidence-based. These are excellent opportunities for collegial consultation and instruction (Van Soeren, Hurlock-Chorostecki, & Reeves, 2011).

Digitizing Evidence Communications

Technological advances have enabled the use of podcasts, videocasts, webinars, social media, and other digital tools to communicate information to targeted audiences (Savel, Goldstein, Perencevich, & Angood, 2007). A *podcast* is an instructional media that can be used "to deliver a web-based audio broadcast via an RSS feed over the Internet to subscribers" (Dictionary.com, 2014). A videocast—terms such as *video podcast* or *vodcast* are used as well—refers to "the online delivery of video on demand, video clip content via Atom or RSS enclosures" (Reference.com, 2009). A *webinar* is an interactive synchronous online presentation with the ability of participants to ask questions or make comments.

The advantage of these electronic tools is that the presentation, whether in audio or video format, can be archived on a specific website for later convenient use by the learner (Abe, 2007; Skiba, 2006). For example, journal clubs and presentations can be audio- and videotaped for later use for those unable to attend at the scheduled time. Podcasts and vodcasts are relatively simple to access by users and inexpensive to produce (Rowell, Corl, Johnson, & Fishman, 2006). PowerPoint presentations can be integrated into podcasts as a means of accompanying the audiotapes (Jham, Duraes, Strassler, & Sensi, 2008). Both podcasts and vodcasts can be downloaded to the user's own mobile device (e.g., iPods, BlackBerry, MP3 players; Abe, 2007).

Disadvantages of these web-based tools are that every user may not have the technology hardware and software and/or the experience to use it. Additionally, unless an interactive feature is integrated into the podcast, the learning is primarily a passive instructional approach (Jham et al., 2008). Refer to Box 18.4 for a listing of websites that provide information on the development of podcasts and vodcasts.

Box 18.4   Helpful Websites for Podcasts

The following websites provide guidance for developing podcasts:

- How to Create Your Own Podcasts—A Step by Step Tutorial
  http://radio.about.com/od/podcastin1/a/aa030805a.htm
- Learning in Hand—Create Podcasts
  http://learninginhand.com/podcasting/create.html
- Online Tools and Software for Creating Podcast Feeds and Posts
  http://radio.about.com/od/onlinepodcastcreation/Online_Tools_and_Software_For_Creating_Podcast_Feeds_and_Posts.htm
- How to Create a Podcast
  http://pharmacy.ucsf.edu/facultyandstaff/podcast/

DISSEMINATING EVIDENCE AT COMMUNITY MEETINGS

Recognized experts in a geographic area may be asked to present evidence-based information in a community setting. This type of presentation can be particularly challenging because community groups may include laypersons and the media, in addition to professionals. This requires that the speaker be able to address all segments of the group in a way that they understand. Before making the presentation, it is important to collaborate with community leaders about the nature of the content to be presented as well as to be culturally sensitive to the potential attendees. Tips for presenting to a mixed audience include the following:

◆ Begin the presentation with a general overview of its purpose, followed by a review of the major points or findings.
◆ Define all abbreviations and acronyms (e.g., the American Academy of Nurse Practitioners, rather than AANP).
◆ Provide definitions as you speak (e.g., "....risk pool, that is, a group of individuals brought together to purchase insurance in order to spread the risk, or cost, among a larger group of people....").
◆ Avoid off-hand remarks that could be misinterpreted or misquoted by any media present. Stick with the facts as you know them or offer your professional, educated opinion when asked.
◆ Offer to answer questions personally after the session for those who might be reluctant to ask a question before a large group.
◆ When offering examples, consider the potentially mixed nature of the audience and offer cases that all members can understand.
◆ Allow ample time for questions and answers as well as general discussion.

The use of slides and corresponding handouts is also useful in keeping all participants interested and focused on the presentation (Bingham & O'Neal, 2013). Refer to the section *Slides to Enhance the Presentation* for guidance on the development of PowerPoint slides to develop effective slides for community presentations. In addition, referral to relevant websites and articles are always appreciated.

DISSEMINATING EVIDENCE AT HOSPITAL/ORGANIZATIONAL AND PROFESSIONAL COMMITTEE MEETINGS

Presenting evidence-based information to a committee of fellow professionals can be a stressful experience. Adequate preparation is again the key to ensure success. Anticipate questions that may reflect not only the information that is being presented but also historical information, because not everyone in the group will be aware of all of the relevant history surrounding a particular issue. Consider the following:

◆ Why is the group interested in the topic?
◆ What is the history of the issue in the particular institution?
◆ Has there been any controversy surrounding the issue that may interfere with the presentation? If so, should it be addressed in an open manner before the presentation begins?
◆ Are there some members of the group who may be more critical than others to the information presented? If it is possible to learn more about concerns ahead of time, they can be addressed more readily during the meeting.
◆ Is there any related information that may need to be discussed during the presentation, and does the presenter have adequate knowledge in the related area?
◆ Is this a group whose meetings are informal, or does the group maintain formal meeting rules?

The most important pieces of information needed before beginning to prepare for a committee presentation are:

◆ What is the composition of the audience?
◆ How much time will there be to share information and answer audience questions?

Whoever invites the presenter to the meeting or is responsible for serving as chairperson should be able to describe the expected attendance, the disciplines represented, and the relevance of the information for the group.

Committee meetings are usually tightly scheduled with little opportunity to go beyond the allotted time for the agenda items. Therefore, it is important to be able to provide key information within the time frame allowed. In addition, if the meeting is held in a hospital or similar facility, staff members may come in and out of the meeting when they are answering pages or attending to patient care responsibilities. This movement in and out of the room can be distracting and unnerving for the speaker, so it is important to prepare mentally for this possibility. In addition, anticipate that some latecomers will ask for information that has already been presented. The best approach is to provide the information in a brief manner and offer to discuss it more fully after the meeting.

After a brief introduction as to its relevance for the group, the presentation can generally follow the format for a journal article on an EBP topic below:

◆ Clinical question
◆ Search for evidence
◆ Critical appraisal
◆ Implications for practice
◆ Evaluation (if the practice change had been implemented)

This should be followed by a discussion period as to the utility of the information for the committee or the facility.

DISSEMINATING EVIDENCE THROUGH JOURNAL CLUBS

The concept of journal clubs has evolved considerably over the years, especially with the use of the Internet as a vehicle for scholarly exchange. One only has to access the World Wide Web by using a search engine with the key words *journal club* to find online journal clubs for many healthcare disciplines, most of which are evidence-based in focus, and appreciate their roles as conduits for the dissemination of clinical care knowledge. Whether journal clubs are offered in the clinical setting, in a more relaxed off site setting, on a website or via the Internet, they serve as another mechanism for disseminating the best evidence on which to base healthcare practice by physicians, nurses and other providers to improve their clinical practice and patient outcomes (Marble, 2009; Silversides, 2011; Steele-Moses, 2013). For example, it may be used as a strategy to foster the goals of the healthcare organization's nursing department to obtain Magnet status or create linkages to nurses who work in isolation, such as school nurses (McLaughlin et al., 2013; Sortedahl, 2012; Tinkham, 2013).

On-Site Journal Clubs

Journal clubs provide an opportunity for clinicians to share and learn about evidence-based approaches in their work settings. An advanced-level clinician can serve as the leader and mentor of a journal club until other colleagues achieve the knowledge and skills necessary to lead a group (Gelling, 2011; Marble, 2009; Steele-Moses, 2013; Tinkham, 2013). The success of the journal club will depend on several factors:

◆ Expertise of the advanced-level clinician in selecting an appropriate review article and other supporting articles that provide substantial sources of evidence
◆ Organizational resources to facilitate the activities of the journal club, such as access to online bibliographic resources that include evidence-based reviews (e.g., Cochrane Controlled Trials Register)
◆ Participation by motivated colleagues/staff
◆ Application to practice resulting in practice changes
◆ Provision of nursing continuing education units
◆ Topics that are of clinical interest and relevance

A journal club is typically led by an advanced-level clinician who understands research design, methods, and statistics. This clinician serves not only as the discussion facilitator but also as an educator because it is likely that colleagues will ask for additional contextual information (McLeod, Steinert, Boudreau, Snell, & Wiseman, 2010). Questions from journal club participants typically focus on the type of research design used, sample selection criteria, instrumentation, and statistical analyses. Therefore, it is essential that the journal club leader have the knowledge to answer these types of questions adequately. Additionally, in order to be effective, the journal club leader needs facilitator skills to encourage members of the club to participate as well as to feel comfortable and supported in sharing input. The facilitation skills for an effective journal club leader include:

◆ Actively listening to questions asked
◆ Using open-ended questions to facilitate discussion
◆ Avoiding the appearance of preference or bias in responding to questions by stating that a particular question is "good," unless equivalent affirming comments are made about all questions
◆ Clearly communicating messages about the purpose and expectations for the club
◆ Coming to the meeting well prepared and organized to conduct the meeting professionally (e.g., ensuring room availability and setup, as well as a sufficient number of handouts and other materials)
◆ Monitoring the flow of discussion to ensure that it is focused on the topic
◆ Interceding when conversation "drift" occurs, redirecting the conversation back to the topic (e.g., "getting back to our point," "as was said before," and "we were talking about …")
◆ Reinforcing responses to questions asked by members with affirming comments in order to encourage group participation
◆ Summarizing major points at the end of the session before concluding the meeting
◆ Demonstrating application to practice

The journal club leader will most likely have the responsibility for selecting the journal article to be discussed by the group participants (O'Nan, 2011). This article should meet the journal club criteria for an evidence-based presentation and should be relevant to the clinical practice of the staff. Selected articles should be on current studies or evidence reviews, use valid and reliable instrumentation, have an adequate number of subjects, and use a research design appropriate for the research question or purpose. Although there may be variations in the format for the journal club, such as including content on the "how to's" for critiquing research articles (Christenbery, 2011), the standard process for the discussion of articles, focusing on the key point and not a reread of the articles, is as follows:

◆ Study objectives/hypotheses
◆ Design and methods, including the setting in which the study was conducted (e.g., the community, the intensive care unit, outpatient clinic, or the home) as well as instruments used along with their validity and reliability for the sample studied
◆ Data analyses, with rationale for the specific tests used
◆ Findings, specifically in terms of the relative significance of the findings, paying careful attention to whether the study had a large enough sample size with power to detect significant findings
◆ Conclusions of the study with clinical implications, such as the clinical procedure related to aseptic management of long-term gastrostomy tubes
◆ Efficient critical appraisal of the study, including its strengths and limitations as well as applicability to practice (e.g., clinicians might be hesitant to change their practice based on the findings from one study that had a very small number of subjects)

Journal clubs are held at regularly scheduled times and locations, enabling participants to plan for meetings. Some journal clubs, held in off-site locations, incorporate social time for members to network (Silversides, 2011). Articles for the journal club should be distributed to members well in advance so that members can read and digest the material. Distribution of forthcoming meetings and identification of the topic to be discussed by e-mail via the institution's targeted mailing list is a convenient and time-efficient method (Christenbery, 2011).

Online Journal Clubs

The Internet provides additional resources and opportunities for developing other types of journal clubs for healthcare professionals. There are numerous online bibliographic databases that can be accessed for obtaining evidence-based answers to questions or accessing substantive articles for a journal club.

For example, an advanced-level clinician on a pediatric unit of a major tertiary medical center wants to find a high-quality article on pediatric pain for next month's journal club. The most effective strategy for finding this article is to access one of several online evidence-based review databases because the most current and rigorously reviewed studies can be found there. These databases include the ACP Journal Club, Evidence-Based Medicine Reviews, Cochrane Database of Systematic Reviews, Cochrane Controlled Trials Register, and Database of Abstracts of Reviews of Effectiveness (DARE). Searching these databases for "pediatric pain" reveals the five citations listed in Box 18.5. Based on the needs of the clinical staff, a clinician selects an article published by Logan et al. in 2013 because it addresses specific clinical practice issues related to pediatric pain.

There are online journal clubs that incorporate the technological advantages available with the Internet. This format enables individual users to access the journal club website at times convenient to personal work schedules, interests, and learning style. Website journal clubs, although highly individualized, are similar to the group meeting format in that an article is reviewed for its applicability for clinical practice (Steenbeek et al., 2009). The difference with the online format is the process, which varies from site to site (e.g., a critical review of a clinical trial initiated by a contributing author and reviewed by website editors, individual efforts of a website editor with feedback from its users). Several online evidence-based websites are listed in Box 18.6.

Additionally, online professional journals may offer a journal club feature enabling feedback from readers. For example, the *American Journal of Critical Care* offers a supplemental section at the end of selected articles for the reader, enabling the review and critique of the study as a preliminary step in considering its application to practice. Discussion of its applicability with other journal readers is available through an online discussion using electronic letters (Kiekkas, Sakellanropoulos, Brkalaki, Manolis, & Samios, 2008).

Institutional-related journal clubs benefit from incorporating an evaluation process. This can be done informally at the conclusion of each of the on-site meetings or at a predetermined end of the online sessions. Evaluation forms can also be used to evaluate the perceived benefit of journal clubs.

Box 18.5 Results of a Search on "Pediatric Pain" in Evidence-Based Review Databases

Aguilar Cordero, M. J., Mur Villaar, N., Padilla Lopez, C. A., Garcia Espinosa, Y., & Garcia Aguilar, R. (2012). Nurse's attitudes to pain in children and their relation to continuing pain management. *Nutricion Hospitalaria (Spain), 27*(6), 2066–2071.

Chiaretti, A., Pierri, F., Valentini, P., Russo, I., Gargiullo, L., & Riccardi, R. (2013). Current practice and recent advances in pediatric pain management. *European Review of Medical Pharmacological Science,* (Suppl 1), *(17)* 112–126.

Gottschling, S., Gronwald, B., Schmitt, S., Schmitt, C., Langler, A., Leidig, E., ... Shamdeen, M. G. (2013). Use of complementary and alternative medicine in healthy children and children with chronic medical conditions in Germany. *Complementary Therapeutic Medicine, 17*(Suppl 1), S61–S69.

Harvey, B. S., Brooks, G., & Hergenroeder, A. (2013). Lumbar injuries of the pediatric population. *Primary Care, 40*(2), 289–311.

Logan, D. E., Williams, S. E., Carullo, V. P., Claar, R.L., Bruehl, S., & Berde, C. B. (2013). Children and adolescents with complex regional pain syndrome: More psychologically distressed than other children in pain. *Pain Resources Management, 18*(2), 87–93.

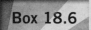

Box 18.6 Examples of Websites Containing Evidence-Based Practice Information

1. **University of Minnesota, Evidenced-Based Nursing (EBN).** This website provides a primer on EBN. Information is provided on what EBN is, models of evidence-based projects, barriers to EBN, evaluating the quality of nursing research, and links to nursing research journals and EBN websites.
   http://evidence.ahc.umn.edu/ebn.htm
2. **Oncology Nursing Society, Evidenced-Based Practice (EBP) Research Center.** This website provides a number of resources on EBP and its application to the specialty of oncology nursing practice. PowerPoint presentations on EBP can be easily accessed.
   http://www.ons.org/Research/PEP/
3. **New York University: Welcome to Nursing Resources: A Self-Paced Tutorial and Refresher.** This online tutorial provides an overview of the online research and evidence-based resources available for nurses. As the title implies, this tutorial provides introductory information for nurses who are unfamiliar with these new approaches to professional nursing practice. Information is also provided on nursing journals.
   http://library.nyu.edu/research/health/tutorial/
4. **John Hopkins Welch Medical Library.** This website is a gateway to a number of nursing resources that include nursing evidence-based sites.
   http://www.welch.jhmi.educhone/Evidence-Based-Medicine
5. **The Center for Transdisciplinary Evidence-based Practice (CTEP) at The Ohio State University College of Nursing.** This website contains a variety of resources on implementing EBP in clinical organizations.
   http://www.nursing.osu.edu/sections/ctep/

There are disadvantages and advantages in using online journal clubs. The user does not have the benefit of hearing the views of colleagues, which may limit learning regarding others' own clinical areas of expertise, critical thinking, and professional attitudes and values. Having the opportunity to participate in open discussion of professional issues is an important activity that promotes group cohesiveness and understanding, often fostering teamwork and group morale. Some learners may benefit more from the group discussion format because it is more suitable to their learning style. Likewise, other staff members may prefer the online format because it is more convenient and accessible. Technical problems associated with security firewall software, problems with the user's computer capacity and connecting to networks are potential barriers (Sortedahl, 2012; Steenbeek et al., 2009).

Journal club meetings enable the moderator to demonstrate professional behavior for other staff members. Professional development is an ongoing process and the journal club is yet another opportunity for leaders to model the importance of using evidence for nursing practice, to demonstrate ways of discussing practice issues in a nonthreatening venue, and to create expectations for professional practice (Marble, 2009; Steele-Moses, 2013).

DISSEMINATING EVIDENCE THROUGH PUBLISHED ARTICLES

Many publishing options are available for individuals who are interested in sharing evidence-based information with colleagues. Typically, writing a journal article or contributing a chapter to a book is the first idea that comes to mind when publishing is considered. Publications of this magnitude may appear overwhelming in terms of time, effort, and lack of prior writing experience. However, there are many other opportunities and options available for individuals who are considering publishing.

Publishing experience can be gained by taking on less ambitious projects, such as serving on a publication committee at work or through a professional organization. Serving on these committees enables professionals to network and learn from each other about the methods and mechanics of publishing. Although the specific purpose of the committee may vary slightly (e.g., a newsletter committee, a publication committee), these committees are not necessarily designed for creating or fostering collective writing efforts. Publication committees may serve as panels to review publication content submitted by prospective authors to an association's newsletter or journal. Other committees may provide oversight to the production of professional materials to ensure that the association or organization's affiliation is properly represented.

Regardless of the specific type of publication committee, membership helps aspiring authors to learn a variety of skill-enhancing efforts on how to write and professionally publish. Ideally, seasoned committee members mentor less experienced committee members in acquiring these skills. For example, reviewing the written work of other colleagues enables one to learn through the editing process, the difference between a well-written manuscript and a poorly written one. Writing a manuscript is not only about sharing expertise concerning evidence-based approaches, it is also about learning how to present information in a manner that enhances readability and understanding by professional audiences. Reading drafts in process is an indirect method of learning to write.

Committee discussions of evidence-based issues and approaches provide an understanding of the processes involved in EBP that include

- Posing the burning clinical question
- Searching for the best and latest evidence
- Critically appraising and synthesizing the evidence
- Clinically implementing a practice change
- Evaluating the change

Also, working with colleagues who have published professionally can influence those who are learning by building their confidence.

Finding a Mentor

Finding a mentor is beneficial for professionals who have had limited publishing experience. This mentor might be found at school or work, on the Internet, with a professional organization, and, in some cases, by asking a nursing journal editor for suggestions. A mentor can guide the novice writer through the process, starting with an idea for a topic and leading to the actual writing and submission process. It is important that the mentor selected be an individual who possesses sufficient publication experience and the willingness to help (Costello, 2012).

There may also be opportunities to collaborate on a joint writing project with a colleague with publication experience. The optimal circumstance for convening a writing team is to locate a co-writer in the same or geographically convenient community. Although the Internet has facilitated working with colleagues in distant locations, the first foray into a writing project with another colleague is best achieved with someone in close proximity. Real-time meetings involving personal contact are a prerequisite for the teaming of professionals with disparate writing experiences. This is yet another form of mentoring with extended hands-on involvement (Baker, 2013; Horstman & Theeke, 2012).

There are advantages to working with a team of colleagues to write and submit a manuscript for publication. The synergistic energy of collective efforts in brainstorming, not only the proposed manuscript outline and its development but also the organizational process for its completion, is significant. Collective and collaborative efforts can be a boon to generating the manuscript in a less burdensome and timelier process. Essential to productive, collaborative publishing efforts is the documented agreement among the authorship team of the roles and responsibilities of each of the members of the writing team. This predetermined agreement involves the specification of individual contribution of each author together with identified benchmarks of progress/completion as well as identification of consequences in the event the author team member does not meet the terms of the agreement. The process of explicating clearly each team members' responsibilities is a critical step to moving forward with the collective publishing endeavor (Baker, 2013).

Although experience and expertise are important, so is compatibility (e.g., writing style, temperament, and personality). A colleague who interacts uncomfortably or arrogantly with a novice writer is a significant detriment. Those who publish must devote extra time and effort beyond their usual workloads; therefore, engaging in an effort that is unpleasant and literally painful is likely to be short lived. Persistence with a specific publishing effort is likely to be brief if these types of negative circumstances exist. Publishing should be both a professionally rewarding and a fun experience (Fowler, 2013; Yoder-Wise & Vlasses, 2012).

Generating the Idea

The first step in getting started with publishing an evidence-based paper is determining the topic. Generating the topic for publication is based on an individual's area of expertise, the clinical question that arises from clinical practice, and the availability of resources to support the initial curiosity and attention to the idea. An idea for an evidence-based publication may have been germinating for some time before it is fully acknowledged as a potential publication topic. For example, a clinician may have noticed that older adult residents in assisted living facilities have extended periods of confusion following hospital admissions. This clinical interest may lead the clinician to search the literature for information on the phenomenon and to find evidence for instituting new interventions. The experience prompts the clinician to believe that other colleagues would benefit from learning about these practices. As a result, the clinician decides to write an article for a gerontology journal.

Brainstorming with other colleagues, including your mentor and/or those with publishing experience, is another approach to generate ideas through a free-association process. The momentum achieved through a rapid exchange of ideas can result in many more ideas that would otherwise not have been identified (Phillips, Sweet, & Blythe, 2009).

The conviction that current practice is inadequate to meet patient needs is another generator of evidence-based publication ideas. For example, health outcome data may demonstrate the need for improvement in selected patient outcomes. A manuscript describing an evidence-based intervention to improve a particular set of patient outcomes is an example of a publication designed to improve both professional practice and patient outcomes (Brennan, Mattick, & Ellis, 2011). Providing the reader with a different slant not previously found in the literature, such as addressing long-term management in community settings, is yet another example of generating ideas for manuscripts (Fowler, 2013).

Planning the Manuscript

Once an idea or a set of ideas has been decided, the prospective author needs to sketch out a plan on how this initial idea or concept can be developed into a manuscript. For evidence-based papers, the formats for writing them do not vary significantly because there is a specified order for presentation of the content; the differences are based more on style rather than substance. Although publication formats vary according to technical specifications and editorial policy of each journal, the standard format for an evidence-based manuscript is title page, abstract, introduction, narrative, and conclusions and clinical applications.

Title Page
The title page is the first page of the manuscript and contains the article's title and all of the authors' names, job titles, affiliations, and contact information. If there are many authors, the corresponding author is indicated. The manuscript title should be succinct, and the key words in the title should be well known and accessible for content bibliographic searches. For example, if the author intends to write an evidenced-based manuscript about adolescents, having the term "children" in the title might mislead readers.

Abstract
An abstract is a brief summary or synopsis of the article. Summaries indicate to the reader whether it is a research or clinical article. The abstract also identifies the major themes or findings and clinical implications. It is important that the abstract adheres to the technical specifications of the journal in terms of word limit and format (Costello, 2012; Happell, 2008).

Introduction
The introduction of the manuscript should be written in a succinct manner and should not be longer than a few paragraphs. It contains information about the purpose of the article, the importance of the topic for the professional audience, and brief supporting evidence as to why this topic is important. Supporting evidence might include prevalence data or demonstration of need. A well-written introduction that is organized and informative will create more interest and motivation for the individual to pursue reading the article (Costello, 2012).

Manuscript Narrative
The narrative, or "middle section" of the manuscript, will differ according to the type of evidence-based paper that is written, journal guidelines, and editorial policy. It is useful to select a couple of examples of articles published in the journal targeted for the submission to obtain a clear idea of how the narrative can be developed. Tables and/or boxes that highlight essential concepts of the narrative are enhancements that improve the readability of the manuscript.

Conclusions and Clinical Implications
The conclusions of the research evidence are presented in a summary form to emphasize the essence or the important "take home" message of the narrative discussion (Costello, 2012). For professionals who are accustomed to reading clinically oriented articles, the format of evidence-based papers may be unfamiliar and more difficult to follow. The conclusion enables the reader to locate the information succinctly if the previous discussion has not been sequenced clearly. The clinical implications section informs the reader about how this evidence can be applied to clinical practice and substantiates the rationale for its use in clinical practice.

Adopting a Positive Attitude

....

**Your living is determined not so much by what life brings to you as by the attitude
you bring to life; not so much by what happens to you as by the way your mind looks
at what happens.
—John Homer Miller**

....

Having a positive attitude toward professional publishing, especially for beginning authors, is an absolute must. When an individual decides to write professionally, she/he needs to develop a resolute attitude that the publication task will be completed regardless of what problems and how many challenges are encountered. First-time authors have the unusual experience of engaging in a very solitary activity that is undertaken by literally hundreds of thousands of people. Yet, there are very few opportunities that enable authors to communicate with one another about the highs and lows of the writing experience (Heinrich, 2007). In 2001, Stephen King wrote a book entitled simply *On Writing* that provides insight into his life as a writer and what he has learned along the way. However, most times authors toil at their computers, writing and deleting what they have written, and rewriting until the words on the page seem to make sense of the ideas they want to convey to their readers.

It is also important for writers to remember that their receipt of request for revisions and rejection letters is the norm for all authors. It is essential not to take the comments personally and put aside the emotional reaction to scholarly criticism. An objective perspective of reviewing comments both negatively and positively is important to writing the revised manuscript draft (Happell, 2011). Reviewer feedback can be very helpful in clarifying portions of the manuscript that are unclear and suggesting additional information to be included. For novice writers, uncertainty about the scope of comments received is best dealt with by reviewing the comments with the mentor or colleagues, who have publication experience.

> **You measure the size of the accomplishment by the obstacles you had to overcome to reach your goals.**
> **—Booker T. Washington**

For many authors, uncertainty and self-doubt can interfere with their writing, resulting in an unfinished manuscript that languishes on the computer's hard drive. For others, perhaps a harsh critique is mailed to them after the review has been completed, releasing feelings of disappointment or anger. For these individuals, the feedback is traumatic and demoralizing. Regrettably some become unwilling to subject themselves to this harrowing experience again. However, it is important to know and appreciate that even the most successful and prominent authors have been subjected to their fair share of rejections. A major difference between those who are successful and those who are not is *persistence*—one of the keys to getting work published (Fowler, 2013).

Sharing the writing responsibilities with other colleagues can mitigate the disappointment of an unfavorable review. Collective review of the manuscript will evoke a more diffuse and divergent response to negative criticism of the paper as compared to the solo author. Having a cohesive team of authors, rather than just one, is more likely to generate the motivation needed to promptly revise the paper. Friction and conflict among members of the author team experienced during the first submission may make it more problematic for writing subsequent drafts (Baker, 2013).

> **Criticism, like rain, should be gentle enough to nourish a man's growth without destroying his roots.**
> **—Frank A. Clark**

Being Organized

Organization is another major factor that contributes to writing success. That is, the process of getting an evidence-based publication submitted and accepted is dependent on creating the circumstances for it to occur. The organizational approach to getting thoughts down on paper in an acceptable professional format will require allocation of time periods for writing and achievement of the steps described in this section on publishing. Therefore, it is useful to remember the following (Baker, 2013; Fowler, 2013; Kiefer, 2010):

- Work on eliminating destructive thinking (e.g., "I can't do this" or "This paper will never get published").
- Remember that every author at some point in his or her career had to start at the beginning.
- Negative manuscript reviews should never be taken personally.
- Some individuals should not serve as reviewers as their critical perspectives are demeaning rather than helpful.
- Manuscript reviews may reflect mixed views wherein one reviewer evaluates the paper favorably in contrast to another who is critical of the manuscript.
- There is a collective experience of feeling confident, unsure, hesitant, weary, excited, bored, and tired that all authors can relate to when writing for publication.

◆ Authors who are successful do not take *no* for an answer easily. They are able to accept criticism, look at it objectively, and revise the paper accordingly, resulting in an improved document that meets the publication readers' needs.

◆ Setting realistic goals for initiating and completing a writing task is essential to prevent the disappointment of unrealistic expectations and possibly abandoning the project entirely.

◆ Setting aside incremental amounts of uninterrupted time for writing on a consistent basis will facilitate the progress needed to achieve the writing goal less painfully.

◆ Developing a plan that specifies a concrete course of action with attainable milestone accomplishments enables an author to feel satisfaction that he/she is achieving their goal.

◆ Goal setting is especially important for the collaborative team, including specification of consequences when a member of the team does not meet delegated writing benchmarks.

Deciding What to Publish

Professional publications on EBP can be found everywhere. The significance of its influence is demonstrated by the number of publications that can be found through bibliographic searches, the number of professional journals that regularly feature columns on EBP, and other publications that address the topic exclusively, such as this book and the journals *Worldviews on Evidence-Based Nursing* and *Evidence-Based Nursing*. Many funders are moving to the reimbursement of EBPs exclusively or preferentially; therefore, it is essential that clinicians are able to identify and interpret such information.

One of the first decisions an author makes in beginning the writing process is the choice of what to write and how it will be written. There are numerous opportunities for publishing that vary from something as straightforward as a letter-to-the-editor to authoring a major nursing textbook. Here is a listing of the wide range of publishing options:

◆ Letters to the editor
◆ Commentaries
◆ Books
◆ Continuing education reviews
◆ Chapters
◆ NCLEX questions
◆ Articles
◆ Evidence-based clinical practice guidelines
◆ Newsletter inserts
◆ Standards of care
◆ Book and media reviews
◆ Policy briefs

Authors with limited publishing experience may want to begin with a more manageable writing project, such as a letter to a journal editor or a review of another's work.

Selecting a Journal

The format and content of a manuscript targeted for an article submission will be dictated by the editorial guidelines and technical specifications of the journal. The author must first target a journal that corresponds to the subject content of the manuscript and reaches the appropriate audience for the information. Authors intending to submit evidence-based papers will need to learn the following typical criteria before making the decision to submit to a particular journal (Polit & Tatano Beck, 2008):

◆ Is the journal peer-reviewed?
◆ What is the journal's impact factor?
◆ What is the profile of the journal's readership?

◆ What is the turnaround cycle for review?
◆ What is the "in press" period (i.e., from time of acceptance to publication)?
◆ What are the technical specifications?
◆ Is this an open or closed access journal?

Manuscripts submitted to peer-reviewed journals are critiqued by a team of reviewers who have expertise in the subject matter of the paper. Any identification of the manuscript's author(s) is removed, and likewise, the anonymity of the reviewers is maintained during the review process. This type of review process is known as the *blind review*. It is believed that the blind review process is the most objective and fair way of judging the significance, technical competence, and contribution to professional literature.

Peer-reviewed journals publish more rigorously reviewed manuscripts than those reviewed by editorial staffs alone. Generally, most authors prefer to have their manuscripts published in peer-reviewed journals for this reason. Manuscripts published in regularly featured columns of peer-reviewed journals may not be peer-reviewed however. Authors need to ascertain this fact before submission. Another useful criterion to use in considering the choice for journal submission is the readership profile. Although the style and format of articles published by journals will be obvious to the author in terms of the type of article (e.g., data-based, clinical, or policy-oriented papers), having other editorial information is useful in terms of understanding the need to insert additional narrative on research methodology or clinical implications (Carroll-Johnson, 2013).

In most instances, information on the review process (e.g., the review period time frame and technical specifications) can be found in the "information for authors" section in each journal. Many authors are concerned about the timeliness in which manuscripts are published. Authors may worry that a research paper that has undergone a lengthy review process will not then be published in a timely manner. Concerns also exist regarding the delay in publishing an in-press manuscript because a lengthy time frame will substantially slow the dissemination and implementation of research findings.

In response to these concerns, several developments in publishing have occurred to facilitate the dissemination of scientific and clinical information. Many journals, including nursing journals, will post manuscripts online on the journal's website as uncorrected or corrected proofs prior to publication as a hard copy version. Each in-press manuscript is assigned a Digital Object Identifier (DOI) number until it is published in the journal issue. This digital string is the unique identification number assigned to electronic versions of manuscripts. The trend in citing references is to continue to include the DOI number after the paper has been published (American Psychological Association [APA], 2013a). The term *in press* in this electronic age of publishing now has several different connotations:

◆ *in press,* accepted manuscript papers that have been accepted by the review panel and journal editor.
◆ *in press,* uncorrected proof manuscripts that have been copyedited as a PDF file by the journal copyeditor; however, the author or team of authors have not reviewed, made necessary corrections, responded to queries from the copyeditor (i.e., missing references) or approved the PDF. A DOI number has been assigned, and the uncorrected proof is available online.
◆ *in press,* corrected proof-all corrections have been made and approved by the authors and the electronic version is available online and will be assigned to a journal issue and number. The manuscript has the same DOI number as assigned as an uncorrected proof.

Answers to these questions can be easily obtained from journal editors. Numerous websites for nursing journals list technical specifications, editorial philosophy, and hyperlinks available to the journal's publisher or editor for convenient access (APA, 2013b). The journal's technical specifications include the following:

◆ Manuscript format depending on type of paper submitted (i.e., research, clinical, column)
◆ Page length, word limits
◆ Reference style format (e.g., APA)
◆ Abstract format and word limit
◆ Declaration of conflict of interests
◆ Acknowledgment that the manuscript is not currently under review by another journal

◆ Margins, font style, and size
◆ Use of graphics, tables, photos, and figures
◆ Face page and author identifying information
◆ Electronic version and software

A noteworthy development with journal publication is the *open access* of electronic journals (Stuber, 2013). These journals are freely available to individuals, in contrast with subscription journals that are based on an annual subscription rate. As with subscription journals, there are peer-reviewed and non-peer-reviewed open-access journals. In some circumstances, an author may be asked to pay a fee to have an article published in an open-access journal, which can run from a nominal fee to several thousand dollars. Open-access journals, which have the institutional support of a university or organization, may not need to charge a fee. It is important for the author to be fully informed as to the reputation of the open-access journal, as with any subscription journal. *Directory of Open Access Journals* (DOAJ) and *Open J-Gate* are online directories of open-access journals.

 Website address of Directory of Open Access Journals is
http://www.doaj.org/

 Website address of Open J-Gate is http://openj-gate.org/

Developing the Manuscript Concept

Developing the manuscript concept depends on the author's area of clinical expertise and a lack of accessible information on which to base clinical practice. A clinician may want to share information with colleagues about an innovative intervention or implementation of a program improvement or may report the findings of testing a new approach to provide clinical services. There is an urgent need to publish articles on the search for and critical appraisal of evidence, as healthcare providers increasingly desire to base their practices on empirically tested approaches, and payers are beginning to demand it.

As the author proceeds with the process of refining the concept for writing an article on EBP, a literature review will assist in organizing the topic into an outline. Reviewing the literature will enable the author to gain an understanding of how to develop this publication uniquely and in a manner that contributes to the body of evidence-based nursing literature (*Science Direct*, n.d.).

Review of the Literature

Throughout this chapter the Internet has been identified as a technology resource. This is also true for publishing efforts. Use of online bibliographic databases enables writers to conduct more comprehensive and better literature searches. The following bibliographic databases will be useful when proceeding with the literature search for writing evidence-based articles and reports:

◆ Cochrane Database of Systematic Reviews (interdisciplinary)
◆ Cochrane Controlled Trials Register (interdisciplinary)
◆ ACP Journal Club (interdisciplinary)
◆ Evidence-Based Medicine Reviews (interdisciplinary)
◆ DARE (interdisciplinary)
◆ Cumulative Index of Nursing and Allied Health Literature (CINAHL, a nursing and allied health literature database that contains international journals from these disciplines)
◆ MEDLINE (a medical literature database of international medical, nursing, and allied health journals that contains primarily medical journals and selected nursing and allied health journals that have met the criteria for inclusion)
◆ Google Scholar
◆ Directory of Open Access Journals
◆ Open J-Gate

A few guidelines need to be considered before starting to write a manuscript. First, a literature review must be conducted to cite references that should be recent, or within the past 3 to 5 years. In some professions, it may be difficult to find current citations from the literature, thereby necessitating accessing the interdisciplinary literature representing not only health-related disciplines but also other disciplines (e.g., education, job development, and rehabilitation). There are also classic references, older than the 3 to 5 years' time frame, from any field that should be included in a publication because these are seminal works on which subsequent publications are based and cannot be ignored.

An author will have completed his or her search for evidence when the author cannot find any new references and is familiar and knowledgeable with the existing literature. Clinicians who write evidence-based articles will rely heavily on empirically based articles as they are searching for evidence. Authors will be less likely to include clinically oriented articles other than to demonstrate the relevance to clinical practice, such as the prevalence of falls among older adults. Textbooks should be referenced sparingly in evidence-based publications unless the books are written on highly specialized topics and are a compilation of perspectives from experts in the field (Heinrich, 2002).

A literature search will inform an author as to the scope of the topic and the evident gaps in the literature. As the literature search proceeds, the author's thinking will be further shaped with new insights and fortified with expert opinion and evidenced based articles that may result in modifications and enhancements of the original article purpose. Uncovering the body of literature in a field of science and practice is a dynamic and evolving intellectual and practice-focused endeavor.

Developing a Timeline

Healthcare professionals are well acquainted with developing and adhering to a work plan that identifies benchmarks of achievement. Having a work plan specifies in a concrete form the necessary tasks the author must undertake to complete the writing goal. The greater the level of specificity, the better chance the author will have for reaching his or her goal. Together with the identified tasks, *realistic* timelines should be listed along with strategies for keeping on track with accomplishing the steps of the writing project. A writing project timeline might look like the one listed below:

- Operationalize the idea/select a topic—June 1
- Develop the outline—June 15
- Locate journals/author guidelines—July 15
- Survey the literature—September 15
- Develop the first draft—November 15
- Review/proofread—December 10
- Make revisions—January 8
- Submit—January 20

Writing Strategies

Content outlines for articles will vary according to the type of manuscript. The generic outline for an evidence-based article, as used in the ongoing evidence-based column in the journal *Pediatric Nursing*, follows this format:

- Introduction to the clinical problem
- The clinical question
- Search for the evidence (i.e., the search strategy used to find the evidence and the results)
- Presentation of the evidence
- Critical appraisal of the evidence with implications for future research
- Application to practice (i.e., based on the evidence reviewed, what should be implemented in clinical practice settings)
- Evaluation (includes outcomes of the practice change if they were measured)

Obviously, writing an article for publication involves much more than just following an outline. The writing process is a slow and tedious effort that is characterized by stops and starts, cutting and pasting, and the frequent use of the delete key. However, writers use several pragmatic tips to help them complete their writing projects. Writing begins with following the manuscript outline at whatever section that can be written, even if it means first writing the simpler portions of the manuscript (e.g., the conclusion and introduction). Placing words on paper is important to "getting words down on paper," meaning to write anything, even if initially the words are awkward sounding and stilted. Inspiration will not necessarily happen spontaneously and requires trial and error and much mental perspiration. Start with any sentence for which there is inspiration, the beginning or the ending of the section can be written later.

Creativity is dependent on discipline and organizational techniques (Issa et al., 2013). These organizational techniques include the following:

- The manuscript outline should be followed as written. If the author discovers the narrative would be better written otherwise, the outline needs revision.
- Writing something is preferable to writing nothing. Awkward-sounding statements can always be edited and/or deleted. Initially, generating loose ideas that are difficult to couple with words can lead to more fluid thinking and word composition.
- Before completing a writing session, leave notes within the document that can be used as prompts for the next writing period. Leaving author notes ensures continuity with the train of thought from the last writing session and helps to facilitate recall and ease with the writing process.
- Write the paper anonymously, meaning there is no self-identification, although there may be exceptions in discussing particular programs. Use the same verb tense throughout, and avoid the use of passive voice. Note the major themes of paragraphs in the margins of the manuscript to discern the discussion sequencing, highlighting potential problems with organization.
- Avoid the use of *should*'s, *must*'s, and other words that are opinionated. Insert information that can be replicated and applied by others by avoiding the use of jargon.

Proofreading the Manuscript

If possible, the optimal proofreading strategy is to have colleagues or friends read the manuscript draft, including individuals who have expertise in the content area as well as those who possess no content expertise. Those without content expertise are specifically helpful in reading the manuscript for clarity, style, and grammatical errors (Fowler, 2013). However, it is essential that whoever proofreads the draft be a good writer with the capacity to provide specific suggestions for editing purposes. Very often, faculty members whose students are writing for publication outside of their course assignments are willing to serve as proofreaders. It is important to provide colleagues with the guidelines for manuscript submission from the targeted journal so that they can review the paper with those guidelines in mind (e.g., formatting, length).

Authors, of course, also serve as their own proofreaders. Setting the manuscript draft aside for a week or two will create the distance needed to read it again with a set of fresh eyes. In this manner, the author can read his or her own work more objectively and potentially pick out flaws with sentence structure, spelling, organization, and content. Once proofreading is completed, the draft is revised based on collegial feedback and the author's own proofing.

In addition to attention to content, the document needs to be well written. A fact-filled manuscript that is choppy or does not flow well, or in which there is poor grammar, will result in a poor review. Reviewers who are distracted by typos or poor writing will not be able to focus adequately on the technical content, and this well be reflected in the review. Students, in particular, may have access to the writing center of their university to help improve their basic writing skills. Writing is more art than science and professionals should not be embarrassed to seek out assistance to improve their writing, irrespective of the subject matter.

Spell checking the document is an absolute must in proofing manuscripts. However, automatic spell checking is not enough because it is not capable of detecting problems with some misspellings. The numbering of tables, graphics, and figures will need to be double-checked to ensure that they are properly matched with the sequence identified in the paper. The citation of references in the text is checked with those in the reference list for correct spelling, dates of publication, and referencing format. Other technical specifications (e.g., pagination, use of headers, margins, fonts) are reviewed to ensure conformity to those listed in the author guidelines. Permissions and transfer of copyright are included with the packet of materials that will be sent to the editorial office.

Once this process is completed, the manuscript can be submitted for review. The information for authors and/or the receipt from the editorial office will indicate the expected turnaround period for the manuscript review. If no feedback has been received after a period of six to eight weeks, it is appropriate to e-mail or call the editorial office to inquire about the status of the review. As mentioned previously, it is important not to take feedback personally. An impassioned approach will serve the author well by moving beyond what might be stinging criticisms to revising the draft based on the reviewers' recommendations. It is at this juncture that the author needs to keep focused on what was and continues to be the original goal—to publish the paper and contribute to the professional literature on EBP (Mee, 2013).

....

**Remember that you never get a second chance to make a great first impression, so make the first submission of the manuscript as flawless as possible.
—Bernadette Melnyk**

....

DISSEMINATING EVIDENCE TO INFLUENCE HEALTH POLICY

Healthcare providers are in an enviable position to advocate for change because they are highly regarded and trusted by the American public. As a leading politician recently remarked to a colleague, "Political endorsements from state nursing organizations are one of the most important endorsements a politician seeks to obtain." In essence, such a testimonial is *evidence* of the potential influence that healthcare providers, individually and collectively, have to impact changes in policy and to be engaged in policy making. The key is not only recognizing this potential but also actively taking advantage of opportunities that arise to be engaged in policy making at all levels of government and within professional organizations and service agencies.

Regrettably, opportunities to affect policy change may not be recognized for their value and importance. A colleague recently witnessed the unpleasant exchange of a legislator's stern rebuke to a nursing administrator from a local nursing education department. This nursing education administrator had been invited to provide testimony on the state's nursing shortage during a legislative hearing on this workforce crisis. Unfortunately, the nursing administrator was unprepared to sufficiently offer legislative testimony. The legislator was angered with her lack of preparation and her inability to answer his questions about the state's nursing shortage and statewide nursing efforts to address this issue. Not only was this an example of inadequate professional preparation, but the circumstances also reflected negatively on the profession as a whole because the policy input on behalf of nurses was not heard.

Similar cases illustrate the range of possibilities for healthcare professionals to influence policy. As healthcare professionals learn to become more involved in policy making, they will be expected to integrate evidence as the basis for policy development. As policy makers, healthcare providers will be "at the table" with key stakeholders, citing evidence to improve healthcare resources and services for national and international populations. Following are specific suggestions for integrating evidence in writing and other policy-making efforts.

Writing Health Policy Issue Briefs

There is growing recognition that current best evidence from research is needed to provide policy-related information to legislators in order to influence policy decisions that improve the quality of health care. Research that informs policy evaluates outcomes that are priorities for patients, healthcare providers, and payers, such as rehospitalizations, quality of life, satisfaction, morbidities, mortality, and costs (Ross & Gross, 2009). In addition to conducting good policy research, there is an urgent need for healthcare professionals to write compelling policy briefs based on findings from sound research that legislators can readily understand. A legislator cannot bring forward legislation without having the necessary substantiation, based on various sources of evidence, as to the need or problem to be addressed (ESRC UK Centre for Evidence-Based Policy and Practice, 2001a, 2001b). However, findings from a survey of a random sample of legislators indicate that they are often overwhelmed by the huge volume of information they receive and need information provided to them to be concise and relevant to current debates (Sorian & Baugh, 2002). Unfortunately, research is often not published in readily digestible form for policy makers and their staff (Health Affairs, 2012). In addition, legislators often rely on their staff to gather information about a topic and provide an overview to them, making legislative staffers a potential audience for evidence-based literature.

One avenue for providing policy makers with sound evidence is by developing issue briefs (see Appendix E for a brief developed by the American Association of Colleges of Nursing to assist policy makers in drafting a bill to enhance the nursing work force). A policy brief is a powerful communication tool that provides current evidence, based on prevalence reports and research by scientists, and/or the opinion of experts that can lead to successful decision making about key policy issues (Health Affairs, 2012).

The key to developing issue briefs is to be succinct and direct in communicating with the intended audience. A well-written issue brief summarizes and clearly communicates to the reader the scope of the policy issue. The reader should be able to scan the document quickly and be able to comprehend the major aspects of the policy issue that is featured. Tips for organizing an issue brief include the following:

◆ Lead with a title on the masthead that clearly conveys the purpose.
◆ Identify the policy issue in the first sentence so that by the end of the opening paragraph, the reader knows the policy issue.
◆ Include background information that highlights the major features of the issue.
◆ Indicate the historical pattern of response to the problem in subsequent statements.
◆ Identify the inherent limitations as well as the problem and why it is still a problem.
◆ Include common opposing views and refute them as well.

Another format for writing policy briefs includes the following components:

◆ Clear statement of the issue
◆ Context and background of the issue/problem, most effectively captured in bullet format
◆ Options: Pros and cons of each recommendation listed
◆ Resources used to prepare the policy brief (Health Affairs, 2012)

An issue brief provides a systematic review and synthesis of literature based on the selected topic addressing the demonstrated clinical outcomes of interventions, cost-effectiveness, and applicability. As the supporting evidence is presented, the reader is led in a logical sequence through the presentation of information that enables a clear understanding of the need for policy change. The concluding remarks of this section provide the links between research, clinical practice, and policy making. It distills for the reader what has been done and how it can be applied to policy making, which may be difficult for elected representatives or stakeholders if they do not have the expertise to "point the way" (Box 18.7).

A review of the literature should be conducted differently for policy makers than for a research audience. The analysis is conducted not only with clinical knowledge in the area but also with an understanding of the practical implications for policy makers. Where the information was obtained (i.e., meaning the type of research studies reviewed and synthesized in the paper; expert opinion of

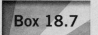

Typical Topics and Components of a Health Policy Issue Brief

Box 18.7

Issue briefs are developed to address issues of interest to policy makers:

TYPICAL TOPICS

Healthcare financing
Quality and safety of patient outcomes
Risk/benefit analysis of cost reduction alternatives
Lower rates of mortality and improved morbidity
The role of technology in health care
Human resource needs
System change to improve services

TYPICAL COMPONENTS

Title
Background of the issue
Historical pattern of response to the problem
Inherent limitations and problems
Why it remains a problem
Review and synthesis of the literature
Clinical outcomes of interventions
Cost-effectiveness
Applicability
Patient Privacy (HIPAA)
Policy implications
System changes
Services proposed
Population outcomes and health disparities

researchers, clinicians, and experts) is incorporated in the brief. Once the strength of the available evidence has been analyzed, conclusions are made about where gaps in the literature exist for which further research is needed. The conclusion will be much briefer than those written for research or review of literature articles.

The healthcare provider who is involved in constructing a policy issue brief will emphasize the application for policy and practice. That is, what is being advocated for policy change? How will the policy result in a change for services, such as treatments, assessment approaches, and evaluation of intervention outcomes (e.g., What clinical outcomes for the target population are expected, such as improved health as evidenced by better cardiovascular status and a higher level of daily functioning)? Policy conclusions should define in detail the possible clinical implications. For example, implications would recommend:

◆ Funding priorities in the treatment of chronic conditions
◆ Projected effects of funding cutbacks (e.g., a decrease in access to care and treatment)
◆ Longitudinal studies of various treatment approaches (e.g., hormone replacement therapy [HRT])
◆ Identification of actual and anticipated population outcomes

In this way, issue briefs assist policy makers in understanding the evidence so that they can create legislation founded on the premise that policy change is based on good science and knowledge.

Design layout of policy briefs helps convey the message to the audience. Obvious requirements in design layout of policy briefs are to ensure that there are graphics to highlight the major propositions, problems, facts, and recommendations. Boxes that contain bulleted, succinct statements are effective. A pullout that defines terminology may be useful if the language or medical terms are unfamiliar to readers. It is important to ensure the graphics are not too busy to be a distraction from the material presented. A case example to illustrate the nature of the problem or the implications of recommendations may be helpful. In a nutshell, policy makers are more likely to use information and evidence from a policy brief if

◆ The issue is clearly stated.
◆ The research evidence in the brief is focused.
◆ The document can be skimmed quickly for salient points.
◆ It is synthesized, conclusion-oriented, and succinct (i.e., no more than 2 to 4 pages)

Use of graphics and visual pointers also enables the reader to navigate through the material easily. To add depth, briefs can be accompanied by other tools, such as slides, spreadsheets, links to articles, websites, and a list of key contacts.

Understanding the Target Audience

Daily, consumers are bombarded with new information about health care that includes promising medications and treatments, hope for medical cures, and new treatment approaches. The barrage of information can be confusing for consumers. The conflicting information on HRT is an excellent example of the confusion women have experienced in understanding what might be the long-term effects of taking hormones. Policy experts have noted that the public seeks information that will enable them to better understand the disease pathophysiology and clinical application of that knowledge. In writing for a particular audience, the author needs to have an awareness of what type of information the audience is looking for and what would be considered most helpful.

Thoughtful and well-referenced issue briefs will be used by professional associations to assist them in the development of critical paths and practice guidelines. For example, the Agency for Healthcare Research and Quality (AHRQ) National Guidelines Clearinghouse contains more than 1,000 clinical practice guidelines that clinicians can access. AHRQ (2013) is currently involved in supporting the implementation efforts of the Affordable Care Act. Additionally, policy makers and other stakeholders can work with clinicians in suggesting topics for evidence review and development.

Writing in Understandable Language

The content and format of a policy brief will vary depending on the knowledge and interest of the intended audience and whether the readers are primarily consumers, policy makers, or professionals. To illustrate, if an issue brief is written for a professional audience, the summary of the research evidence can be presented using research terminology. If issue briefs are written for non-health professional audiences (e.g., legislators), research terminology is presented in more general terms to aid comprehension. Generally speaking, the reading level for widespread consumer distribution should be for a sixth-grade reading level (using the Flesch Kineard Reading Level found in software tools to assess reading level is most helpful). For policy makers, the format needs to emphasize practical information that is easy to read, although the content may also be adapted to the interests of individual legislators.

....

"Don't write so that you can be understood...write so you can't be misunderstood."
—President William Howard Taft

....

Health literacy is now recognized as a major public health concern affecting Americans. The U.S. digital brochure entitled *Healthy People 2020* identifies the following objective to increase health awareness among

Americans: Increase public awareness and understanding of the determinants of health, disease, and disability, and the opportunities for progress (U.S. Department of Health and Human Services, 2013). As national surveys and research studies demonstrate, the majority of the U.S. public have limited and inadequate understanding of the health information they receive to care for themselves and their families (Flores, Abreu, & Tomany-Korman, 2005; Kutner, Greenberg, Jin, & Paulsen, 2006; Leyva, Sharif, & Ozuah, 2005).

It is the writer's responsibility to apply or translate for the reader the synthesis of research for policy (i.e., how a particular practice can be improved and what the expected outcomes are for the targeted underserved populations). Authors need to keep in mind the targeted readership and the change that is being advocated. Based on these two primary criteria, the issue brief will be written in the style and format appropriate for the audience. All knowledge must have local application in order to be used. Briefs that are effective need to be written in a matter that policy makers see the relevance and impact for application at the local, state, and/or national levels. Lastly, the constant stream of information available today can lead to overload and be a barrier to accessing and using evidence. Having an existing relationship or intending to develop one with policy makers is important. It was found that seeking the advice and expertise of colleagues related to medical issues was preferable to seeking information from the literature. This model would likely apply to working with policy makers as well. Relationships and other methods of contact will strengthen the ties with policy makers, such as bulletins for decision makers that focus on a particular issue. Additionally, healthcare provider experts aware of the organizational barriers of workload, time constraints, and authority to implement change associated with projected change will be in a position to address these concerns directly through personal contacts with policy makers (Fatemah, R, 2012). Policy briefs are designed to inform readers with analyses of research results that have policy relevance. Issue briefs are effective tools for use by nursing professionals to describe, discuss, and recommend the need for policy changes.

WORKING WITH THE MEDIA TO DISSEMINATE EVIDENCE

Healthcare professionals need to think realistically about reasons the news media might want to report about their evidence-based story. Professionals who are serious about disseminating evidence need to understand how to work best with news media and what attracts their interest to writing or producing a story. The knowledge may mean the difference between a successful or a fruitless effort.

This section provides general guidance for talking to the media about findings from research and evidence-based implementation projects. Emphasis is placed on the dynamic nature of news, factors influencing why reporters cover certain stories, and information about how to influence the process for the best chances for success.

The Basics

The Internet and digital revolution have changed the media dynamically in the past decade. Web-based or digital media outlets have increased exponentially with the various delivery technologies, such as Twitter, Facebook, blogs, and other social media. The control over news of the established mass media, especially metropolitan newspapers and consumer magazines, has been reduced. While opportunities abound, competition for media space and time has also increased. There are many newsworthy stories to tell in health care in many more media outlets. However, there are also a plethora of other stories in other areas that are competing for coverage.

The media and its audiences are on information overload. At any instant, people can choose from hundreds of channels broadcast into living rooms, select from millions of websites, read news in a multitude of specialty professional publications, and obtain byte-size news from social media such as Pinterest, Instagram, Facebook, and Twitter, as well as blogs and wikis. A healthcare provider's story on research findings has to compete for attention and space and time in all these media.

The first step in gaining media attention is to have a clear and newsworthy message that is easy to understand. What is the importance of your message to the public? Have you developed a new method for identifying children at risk of abuse? Does your work inspire young people to explore education and careers in research or the healthcare professions? Have you developed a new method to prevent obesity and cardiovascular disease?

Second, you must determine the audience that you want to reach to decide which media to target to reach it. Specifically, knowing which audience you need to reach is essential to disseminating your information effectively. You need to identify the media outlet's readers, viewers, and listeners.

Finally, it is important to conduct a reality check to assess the competition. There is a multitude of information-rich websites, libraries full of books, research magazines for most disciplines, all of which compete for the public's attention and time. The bottom line is that just because you want a reporter to listen to what you have to say about the evidence on a particular topic does not mean the reporter will be interested in writing a story or article. This may be the most common mistake of healthcare providers in working with media.

When contacting news media, you often find a highly intelligent person working at a frenzied pace because of multiple deadlines and time pressures. Be prepared to state your message concisely and quickly, and be ready to engage that reporter or editor's news interest. Never presume that because you have something that is important to you to say that the editor or reporter will or can provide his/her time to listen. You probably are one of dozens who contact the reporter on that day in the midst of a multitude of demanding tasks that need to be accomplished in a hectic setting.

Make your case quickly for why the media should cover your story and place yourself and your story through scrutiny that mirrors a review from a top journal. You should know who has done or is doing similar work to yours and how your work differs. Be prepared to justify why funding was provided for your research or project. Be ready to explain the significance of your work in a way that the reporter can understand, which may result in an explanation unlike one you have ever given to other colleagues. It is important to first ask yourself this question: Why should my story be published on a day when many major health news stories are also breaking?

News Is Dynamic

Once you have refined your story pitch and defined the audience that you would like to reach, you need to recognize the inherent power of the media. When people turn to the Internet, cable TV, or the radio, they simply hit a key. They are hit with a burst of information. Most of us simply tend to listen to what we hear—not quite unquestioningly, but certainly passively. For example, people turn on the radio, hear the day's top news, and retain the stories that most interest them. However, there is truthfully no central repository of developments and events deemed to be "news" from which the media selects systematically. Instead, editors make fast intuitive decisions on the news they think interests the majority of their readers. Consequently, the public's interest, events, and your efforts to tell your story in part determine what gets covered.

As a receiver of news, you permit your views to be influenced by a journalist or editor in the media. Whether it is a radio announcer in Albuquerque, a TV news producer shouting across a newsroom in Los Angeles, or a well-known blogger writing content from his computer in his home office, you are subjecting yourself to others' choices about what you should and should not hear. People make these choices every day (i.e., which information to pass along and which to ignore). You often tell your neighbors about the stories that most interested you on a given day so, in a sense, we are all editors.

There is no single body of facts that constitute news and another set of facts that constitutes non-news. Deciding the news is an incredibly dynamic and intuitive process, and becoming aware of this is a huge step toward working with the media effectively (Figure 18.1). Prepare carefully first, then pursue your share of media attention as there are certainly many competitors trying to "sell" their messages or stories on any given day. The winner of the race is often the one who is proactive and convincing in "messaging" the value of their story to the media.

In addition to the specifics of your story, there is a multitude of factors that will decide whether your news is the media's news on any given day (Box 18.8). Being aware of these and other factors is important if your story is to make the news.

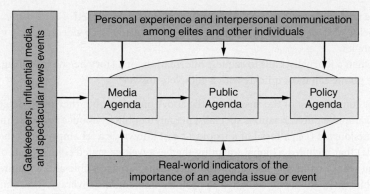

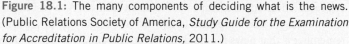

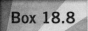

Figure 18.1: The many components of deciding what is the news. (Public Relations Society of America, *Study Guide for the Examination for Accreditation in Public Relations,* 2011.)

- What categories of news does the media outlet cover most often?
- Consider the reporter's deadline time when contacting him or her?
- What else is happening in the community, state, nation, or world today? Has there been a big layoff locally? A major accident with fatalities?
- Which other staff reporters cover your healthcare evidence topic when the regular editor is unavailable?
- What is the editorial approach or policy of the news outlet? Aggressive or conservative?

Box 18.8 Factors That Help Determine the News Value of Research Evidence

- *Interest*—Is it interesting and newsworthy?
- *Relevance*—Is it relevant? How could the findings make a difference in anyone's life and health?
- *Other events*—What else is happening in the nation, state, or local community this day or week (e.g., a hospital closing, impeachment proceedings, a war)?
- *Availability*—How available or reachable is the healthcare provider?
- *Exceptionality*—Is the evidence-based research extraordinary in a measurable sense? Is the research funding an unusually large amount?
- *Compatibilities*—How does the development fit into the overall strategy of the institution?
- *Quotability*—Is the healthcare provider quotable? Does he or she speak in a relatable, nontechnical language? Is the spokesperson experienced and/or comfortable talking with news media?
- *Visual appeal*—Are good photos or graphic artwork available quickly?
- *High-profile affiliations*—Are the study's findings being announced through a major journal or at a major conference?
- *Human interest*—Is a patient who was included in the study available so that human experience can be included in the story?
- *Clarity and applicability*—Is the take-home message clear and applicable to people's lives?
- *Cost*—What is the total amount of funding involved?

◆ What are the reader/viewer/listener demographics of the media outlet?

◆ Can you quickly provide or offer the best opportunity for artwork or videotape or a visually interesting angle?

◆ In the case when a journalist calls to request information for a story he/she is writing, which source returned the phone call most quickly with a complete answer?

You cannot control most of the answers to the above questions, but they often determine coverage of stories. For example, a public relations specialist prepared publicity about a research finding published in a top scientific journal (i.e., a fossil of a tropical beast known as a "champsosaur" that was found in the Arctic Circle) that included a global warming theme, a well-executed color sketch of an interesting beast, an animal whose name sounded like "champosaurus," an accessible and engaging scientist, and a top-notch publication. All of these aligned to promise tremendous coverage. That same day, though, the U.S. House of Representatives voted to impeach President Clinton. As a result, the "champosaurus" story was not published owing to a development over which the researcher or reporter had no control.

The point to remember is that news is a fluid, unpredictable medium. There are all sorts of people influencing events to determine what is read, heard, viewed, or tweeted. You can compete successfully for media attention if you follow the above points, take a realistic approach, and have a positive attitude.

You will also find that many others may attempt to use your communications program from your evidence findings story. Box 18.9 provides some examples of the people who might become involved in an ordinary healthcare or research story. Your graduate student may seek to turn the findings into a job offer. The public relations (PR) department may tout the results to the media, seeking positive publicity for the institution. The fundraising office may meet with a prominent donor who might give millions of dollars, based on work just like yours. Your competitors will comb through the article, seeking weak spots. The company funding your pharmaceutical research may be thrilled with the results and will promote them to investors. Also, politicians may claim credit for approving the funding that resulted in such important knowledge. The list goes on and on.

| **Box 18.9** | Who Can Help Disseminate Evidence? |

◆ Your graduate students
◆ Your postdoctoral fellows
◆ Your department chair
◆ Your dean
◆ Your colleagues
◆ PR staff
◆ Development office
◆ Technology-transfer office
◆ Alumni office
◆ Funding organization/agency
◆ Journals that publish findings
◆ Professional organizations/associations
◆ Manufacturer of the product you tested
◆ PR firm hired by manufacturer
◆ PR firm hired by journal
◆ Political leaders in states and cities impacted most
◆ Patient advocacy groups
◆ Collaborators at other institutions

Much of the competition for news space and its interpretation is invisible to the typical healthcare professional, who usually spends years immersed in his or her work, compared with time spent with an actual media representative. Thus, many healthcare professionals approach the media with over-confidence or naivety. Although anyone who works with the media ought to be prepared for a negative response, healthcare providers seem to be particularly vulnerable to being caught off-guard when a supposedly straightforward process of communication goes poorly.

The Up- and Downside of Working With Media

Working with the media to get out your evidence story may produce many surprises. There are a great many pitfalls about working with the media so a cost-versus-benefit analysis needs to be done before deciding to pursue this avenue of dissemination.

Media may really scrutinize your claim that your project is the first or only one with certain findings as you sincerely believed to be the case. Researchers at other universities may dispute your findings to protect their proprietary evidence-based research data. Your colleagues down the hall in the college may be jealous of your work because prospective graduate students want to visit your team, not theirs. Simply put, working with the media may consume large amounts of time and energy with minimal returns.

However, media attention can be extremely beneficial as well. You might be invited to speak at a national conference based on an organizer's Internet search of a topic. After reading about your work, a representative from a large company may contact you about funding your work. The article may help fuel perceived momentum around an expansion of research or a healthcare topic, resulting in a spike in donations that will fund future initiatives. There may also be a boost in coverage by other media that helps strengthen your institution's reputation or brand and recruit and retain the best and brightest individuals. News coverage about the findings from a clinical trial can also speed research and fuel initiatives to better health outcomes for the public. Researchers and clinicians who promote their research findings have witnessed all these results and more. News coverage about a nurse's study of rocking-chair therapy to treat dementia was covered by major publications around the world and is now used by dozens of nursing homes, thanks to some basic PR. Before that story was widely publicized, it was rejected by dozens of reporters. However, a single news story by a reporter at *The Boston Globe* launched the story into popularity and the research into use worldwide. Publicity about a finding on vaccines and thimerosal resulted in editorials in *The New York Times* and *The Wall Street Journal*. Also, research shows that coverage in the general press has a positive impact on the number of times a research article is cited in the scientific press. Increased citations in the scientific press, more funding, greater collaboration, jobs for students, and research making a difference in public health—these are all important outcomes to healthcare providers.

Frequently, the first step toward disseminating these outcomes after careful preparation is conducted as outlined above is simply calling or contacting a reporter. Many healthcare professionals are hesitant to take this simple action for fear that the mere act of informing a person outside of their communities may be construed as "hyping" the results. However, many individuals forget that much of the funding for their work came from taxpayers and that they have an obligation to report back to the people who paid for their work.

Some Sound Advice

Even when reluctant to call the media, chances are that you will have contact with a reporter about your study's findings eventually. When this occurs, you might want to have Box 18.10 posted nearby as a starting point or simply have handy the phone number of your PR person, who should work as your advocate. Frequently, a PR representative can clarify a reporter's questions for you or provide you with their background. It is not uncommon for a local reporter to know nothing about research or the health area it affects. On the other hand, journalists at prestigious media might have doctorates and the knowledge and ability to talk in-depth about your evidence findings. A PR staff member can also redirect a

> **Box 18.10** When a Reporter Calls: A Quick Guide to Action
>
> ◆ Call your PR person for advice, background information on the journalist, support, and backup.
> ◆ Relax and talk with the reporter in a calm and confident tone.
> ◆ Think of the messages that want to communicate in advance? Focus on two or three main messages that you want to convey, and be ready to work those into your answers to the reporter's questions.
> ◆ Before the interview, have background materials ready, and offer to provide them to the reporter.
> ◆ Think before you answer and do not be pressured to provide immediate answers. Offer to call the reporter back, and use time to collect your thoughts. In many cases, when a person claims to have been misquoted, they are simply unhappy about what they said to the reporter.
> ◆ Give the reporter your phone numbers (including home number), and say you would be happy to take calls anytime if he or she has any more questions or would like further clarification.
> ◆ Do not ask to see the story in advance because you are not the reporter's boss, do not own the publication, station or online news site, and do not determine what is covered and how. Instead, offer to be a resource and encourage the reporter to contact you with further questions.

call to someone else in the organization that is more appropriate or provide you the happenings within your organization that might influence the reporter's approach. Occasionally, a PR representative might also help you to provide minimal information and be cautious working with certain reporters because of their editorial biases or negative experiences.

If a PR professional supports your work, you must remain aware that he or she is also interpreting the story to some extent and placing your work in a particular context to have the best chance for coverage. For instance, after a PR specialist conducts a careful interview and does some reading about the topic, he or she attempts to write a summary of the healthcare professional's work in approximately 800 words (see Appendix F for an example of a news release draft provided for review). Typically, a physician, nurse, or researcher will read what is written, change a couple of lowercase letters to uppercase, and perhaps correct an error or two or insert some jargon. They typically limit their comments to the words presented to them in the summary. It rarely occurs to many professionals that they have left the entire interpretation of their work (e.g., the context, the emphasis) up to the PR specialist. If the words are accurate, they approve the overall theme. It is great when that happens, but healthcare professionals should consider whether the PR person's version is accurate or in context.

A PR practitioner who specializes in supporting research can also advise you about a host of other issues that may arise when disseminating evidence to the media. Some of these issues include the following.

Embargoes

A **news embargo** (i.e., a restriction on the release of any media information about the findings from a study before they are published in a journal article) is often used by some journals or science organizations to give reporters time to develop a story on a complex or exciting topic. However, not all reporters agree to embargoes; many see them as authorized or misguided attempts to "manage" the news—and not all embargoes have legitimate reasons. To be safe, if you are part of an embargoed story, you need to clarify this up front with the reporter before you say anything of substance. Hundreds of research stories are embargoed every week, and rarely does anything go wrong. If you and the reporter agree on the embargo, it is fine to speak to the reporter, and the story will appear after the embargo expires.

Off-the-Record Comments

Do not go there. Anything you say is on the record, and if you talk and then say afterward, "That was off the record," the reporter has no obligation to regard those comments as not to be published. You have to establish that *before* the interview. Even then, it is risky and better to avoid.

Peer Review

Peer review is crucial to experienced research reporters, and as crucial to them as it is to researchers. If you are making a claim, you need to have evidence that has been reviewed by someone else. Stories claiming any type of medical or scientific progress in detail usually rely on a publication in a journal or at least a presentation at a professional meeting. Even so, the rules are not always clear. A journal article almost always has much more detailed evidence and has been more rigorously reviewed than an abstract for a poster presentation, so the timing can be delicate. So, too, can the news about a paper or presentation. For instance, some journals reject manuscripts if you or your institution has actively promoted the results in other media, but they might accept them even if you can prove that other media initiated the coverage.

News Conferences

Professionals from most health disciplines tend to be nervous when speaking or being interviewed during a news conference. The use of charts and photos can help to emphasize or better explain major or complex points and reduce anxiety. Keeping comments short also puts the speaker at ease. Select speakers for the news value they contribute and their presentation skills. If you are talking about research results, make sure you have presented at a meeting or published in a journal before the conference. Healthcare professionals who make claims and present study findings at a news conference without supporting evidence that has been peer-reviewed place their careers at risk.

It is also important to remember technology-transfer issues. In other words, contact your technology-transfer department, and consider filing a patent application on any research/program products *before* you publish or present your results.

....
Never argue with anyone who buys ink by the barrel.
—Congressman Bruce Brownson, 1964
....

Reporters come with a variety of interests and abilities, but all have the power to reach out to more people with your message than you can possibly reach without them. When dealing with a reporter on a deadline, spending 5 minutes explaining a complex point will save the journalist 45 minutes to conduct research on their own as well as lessen the risk of errors. Avoiding the temptation to send them to the library, along with the other "don'ts" listed in Box 18.11, will go a long way toward building your effectiveness as a reliable media source.

You may not want to work with certain reporters because of their reputation for inaccuracy or bias on certain topics. There are reporters who have no interest in looking objectively at news and who instead are seeking a human face to place on a story already written. Additionally, there are reporters who will try to have you report their version of a story instead of the facts. In a story about why people were volunteering to be vaccinated against smallpox, a representative from a major TV network was not satisfied with the answer provided by one participant. The answer did not match the producer's preconceived notion of why people were volunteering, so he instructed the participant to use the word *patriotism* in his answer. Because the young man had been prepared for the pressure exerted by reporters, he disregarded the advice and provided an honest answer. The story was a success, in addition to being truthful.

Box 18.11 Some "Don'ts" When Working With Reporters

◆ Don't use scientific jargon.
◆ Don't assume you are a media expert.
◆ Don't wait hours to return a call; call back immediately.
◆ Don't expect a story to name every contributor or collaborator.
◆ Don't assume the reporter is familiar with the details of your project or discipline—ask.
◆ Don't dictate the "proper" questions or the story angle.
◆ Don't talk about just the positive aspects of your research findings; also discuss the limitations.
◆ Don't ask to see a copy of the story before it is published.

Fast Facts to Communicating EBP to Media

◆ Inform your public relations staff of your plan to contact the media and ask for relevant information and advice.
◆ Establish a relationship of mutual respect when working with journalists.
◆ Research what stories or articles the reporter has written recently to increase your credibility in working with them.
◆ Be ready to define EBP when working with general reporters who do not cover healthcare stories regularly.
◆ Develop three major messages or points about why your EBP story is of interest to the news outlet's readers, viewers, or listeners; write them on an index card before you talk with the reporter or editor. Tell the reporter that you will call back in 5 to 10 minutes if you do not have these points prepared.
◆ Always respect journalists' time and preferences for communicating with them.
◆ Never demand that an "error" be corrected; explain that you would like to provide more accurate information for future coverage of the topic.
◆ Avoid arguing with a journalist during an interview or after a story is published; always discuss points of disagreement in a professional manner.

The payoff from working effectively with print and electronic media can be enormous but the work to accomplish it daunting. It is important to prepare thoroughly, seek the assistance of an experienced PR advisor, be patient but persistent, and do your best. Although it would be simpler if quality work attracted attention on its own, the reality is that news is a competitive game and you should prepare a game plan and practice to play your best.

EBP FAST FACTS

◆ New evidence will not achieve its maximum value to clinical practice and better patient outcomes unless it is communicated effectively.
◆ The primary goal of disseminating evidence, whether it is presentations or publications, is to facilitate the transfer and adoption of research findings into clinical practice.
◆ Excellent preparation for dissemination reduces performance anxiety, builds confidence, and enhances the success of any communications initiative. Remember, you never get a second chance to make a great first impression.

◆ An effective presentation begins with an understanding of audience characteristics and needs, conference characteristics, and topical focus.

◆ Follow journal guidelines meticulously when submitting a manuscript.

◆ Set a goal to turn a presentation into a manuscript for publication within 90 days of the presentation.

◆ Target the media and policy makers as outstanding venues for evidence dissemination in addition to more traditional routes of dissemination (presentations and publications).

References

Abe, D. (2007). Teacher upgrade: Podcasts uploading your childbirth class. *International Journal of Childbirth Education, 22*, 38.

American Psychological Association. (2013a). What is a digital object identifier, or DOI? Retrieved July 10, 2013, from http://www.apastyle.org/learn/faqs/what-is-doi.aspx

American Psychological Association. (2013b). *Publication manual of the American Psychological Association* (6th ed.). Washington, DC.

Baker, J. D. (2013). Collaborative writing. *AORN Journal, 97*(1), 4–6.

Billings, D. M., & Kowalski, K. (2009a). Strategies for making oral presentations about clinical issues: Part 1. At the workplace. *The Journal of Continuing Education in Nursing, 40*(4), 152–153.

Billings, D. M., & Kowalski, K. (2009b). Strategies for making oral presentations about clinical issues: Part 1. At professional conferences. *The Journal of Continuing Education in Nursing, 40*(5), 198–199.

Billings, D. M., & Kowalski, K. (2010). Don't ignore that call for posters! *The Journal of Continuing Education in Nursing, 41*(9), 392–393.

Bingham, R., & O'Neal, D. (2013). Developing great abstracts and posters: How to use the tools of science communication, *Nursing Women's Health, 17*(2), 131–138.

Brennan, N., Mattick, K., & Ellis, T. (2011).The map of medicine: A review of evidence for its impact on healthcare. *Health Information Library Journal, 28*(2), 93–100.

Carroll-Johnson, R. M. (2013). Submitting a manuscript for review. *Clinical Journal of Oncology Nursing, 5*(3 Suppl), 13–16. Retrieved May 7, 2013, from http://www.ons.org/Publications/CJON/AuthorInfo/WritingSupp/Submitting/

Christenbery, T. (2011). Manuscript peer review: A guide for advanced practice nurses. *Journal of the American Academy of Nurse Practitioners, 23*(1), 15–22.

Christenbery, T. L., & Latham, T. G. (2013). Creating effective scholarly posters: A guide for DNP students. *Journal of the American Academy of Nurse Practitioner, 25*(1), 16–23.

Cleary, M., Happell, B., Lau, S. T., & Mackey, S. (2013). Student feedback on teaching: Some issues for consideration for nurse educators. *International Journal of Nursing Practice, 19*(Suppl 1), 62–66.

Costello, J. (2012). Publish or perish: Getting yourself published. *British Journal of Cardiac Nursing, 7*(11), 549–551.

Coumoyer, B. (2012). *How to project PowerPoint slides via iPad, iPhone or iPod touch.* Retrieved May 9, 2013, from www.brainshark.com/ideas/

DeSilets, L. D. (2010). Poster presentations. *The Journal of Continuing Education in Nursing, 41*(10), 437–438.

Dictionary.com. (2014). Vodcast. Retrieved May 27, 2014, from http://dictionary.reference.com/browse/vodcast

ESRC UK Centre for Evidence-Based Policy and Practice. (2001a). *Working Paper 1.* London: University of London, Department of Politics.

ESRC UK Centre for Evidence-Based Policy and Practice. (2001b). *Working Paper 6.* London: University of London, Department of Politics.

Fatemah, R. (2012). Evidence-informed health policy making: The role of the policy brief. *International Journal of Preventive Medicine, 3*(9), 596–598.

Flores, G., Abreu, M., & Tomany-Korman, S. C. (2005). Limited English proficiency, primary language at home, and disparities in children's health care: How language barriers are measured matters. *Public Health Reports, 120*, 418–430.

Fowler, J. (2013). Advancing practice: From staff nurse to nurse consultant. Part 8 publication. *British Journal of Nursing, 22*(8), 490.

Gelling, L. (2011). Welcome to the club. *Nursing Standard, 26*(1), 61.

Griffin, I., Buccino, R., Klein, D., & Thaler-Carter, R. E. (2010). Profession speaking: 10 tips on moderating a panel discussion, *Executive Communications.* Retrieved August 2, from www.exec-comms.com/blog/2010/08/02/10/

Hamilton, C. W. (2008). At a glance: A stepwise approach to successful poster presentations. *Chest, 134*, 457–459.

Happell, B. (2008). Conference presentations: A guide to writing the abstract. *Nurse Researcher, 15*, 79–87.

Happell, B. (2011). Responding to reviewers' comments as part of writing for publication. *Nurse Research, 18*(40), 23–27.

Health Affairs Editorial Staff. (2012). Health policy brief: Basic health programs. *Health Affairs,* November 15.

Health Care Transition Research Consortium. (2013). *Health Care Transition Research Consortium 5th Annual Research Symposium.* Retrieved July 7, 2013, from https://sites.google.com/site/healthcaretransition/presentations

Heinrich, K. T. (2002). Manuscript development. Slant, style, and synthesis: 3 keys to a strong literature review. *Nurse Author and Editor, 12*(1), 1–3.

Heinrich, K. T. (2007). Dare to share: A unique approach to presenting and publishing. *Nurse Educator, 32,* 269–273.

HLWIKI International. (2013). *BOPPPS model.* Retrieved July 7, 2013, from http://hlwiki.slais.ubc.ca/index.php/BOPPPS_Model

Horstman, P., & Theeke, L. (2012). Using a professional writing retreat to enhance professional publications, presentations, and research development with staff nurses. *Journal of Nurse Staff Development, 28*(2), 66–68.

Issa, N., Mayer, R. E., Schuller, M., Wang, E., Shapiro, M. B., & DaRosa, D. A. (2013). Teaching for understanding in medical classrooms using multimedia design principles. *Medical Education, 47*(4), 388–396.

Jham, B. C., Duraes, G. V., Strassler, H. E., & Sensi, L. G. (2008). Joining the podcast revolution. *Journal of Dental Education, 72,* 278–281.

Kiekkas, P., Sakellanropoulos, G. C., Brkalaki, H., Manolis, E., & Samios, A. (2008). Nursing workload associated with fever in the general intensive care unit. *American Journal of Critical Care, 17,* 522–533.

King, S. (2001). *On writing.* New York: Pocket Books.

Kutner, M., Greenberg, E., Jin, Y., & Paulsen, C. (2006). *The health literacy of America's adults: Results from the 2003 National Assessment of Adult Literacy* (NCES 2006-483). Washington, DC: National Center for Education Statistics.

Lannon, J., Gurak, L., & Daemon, D. (2012). *Technical communication* (12th ed.). Boston, MA: Longman.

Larkin, M. E., Griffith, C. A., Pitler, L., Donahue, L., & Sbrolla, A. (2012). Building communities of practice: The research nurse round table. *Clinical and Translational Science, 5*(5), 428–431.

Leyva, M., Sharif, I., & Ozuah, O. (2005). Health literacy among Spanish-speaking Latino parents with limited English proficiency. *Ambulatory Pediatrics, 5,* 56–59.

Majid, S., Foo, S., Luyt, B., Zhang, X., Theng, Y., Chang, Y., & Mokhtar, I. (2011). Adopting evidence-based practice in clinical decision making: Nurses' perceptions, knowledge, and barriers. *Journal of the Medical Library Association, 99*(3), 229–236.

Marble, S. G. (2009). Five-step model of professional excellence. *Clinical Journal of Oncology Nursing, 13*(3), 310–315.

McLeod, P., Steinert, Y., Boudreau, D., Snell, L., & Wiseman, J. (2010). Twelve tips for conducting a medical education journal club. *Medical Teaching, 32*(5), 368–370.

Mee, C. L. (2013). Ten lessons on writing for publication. *Clinical Journal of Oncology Nursing,* Retrieved May 7, 2013, from http://www.ons.org/Publications/CJON/AuthorInfo/WritingSupp/TenLessons/

Miracle, V. A. (2008). Effective poster presentations. *Dimensions of Critical Care Nursing, 27,* 122–124.

Phillips, W. L., Sweet, C. A., & Blythe, H. R. (2009). Collaborating on writing. *Academe, Sep–Oct* Retrieved on May 27, 2014 from *http://www.aaup.org/article/collaborating-writing#.U4Uq_vldXOM.*

Polit, D. F., & Tatano Beck, C. T. (2008). *Nursing research: Generating and assessing evidence for nursing practice* (8th ed.). Philadelphia, PA: Lippincott Williams & Wilkins.

Ranse, J., & Haynes, C. (2009). A novice's guide to preparing and presenting an oral presentation at a scientific conference. *Journal of Emergency Primary Health Care, 7*(1), Article 5.

Reference.com. (2009). *Vodcast.* Retrieved January 19, 2009, from http://www.reference.com/search?q = Vodcast

Rogoschewsky, T. L. (2011). Developing a conference presentation: A primer for new library professionals. *Partnership: The Canadian Journal of Library and Information Practice and Research, 6*(2). Retrieved July 7, 2013, from https://journal.lib.uoguelph.ca/index.php/perj/article/view/1573/2284

Ross, J. S., & Gross, C. P. (2009). Policy research: Using evidence to improve healthcare delivery systems. *Circulation, 119,* 891–898.

Rowell, M. R., Corl, F. M., Johnson, P. T., & Fishman, E. K. (2006). Internet-based dissemination of educational audiocasts: A primer in podcasting-How to do it. *American Journal of Radiology, 186,* 1792–1796.

Savel, R. H., Goldstein, E. B., Perencevich, E. N., & Angood, P. B. (2007). The critical care podcast: A novel medium for critical care communication and education. *Journal of American Medical Informatics Association, 14,* 94–99.

Sawatzky, J. V. (2011). My abstract was accepted, now what? A guide to effective conference presentations. *Canadian Journal of Cardiovascular Nursing, 21*(2), 37–41.

Science Direct. (n.d.) Articles in press. Retrieved on July 10, 2013, from http://www.sciencedirect.com/science/journal/aip/08825963#FCANote

Sherman, R. O. (2010). How to create an effective poster presentation, *American Nurse Today,* September 2010, p. 13.

Silversides, A. (2011). Journal clubs: A forum for discussion and professional development. *Canadian.NURSE.com,* February, 19–23.

Skiba, D. J. (2006). Emerging technologies center: The 2005 word of the year: Podcast. *Nursing Education Perspectives, 27,* 54–55.

Sorian, R., & Baugh, T. (2002). Power of information: Closing the gap between research and policy. *Health Affairs, 21*(2), 264–268.

Sortedahl, C. (2012). Effect of online journal club on evidence-based practice knowledge, intent, and utilization in school nurses. *Worldviews on Evidence-Based Nursing, Second Quarter,* 117–125. doi: 10.1111/j.1741 -6787.2012.00249.x

Steele-Moses, S. K. (2013). Developing a journal club at your institution. *Clinical Journal of Oncology Nursing, 13*(1), 109–112.

Steenbeek, A., Edgecombe, N., Durling, J., LeBlanc, A., Anderson, R., & Bainbridge, R. (2009).Using an interactive journal club to enhance nursing research knowledge acquisition, appraisal, and application. *International Journal of Nursing Education Scholarship, 6*(1), 1–8. doi:10.2202/1548-923X.1673

Stuber, P. (2013). *Open access overview: Focusing on open access to peer-reviewed research articles and their preprints.* Retrieved July 10, 2013, from http://legacy.earlham.edu/˜peters/fos/overview.htm

Tinkham, M. R. (2013). The road to Magnet: Implementing new knowledge, innovations, and improvements. *AORN, 97*(5), 579–581.

U.S. Department of Health and Human Services. (2013). *Healthy People 2020: Understanding and improving health* (2nd ed.). Washington, DC: U.S. Government Printing Office.

Van Soeren, M., Hurlock-Chorostecki, C., & Reeves, S. (2011). The role of nurse practitioners in hospital settings: Implications for interprofessional practice. *Journal of Interprofessional Care, 25*(4), 245–251.

Winters, J. M., Walker, S. N., Larson, J. L., & Lanuza, D. M. (2006). True tales from publishing research. *Western Journal of Nursing Research, 28,* 751–753.

Yoder-Wise, P. S., & Vlasses, F. R. (2012). Pathways to a leadership legacy: Pursuing professional publication. *Nurse Leader, 10*(5), 36–38.

Faculty Research Projects Receive Worldwide Coverage

Written by Emily Caldwell, Assistant Director of Research Communications, The Ohio State University. Reprinted with permission from The Ohio State University.

Two recent research projects by Drs. Bernadette Melnyk and Linda Chlan of The Ohio State University have been covered by media outlets from all over the globe and continue to generate interest. What follows is an account of the studies' research findings and examples of the attention following their papers being published in major medical journals.[1]

Example 1: The COPE Program[2]

Adding a mental health component to school-based lifestyle programs for teens could be key to lowering obesity, improving grades, alleviating severe depression, and reducing substance use, a new study suggests.

As a group, high-school students who participated in an intervention that emphasized cognitive behavioral skills building in addition to nutrition and physical activity had a lower average body mass index (BMI), drank less alcohol, and had better social behaviors and higher health class grades than did teenagers in a class with standard health lessons.

Symptoms in teens who were severely depressed also dropped to normal levels at the end of the semester compared with the control group, whose symptoms remained elevated. Most of the positive outcomes of the program, called COPE, were sustained for 6 months.

Thirty-two percent of youths in the United States are overweight or obese, and suicide is the third leading cause of death among young people aged 14 to 24 years, according to the Centers for Disease Control and Prevention. Yet most school-based interventions don't take on both public health problems simultaneously or measure the effects of programs on multiple outcomes, said Bernadette Melnyk, PhD, RN, CPNP/PMHNP, FAANP, FNAP, FAAN, creator of the COPE program, dean of The Ohio State University College of Nursing and lead author of the study. "This is what has been missing from prior healthy lifestyle programs with teens—getting to the thinking piece. We teach the adolescents that how they think directly relates to how they feel and how they behave," says Melnyk, also Ohio State's chief wellness officer. The study is published in the *American Journal of Preventive Medicine*.

A total of 779 high-school students aged 14 to 16 years in the Southwestern United States participated in the study. Half attended a control class that covered standard health topics such as road safety, dental care, and immunizations. The others were enrolled in the intervention Melnyk and colleagues were testing for its effectiveness—a program called COPE (Creating Opportunities for Personal Empowerment) Healthy Lifestyles TEEN (Thinking, Emotions, Exercise, Nutrition).

---

[1] The National Institute of Nursing Research supported this research (#1R01NR012171; Principal Investigator—Bernadette Melnyk). Coauthors include Diana Jacobson, Stephanie Kelly, Michael Belyea, Gabriel Shaibi, Leigh Small, Judith O'Haver, and Flavio Marsiglia of Arizona State University.

432

Melnyk began developing COPE more than 20 years ago while she was a nurse practitioner at an inpatient psychiatric unit for children and adolescents. The program is based on the concepts of cognitive behavioral therapy, with an emphasis on skills building.

It's not counseling in the classroom, however. The entire COPE curriculum, a blend of weekly 50-minute behavioral skills sessions, nutrition information, and physical activity over the course of 15 weeks, is spelled out for instructors in manuals and PowerPoint presentations.

"These are skills that I can teach a variety of professionals how to deliver, and they don't have to be certified therapists," says Melnyk, also a professor of pediatrics and psychiatry in the College of Medicine.

At its core, the COPE program emphasizes the link between thinking patterns, emotions, and behavior as well as the ABCs of cognitive behavioral skills building: activator events that trigger negative thoughts, negative beliefs teens may have about themselves based on the triggering event, and the consequences of feeling bad and engaging in negative behavior as a result.

"We teach kids how to monitor for activator events and show them that instead of embracing a negative belief, they can turn that around to a positive belief about themselves," Melnyk says. "Schools are great at teaching math and social studies, but we aren't giving teens the life skills they need to successfully deal with stress, how to problem-solve, how to set goals, and those are key elements in this healthy lifestyle intervention."

COPE includes also nutrition lessons on such topics as portion sizes and social eating and 20 minutes of movement—dance, dodge ball, taking a walk, anything to keep the students out of their seats.

Immediately after the programs ended, and 6 months afterward, COPE students' outcomes exceeded the control group's, on average, in several areas: 4,061 more steps per day; a significantly lower average BMI; better scores in cooperation, assertion, and academic competence; and a trend toward lower alcohol use among the COPE teens. In addition, 97.3% of COPE teens who started at a healthy weight remained in that category.

Melnyk noted that it's not possible to tease out exactly which component of the program has the most profound effect on teens, but it's likely to be the combination of all of them together.

Six school districts and a YMCA chapter in Ohio have already adopted COPE. Melnyk plans to continue testing an adapted version of the program for younger children in schools and community settings. See Box 1 for a list of publications in which stories about COPE have appeared.

Example 2: Anxiety and ICU Patients on Mechanical Ventilators[3]

Chlan, who joined Ohio State in January, led this study while a member of the faculty at the University of Minnesota. Coauthors include Craig Weinert, Annie Heiderscheit, Mary Fran Tracy, Debra Skaar, and Kay Savik, all of the University of Minnesota and Jill Guttormson of Marquette University.

New research suggests that for some hospitalized intensive care unit (ICU) patients on mechanical ventilators, using headphones to listen to their favorite types of music could lower anxiety and reduce their need for sedative medications.

In a clinical trial, the option to listen to music lowered anxiety, on average, by 36.5%, and reduced the number of sedative doses by 38% and the intensity of sedation by 36% compared with ventilated ICU patients who did not receive the music intervention. These effects were seen, on average, 5 days into the study.

The research is published online in the *Journal of the American Medical Association*.

Researchers first assessed the patients' musical preferences and kept a continuous loop of music running on bedside CD players. When patients wished to listen to music, they were

[2] This research was funded by a grant from the National Institute of Nursing Research.

Box 1 COPE Study Media Coverage

Stories about Bernadette Melnyk's research originally published in the *American Journal of Preventive Medicine* have appeared in or on:

TIME Health
US News & World Report
Reuter's Health
WTOP 103.5FM DC
KPTV Fox12 Oregon
Health.com
DailyRX
MedicalXpress
Philly.com
KVVU Fox5 Las Vegas
Guardian Express
National Post
Counsel & Heal
eNews Park Forest
WOSU 89.7 FM—All Sides with Ann Fisher
National Academies of Practice newsletter
American Association of Nurse Practitioners
RedOrbit
WTTG Fox5 DC
PsychCentral
Phoenix Health News Examiner
EmpowHER
The Globe and Mail
NIH Medline
Medicine Online
MedCity News

able to put on headphones that were equipped with a system that time- and date-stamped and recorded each use.

Professional guidelines recommend that pain, agitation, and delirium be carefully managed in the ICU, with the goal of keeping mechanically ventilated patients comfortable and awake. However, the researchers acknowledged that oversedation is common in these patients, which can lead to both physiologic problems linked to prolonged immobility and psychological issues that include fear and frustration over not being able to communicate, and even posttraumatic stress disorder.

"We're trying to address the problem of oversedation from a very different perspective, by empowering patients. Some patients do not want control, but many patients want to know what is going on with their care," says Linda Chlan, PhD, RN, FAAN, distinguished professor of symptom management research in The Ohio State University's College of Nursing and lead author of the study.

"But I'm not talking about using music in place of the medical plan of care. These findings do not suggest that clinicians should place headphones on just any ICU patient. For the intervention to have the most impact and to have the desired effect of reducing anxiety, the music has to be familiar and comforting to the patient—which is why tailoring the music collection for the patient to listen to was key to the success of this study."

Chlan and colleagues conducted the study with 373 patients in 12 ICUs at five hospitals in the Minneapolis-St. Paul area. Of those, 126 patients were randomized to receive the patient-directed music intervention, 125 received usual care, and 122 were in an active control group and could self-initiate the use of noise-canceling headphones. All patients had to be alert enough to give their own consent to participate.

A music therapist assessed each patient in the music group to develop a collection that met the patient's preferences. This was no easy task, as the patients are not able to speak when they are on a ventilator.

Researchers instructed patients to use the intervention if they were feeling anxious, wanted to relax, or needed quiet time. Nurses were asked to prompt patients twice during each shift about their interest in listening to music.

In all patients, researchers performed daily assessments of anxiety and two measures of sedative exposure to any of eight commonly used medications. Anxiety was measured with a visual analog scale that asked patients to describe their anxiety by pointing to a chart anchored by the statements "not anxious at all" and "most anxious ever." Patients remained in the study as long as they were on ventilators, up to a maximum of 30 days.

A complex statistical analysis of the data showed that significant reductions in anxiety and sedation could be seen in patients in the music intervention within 5 days when they were compared with patients who received usual care. Patients using noise-canceling headphones showed some improvements in anxiety and lower sedation intensity, but the effects were not as strong as those seen in the music group.

"There is something there with noise-canceling headphones, but the music is so much more powerful. With the music, we were able to show a simultaneous reduction in anxiety and in sedation," Chlan said. "When we listen to music, our entire brain lights up. We want to capitalize on the pleasant, comforting memories associated with music because it occupies brain channels that otherwise would be occupied by an anxiety-producing stimulus. That's why music is so much more than just something nice to listen to."

A former medical ICU nurse, Chlan now leads a research program that emphasizes testing treatment strategies that complement traditional medical approaches to ICU care.

"I think about tackling the modifiable risk factors. And sedation is directly modifiable because it is controlled by the clinician. Nonpharmacologic, integrative interventions like music bring in a piece that does not induce adverse side effects and does not contribute to ICU-acquired problems," she says.

She and her colleagues now are working on making the highly controlled research protocol more friendly to standard hospital practices. "If this is going to have wide clinical impact, that really has to be done," she says. See Box 2 for a list of publications in which stories about the music study have appeared.

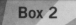 Box 2   Music Study Media Coverage

Media placements about Linda Chlan's research originally published in the *Journal of the American Medical Association* have appeared in or on:

CBS Radio
The Globe and Mail
MedPage Today
State of Health blog
AACN Critical Care
American Thoracic Society News
UPI wire services
MDLinx
US News & World Report
Philadelphia Inquirer
Huffington Post
Nurse Practitioner News
Critical Care SmartBrief
WOSU—Music in Mid-Ohio
WOSU—All Sides with Ann Fisher
MENAFN News (Middle East North Africa Financial Network)
American College of Physicians Hospitalist magazine
Psychiatric News
Reader's Digest

Chlan also served as an expert source in a story about music reducing the amount of stress children have over IV needles, which was covered in the *Chicago Tribune, Baltimore Sun,* and Fox News.

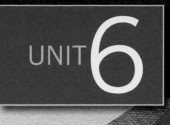

Next Steps: Generating External Evidence and Writing Successful Funding Proposals

Start by doing what is necessary, then do what is possible, and suddenly you are doing the impossible

—St. Francis of Assisi

Chapter 19
Generating Evidence through Quantitative Research

Bernadette Mazurek Melnyk, Dianne Morrison-Beedy, and Robert Cole

Man's mind, stretched to a new idea, never goes back to its original dimensions.

—Oliver Wendell Holmes

When there is a lack of research reported in the literature to guide clinical practice, it becomes necessary to design and conduct studies to generate **external evidence** (i.e., evidence generated through rigorous research that is intended to be used outside of one's own clinical practice setting). There are many areas in clinical practice that do not have a sufficient evidence base (e.g., care for dying children). As a result, there is an urgent need to conduct studies so that healthcare providers can base their treatment decisions on sound evidence from well-designed studies instead of continuing to make decisions that are steeped solely in tradition or opinion.

THE IMPORTANCE OF GENERATING EXTERNAL EVIDENCE

This chapter provides a general overview and practical guide for formulating clinical research questions and designing studies to answer these questions. It also includes suggestions on when a quantitative approach would be more appropriate to answer a specific question. A variety of quantitative research designs are discussed, from **descriptive studies** to **randomized controlled trials** (RCTs). Descriptive studies are designed to explore or predict relationships between variables. RCTs are rigorous studies designed to test the effect of interventions or treatments. Descriptive studies serve as the building blocks for RCTs. Techniques to enhance the rigor of quantitative research designs are highlighted, including strategies to strengthen **internal validity** (i.e., the ability to say that it was the independent variable or intervention that caused a change in the dependent variable or outcome, not other extraneous variables), as well as **external validity** (i.e., generalizability, which is the ability to generalize findings from a study's sample to the larger population). Specific principles of conducting *qualitative studies* are detailed in Chapter 20.

Getting Started: From Idea to Reality

We are told never to cross a bridge until we come to it, but the world is owned by men who have 'crossed bridges' in their imagination far ahead of the crowd.
—Speakers Library

Many ideas for studies come from clinical practice situations in which questions arise regarding best practices or evolve from a search for evidence on a particular topic (e.g., Is music or relaxation therapy more effective in reducing the stress of patients after surgery? What are the major variables that predict the development of posttraumatic stress disorder in adults after motor vehicle accidents?). However, these ideas are often not studied by practitioners due to competing demands or inadequate knowledge, skills, or resources to complete the project successfully. However, clinical ideas or research questions can be shared with doctorally prepared clinicians or researchers who can partner with the practitioner to launch a study. Thus, the person who had the idea or question can assume an active role on the study team but need not take on the role of the lead person, or **principal investigator (PI)**, who is responsible and accountable for overseeing all elements of the research project.

....

The greatest successful people of the world have used their imagination.... They think ahead and create their mental picture, and then go to work materializing that picture in all its details, filling in here, adding a little there, altering this a bit and that a bit, but steadily building—steadily building.
—Robert Collier

....

After an idea is generated for a study and a search for and critical appraisal of the literature has been conducted, a collaborative team can be established to be part of the planning process from the outset. Because clinicians often have many crucial clinical questions but typically need assistance with details of study design, methods, and analysis, formulating a team comprised of seasoned clinicians and research experts (e.g., doctorally prepared clinical researchers) will usually lead to the best outcomes. Increasingly, teams of transdisciplinary professionals are brought together adding value to the project by broadening perspectives and approaches applied, especially during the study design and interpretation of findings. Many funding agencies often expect transdisciplinary collaboration on research projects. Convening this collaborative team for a **research design meeting** at the outset of a project is exceedingly beneficial in developing the study's design and methods.

Approximately 1 to 2 weeks before the research design meeting is conducted, a concise, two-page study draft should be prepared and disseminated. This draft acts as an outline or overview of the clinical problem and includes the research question and a brief description of the proposed methods (Box 19.1 for an example of a study outline and Boxes 19.2 and 19.3 for completed examples of study outlines for different types of clinical studies). As the study outline develops, a list of questions related to the project should be answered:

Box 19.1   Outlining Important Elements of a Clinical Study

Before developing a study protocol, it is extremely beneficial to develop a one- to two-page outline of the elements of a study.

  I. Significance of the Problem and the "So What?" Factor
 II. Specific Aim of the Study
    A. Research Question(s) or
    B. Hypotheses
III. Theoretical/Conceptual Framework
 IV. Study Design
  V. Subjects
    A. Sampling Design
    B. Sampling Criteria
        1. Inclusion Criteria
        2. Exclusion Criteria
 VI. Variables
    A. Independent Variable(s) (in an experimental study, the intervention being proposed)

(continued)

> B. Dependent Variable(s) (the "so what" outcomes) and Measures
> C. Mediating Variable, if applicable (e.g., the variable through which the intervention will most likely exert its effects)
> D. Confounding or Extraneous Variable(s) with potential control strategies
> VII. Statistical Issues
> 　A. Sample Size
> 　B. Approach to Analyses

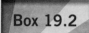

Box 19.2　Example of a Completed Study Outline for a Descriptive Correlational Study

A nonexperimental study entitled "Relationship between Depressive Symptoms and Motivation to Lose Weight in Overweight Teens."

I. Significance of the Problem

Data from the Centers for Disease Control indicate that 18% of adolescents are overweight. The major negative consequences associated with obesity in adolescence include premature death, type 2 diabetes, hyperlipidemia, hypertension, and depression. It is known that motivation to lose weight is a key factor in weight loss, but the relationship between depressive symptoms and motivation to lose weight in adolescence has not been studied.

II. Specific Aim of the Study with Research Question(s) or Hypotheses

The aim of this study is to answer the following research question: What is the relationship between depressive symptoms and motivation to lose weight in overweight adolescents?

III. Theoretical/Conceptual Framework

Control theory contends that, when there is a discrepancy between a standard or goal (e.g., perceived ideal weight), this discrepancy should motivate individuals to initiate behaviors (e.g., exercise, healthy eating) that allow them to achieve their goal. However, there are often barriers that may inhibit an individual in being motivated to initiate these behaviors. In this study, depression is viewed as a barrier to motivation and behaviors that would allow teens to achieve their ideal weight.

IV. Study Design

A descriptive correlational design will be used.

V. Subjects

A. *Sampling Design*: A random sample of 80 overweight adolescents will be drawn from two randomly selected high schools in Columbus, Ohio; one from the city school district and one from the suburban area.

(continued)

B. *Sampling Criteria*
   1. *Inclusion Criteria*: Adolescents with a body mass index of 25 or greater enrolled in the two high schools.
   2. *Exclusion Criteria*: Adolescents with a current diagnosis of major depression and/or suicidal ideation.

VI. **Variables**
   A. *Independent Variable(s)*: Depressive symptoms will be measured with the well known, valid, and reliable Beck Depression Inventory (BDI-II).
   B. *Dependent Variable(s)*: Motivation to lose weight will be measured with a newly constructed scale that has been reviewed for content validity with experts in the field. This new scale has been pilot tested with 15 overweight teens and found to have a Cronbach's alpha of 0.80.
   C. *Mediating Variable, if Applicable*: Not applicable.
   D. *Confounding or Extraneous Variable(s) with Potential Control Strategies*: Gender is a potential confounding variable, because there is a higher incidence of depression in adolescent females than males documented in the literature. Therefore, stratified random sampling will be used so that an equal number of males and females will be drawn for the sample.

VII. **Statistical Issues**
   A. *Sample Size*: To obtain a power of 0.8 and medium effect size at the 0.05 level of significance, a total of 80 adolescents will be needed.
   B. *Approach to Analyses*: A Pearson's r correlation coefficient will be used to determine if a relationship exists between the number of depressive symptoms and motivation to lose weight in this sample.

Box 19.3   Example of a Completed Study Outline for a Randomized Controlled Trial

A Randomized Clinical Trial entitled "Maintaining HIV Prevention Gains in Female Adolescents" (Morrison-Beedy, D., funded by the National Institutes of Health/National Institute of Nursing Research, R01-NR008194-01A1, 2004–2009.)

I. **Significance of the Problem**

Reducing the number of HIV infections in adolescents is a critical adolescent objective in *Healthy People 2020* and the highest priority on the national HIV agenda. Year 2000 data indicate that adolescents, persons 13 to 19 years of age, are the only age category where the number of females infected with HIV or with AIDS outnumber the number of males. The majority of these cases were a result of transmission of HIV through heterosexual contact. STIs such as chlamydia and gonorrhea also facilitate the transmission of HIV and in 1998 young women ages 15 to 19 years had higher reported rates of these diseases than adolescent males

(continued)

or older persons of either gender. Prevention interventions to reduce risk behaviors remain the foremost means to curtail the AIDS epidemic, yet very few randomized controlled trials are targeted to adolescent females.

II. Specific Aim with Research Question/Hypothesis

The purpose of this randomized controlled trial is to test the short- and long-term efficacy of a theoretically based, manualized HIV-prevention intervention in sexually active adolescent girls aged 15 to 19. We hypothesized that participants of the theoretically based intervention will increase (a) HIV-related knowledge, (b) motivation to reduce risk, (c) HIV-preventive behavioral skills, and (d) decrease the frequency of risky sexual practices as compared to control participants *in a structurally equivalent health promotion intervention at postintervention, and at 3, 6, and 12 months.*

III. Theoretical/Conceptual Framework

The theoretical framework for this study is derived from Fisher and Fisher's Information-Motivation-Behavioral Skills Model (IMB). The IMB combines elements from several health behavior models to specify several critical determinants of HIV-related behavioral change. They posit that initiating and maintaining these behaviors result from **information** about HIV prevention and transmission, the **motivation** to reduce risk, and the **behavioral skills** specific to HIV prevention. Using the IMB to guide intervention development for adult women, we have extended information-only and information-and-skills-based programs by enhancing the motivational components of an HIV risk reduction program for women. We included aspects of both immediate (behavior-focused) motivation and broader-based motivation related to life goals, personal and community values, and other trans-situational influences. Designed to increase the participant's collaboration and avoid resistance to change, this client-centered but directive style differs from purely didactic or confrontational approaches. Our team subsequently conducted elicitation research with sexually active girls 15 to 19 years and modified the intervention to address the needs of this age group. A pilot test of this intervention suggests that this approach may be particularly useful when developing HIV prevention interventions for adolescent females as well. *The study allows us to explore important gender-related moderators of behavior change in adolescent girls (e.g., sexual assertiveness, self management skills),* an important omission in prior studies of adolescent girls.

IV. Study Design

An RCT will be used with random assignment of subjects to either the experimental intervention group or the control group.

V. Participants

A. *Sampling Criteria*: Adolescent girls who meet the following criteria will be eligible for study participation:
   1. Aged 15 to 19
   2. Neither pregnant nor actively trying to become pregnant
   3. No births within the past 3 months
   4. Heterosexually active within the past 3 months
   5. English-speaking

(continued)

B. *Sampling Design*: A convenience sample of adolescent girls who meet the inclusion criteria and agreed to participate in the study.

VI. Variables

A. *Independent Variable(s)*: The experimental and control group both participated in interventions that were theoretically and empirically guided, gender-focused, and developmentally appropriate for adolescents aged 15 to 19 and included content that addressed the following variables:
  1. Information regarding HIV in the experimental group or health information in the control group
  2. Motivation to change behaviors improve health
  3. Behavioral skills such as assertive communication in both groups

B. *Dependent Variable(s)*: The frequency of unprotected and protected vaginal, oral, and anal intercourse in the past 3 months will be assessed at baseline, postintervention and at 3, 6, and 12 months. Number and type of sexual partner(s) will also be assessed (i.e., steady vs. nonsteady partner).

C. *Confounding or Extraneous Variable(s) with Potential Control Strategies*: Results could be confounded if participants brought up topics within the control group that were related to the experimental intervention. However, facilitators were trained, and the manual provided specific instructions on how to steer the conversation back to control topics. Other concerns were that there might be "crosstalk", that is cross-contamination between girls randomized to different groups who might come together in social or school settings. However, researchers believed that as the trained interventionists used motivational interviewing strategies, the content could not be duplicated simply by conversations between the groups.

VII. Statistical Issues

A. *Sample Size*: The sample size of 738 was based on the expected small effect size anticipated for change in STI rates (biologically documented) lab tests.

B. *Approach to Analyses*: Cronbach's alpha will be used to determine internal consistency reliability of the study instruments. Baseline characteristics of the intervention groups will be tabulated and any significant differences between groups and between sites will be noted. Additionally, we will conduct analyses to identify the correlates of program attendance to determine whether any baseline characteristic is associated with program completion or attrition. Formal analyses will use the intent-to-treat principle, that is, keeping all study subjects in their assigned randomization group for analysis and will require a two-sided alpha level of 0.05 for statistical significance. To test the study hypotheses, we will use zero-inflated Poisson (ZIP) regression analyses for frequency of sexual behavior. We will also analyze impact of the intervention on the number of sex partners, by categorizing number of partners and then modeling using generalized logit regression to assess differences between participants based on number of partners. The ZIP model will be evaluated with 3-, 6-, and 12-month postintervention outcome data.

◆ Is this idea feasible and clinically important?

◆ What is the **"so what" factor?** (i.e., the conduct of research with high-impact potential to improve outcomes that the current healthcare system is focused on, such as patient complications, readmission rates, length of stay, cost) (Melnyk & Morrison-Beedy, 2012)

◆ What is the aim of the study, along with the research question(s) or hypotheses?

◆ What is the best design to answer the study question(s) or test the hypotheses?

◆ What are the "so what" outcomes that are important to measure and potential sources of data? Are there valid and reliable instruments to measure the desired outcomes?

◆ What should be the **inclusion** and **exclusion criteria** for the potential study participants?

◆ What are the essential elements of the intervention, if applicable, and how will **integrity of the intervention** be maintained (i.e., assurance that the intervention is being delivered exactly in the manner in which it was intended to be delivered)?

The research design planning session needs to foster an environment in which constructive critique and candid discussion will promote a finely tuned study design. It is important to define the roles for each of the study team members (e.g., percentage of effort on the study, specific functions, availability, and order of authorship once the study is published). In addition, potential funding sources for the study should be discussed, as well as who will assume specific responsibilities in writing a grant proposal if funding is necessary to conduct the project (see Chapter 21 for specific steps in writing a successful grant proposal and Box 19.4 for a summary of initial steps in designing a clinical study).

Designing a Clinical Quantitative Study

Box 19.5 identifies several factors to consider in developing a quantitative study. Understanding prior work in the area of study builds the initial case for need. This is followed closely by significance of the problem and feasibility of investigating the issue. Once an important question has been identified and it is likely that a study to investigate the problem can be carried out, the building blocks have been laid for designing the study.

Box 19.4 Initial Steps in Designing a Clinical Study

◆ Cultivate a spirit of inquiry as you deliver care to patients in your practice setting.

◆ Ask questions about best practices for specific clinical problems.

◆ Develop a "creative ideas" file as thoughts for studies emerge.

◆ Pursue a clinical research question that you care about and that is an important "so what?" factor.

◆ Search for, critically appraise, and synthesize systematic reviews and prior studies in the area of interest.

◆ Establish a potential collaborative team for the project.

◆ Plan a research design meeting.

◆ Prepare and disseminate a concise two-page study outline.

◆ Conduct the research design meeting to plan specific details of the clinical study, decide on the roles of team members, and plan the writing of a grant proposal for funding if needed.

◆ Incorporate feedback and input from team members and other experts to improve the study design.

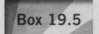

Box 19.5 Major Factors to Consider When Designing a Quantitative Study

◆ Prior studies in the area
◆ Significance of the problem and the "so what" factor
◆ Innovation of the project
◆ Feasibility
◆ Setting for the study and access to potential subjects
◆ Study team
◆ Ethics of the study

Critical Analysis and Synthesis of Prior Data

If this critical analysis reveals numerous studies that describe a particular construct or phenomenon, such as stressors of family caregivers of hospitalized elders, as well as studies that identify the major predictors of caregiver stress during hospitalization (e.g., uncertainty regarding the caregiving role in the hospital, lack of knowledge regarding how best to enhance outcomes in the hospitalized elder), another descriptive study in the field may not be needed. Instead, the next logical step in this example (based on the descriptive and predictive evidence already generated from prior studies) would be to design and test an educational intervention that informs family caregivers of the functions they can perform to improve their hospitalized elder's health outcomes. In contrast, if the phenomenon of caregiver stress is not well understood or adequately measured in the literature, conducting a qualitative or descriptive study may be the most appropriate step in conducting research in this area. This type of study might begin with open-ended questions to allow participants to respond in their own words to such questions as, How would you describe what it is like for you to care for your partner or parent? or How have things changed for you now, while your family member is in the hospital? Research in a particular area frequently begins with qualitative work in which a phenomenon or construct is explored with heavy emphasis on interview or observation data (see Chapter 22). When more is known about the nature of the phenomenon through qualitative work, quantitative research is usually undertaken in which the construct of interest is described using measurement scales, test scores, and statistical approaches (Figure 19.1). Oftentimes, descriptive, quantitative, qualitative, and formative work is conducted in parallel or alternating steps, and these findings build the case for, and ultimately design of, interventions that impact health outcomes.

As Figure 19.1 shows, quantitative research designs range from descriptive and correlational descriptive/predictive studies to RCTs. **Correlational descriptive** and **correlational predictive** designs examine the relationships between two or more variables (e.g., What is the relationship between smoking and lung cancer in adults? or What maternal factors in the first month of life predict infant cognitive development at 1 year of age?). These designs are the study of choice when the **independent variable** cannot be manipulated experimentally because of some individual characteristic or ethical consideration (e.g., individuals cannot be assigned to smoke or not smoke). The goal in correlational descriptive or correlational predictive studies is to provide an indication of how likely it is that a cause-and-effect relationship might exist (Powers & Knapp, 2010).

Although RCTs, or *experiments*, are the strongest designs for testing cause-and-effect relationships (i.e., testing the effects of certain clinical practices or interventions on patient outcomes), only a small

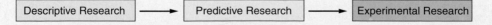

Figure 19.1: Progression of quantitative research.

percentage of studies conducted in many of the health professions are experimental studies or clinical trials. Additionally, of those intervention studies reported in the literature, many have limitations that weaken the evidence that is generated from them, including:

◆ Lack of random assignment to study groups
◆ Lack of or underdeveloped theoretical frameworks to guide the interventions
◆ Small sample sizes that lead to inadequate **power** to detect significant differences in outcomes between the experimental and control groups
◆ Limited attention to maintaining the fidelity of the intervention so that all participants receive a similar treatment
◆ Omission of **manipulation checks**, which are assessments verifying that subjects have actually processed the experimental information that they have received or followed through with prescribed intervention activities
◆ Failure to limit **confounding** or **extraneous variables** (i.e., those factors that interfere with the relationship between the independent and dependent variables)
◆ Lack of more long-term follow-up to assess the sustainability of the treatment or intervention

Therefore, because a **true experiment** (i.e., one that has an intervention, a comparison or attention control group, and random assignment) is the strongest design for the testing of cause-and-effect relationships and provides strong, or **Level II evidence** (i.e., evidence generated from an RCT, the next strongest evidence behind systematic reviews of RCTs; see Chapter 1) on which to change or improve practice, there is an urgent need for healthcare professionals to move beyond descriptive and correlational studies in order to build higher level evidence. For a description of the process of building the foundation for an RCT beginning with description and predictive studies, refer to the case study in the resources that accompany this book.

Significance of the Question

A second critical factor to consider when designing studies is the significance of the problem or research question, or otherwise known as the "so what?" factor. There may be research questions that are interesting (e.g., Do pink or blue scrubs worn by intensive care unit nurses have an impact on the mood of unit secretaries?), but answering them will not significantly improve care or patient outcomes. Therefore, a funding agency is not likely to rate the significance of the problem as important. Problems that are significant for study are usually those that affect a large percentage of the population or those that frequently affect the process, outcomes, or cost of patient care.

Feasibility

The third factor to consider when designing a study is feasibility. Before embarking on a study, important questions to ask regarding feasibility are

◆ Can the study be conducted in a reasonable amount of time?
◆ Are there an adequate number of potential subjects to recruit into the study?
◆ Have the settings for recruitment been identified and is accessibility a concern?
◆ Does the lead person (PI) have sufficient time and expertise to spearhead the effort?
◆ Are there major ethical or legal constraints to undertaking this study?
◆ Are there adequate resources available at the institution or clinical site to conduct the study? If the answer is no, what is the potential for obtaining funding?

If the answer to any of these questions is no, further consideration should be given to the feasibility of the project.

As a general rule, it typically takes more time to carry out a clinical study than is originally projected. Even when participant numbers are projected to be sufficient for the time allotted for data collection when planning a study, it is wise to incorporate a buffer period (i.e., extra time) in case **institutional review board (IRB)** approval is delayed, access to recruitment settings is more time-consuming, or subject recruitment takes longer than anticipated. Also, certain times of the year are more conducive for data collection than others (e.g., in conducting a study with elementary school students, data collection will be possible only when school is in session). Certain settings are more conducive to the conduct of clinical research than others. Settings that tend to facilitate research are those in which there is administrative approval and staff "buy-in" regarding clinical studies. Settings in which staff members perceive research as burdensome to them or their patients may confound study results as well as hamper a study's progress. Obtaining administrative approval to conduct a study and getting a sense of staff support for a project is an early and critical preparatory step for a clinical research project.

....
Alone we can do so little; together we can do so much.
—Helen Keller
....

It is important to consider the experience, skills, interest, and commitment of each member of the team. Study team members should possess the skills needed to plan, implement, analyze, and interpret the research data. For a novice researcher, the addition of seasoned researchers to the project will be important for its success, especially as challenges are encountered in the course of the initiative.

....
It is literally true that you can succeed best and quickest by helping others to succeed.
—Napoleon Hill
....

Ethical considerations include the need to assess burden to study participants as well as whether the benefits of participation in the study will exceed the risks. Serious consideration must also be given to the gender, age, and racial/ethnic composition of the sample. For federal grant applications, strong rationale must be provided if women, children, and minority subjects will be excluded from the research project. All study team members need to be knowledgeable regarding the ethics of conducting the study and the rights of participant subjects. Further discussion about obtaining research subjects' review approval for a clinical study appears later in this chapter and in Chapter 22.

Ultimately, feasibility rests on the financial support available for conducting the study. Even the smallest of studies require resources, even if only in the time and energy of the person serving as PI. The study can be supported by grants through internal or external agencies or by in-kind support of personal efforts and materials. Careful attention to various factors affecting study feasibility sets the stage for successful research investigations.

SPECIFIC STEPS IN DESIGNING A QUANTITATIVE STUDY

When designing a quantitative clinical research study, there is a specific series of orderly steps that are typically followed (Box 19.6). This is referred to as the *scientific approach to inquiry*.

Step 1: Formulate the Study Question

The first step in the design of a study is developing an innovative, yet answerable study question. Hulley, Cummings, Browner, Grady, and Newman (2006) use the acronym FINER (feasible, interesting, novel, ethical, relevant) to determine the quality of the research question. Feasibility is an important issue when formulating a research question. Although a research question may be interesting (e.g., What is the effect of a therapeutic intervention program on depression in women whose spouses have been murdered?), it could take years to collect an adequate number of participants to conduct the statistical analysis to answer the question.

Box 19.6 Specific Steps in Designing a Quantitative Clinical Study

1. Formulate the study question.
2. Establish the significance of the problem and the "so what" factor.
3. Search for, critically appraise, and synthesize available evidence.
4. Develop the theoretical/conceptual framework.
5. Generate hypotheses when appropriate.
6. Select the appropriate research design.
7. Identify the population/sampling plan and implement strategies to enhance external validity.
8. Determine the measures that will be used.
9. Outline the data collection plan.
10. Apply for human subjects' approval.
11. Implement the study.
12. Prepare and analyze the data.
13. Interpret the results.
14. Disseminate the findings.
15. Incorporate the findings in EBP and evaluate the outcomes.

On the other hand, if a research question is not interesting to the investigator, there is a chance that the project may never reach completion, especially when challenges arise that make data collection difficult. Other feasibility issues include the amount of time and funding needed to conduct the project, as well as the scope of the study. Studies that are very broad and that contain too many goals are often not feasible or manageable.

Research questions should be novel, meaning that obtaining the answer to them should add to, confirm, or refute what is already known, or they should extend prior research findings. Replication studies (studies that use the same methods but with different subjects) are important, especially if they address major limitations of prior work.

Research questions should be ethical in that they do not present unacceptable physical or psychological risks to the subjects in the study. The institution of strict federal regulations surrounding research with human subjects has curtailed studies in which the risks exceed the benefits of participation in a study. Before a research study is conducted, review of the entire protocol by a **research subjects review board** (RSRB), sometimes referred to as an Institutional Review Board (IRB), is necessary.

 Many universities and clinical agencies have websites that provide comprehensive information on (a) how to submit studies for review; (b) answers to frequently asked questions; and (c) information about regulations regarding research, including specific details related to HIPAA (Health Insurance Portability and Accountability Act) (see http://orrp.osu.edu/irb/)

In institutions where a formal RSRB is not in existence, there should be some type of ethics committee that reviews and approves research proposals. The institutions partner with those that have a formal RSRB for such purposes.

Finally, research questions should be relevant to science and/or clinical practice. They should also have the potential to have an impact on health policy and guide further research (Hulley et al., 2006; Box 19.7).

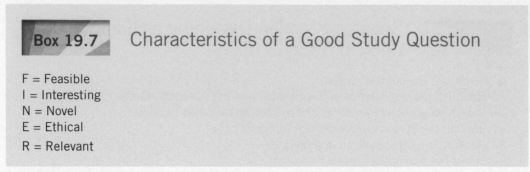

Box 19.7 Characteristics of a Good Study Question

F = Feasible
I = Interesting
N = Novel
E = Ethical
R = Relevant

From Hulley, S. B., Cummings, S. R., Browner, W. S., Grady, D., & Newman, T. B. (2006). *Designing clinical research* (3rd ed.). Philadelphia, PA: Lippincott Williams & Wilkins.

Step 2: Establish Significance of the Problem and the "So What?" Factor

The problem of interest should be one that is clinically important or that will extend the science in an area and have an impact on important outcomes (Melnyk & Morrison-Beedy, 2012). When embarking on a study, it is imperative to ask questions about why the clinical problem is important, including:

- What is the incidence of this particular problem?
- How many individuals are affected by this problem?
- Will studying this problem potentially improve the care that is delivered to patients?
- Will studying this problem potentially influence health policy?
- Will studying this intervention lead to better health outcomes in patients?
- Will studying this problem assist clinicians in gaining a better understanding of the area so that more sensitive clinical care can be delivered?
- "So what" will be the end outcome of the study?

Step 3: Search, Critically Appraise, and Synthesize Evidence

A thorough search for, critical appraisal of, and synthesis of all relevant studies in the area are essential (see Chapters 3 to 6) before the study design is planned. It is beneficial to begin first with a search for **systematic reviews** on the topic. A systematic review is a summary of evidence in a particular topic area that attempts to answer a specific clinical question using methods that reduce bias, usually conducted by an expert or expert panel on a particular topic (Melnyk & Fineout-Overholt, 2011). When it is conducted properly, a systematic review uses a rigorous process for identifying, critically appraising, and synthesizing studies for the purpose of answering a specific clinical question and drawing conclusions about the evidence gathered (e.g., How effective are educational interventions in reducing sexual risk-taking behaviors in teenagers? What factors predict osteoporosis in women?). In using a rigorous process to determine which types of studies will be included in a systematic review, author bias is usually eliminated and greater credibility can be placed in the findings from the review.

In systematic reviews, methodological strengths and limitations of each study included in the review are discussed and recommendations for clinical practice as well as further research are presented (Guyatt & Rennie, 2008). The availability of a systematic review in a particular topic area can provide quick access to the status of interventions or clinical studies in a particular area as well as recommendations for further study. If a systematic review in the area of interest is not available, the search for and critical appraisal of individual studies should begin. In reading prior studies, it is helpful to develop a table of the following information so that a critical analysis of the body of prior work can be conducted:

◆ Demographic characteristics and size of the sample
◆ Study setting
◆ Research design used (e.g., descriptive correlational study, RCT), including the type of intervention (if applicable)
◆ Outcome variables measured, including instruments used
◆ Major findings
◆ Strengths and limitations

Once a table such as this is developed, it will be easier to identify strengths as well as gaps in prior work that could be addressed by the proposed study.

Step 4: Identify a Theoretical/Conceptual Framework

A **theoretical** or **conceptual framework** is comprised of a number of interrelated statements that attempt to describe, explain, and/or predict a phenomenon. Identifying a conceptual or theoretical framework is an important step in designing a clinical study. Its purpose is to provide a framework for selecting the study's variables, including how they relate to one another, as well as to guide the development of the intervention(s) in experimental studies. Without a well-developed theoretical framework, explanations for the findings from a study may be weak and speculative (Melnyk & Feinstein, 2001).

As an example, self-regulation theory (Johnson, Fieler, Jones, Wlasowicz, & Mitchell, 1997; Leventhal & Johnson, 1983) has provided an excellent theoretical framework for providing educational interventions to patients undergoing intrusive procedures (e.g., endoscopy) and chemotherapy/radiation. The basic premise of this theory is that the provision of concrete objective information to an individual who is confronting a stressful situation or procedure will facilitate a cognitive schema or representation of what will happen that is similar to the real-life event. As a result of an individual knowing what he or she is likely to experience, there is an increase in understanding, predictability, and confidence in dealing with the situation as it unfolds (Johnson et al., 1997), which leads to improved coping outcomes.

Through a series of experimental studies, Melnyk and colleagues extended the use of self-regulation theory to guide interventions with parents of hospitalized and critically ill children (Melnyk, 1994; Melnyk et al., 2004; Melnyk, Alpert-Gillis, Hensel, Cable-Beiling, & Rubenstein, 1997), parents of low-birth-weight premature infants (Melnyk et al., 2001, 2006), and parents with young children experiencing marital separation and divorce (Melnyk & Alpert-Gillis, 1996). Extensive evidence in the literature from descriptive studies indicated that a major source of stress for parents of hospitalized and critically ill children is their children's emotional and behavioral responses to hospitalization. Thus, it was hypothesized that parents who receive the COPE (Creating Opportunities for Parent Empowerment) intervention program, which contains educational information about children's likely behavioral and emotional changes during and following hospitalization, would have stronger beliefs about their children's responses to the stressful event. It was also hypothesized that the COPE program would work through parental beliefs about their children and their role—the proposed **mediating variable** (i.e., the variable or mechanism through which the intervention works)—to positively influence parent and child outcomes. As a result of them knowing what to expect of their children's emotions and behaviors during and following hospitalization, it was predicted that parents who receive the COPE program would have better emotional and functional coping outcomes (i.e., a decreased negative mood state and increased participation in their children's care) than would parents who did not receive this information. Ultimately, because the emotional contagion hypothesis (Jimmerson, 1982; VanderVeer, 1949) states that heightened parental anxiety leads to heightened child anxiety, it was expected that the children of parents who received the COPE program would have better coping outcomes than would those whose parents did not receive this educational information. Thus, through this series of clinical trials, empirical

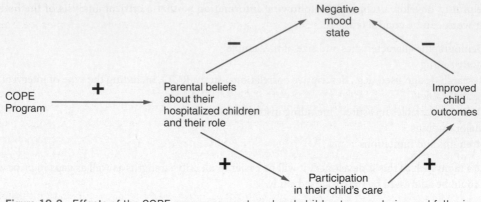

Figure 19.2: Effects of the COPE program on maternal and child outcomes during and following critical care hospitalization.

support for the effectiveness of the COPE program was generated in addition to data that explain how the intervention actually works to affect patient and family outcomes (Figure 19.2).

Step 5: Generate Hypotheses When Appropriate

Hypotheses are predictions about the relationships between study variables. For example, when using self-regulation theory, a hypothesis that would logically emerge from the theory would be that parents who receive concrete objective information about their children's likely responses to hospitalization (i.e., the independent variable) would report less anxiety (i.e., the **dependent** or **outcome variable**) than would parents who do not receive this information. To include hypotheses in a clinical study, there should be either a theory or conceptual framework to guide the formulation of these predictions or enough evidence from prior work to provide a sufficient foundation on which to make predictive statements. In situations where the evidence on which to base predictive statements is insufficient or where an investigator chooses not to use a theoretical or conceptual framework to guide his or her work (which is not advised), research questions should be developed so that the problem might be more fully understood rather than predicting how variables will change.

Step 6: Select the Appropriate Research Design

The **design** of a clinical study is its foundation. It is the overall plan (i.e., the study protocol for testing the study hypotheses or questions) that includes the following:

- Strategies for controlling confounding or extraneous variables
- Strategies for when and how the intervention will be delivered (in experimental studies)
- How often and when the data will be collected

A good quantitative design is one that

- Appropriately tests the hypotheses or answers the research questions
- Lacks bias
- Controls extraneous or confounding variables
- Has sufficient **power** (i.e., the ability to detect statistically significant findings)

If the research question or hypothesis concerns itself with testing the effects of an intervention or treatment on patient outcomes, the study calls for an **experimental design**. In contrast, if the hypothesis/research question is interested in quantitatively describing a selected variable or is interested in the relationship between two or more variables (e.g., What is the relationship between the average amount of sleep and test performance in college students? What presurgery demographic variables predict successful recovery from open heart surgery?), a **nonexperimental study design** would be the most appropriate. The next section of this chapter reviews the most common designs for nonexperimental as well as experimental studies.

Nonexperimental Study Designs

Typically, nonexperimental designs are used to describe, explain, or predict a phenomenon. These types of designs are also undertaken when it is undesirable or unethical to manipulate the independent variable or, in other words, to impose a treatment. For example, it would be unethical to assign underage teenagers randomly to drink alcohol in order to study its effects on sexual risk-taking behaviors. Therefore, an alternative design would be a nonexperimental study in which sexual risk-taking behaviors are measured in a group of adolescents who report alcohol use, compared with a group who does not report use.

Descriptive Studies. The purpose of descriptive studies is to describe, observe, or document a phenomenon that can serve as a foundation for developing hypotheses or testing theory. For example, a descriptive study design would be appropriate to answer each of the following clinical questions:

◆ What is the incidence of complications in women who are on bed rest with preterm labor?
◆ What is the average number of depressive symptoms experienced by teenagers after a critical care hospitalization?
◆ In adults with type 2 diabetes, what are the most common physical comorbidities?

Survey Research. Surveys provide a way to obtain descriptive information using self-report data and are typically collected to assess a certain condition or status. Most survey research is **cross-sectional** (i.e., all measurements are collected at the same point in time) versus research that is conducted over time (e.g., **cohort studies**, which follow the same sample longitudinally).

Survey data can be collected via multiple strategies; in addition to personal or telephone interviews and mailed or in-person questionnaires, data can also be obtained using technology such as computers or cell phones. For example, a group of healthcare providers might be surveyed with a questionnaire designed to measure their knowledge and attitudes about evidence-based practice (EBP). Data gained from this survey might then be used to design inservice education workshops to enhance the providers' knowledge and skills in this area.

Major advantages of survey research include rapid data collection and flexibility. Disadvantages of survey research include low response rates—especially if the surveys are mailed—and gathering information that is fairly superficial.

Correlational Studies. Correlational research designs are used when there is an interest in describing the relationship between or among two or more variables. In this type of design, even when there is a strong relationship that is discovered between the variables under consideration, it is not substantiated to say that one variable caused the other to happen. For example, if a study found a positive relationship between adolescent smoking and drug use (e.g., as smoking increases, drug use increases), it would not be appropriate to state that smoking causes drug use. The only conclusion that could be drawn from these data is that these variables **covary** (i.e., as one changes, the other variable changes as well).

Correlational Descriptive Research. When there is interest in describing the relationship between two variables, a correlational descriptive study design would be most appropriate. For example, the following two research questions would be best answered with correlational designs:

◆ What is the relationship between number of days that a person is on bed rest after a severe motor vehicle accident (the independent variable) and the incidence of decubiti ulcers (the dependent variable)?
◆ What is the relationship between smoking marijuana (the independent variable) and the incidence of sexually transmitted infections in female adolescents (the dependent variable)?

Correlational Predictive Research. When an investigator is interested in whether one variable that occurs earlier in time predicts another variable that occurs later in time, a correlational predictive study

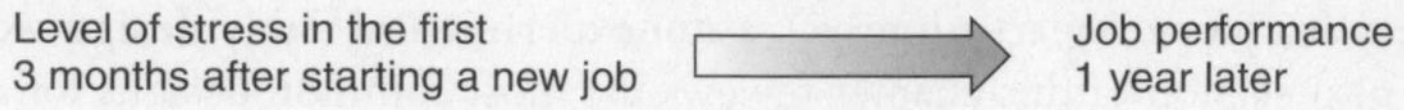

Level of stress in the first
3 months after starting a new job   ➜   Job performance
1 year later

Figure 19.3: A correlational predictive study.

should be undertaken. For example, the following research questions would best lend themselves to this type of study (Figure 19.3):

- Does maternal anxiety shortly after a child's admission to the intensive care unit (the independent variable) predict posttraumatic stress symptoms 6 months after hospitalization (the dependent variable)?
- Does the level of stress during the first 3 months after starting a new job (the independent variable) predict performance 1 year later?

Establishing a strong relationship between variables in correlational predictive studies provides evidence for the need to influence the independent variable in a future intervention study. For example, if findings from research indicated that job stress in the initial months after starting a new position as a practitioner predicted later job performance, a future study might evaluate the effects of a training program on reducing early job stress with the expectation that a successful intervention program would improve later job performance. Although it should never be stated that a cause-and-effect relationship is supported with a correlational study, a predictive correlational design is stronger than a descriptive one with regard to making a causal inference because the independent variable occurs before the dependent variable in time sequence (Polit & Beck, 2008).

Case–Control Studies. Case–control studies are those in which one group of individuals (i.e., cases) with a certain condition (e.g., migraine headaches) is studied at the same time as another group of individuals who do not have the condition (i.e., controls) to determine an association between one or more predictor variables (e.g., family history of migraine headaches, consumption of red wine) and the condition (i.e., migraine headaches). Case–control studies are usually retrospective or *ex post facto* (i.e., they look back in time to reveal predictor variables that might explain why the cases contracted the disease or problem and the controls did not).

Advantages of this type of research design include an ability to determine associations with a small number of subjects, which is especially useful in the study of rare types of diseases, and an ability to generate hypotheses for future studies (Hulley et al., 2006). One of the major limitations to using this study design is **bias** (i.e., an inability to control confounding variables that may influence the outcome). For example, the two groups of individuals previously presented (i.e., those with migraines and those without migraines) may be different on certain variables (e.g., amount of sleep and stress) that may also influence the development of migraine headaches. Another limitation is that because case–control studies are usually retrospective, one is limited to data available at a prior time. Often, data on interesting variables were not thought to be important and not collected.

Cohort Studies. A cohort study follows a group of subjects longitudinally over a period of time to describe the incidence of a problem or to determine the relationship between a predictor variable and an outcome. An example would be finding out if daughters of mothers who had breast cancer have a higher incidence of the disease versus those whose mothers did not have breast cancer. Two groups of daughters (i.e., those with and without a mother with breast cancer) would be studied over time to determine the incidence of breast cancer in each group. A major strength (advantage) of prospective cohort studies includes being able to determine the incidence of a problem and its possible cause(s). A major limitation (disadvantage) is the lengthy nature of this type of study, the costs of which often become prohibitive.

Experimental Study Designs

A true experiment, or RCT, is the strongest design for testing cause-and-effect relationships (e.g., whether an intervention or treatment affects patient outcomes) and provides strong evidence on which to change and improve clinical practice. For evidence to support causality (i.e., cause-and-effect relationships), three criteria must be met:

1. The independent variable (i.e., the intervention or treatment) must precede the dependent variable (i.e., the outcome) in terms of time sequence.
2. There must be a strong relationship between the independent and dependent variables.
3. The relationship between the independent and dependent variables cannot be explained as being due to the influence of other variables (i.e., all possible alternate explanations of the relationship must be eliminated).

Although true experiments are the best designs to control for the influence of confounding variables, it must be recognized that control of potential confounding or extraneous variables is very challenging when conducting studies in the real world—not in the laboratory. Other limitations of experiments include the fact that they are usually time consuming and expensive.

Intervention studies or clinical trials typically follow a five-phase development sequence:

- **Phase I: Basic research** that is exploratory and descriptive in nature and that establishes the variables that may be amenable to intervention or in which the content, strength, and timing of the intervention are developed, along with the outcome measures for the study.
- **Phase II: Pilot research** (i.e., a small-scale study in which the intervention is tested with a small number of subjects so that the feasibility of a large-scale study is determined and alternative strategies are developed for potential problems).
- **Phase III: Efficacy trials** in which evaluation of the intervention takes place in an ideal setting and clinical efficacy is determined (in this stage, much emphasis is placed on internal validity of the study and preliminary *cost-effectiveness* of the intervention).
- **Phase IV: Effectiveness of clinical trials** in which analysis of the intervention effect is conducted in clinical practice and clinical effectiveness is determined, as is cost-effectiveness (in this stage, much emphasis is placed on external validity or generalizability of the study).
- **Phase V: Effects on public health** in which wide-scale implementation of the intervention is conducted to determine its effects on public health (Whittemore & Grey, 2002).

Many practitioners assume a leadership role in Phases I and II of this sequence and more of a collaborative role as a member of a research team in Phases III through V.

Randomized Controlled Trial or True Experiment. The best type of study design or gold standard for evaluating the effects of a treatment or intervention is an RCT or true experiment, in that it is the strongest design for testing cause-and-effect relationships. True experiments or RCTs possess three characteristics:

1. An experimental group that receives the treatment or intervention
2. A control or comparison group that receives standard care or a comparison intervention that is different from the experimental intervention
3. **Randomization** or **random assignment**, which is the use of a strategy to randomly assign subjects to the experimental or control groups (e.g., tossing a coin)

Random assignment is the strongest method to help ensure that the study groups are similar on demographic or clinical variables at baseline (i.e., before the treatment is delivered). Similarity between groups at the beginning of an experiment is very important in that if findings reveal a positive effect on the dependent variable, it can be concluded that the treatment, not other extraneous variables, is what affected the outcome. For example, results from an RCT might reveal that a cognitive behavioral intervention reduced depressive symptoms in adults. However, if the adults in the experimental and control groups were not similar on certain characteristics prior to the start of the intervention (e.g., level of social support, number of current stressful life events), it could be that differences between the groups on these variables accounted for the change in depressive symptoms at the end of the study, instead of the change being due to the positive impact of the intervention itself.

R	O_1	X_1	O_2
R	O_1	X_2	O_2

Figure 19.4: Two-group RCT with pretest/posttest design and structurally equivalent comparison group. R, random assignment; X, intervention/treatment, with X_1 being the experimental intervention and X_2 being the comparison/control intervention; O, observation/measurement, with O_1 being the first time the variable is measured (at baseline) and O_2 being the second time that it is measured (after the intervention).

Examples of true experimental designs along with advantages and disadvantages of each are presented in Figures 19.4 through 19.9. The symbol designations in the figures have been used for years in the literature since the publishing of a landmark book on experimental designs by Campbell and Stanley (1963). Note that time moves from left to right, and subscripts can be used to designate different groups if necessary.

Two-Group RCT with Pretest/Posttest Design and Structurally Equivalent Comparison Group. The major advantage of the design illustrated in Figure 19.4 is that it is a true experiment, the strongest design for testing cause-and-effect relationships. As seen in Figure 19.4, the inclusion of a comparison group in the design that receives a different or "attention control" intervention similar in length to the experimental intervention is important. This control group helps to provide evidence that any effects of the experimental intervention are not just the result of giving participants "something" instead of "nothing" but are actually due to the effect of the experimental intervention itself. At the same time, including a comparison intervention may dilute some of the positive effects of the experimental intervention. This is especially true if a study outcome being measured is tapping a psychosocial variable, such as anxiety (e.g., giving participants something instead of nothing, as would be the case with a pure control group, might reduce anxiety simply because someone spent time with the participant). The benefits of this design (i.e., including an attention control or comparison intervention) outweigh the risk of diluting the positive effects of the experimental intervention. Although pretesting the subjects on the same measure that is being used as the outcome for the study (e.g., state anxiety) may, in itself, sensitize them to respond differently when answering questions on the anxiety measure the second time, this approach allows the investigator to determine whether subjects are similar on anxiety at the beginning of the study. A disadvantage of this design, as with all experiments, is that it is typically more expensive and time consuming than nonexperimental designs.

Two-Group RCT with Posttest Only Design. The advantage of conducting a two-group RCT with a posttest-only design is that there is no pretesting effect (Figure 19.5). For example, if you were interested in evaluating the effects of a HIV/STI educational program on adolescent girls' knowledge of sexual-risk reduction, you may not want to pretest the participants by asking them questions such as, "Can a person get HIV from a toilet seat?" or "Can using a latex condom or rubber lower a person's chance of getting HIV?" Despite the fact that they did not receive the educational program, the administration of a pretest

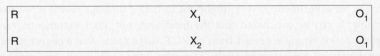

R	X_1	O_1
R	X_2	O_1

Figure 19.5: Two-group RCT with posttest design only. R, random assignment; X, intervention/treatment, with X_1 being the experimental intervention and X_2 being the comparison/control intervention; O, observation/measurement.

| R | X_1 | O_1 | O_2 | O_3 |
| R | X_2 | O_1 | O_2 | O_3 |

Figure 19.6: Two-group RCT with long-term repeated measures follow-up. R, random assignment; X, intervention/treatment, with X_1 being the experimental intervention and X_2 being the comparison intervention; O, observation/measurement, which will occur at three different time points (i.e., O_1, O_2, and O_3) after the intervention/treatment is delivered.

itself may lead the girls in the control group to ask their healthcare providers about HIV risk. As a result, findings may reveal no difference in knowledge between the two study groups at the end of the study—not necessarily because the intervention did not work but due to the strong influence of pretesting effects on the outcome.

The main disadvantage of a posttest-only design is that baseline differences on the study groups are unknown. Even though random assignment is used (see Figure 19.5), to control for extraneous or confounding variables, there is still a chance that the two groups may be unequal or different at the start of the study. Differences in important baseline study measures between experimental groups may then negatively affect a study's outcomes or interfere with the ability to say that it was the intervention itself that caused a change in the dependent variable(s). For example, in an intervention to control postoperative pain in patients following surgery, differing levels of anxiety prior to the intervention between both groups may alter the impact of the pain-reduction intervention. Without assessing these differences before the intervention, the investigator will be limited in the ability to say whether posttest data provide support for the utility of the intervention.

Two-Group RCT with Long-Term Repeated Measures Follow-Up. If an investigator is interested in whether an intervention produces both short-term and long-term effects on an outcome, it is important for a study to build into its design repeated measurements of the outcome variable of interest (Figure 19.6). The advantage of this type of design is that repeated assessments of an outcome variable over time allow an investigator to determine the sustainability of an intervention's effects. A disadvantage of this type of design is that *study attrition* (i.e., loss of subjects) may be a threat to the internal validity (control) of the study. Another disadvantage of this design is that it is costly to follow subjects for longer periods of time. In addition, repeated follow-up on the same measures may also have the disadvantage of introducing testing effects that influence the outcome. For example, individuals may think about their answers and change their beliefs as part of the repeated follow-up sessions, not as the result of the intervention. Also, subjects may learn how repeated follow-up assessments work, and, if the study entails extensive questioning when individuals admit to certain things (e.g., being depressed or taking drugs), they may learn to respond in a way to avoid these lengthy follow-up questions or interviews.

Two-Group RCT with True Control Group That Receives No Intervention. The real disadvantage to conducting an RCT with a true control group that receives no attention or intervention whatsoever (Figure 19.7) is that any positive intervention effects that are found may be solely related to participants in the intervention group "receiving something versus nothing." For example, if a healthcare provider was studying the effects of a stress reduction program on college students experiencing test anxiety, simply having someone spend extra time with the students could reduce their anxiety, regardless of whether the intervention itself was helpful.

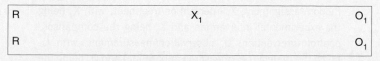

| R | X_1 | O_1 |
| R | | O_1 |

Figure 19.7: Two-group RCT with true control group that receives no intervention. R, random assignment; X, intervention/treatment, with X_1 being the experimental intervention; O, observation/measurement.

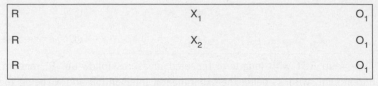

Figure 19.8: Three-group RCT (i.e., one group who receives one type of experimental intervention, one group who receives a different or comparison intervention, and a pure control group who receives no intervention or standard care). R, random assignment; X, intervention/treatment, with X_1 being the experimental intervention and X_2 being the comparison intervention; O, observation/measurement, which only occurs once (i.e., postintervention).

Three-Group RCT. The inclusion of a third group, as shown in Figure 19.8, allows an investigator to separate the effects of giving something (i.e., a comparison or attention control intervention) from a pure control group (i.e., a group who receives nothing or standard care)—a very strong experimental design. Disadvantages typically include the need to recruit additional subjects for the three conditions and increased costs to conduct the study.

Solomon Four-Group Design. The main advantage to conducting an experimental study that employs a **Solomon four-group design** (i.e., an experiment that uses a before-after design for the first experimental and control groups and an after-only design for the second experimental and control groups; Polit & Beck, 2008) is that it can separate the effects of pretesting the subjects (i.e., gathering baseline measures) on the outcome measure(s) (Figure 19.9). Disadvantages include the need for additional participants as well as costs for increasing the size of the sample.

Factorial Design. A **factorial design** (Figure 19.10) is an experiment that has two or more interventions or treatments. A major advantage of this type of design is that it allows an investigator to study the separate and combined effects of different types of interventions. For example, if a healthcare provider were interested in the separate and combined effects of two different interventions (i.e., educational information and an exercise program) on reducing blood pressure in adults with hypertension, this type of design would result in four groups:

R	O_1		X_1	O_2
R			X_1	O_2
R	O_1		X_2	O_2
R			X_2	O_2

Figure 19.9: Solomon four-group design in which a pair of experimental and control groups receive pretesting as depicted by O_1 and a pair who do not receive pretesting. R, random assignment; X, intervention/treatment, with X_1 being the experimental intervention and X_2 being the comparison/control intervention; O, observation/measurement, with O_1 being the pretest (i.e., measured at baseline) and O_2 being the posttest (i.e., measured after the intervention is delivered).

EDUCATIONAL INFORMATION

	Yes	No
EXERCISE Yes	Education and exercise	Exercise only
No	Education only	Neither education nor exercise

Figure 19.10: 2 × 2 factorial experiment that generates four study groups. **(A)** A group who receives both education and exercise. **(B)** A group who receives education only. **(C)** A group who receives exercise only. **(D)** A control group who receives neither education nor exercise.

1. A group of subjects who would receive educational information only
2. A group of subjects who would receive an exercise program only
3. A group of subjects who would receive both educational information and an exercise program
4. A group of subjects who would receive neither information nor exercise

A major strength of this design is that it could be determined whether education or exercise alone positively affects blood pressure or whether a combination of the two treatments is more effective than either intervention alone. Disadvantages to this design typically include additional subjects and costs.

Quasi-Experimental Studies. Designs in which the independent variable (i.e., a treatment) is manipulated or introduced but where there is a lack of random assignment or a control group are called **quasi-experimental designs.**

Although **quasi-experiments** may be more practical and feasible, they are weaker than true experimental designs in the ability to establish cause-and-effect inferences (i.e., to say that the independent variable or treatment was responsible for a change in the dependent variable and that the change was not due to other extraneous factors).

There are times when quasi-experiments need to be conducted because random assignment is not always possible. For example, individuals cannot be assigned to smoking and nonsmoking conditions. Even when it is ethically feasible to use random assignment, the study setting might preclude it. For example, school principals frequently resist assigning children to programs based on random assignment. In addition, random assignment can be disruptive in schools (e.g., taking children out of their regular classrooms for special programs). Quasi-experiments, that is, designs that compare groups created by some method other than random assignment, provide an alternative to true experiments. Despite their limitations, some of these designs can be quite powerful in their ability to eliminate alternative explanations for the relationship between an intervention and the outcomes in a study. Two examples of quasi-experimental designs are shown in Figures 19.11 and 19.12.

Quasi-Experiment with Pretest and Posttest Design, Comparison/Control Group, No Random Assignment. In Figure 19.11, there is an experimental group and an attention control group that both receive a

O_1	X_1	O_2
O_1	X_2	O_2

Figure 19.11: A quasi-experiment with pretest and posttest design and a comparison/control group but lacking random assignment. X, intervention, with X_1 being the experimental intervention and X_2 being the comparison/control intervention; O, observation, with O_1 indicating measurement at baseline and O_2 indicating measurement after the intervention is delivered.

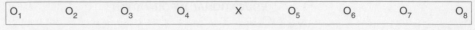

Figure 19.12: Time series design.

treatment, but the subjects have not been randomly assigned to the two study groups so the probability of equal study groups cannot be assured. Therefore, a pretest is administered so that it can be determined whether the two study groups are equal at baseline before the intervention is delivered. In quasi-experiments, pretesting is especially important to assess whether the subjects are similar at baseline on the variable(s) that will be used as the outcome(s) in the study. However, even with pretesting that shows no preintervention differences, a quasi-experiment is still not as strong as a true experiment that uses random assignment. Because the groups are preexisting or created by a means other than random assignment in a quasi-experiment, there could be other unexplored differences between them that might account for any differences found on the outcome variables. If only posttesting is conducted in a quasi-experimental design in which random assignment was not used, it would be very difficult to have confidence in the findings because it would not be known whether the study groups were similar on key variables at the beginning of the study. In contrast, when random assignment is used in true experimental designs, it is very likely that the study groups will be equivalent on pretest measures.

Interrupted Time Series Design. Another example of a quasi-experimental study is the interrupted time series design (Figure 19.12). In this study, there is no random assignment or comparison/attention control group. This design incorporates a long series of pretest observations, an intervention, and a long series of posttest observations.

The time series design is used most frequently in communities or agencies that maintain careful archival records. It can also be used with community survey data if the survey questions and sample remain constant over time. An intervention effect is evidenced if a stable pattern of observations over a long period of time is found, followed by a marked change at the point of the intervention, then a stable pattern again over a long time after the intervention. For example, adolescent truancy rates might be tracked over several years, followed by an intervention with the tracking of truancy rates for several additional years. If there is a marked drop in truancy rates at the point of the intervention, there is reasonable evidence for a program's effect. Even though this is a single-group design, this is often sufficient to rule out a variety of alternative explanations.

One frequent challenge to single-group designs is the threat of **history**, which involves the occurrence of some event or program unrelated to the intervention that might account for the change observed. History remains a viable alternate explanation for a change in the dependent variable only if the event happens at the same time point as the intervention. If the event occurs earlier or later than the experimental intervention, it cannot explain a change in outcome that occurs at or around the time of the intervention.

Another possible alternate explanation for observed changes in a single-group design is the **maturation** threat. Maturation is a developmental change that occurs even in the absence of the intervention. A true maturation effect will occur gradually throughout the pretest and posttest periods and thus could not account for sharp changes that occur at the point of the intervention.

Observed changes might also occur because of repeated testing or changes in instrumentation. Repeat testing of individuals typically influences their subsequent scores. In addition, performance on skills-based tests should increase over time simply due to practice. Finally, mortality as well as attrition or movement into and out of a community could also influence the outcome data, but they offer an alternate explanation only if it started at the point of treatment.

Tamburro et al. (2002) employed an interrupted time series design in their evaluation of the impact of the Mid-South Safe Kids Coalition on rates of serious unintentional injuries (i.e., those leading to hospitalization or death). Consistent data were available for 1990 and 1991, 2 years prior to the implementation of the coalition, and for 1993 through 1997, about 6 years following the implementation. All children in the county younger than 10 years who were treated in a single hospital were included in the sample. Analyses showed a statistically significant drop in the rates of targeted injuries from 3.5 to 2.0 per 1,000 children, beginning precisely at the point the coalition was formed.

X	O_1

Figure 19.13: Preexperiment in which there is no random assignment or no comparison/control group. X, intervention; O, observation.

Preexperimental Studies. Preexperiments lack both random assignment and a comparison/attention control group (Figure 19.13). As such, they are very weak in internal validity and allow too many competing explanations for a study's findings.

Other Important Experimental Design Factors. Methods to ensure quality and consistency in the delivery of the intervention (i.e., maintenance of integrity) are crucial for being able to determine whether and how well an intervention works. Preexperimental designs are more appropriately used in early intervention development and pilot testing phases.

Integrity and Reproducibility. Frequently, investigators spend inordinate amounts of time paying particular attention to the dependent variable(s) or measure(s) to be used in a study and do not give sufficient time and attention to how an intervention is delivered. In addition, at the outset of an intervention study, it is critical to give thought to whether the intervention will be able to be reproduced by others in different settings. Reproducibility is critical if translation of the intervention into real-life practice settings is going to occur. As such, it is important to manualize or create standardized materials that specifically outline the content of the intervention so that others can replicate it and expect the same results in their practice settings. Use of videotapes, audio tapes, DVDs, or other types of reproducible materials to deliver an intervention ensures that each subject will receive all of the intervention content in exactly the same manner. However, this type of delivery is not always best suited to a particular clinical population. For example, groups may be the best strategy to deliver interventions to teens at high risk for STIs because they allow for the teaching of refusal skills through role-playing.

In a study conducted by Morrison-Beedy and colleagues (2012), several healthcare providers were used to deliver an information/motivation/behavioral skills training program in four 2-hour group sessions to urban minority female adolescents. The content of the program and necessary skills to be taught for each of the sessions were detailed in a written manual. However, before the actual study commenced, intensive training of the interventionists occurred (e.g., practice groups and role-playing) to ensure that each of them would deliver the content of the program and the teaching of behavioral skills in the same manner. Once the study started, sessions were audiotaped and reviewed by the investigators to ensure quality and completeness in the delivery of the educational information and behavioral skills.

If rigorous standards to ensure the integrity of an intervention do not occur in a study, it would be difficult to know whether the findings generated were the result of the intervention itself or other extraneous variables (Melnyk & Fineout-Overholt, 2011). When integrity of an intervention is maintained, greater confidence can be placed in a study's findings.

Pilot Study. Before conducting a large experimental study, it is extremely beneficial to first conduct a pilot study, which is a preliminary study that is conducted with a small number of subjects (e.g., 30 to 40) versus a full-scale clinical trial with large numbers of subjects. A pilot study is critical in determining the feasibility of subject enrollment, the intervention, the protocol or data collection plan for the study, and the likelihood that subjects will complete follow-up measures. With the development and implementation of new study measures, it is also essential to pilot them before use in a full-scale study to determine their validity and reliability. Pilot work enables investigators to identify weaknesses in their study design so that they can be corrected for the full-scale study. Subjects used for the pilot study should match those individuals who will be participating in the full-scale clinical trial.

Pilot studies are frequently conducted by advanced practice nurses and other master's prepared clinicians and often lead the way to full-scale clinical trials. Working through the details for a large-scale intervention trial with a pilot study saves much time, energy, and prevents frustration as well as provides convincing evidence that a large-scale clinical trial is feasible and well worth the effort. Pilot studies can be used both to develop the intervention and to trial the intervention and control conditions in a smaller-scale version of the full-scale study (Morrison-Beedy, Carey, Kowalski, & Tu, 2005; Morrison-Beedy, Nelson, & Volpe, 2005).

Manipulation Checks. Manipulation checks are important assessments to determine whether the intervention was successfully conducted. For example, if an investigator was delivering an educational intervention intended to teach healthcare providers about a disease and its treatment in order to improve patient outcomes, a manipulation check might be a test given to participants with a number of multiple-choice questions about the content of the intervention. Answering a certain percentage of these questions correctly would indicate that the subjects successfully processed the educational information. As another example, an investigator may be interested in the effects of a new aerobic exercise program on weight loss in young adults. Participants in the experimental group could be taught this program and instructed to complete the prescribed activities three times per week. A manipulation check to ensure that subjects actually adhered to the prescribed exercise exercises may involve keeping a log that lists the dates and number of minutes spent following the program. These types of assessments are critical in order to verify that manipulation of the independent variable or completion of the treatment was achieved. If manipulation checks are not included in an experimental study and results indicate no differences between the experimental and attention control/comparison groups, it would be very difficult to explain whether it was a lack of intervention potency or the fact that subjects did not attend to or adhere to the intervention that was responsible for a lack of intervention effects.

Intervention Processes. When preparing to conduct an intervention study, it is important to think not only about the dependent variables or outcomes that the intervention might affect, but also about the process through which the intervention will exert its effects. The explanations about how an intervention works are important in facilitating its implementation into practice settings (Melnyk, Crean, Feinstein, & Alpert-Gillis, 2007; Melnyk & Feinstein, 2001). For example, an investigator proposes that a cognitive behavioral intervention (the independent variable) will reduce depressive symptoms (the dependent variable) in adults with low self-esteem. At the same time, however, the investigator proposes the mechanism of action (i.e., the mediating variable) through which the intervention will work. Therefore, it is hypothesized that the experimental intervention will enhance cognitive beliefs about one's ability to engage in positive coping strategies, which in turn will result in a decrease in depressive symptoms (Figure 19.14). Conceptualization of a well-defined theoretical framework at the outset of designing an intervention study will facilitate explanations of how an intervention program may influence a study's outcomes.

Control Strategies. When conducting experimental studies, it is critical to strategize about how to control for extraneous factors that may influence the outcome(s) so that the effects of the intervention itself can be determined. These extraneous factors include those internal or intrinsic to the individuals who participate in a study (e.g., fatigue and level of maturity) and those external to the participants (e.g., the environment in which the study is conducted).

As explained earlier, the best strategy to control for extraneous variables is randomization or random assignment. By randomly assigning subjects to study groups, there is a good probability that the subjects in the groups will be similar on important characteristics at the beginning of a study.

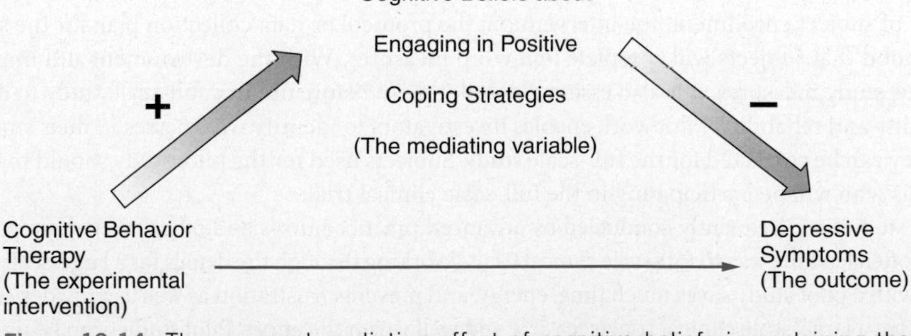

Figure 19.14: The proposed mediating effect of cognitive beliefs in explaining the effects of cognitive behavioral therapy on depressive symptoms.

When random assignment is not possible, other methods may be used to control extraneous or confounding variables. One of these strategies is **homogeneity**, or using subjects who are similar on the characteristics that may affect the outcome variable(s). For example, if a study were evaluating the effects of an intervention on parental stress during the critical care hospitalization of children, it may include only parents from intact marriages because divorced parents may have higher stress levels than nondivorced parents. In addition, very young mothers may have high stress levels. Therefore, this study's inclusion criteria may include only those parents who are from intact marriages as well as those who are older than 21 years. A limitation of this strategy is that at the end of the study, findings can be generalized only to married parents older than 21 years.

Another strategy to control intrinsic factors in a study is **blocking**. Blocking entails deliberately including a potential extraneous intrinsic or confounding variable in a study's design. For example, if there were a concern that level of motivation would affect the results of a study to determine the effects of aerobic exercise (i.e., the treatment) on weight loss in young adults, an investigator may choose to include motivation as another independent variable in the study, aside from the exercise program itself. In doing so, the effects of both motivation and exercise on weight loss could be studied in a 2 × 2 **randomized block design** (Figure 19.15) involving two independent variables with two levels: (a) exercise and no exercise and (b) high motivation and low motivation. The benefit of this type of design is that the interaction between motivation and exercise on weight loss could also be determined (i.e., Do individuals with high levels of motivation have greater weight loss than those with low motivation?).

Threats to Internal Validity. **Internal validity** is the extent to which it can be said that the independent variable (i.e., the intervention) causes a change in the dependent variable (i.e., outcome) and that the results are not due to other factors or alternative explanations. There are a number of major threats to the internal validity of a study that should be addressed in the planning process.

Attrition. The first threat to internal validity is **attrition**, or dropout of study participants, which may result in nonequivalent study groups (i.e., more individuals lost from the study in the attention control group than from the experimental group or more individuals with a certain characteristic withdrawing from participation). As a result of losing more subjects from the control group than from the experimental group or more subjects with a certain characteristic (e.g., high anxiety), the study findings may be different than if those individuals had remained in the study. For example, if individuals with the poorest outcomes felt that they were not gaining any benefit from the study, which led them to drop out of a study, differences between the two study groups may not surface during statistical analyses.

One strategy for preventing differential attrition is not to overly persuade potential subjects to participate in a study. There is a fine line between encouraging a potential subject to participate in a study and overly persuading him or her to participate. If someone decides to participate only after much encouragement, there is an increased probability that he or she may drop from the study.

Another strategy for preventing attrition is to offer research subjects a small honorarium for participating in a study. Some studies provide an honorarium during each time point that a subject completes a specific phase of a study protocol (e.g., completing a set of questionnaires or receiving an intervention), whereas others provide an honorarium when the subjects complete the entire study protocol. Providing an honorarium sends the message that an individual's time for participating in a study is valued.

AEROBIC EXERCISE

		Yes	No
MOTIVATION	High	High motivation and exercise	High motivation and no exercise
	Low	Low motivation and exercise	Low motivation and no exercise

Figure 19.15: A 2 × 2 randomized block design, blocking on motivation.

If there will be substantial time between contacts in a study, it is important to maintain periodic communication through cards or telephone calls. Lengthy lapses in communication with subjects make it easier for them not to return phone calls and questionnaires as well as to miss follow-up appointments. To prevent attrition, another helpful strategy is to maintain consistency in who provides follow-up with the participants. One consistent person on the research team who follows a subject longitudinally over time will enhance the chances of successfully obtaining repeated follow-up data.

Finally, it is important to reduce subject burden to prevent attrition from a study. Participants can become easily overwhelmed if each contact involves the completion of several questionnaires that require a lot of time. An important question to ask for each proposed dependent variable is: How key is the measurement of this outcome or is it just a nice additional piece of data to include in the study? As a general rule of thumb, the easier and less time consuming it is to participate in a study, the greater will be the probability of completion. It is also more valuable to have complete data on a few key variables than having partial data on an extensive list of variables that are of interest.

Confounding Variables/Selection. The best strategy to control for or minimize the influence of confounding variables is to randomly assign subjects to study groups. Another strategy for controlling potential confounding variables is to establish thoughtful inclusion and exclusion criteria. Maintaining consistent study conditions for all participants is another strategy for controlling potential confounding variables. One way to ensure consistency is to establish clearly written study protocols so that every individual on the team understands the intricacies of when and how the interventions will be delivered, as well as the specific steps of data collection.

Nonadherence and Failure to Complete the Intervention Protocol. Designing a realistic intervention is important so that it will eventually be transportable to the real clinical practice world. There is a delicate balance between designing an intervention that will produce sustainable **effects** versus one that will be easy to implement in practice. As such, much consideration should be given to the logistics of the intervention (e.g., feasibility and user-friendliness).

If there are multiple sessions with ongoing phases of the intervention, it is important to record which and how many sessions are attended and completed by study participants because this will facilitate the evaluation of whether a dose response exists (i.e., the greater the number of sessions one attends, the larger the effect of the intervention).

Measurement of Change in Outcome Variables. In intervention studies where it is important to demonstrate a change in key dependent variables that the treatment will impact, it is critical to use measures that are sensitive to change over time. For example, if a certain measure has high **test–retest reliability** (i.e., it is stable over time, such as an individual's personality), there will be little opportunity to affect a change in that measure. This is in contrast to other types of studies in which high test–retest reliabilities on certain measures are desirable (e.g., cohort studies that do not employ interventions in which you are following certain variables over time). For example, an individual's trait anxiety is the general predisposition to anxiety over time, which has been empirically shown to be a stable construct. In contrast, an individual's state anxiety fluctuates, depending on the situation. Therefore, an intervention would most likely affect state, not trait anxiety. Therefore, state anxiety would be a better outcome measure in an intervention study than would trait anxiety.

In conducting intervention studies, it is important to use the same measures longitudinally so that intervention effects over time can be determined. Carefully planning the timing of assessments is critical, especially if there is interest in both the short-term and long-term effects of an intervention. It is also important to use measures that assess variability and that have been tested in the population of interest to avoid **ceiling** and **floor** effects (i.e., participant scores that cluster toward the low end or high-end score of a measure).

In addition to measuring the outcomes of interventions with quantitative scales, it is important to administer an evaluation questionnaire at the end of a study so that subjects can provide open-ended responses to whether and how they believed the intervention was helpful. These types of responses are especially important if, by chance, the quantitative measures in the study reveal no statistically significant differences between study groups on key outcome variables.

It is also important to assess both clinical meaningfulness and statistical significance when determining whether an intervention has been successful. For example, the greater the number of subjects that are included in a study, the more statistical *power* there will be to detect statistically significant differences between groups. In contrast, the smaller the sample size, the lower the power and the more difficult it will be to detect statistically significant findings. For example, in one hypothetical study with 1,000 subjects, an investigator found that teens who were enrolled in an expensive smoking cessation program smoked two cigarettes less per day than did teens who did not receive the program. This finding was statistically significant at the 0.05 level. As a result of this significant finding, the costly smoking cessation program was widely implemented. Although the finding was statistically significant, the clinical meaningfulness of this finding is weak. In contrast, another investigator conducted the same study with 50 adolescents and found that the experimental group teens smoked 10 cigarettes less per day than did teens who did not receive the smoking cessation program. This difference, however, was not statistically significant due to a small number of subjects and low statistical power. Therefore, a decision was made not to implement the program routinely because there was not a statistically significant difference between the study groups. However, a 10-cigarette difference between groups is more clinically meaningful than a 2-cigarette difference. This is a good example of how faulty decisions can be made if only statistically significant findings are considered important and their clinical meaningfulness is ignored, and conversely if statically and clinically relevant results cannot be assessed because the study was "underpowered."

History. History is another major threat to the internal validity of a study. This condition happens when external events take place concurrently with the treatment that may influence the outcome variables. For example, if a study were being conducted to determine the effects of a violence prevention intervention on anxiety in school-age children and a school shooting occurred that received extensive media attention during the course of the trial, children's anxiety levels at the end of the study could be high despite any positive effects of the intervention. The best way to minimize the threat of history is random assignment because at least both groups then should be equally affected by the external event.

Maturation. The passage of time alone can have an impact on the outcomes of a study. For example, when studying infants who are growing rapidly, an acceleration in cognitive development may occur, regardless of the effects of an intervention that is aimed at enhancing cognition. The best way to deal with the threat of maturation is to use random assignment to allocate subjects to experimental and control groups as well as to recognize it as a potential alternative explanation for a study's findings.

Testing. Completing measures repeatedly could influence an individual's responses the next time a measure is completed. For example, answering the same depression scale three or four times could program someone to respond in the same way on subsequent administrations of the scale.

On the other hand, lengthy lapses in the administration of an instrument may result in a failure to detect important changes over time. Therefore, the best way to deal with this threat to internal validity is to think very carefully about how many times subjects are being asked to complete study measures and provide a strong rationale for these decisions.

Step 7: Identify the Sample and Enhance External Validity

External validity addresses the **generalizability** of research results (i.e., our ability to apply what we learn from a study sample to the larger population from which the sample was drawn). Clearly, a great deal is learned from the samples we study. However, there is always interest in applying that knowledge to a broader population (e.g., to the next 100,000 patients, not just the 100 in a particular study).

The key to external validity is the degree to which the sample that is being studied is representative of the population from which it was drawn. Creating a representative sample is a complex and challenging task. Samples are rarely if ever perfectly representative of the populations of interest, but there can be reasonable approximations.

There are four steps to consider when building a sample (Trochim, 2006):

1. Carefully define the theoretical population. The theoretical population is the population to which you wish to generalize your results (e.g., all 3-year-old children).
2. Describe the population to which you have access (i.e., the study population). Continuing with our example, this might include all 3-year-old children in the county in which you work, or perhaps in all of the counties in which your collaborators work. At this point, it is necessary to consider how similar the study population is to the theoretical population. Typically, if the county is large and diverse, it is reasonable to assume that the study population is an acceptable substitute for the theoretical population. However, if the focus of your work is strongly influenced by regional factors, such as climate, culture, or access to services, the choice of a study population could severely limit generalizability to the theoretical population.
3. Describe the method you will use to access the population; in other words, define the sampling frame. It is highly unlikely that there will be a single comprehensive list of all 3-year-old children living in any one region at a particular time. You must find some practical method of identifying eligible children; then assess how the available methods might introduce bias or nonrepresentativeness. One strategy might be to approach the day care programs in the region. This would certainly be efficient, but not all 3-year-olds attend day care, and those who do are unlikely to be fully representative of the study population. For example, children whose mothers do not work outside the home are less likely to attend day care. Another approach might be to contact all of the pediatric offices in the region and solicit their cooperation in identifying the 3-year-olds under their care. Certainly, all young children see a pediatrician or nurse practitioner from time to time, even if they do not regularly keep their well child appointments. However, not all children in the region may receive care at the local pediatric offices. Perhaps families at one or both ends of the socioeconomic spectrum travel outside of the region for their care; perhaps others avoid care because of a lack of insurance and use only the emergency department on an as-needed basis. Finally, the records at the pediatric offices might be out of date. A child may have come in for a 2-year visit, then moved away. Each of these possible alternatives needs to be reviewed and evaluated. *The method that balances efficiency with representativeness will be the best choice.* If there are more sites (day care centers and pediatric offices) than one can efficiently work with, a mechanism to choose a portion of the sites must be selected. The options will be described in the next section, along with mechanisms for selecting actual subjects from the sampling frame.
4. Typically, the sampling frame will include many more potential subjects than are required for the study. Thus, the fourth step in the process is identifying a method to select those individuals who will be invited to participate. Once again, the method chosen should balance efficiency and representativeness.

Random Sampling

Randomly selecting both study sites (e.g., clinics or day care centers) and subjects within these sites is the method most likely to avoid bias. In **random sampling**, every potential subject has an equal chance of being selected. The most straightforward way to think about random sampling is to imagine taking the list of everyone in the sampling frame, cutting it into small pieces with one name on each piece, placing all the names in a bowl, and drawing from the bowl the number of names required for the study design. This might work for selecting 6 day care programs from a list of 25, but in practice, it is an inefficient way to draw a sample of 200 children from a sampling frame of 10,000. That is quite a bit of cutting!

A more efficient method is to assign everyone in the sampling frame a unique number, then, reading down the columns of a random number table or a list of random numbers generated by a computer algorithm, select those cases whose identifiers are included in the list of random numbers. If the entire sampling frame is available electronically, most computer database programs will draw random samples of cases of any specified number. A major limitation with random sampling is that the full list of members of a population (e.g., women with cervical cancer) rarely exists.

Random sampling is an efficient way in which to create a representative sample, but it does not guarantee representativeness. By definition, the process is random. However, it is possible, although quite unlikely, that a very atypical sample might emerge. In using random sampling to create a sample of 200 from 10,000 children, every possible sample of 200 has an equal chance of being drawn. It is possible, although very unlikely, that the sample drawn will contain 200 boys and no girls. More realistically, smaller (proportionately) subgroups might be underrepresented or entirely absent. If the research involves handedness or physical stature, it is possible that the selected sample will have no left-handed children or no children below or above a given height. To avoid this possibility, sampling procedures frequently incorporate **stratification**.

Stratified Sampling

Stratification involves dividing the study population into two or more subpopulations, then sampling separately from each. For example, if you would like to ensure that exactly 50% of the 200 children in the study sample are male, you would divide the study population into male and female groups and randomly sample 100 from each. This type of simple stratification works only if information about the stratification variable is included in the sampling frame data, that is, in the day care center or pediatric office records. It is unlikely that you would be able to stratify by handedness using this simple strategy. Similarly, it would be unlikely that you would be able to stratify on measures such as depression, self-esteem, or life stress because information about these variables is unlikely to be included in any accessible preexisting database.

A variation on this theme involves a second stage of information gathering and sampling. Once the initial sampling frame is identified, a brief survey is conducted with a large random sample. The survey includes questions about variables on which you would like to stratify. A second random sample can now be drawn from the sample of completed surveys. This second-stage sampling can be stratified based on this new information. Such sampling designs are somewhat more complex to analyze, but they do ensure that all of the subgroups of interest are included in adequate numbers.

Cluster (Area) Random Sampling

If the study population is spread over a wide geographical area, you can use another variation of two-stage sampling. First, you divide the large area into regions or clusters (e.g., counties or census tracts). From the full list of clusters, you can randomly sample a sufficiently manageable number of clusters. Then individual subjects from each cluster can be randomly sampled. Clearly, it is best to have the same sampling strategy and the same sampling frame within each cluster. Like the other two-stage strategies, this requires somewhat more complex approaches to data analysis, but it makes collecting data across large geographic regions economical. If, for example, your sample population is all women in a state and you randomly sample from that population (e.g., from state motor vehicle or telephone records), you then must drive all over the state to collect your data. If you divide the state into counties and randomly sample six counties, the logistics of data collection become manageable as long as you believe that these six counties fairly reflect the overall state profile.

Nonprobability or Purposive Samples

There are occasions when it is not feasible to use random sampling. Nevertheless, you should make every effort to develop a representative sample and to employ a systematic approach that can be well described. This is purposive sampling (Trochim, 2006). A good description of your sampling strategy, whether random or not, permits the readers of your work to judge for themselves the representativeness of your sample and the generalizability of your results. Simply characterizing the sampling strategy as one of "convenience" with no further discussion leaves the reader with the impression that no thought whatsoever was given to external validity and no judgment can be made about generalizability. The reader is left to believe that you are assuming that your findings are invariant across all people and all places.

Heterogeneity Sampling

With this approach, instead of sampling just the modal or typical case, you take care to sample heterogeneously (select a sample of people unlike each other) to ensure a broad spectrum of subjects. In the example involving counties described previously, rather than sampling just the modal rural counties, you would sample rural, urban, and suburban counties. With respect to schools, you might select comprehensive, magnet, and some specialized school programs. With respect to individual children, you might sample college-bound students, those in vocational programs, and perhaps even some who have dropped out or are about to drop out of school.

Snowball Sampling

Snowball sampling is helpful when assembling a sample of infrequent or hard-to-find cases. With snowball sampling, each subject is asked to recommend other potential subjects or to inform other possible subjects about the opportunity to participate in the study. For example, if one is studying older adults with relatively rare diseases or conditions, the spouses of one case will be likely to know or at least to have met other individuals whose spouses have the same condition. In snowball sampling, the investigator is less concerned with the broad representation of a large study population and more concerned with finding the relatively few members of that population who exist.

Respondent-Driven Sampling

When studying a population that is generally "hidden" or otherwise difficult to reach, respondent-driven sampling (RDS) can be employed to recruit individuals who might otherwise have been unobserved, such as prostitutes or drug users. RDS is derived from snowball sampling; once an individual is accepted into the study, he or she is given a set number of vouchers with unique serial numbers and is then incentivized to recruit additional persons with similar inclusion criteria (Heckathorn, 1997). The original group of participants is recruited, generally, from locations that may be more accessible to researchers. For example, for a study on intravenous drug users, researchers could recruit their original cohort from locations where needles are exchanged. Mathematical models based on Markov chain theory and biased network theory are applied to compensate for nonrandomized recruitment methods (Volz & Heckathorne, 2008). RDS methodology has demonstrated that this method can result in samples, wholly independent of the original set of participants (Heckathorn, 1997). Nelson (2009) utilized RDS to recruit Black adolescent mothers for his study on the influence of sexual partner type on condom-use decision making. The first participants were recruited from a sexual-health clinic or through response to marketing materials and were identified as the "seed." This seed group launched a growing chain of peer referrals, with participants from each subsequent group (or "wave") referring additional peers for recruitment waves. A visual representation of this process is illustrated in Figure 19.16.

Determination of Sample Size

Determining adequate sample size is a critical step and should be done early in the process of designing a study. It is important to remember that the sample size estimate should be calculated on how many subjects need to be enrolled at the last data collection period, not just enrolled at the start of the study (Browner, Newman, Cummings, & Hulley, 2001). It is important to build in anticipated study attrition (the rate of dropout of participants) to determine the sample size needed. For some studies, 20% or greater attrition is not unexpected depending on characteristics of the sample (e.g., children, the very ill) and what is required of participants to enroll in the study (e.g. multiple data collections, invasive procedures). Examining prior studies with similar participants or interventions should provide insight into approximate attrition rates that can be used in designing your study and estimating sample size. Too few subjects will result in low statistical power and the inability to detect significant findings in a study when they truly do exist (i.e., making a *type II error*, such as when an investigator accepts a false null hypothesis, which states there is no relationship between the independent and dependent variables). Many studies conducted in the health professions result in nonsignificant findings as a result of samples that are too small. On the other hand, enrolling more subjects than needed will result in greater costs to a study than necessary. When estimating sample size, it is important to obtain the statistics on the number of patients who would have met your study criteria who were available in the clinical setting during the prior year where the study will be conducted. These data will allow you to determine the feasibility of recruiting the necessary number of subjects during the course of your study.

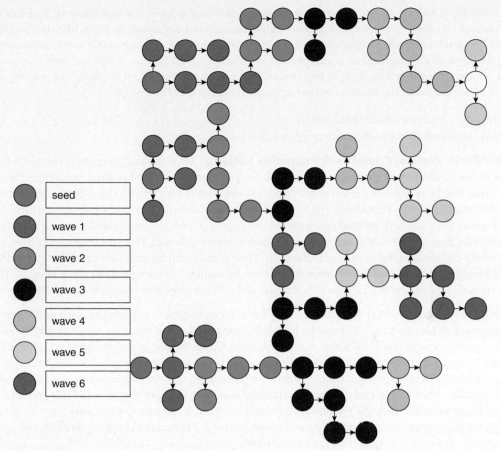

Figure 19.16: Respondent-driven sample network.

Power analysis is a procedure used for determining the sample size needed for a study and helps to reduce type II errors (Polit & Beck, 2008). Readers are encouraged to refer to available resources to assist with the process of power analysis and calculation of sample size (Cohen, 1988, 1992; Jaccard & Becker, 2009).

Refusal to Participate and Study Attrition

The actual generalizability of the results depends not on who is approached to participate in a study but on who actually completes the study and is not lost to study attrition. Not everyone who is approached agrees to participate, and not everyone who agrees to participate completes the study. If the number of people who refuse or who drop out is relatively small and there is no reason to believe that any subgroup of subjects was more likely to drop out than any other (i.e., the pattern of refusals and dropouts was random), the final sample will still be representative of the study population. Quite frequently, however, those who refuse to participate and those who drop out are not a random subset.

People with exhibitionist tendencies (i.e., those who like to talk about themselves), hypochondriacs (i.e., always in need of confirmation of their illness or looking for free services), people with a strong social conscience, and those generally willing to volunteer are less likely to refuse. Thus, they will be overrepresented in any sample in which there is a substantial degree of refusal or dropout (Rosenthal & Rosnow, 2008). People who volunteer may be more likely to be affluent and well educated. Excessive study incentives, especially for enrollment, can lead to an enthusiastic group of persons who consent but then drop out along the way.

The best strategy to enhance external validity is to minimize refusal and dropout rates. To assess the potential impact of these threats, it is essential to have a clear sampling frame and to keep records of who is approached, who agrees to participate, who refuses, and ultimately who completes the study.

If anything is known about those who were approached and refused, the possibility of bias can be addressed by comparing those who refused with those who did not as well as those who dropped out with those who did not. Understanding the impact of refusal rates is not possible using convenience sampling in which advertisements are placed in the newspaper or signs are posted and only those who are interested are identified. Such strategies must assume that the findings of the study (e.g., the impact of the intervention or the beliefs of the participants) are invariant across people.

Strategies to Promote Participation

There are several strategies that encourage participation in a study.

Have Direct, Personal Contacts with Prospective Subjects. Avoid making potential participants take any action or demonstrate any initiative to enroll, such as requiring them to complete enrollment forms or make telephone calls. Be persistent but respectful when contacting prospective subjects. Send letters of introduction on official stationery introducing the study and stating who and when someone will call to explain the study further. Use high-powered mailings (e.g., special delivery and/or hand-addressed envelopes) because individuals are much more likely to open such mail. Have the letters come from the PI whose credentials lend credibility to the study. Finally, communicate that volunteering is normative, not unusual behavior. You do not want to start out by saying, "You are probably quite busy...." This conveys an expectation that the person will refuse and actually gives them a socially acceptable reason.

Make Participation As Easy As Possible. Do what you can to remove any barriers, such as the cost of babysitting or transportation. If possible, have babysitting available at the study site. If that is not possible, provide a sufficient honorarium to cover the cost. Cover the cost of transportation or send a cab to transport individuals to the study site. Make the study as nonthreatening, stress free, and brief as possible, given the research design. Lengthy interviews covering a number of personal topics will burden subjects. Be certain each section is essential. Train the recruiters and interviewers well. Make certain that they are comfortable with the recruitment protocol, script, and interview before working with actual subjects. Interviewers must be accepting and nonjudgmental. They must not appear shocked, awkward, or unprepared during any conversation or interview.

Make Participation Worthwhile. Carefully and clearly explain the importance of the work and the manner in which the study results might improve care or services to patients and/or families like theirs. Make participation sound interesting. Emphasize what the subjects might learn about themselves or their families. Tell them about any activities they might actually enjoy.

Step 8: Determine Measures

Selection of measures or instruments to assess or observe a study's variables is a critical step in designing a clinical study. As a rule, it is best to choose measures that yield the highest level of data (i.e., *interval* or *ratio data*, otherwise known as *continuous variables*) because these types of measures will allow fuller assessments of the study's variables as well as permit the use of more robust statistical tests. Examples of interval- or ratio-level data that have quantified intervals on an infinite scale of values are weight in pounds, number of glasses of beverages consumed a day, and age. **Ordinal data** are those that have ordered categories with intervals that cannot be quantified (e.g., none, a little, some, a lot, and very much so). Finally, **categorical data** have unordered categories in which one category is not considered higher or better than another (e.g., sex, gender, and race).

Measures should be both **valid** (i.e., they measure what they are intended to measure) and **reliable** (i.e., they consistently and accurately measure the construct of interest). If possible, it is best to use measures that have been used with similar samples as the study being planned, as well as those that are reported to have **reliability coefficients** of at least 0.70 or better instead of measures that have not been previously tested in prior work or have been tested with samples very different from the proposed study. It is very difficult to place confidence in a study's findings if the measures used did not have established validity or the **internal consistency reliability** of the measures was less than 0.70.

It is also important to recognize that obtaining two forms of assessment on a particular variable (e.g., self-report and observation) enhances credibility of the findings when the data from these different sources converge. For example, if a parent reports that his or her child is high on externalizing behaviors (i.e., acting-out behaviors) on an instrument that measures these behaviors, and the child's teacher also completes a teacher version of the same instrument that yields high scores, the convergence of these findings produces a convincing case for the child being high on externalizing behaviors.

If observation data are being gathered, it is important to train observers on the instrument that will be used in a study so that there is an **interrater reliability** or agreement on the construct that is being observed (e.g., maternal–infant interaction) at least 90% of the time. In addition, for intervention studies, it is important that observers be blind to the study group (i.e., unaware as to whether the subjects are in the experimental or control groups) to avoid bias in their ratings.

Step 9: Outline Data Collection Plan

The data collection plan typically specifies when and where each phase of the study (e.g., subject enrollment, intervention sessions, and completion of measures) will be completed and exactly when all the measures will be obtained. Careful planning of these details is essential before the study commences. A timetable is often helpful to outline the study procedures so that each member of the team is aware of the specific plan for data collection (Table 19.1).

Step 10: Apply for Human Subjects Approval

Before the commencement of research, it is essential to have the study approved by an RSRB that will evaluate the study for protection of human subjects. Federal regulations (Code of Federal Regulations, 2009) now mandate that any research conducted be reviewed to ensure the following:

Table 19.1 Timetable for a Study's Data Collection Plan

Year	2008	2008–2009	2009–2012	2012
Months	1–5	6–20	21–51	52–60
Setup/logistics	*			
Buy equipment	*			
Hire and train staff	*			
Meet with consultants	*			
Refine procedures	*			
Pilot group training (6/04)		*		
Recruit participants/preassess (start 7/04)		*	*	
Intervention sessions		*	*	
Postassessment		*	*	
Data analysis (4/08)				*
Final reports				*
Prepare presentations & manuscripts (12/08)				*

◆ Risks to subjects are minimized.
◆ Selection of subjects is equitable (e.g., women, children, and individuals of a certain race/ethnicity are not excluded).
◆ Informed consent is obtained and documented if indicated (see Appendix H for an example of an approved consent form).
◆ A data and safety monitoring plan is implemented when indicated (e.g., for clinical trials; see this book's companion website at http://thepoint.lww.com/melnyk3e for an example of a data safety and monitoring plan).

In addition, any individual involved in a study as an investigator, subinvestigator, study coordinator, or enroller of human subjects must pass a required test on the protection of human subjects, based on the Belmont Report. The Belmont Report was issued in 1978 by the National Commission of the Protection of Human Subjects of Biomedical and Behavioral Research and outlined three principles on which standards of ethical conduct in research are to be based:

1. Beneficence (i.e., no harm to subjects)
2. Respect for human dignity (e.g., the right for self-determination, as in providing voluntary consent to participate in a study)
3. Justice (e.g., fair treatment and nondiscriminatory selection of human subjects)

Guidelines for RSRB application and review should be obtained from the institution(s) in which the study will be conducted.

 See The Ohio State University's website at **http://orrp.osu.edu/irb/** for one example of required guidelines and forms for submission of a research study for human subjects' review.

Step 11: Implement the Study

Once human subjects' approval for the study is obtained, data collection can begin. Particular detail and attention should be paid to the process of data collection for the first 5 to 10 subjects regarding the ease of enrollment and completion of study questionnaires.

These first 5 or 10 cases can be considered a pilot phase used to identify problems in the intervention, recruitment, or data gathering so that changes can be made if needed. This is a good time for the research team to work through any challenges encountered and to implement strategies to overcome them. Once the main study begins, no changes should be made. If changes are made, subjects evaluated before the changes cannot be analyzed along with subjects evaluated afterward.

During the conduct of the study, emphasis should be placed on the review of questionnaires after completion by study participants to prevent missing data that pose challenges for data analysis as well as to determine whether subjects meet clinical criteria on sensitive measures or those that identify them as at risk for certain conditions (e.g., major depression, suicide). Weekly or biweekly team meetings are very beneficial for the research team to overcome challenges in data collection and to maintain cohesiveness during the conduct of the study.

Step 12: Prepare and Analyze Data

In the preparation phase of data analysis, it is important to assess study measures for completeness and to make determinations about what strategies will be used to handle missing data. For example, if less than 30% of the data are missing on a questionnaire, it is acceptable practice to impute the mean for missing items. If, on the other hand, more than 30% of the data are missing on a questionnaire, investigators commonly eliminate it from data analysis. There is a growing body of literature on handling missing data, and researchers should document the details of missing data and the methods for dealing with the missing values into their data analysis (Penny & Atkinson, 2012).

Creating a codebook regarding how certain responses will be translated into numerical form is important before data can be entered into a statistical program, such as SPSS (Statistical Package for the Social Sciences). For example, marital status could be coded as "1" married, "2" not married, "3" divorced, or "4" married for the second or third time. Verifying all entered data is also a critical step in preparing to analyze the data.

Multiple statistical tests can be conducted to answer research questions and to test hypotheses generated in quantitative studies, and readers are encouraged to consult a statistical resource for detailed information on these specific tests. For example, Munro's text *Statistical methods for healthcare research, 6th edition* (2012) is a user-friendly book that provides excellent information and examples of common statistical analyses for quantitative studies.

Step 13: Interpret the Results

Careful interpretation of the results of a study (i.e., explaining the study results) is important and should be based on the theoretical/conceptual framework that guided the study as well as prior work in the area. Alternative explanations for the findings should always be considered in the discussion. In addition, it is important to discuss findings from prior research that relate to the current study as well as the study's implications for clinical practice and/or policy.

Step 14: Disseminate the Findings

Once a study is completed, it is imperative to disseminate the findings to both researchers and clinicians who will use the evidence in guiding further research in the area or in making decisions about patient care. The vehicles for dissemination should include both conferences in the form of oral and/or poster presentations and publications (see Chapter 18 for helpful strategies on preparing oral and poster presentations, as well as writing for publication). In addition, the findings of a study should also be disseminated to the media, healthcare policy makers, and the public (see Chapter 18).

Step 15: Incorporate Findings into Evidence-Based Practice and Evaluate Outcomes

Once evidence from a study is generated, it is important to factor that evidence into a decision regarding whether it should be incorporated into patient care. Studies should be critically appraised with respect to three key questions:

1. Are the findings valid (i.e., as close to the truth as possible)?
2. Are the findings important (e.g., strength and preciseness of the intervention)?
3. Are the findings applicable to your patients? (See Unit 2.)

Once a decision is made to incorporate the findings of a study into practice, an outcomes evaluation should be conducted to determine the impact of the change on the process or outcomes of clinical care (see Chapter 10).

EBP FAST FACTS

- ◆ Descriptive and predictive studies lay the foundation for developing interventions.
- ◆ True experiments or RCTs are the strongest designs to support cause and effect (i.e., the independent variable or intervention causes a change in the dependent or outcome variable).
- ◆ Study feasibility addresses factors including adequate time and resources, access to participants, team member expertise, and ethical and legal constraints.

◆ Threats to internal validity (the ability to say that it was the intervention or treatment that caused a change in outcome) and external validity (generalizability) require a balanced approach because increasing strategies to lessen one usually decreases strategies to minimize the other.

◆ Success of transferring the evidence generated by a quantitative study largely depends on developing an innovative yet answerable research question that addresses a "so what" factor and measures outcomes that matter in real-world healthcare settings (e.g., patient complications, length of stay, rehospitalizations, cost).

References

Browner, W. S., Newman, T. B., Cummings, S. R., & Hulley, S. B. (2001). Estimating sample size and power: The nitty-gritty. In S. B. Hulley, S. R. Cummings, W. S. Browner, D. Grady, N. Hearst, & T. B. Newman (Eds.), *Designing clinical research: An epidemiologic approach* (2nd ed., pp. 65–85). Philadelphia, PA: Lippincott Williams & Wilkins.

Campbell, D. T., & Stanley, J. C. (1963). *Experimental and quasi-experimental designs for research*. Chicago: Rand McNally.

Code of Federal Regulations. (2009). *Protection of human subjects*: 45CFR46 (Rev. January 15, 2009). Washington, DC: Department of Health and Human Services. Retrieved from http://www.hhs.gov/ohrp/humansubjects/guidance/45cfr46.html

Cohen, J. (1988). *Statistical power analysis for the behavioral sciences* (2nd ed.). Mahwah, NJ: Lawrence Erlbaum.

Cohen, J. (1992). *A power primer: Psychological bulletin*. Washington, DC: American Psychological Association.

Guyatt, G., & Rennie, D. (2008). *Users' guides to the medical literature: Essentials of evidence-based clinical practice*. Chicago: American Medical Association.

Heckathorn, D. (1997). Respondent-driving sampling: A new approach to the study of hidden populations. *Social Problems, 44*(2), 174–199.

Hulley, S. B., Cummings, S. R., Browner, W. S., Grady, D., & Newman, T. B. (2006). *Designing clinical research* (3rd ed.). Philadelphia, PA: Lippincott Williams & Wilkins.

Jaccard, J., & Becker, M. A. (2009). *Statistics for the behavioral sciences* (5th ed.). Belmont, CA: Wadsworth.

Jimmerson, S. (1982). Anxiety. In J. Haber, A. Leach, & B. Sideleau (Eds.), *Comprehensive psychiatric nursing*. New York: McGraw-Hill.

Johnson, J. E., Fieler, V. K., Jones, L. S., Wlasowicz, G. S., & Mitchell, M. L. (1997). *Self-regulation theory: Applying theory to your practice*. Pittsburgh, PA: Oncology Nursing Press.

Leventhal, H., & Johnson, J. E. (1983). Laboratory and field experimentation: Development of a theory of self-regulation. In P. J. Woolridge, M. H. Schmitt, J. K. Skipper, Jr., & R. C. Leonard (Eds.), *Behavioral science and nursing theory* (pp. 189–262). St. Louis, MO: Mosby.

Melnyk, B. M. (1994). Coping with unplanned childhood hospitalization: Effects of informational interventions on mothers and children. *Nursing Research, 43*, 50–55.

Melnyk, B. M., Alpert-Gillis, L., Feinstein, N. F., Crean, H., Johnson, J., Fairbanks, E., … Corbo-Richert, B. (2004). Creating opportunities for parent empowerment (COPE): Program effects on the mental health/coping outcomes of critically ill young children and their mothers. *Pediatrics, 113*(6), e597–e606.

Melnyk, B. M., Alpert-Gillis, L., Feinstein, N. F., Fairbanks, E., Schultz-Czarniak, J. Hust, D., … Sinkin, R. A. (2001). Improving cognitive development of LBW premature infants with the COPE program: A pilot study of the benefit of early NICU intervention with mothers. *Research in Nursing and Health, 24*, 373–389.

Melnyk, B. M., & Alpert-Gillis, L. J. (1996). Enhancing coping outcomes of mothers and young children following marital separation: A pilot study. *Journal of Family Nursing, 2*(3), 266–285.

Melnyk, B. M., Alpert-Gillis, L. J., Hensel, P. B., Cable-Beiling, R. C., & Rubenstein, J. S. (1997). Helping mothers cope with a critically ill child: A pilot test of the COPE intervention. *Research in Nursing & Health, 20*, 3–14.

Melnyk, B. M., Crean, H. F., Feinstein, N. F., & Alpert-Gillis, L. (2007). Testing the theoretical framework of the COPE program for mothers of critically ill children: An integrative model of young children's post-hospital adjustment behaviors. *Journal of Pediatric Psychology, 32*(4), 463–474.

Melnyk, B. M., & Feinstein, N. F. (2001). Mediating functions of maternal anxiety and participation in care on young children's posthospital adjustment. *Research in Nursing & Health, 24*, 18–26.

Melnyk, B. M., Feinstein, N. F., Alpert-Gillis, L., Fairbanks, E., Crean, H. F., Sinkin, R., … Gross, S. J. (2006). Reducing premature infants' length of stay and improving parents' mental health outcomes with the COPE NICU program: A randomized clinical trial. *Pediatrics, 118*(5), 1414–1427.

Melnyk, B. M., & Fineout-Overholt, E. (2011). *Evidence-based practice in nursing and healthcare: A guide to best practice* (2nd ed.). Philadelphia, PA: Lippincott, Williams & Wilkins.

Melnyk, B. M., & Morrison-Beedy, D. (2012). Setting the stage for intervention research: The "so what" factor. In B. M. Melnyk & D. Morrison-Beedy (Eds.), *Intervention research: Designing, conducting, analyzing and funding.* New York: Springer Publishing Company.

Morrison-Beedy, D., Carey, M. P., Kowalski, J., & Tu, X. (2005). Group-based HIV risk reduction intervention for adolescent girls: Evidence of feasibility and efficacy. *Research in Nursing and Health, 28*(1), 3–15.

Morrison-Beedy, D., Jones, S., Xia, Y., Tu, X., Crean, H., & Carey, M. (2012). Reducing sexual risk behavior in adolescent girls: Results from a randomized controlled trial. *Journal of Adolescent Health 52*(3), 314-321. doi:10.1016/j.jadohealth.2012.07.005

Morrison-Beedy, D., Nelson, L. E., & Volpe, E. (2005). HIV risk behaviors and testing rates in adolescent girls: Evidence to guide clinical practice. *Pediatric Nursing, 31*(6), 508–512.

Munro, B. H. (2012). *Statistical methods for health care research* (6th ed.). Philadelphia, PA: Lippincott, Williams & Wilkins.

National Commission for the Protection of Human Subjects of Biomedical and Behavioral Research. (1978). *Belmont report: Ethical principles and guidelines for research involving human subjects.* Washington, DC: U.S. Government Printing Office.

Nelson, L. (2009). *Influence of sexual partner type on condom-use decision making by Black adolescent mothers* (ProQuest dissertations and theses 361-n/a). University of Rochester School of Nursing. Retrieved from http://search.proquest.com/docview/accountid=14745.

Penny, K. I., & Atkinson, I. (2012). Approaches for dealing with missing data in health care studies. *Journal of Clinical Nursing, 21*(19–20), 2722–2729. doi:10.1111/j.1365-2702.2011.03854.x

Polit, D. F., & Beck, C. T. (2008). *Nursing research: Generating and assessing evidence for nursing practice* (8th ed.). Philadelphia, PA: Lippincott, Williams & Wilkins.

Powers, B. A., & Knapp, T. R. (2010). *A dictionary of nursing theory and research* (4th ed.). New York: Springer.

Rosenthal, R., & Rosnow, R. L. (2008). *Essential of behavioral research: Methods and data analysis* (3rd ed.). New York: McGraw-Hill.

Tamburro, R. F., Shorr, R. I., Bush, A. J., Kritchevsky, S. B., Stidham, G. L., & Helms, S. A. (2002). Association between the inception of a SAFE KIDS Coalition and changes in pediatric unintentional injury. *Injury Prevention, 8,* 242–245.

Trochim, W. M. (2006). *The research methods knowledge base* (3rd ed.). Cincinnati, OH: Atomic Dog Publishing.

VanderVeer, A. H. (1949). The psychopathology of physical illness and hospital residence. *Quarterly Journal of Child Behavior, 1,* 55–79.

Volz, F., & Heckathorne, D. (2008). Probability based estimation theory for respondent driven sampling. *Journal of Official Statistics, 24*(1), 79–97.

Whittemore, R., & Grey, M. (2002). The systematic development of nursing interventions. *Journal of Nursing Scholarship, 34*(2), 115–120.

Chapter 20

Generating Evidence Through Qualitative Research

Bethel Ann Powers

The future depends on what we do in the present.

          —Mahatma Gandhi

This chapter introduces general characteristics of qualitative research. It also, by means of explanation and illustration, takes the reader through a series of steps employed by researchers to design qualitative studies. A single chapter cannot adequately provide a tutorial on how to do qualitative research. Instead, the intent of this work is to enable readers to appreciate what is necessary to generate qualitative evidence.

Qualitative studies are helpful in answering particular kinds of research questions concerned with human responses in a particular situation and context and the meanings that humans bring to those situations. The choice to study human response and meaning from a qualitative perspective involves the researchers' commitment to certain philosophical assumptions within this field of research. The belief that human experience is made up of multiple realities directs researchers to designs and approaches that take these multiple realities of study participants into account. This leads to researchers' perceived need to spend time and develop close relationships with participants to observe and gain direct firsthand information from them about their experiences. See Creswell (2007) for a more detailed explication of philosophical, paradigm (i.e., worldview), and interpretive frameworks that characterize qualitative research (e.g., ontological, epistemological, theoretical, methodological). Also, for a more detailed understanding of how research questions arising from qualitative research traditions fit within the different hierarchies of best evidence, readers are invited to refer to the article in *Nursing Outlook* by Grace and Powers (2009) entitled "Claiming our core: Appraising qualitative evidence for nursing questions about human response and meaning."

Once the decision is made to adopt such a philosophical stance, a wide array of theoretical perspectives and technical approaches are available to qualitatively address various types of research questions about human experience. For example, when a concept or phenomenon is not well understood or is inadequately covered in the literature, conducting qualitative studies may be a good way to develop knowledge in this area. Examples of such studies include the exploration of women's expectations of childbirth and the sources of information that first-time moms use to find out about motherhood (Martin, Bulmer, & Pettker, 2013) and the exploration of the personal meaning that "coping" has for people who have been disabled on the job who are in pain (Carroll, Rothe, & Ozegovic, 2013).

Qualitative studies are also helpful when much is known about a phenomenon, but what is known in certain areas is deficient in quality, depth, or detail. Thus, qualitative studies may explore specific concepts or variables, such as the following.

- The inner experiences of nonphysical suffering and trust for chronically ill individuals nearing the end of life (Sacks & Nelson, 2007)
- The influence of multiple chronic conditions on body image in later life (Clarke, Griffin, & PACC Research Team, 2008)
- Vulnerability and suffering in a study exploring vulnerability in health care as it is encountered in every day practice (Gjengedal et al., 2013).

Qualitative researchers may develop theories or offer insights that explain the processes individuals go through when dealing with an issue. An example of such explanations are the ethical challenges and possibilities in the relationship with patients suffering from dementia and its impact on quality care (Sellevold, Egede-Nissen, Jakobsen, & Sørlie, 2013), the process of parenting a child with life-threatening heart disease (Rempel & Harrison, 2007) and the interpretation of the nature of hope in the context of AIDS dementia in the era of HAART (highly active antiretroviral therapies; Kelly, 2007).

Qualitative studies may provide comprehensive views on topics from a sociocultural perspective. Some specific examples of this focus include the study of how local Somali Bantu refugee mothers perceived the educational and/or health needs of their children with disabilities (Beatson, 2013), discovering how cultural and ethnic beliefs influence healthcare access and outcomes of pregnant Sudanese women in Canada (Higginbotham et al., 2013), the study of recently arrived refugees' perceptions of community-level support (Barnes & Aguilar, 2007), and discovering the disparities in health care for rural Hispanic immigrants in the Midwest United States (Cristancho, Garces, Peters, & Mueller, 2008).

All qualitative studies aim to increase sensitivity to human experiences in order to enhance understanding or stimulate social action. Examples include gaining insight and increased understanding about how living with chronic non-cancer-related lymphedema affects individuals' lives (Bogan, Powell, & Dudgeon, 2007), gaining understanding of potential issues and concerns related to the impact of childhood leukemia on survivors' career, family, and future expectations (Brown, Pikler, Lavish, Keune, & Hutto, 2008), how it is to live and cope with a malignant fungating wound (Probst, Arber, & Faithfull, 2013) and gaining understanding of potential issues and concerns related to the impact of the diagnosis of leukemia on adults (Papadopoulou, Johnston, & Themessl-Huber, 2013).

BASIC UNDERSTANDINGS ABOUT QUALITATIVE RESEARCH

Before discussing specific considerations in designing a qualitative study, it is important to address some common misunderstandings (see Box 20.1). First, the terms *qualitative* and *descriptive* are often used interchangeably and applied indistinguishably, so it is important to understand that this can create confusion. For example, referring to all nonnumerical data as descriptive or qualitative data to distinguish them from numerical or quantitative data confuses the nature of the data with the research processes that produce them. Any type of study design can produce numerical and nonnumerical data, but only qualitative studies produce qualitative data. Similarly, both quantitative and qualitative research traditions have distinct types of descriptive research designs. Therefore, it is important to distinguish between the two. Qualitative descriptive studies are not equivalent to quantitative types of descriptive research. Their purposes and underlying assumptions are very different.

Second, a single set of procedural steps for designing qualitative research studies is not possible because of the diversity and complexity of the field. Reading Chapter 6 will help readers understand the emphasis on general principles that apply to qualitative research design.

Box 20.1 Basic Understandings About Qualitative Research

◆ Not all descriptive research is qualitative.
◆ Not all qualitative research is descriptive.
◆ There is no single set of procedural steps for designing qualitative research studies.
◆ Researchers who have been mentored in the qualitative approach their research question requires have comparative advantages over "those who try to do qualitative research by reading manuals" (Morse, 1997, p. 181).

Finally, mentored experiences are important in developing expertise in all areas of research—quantitative as well as qualitative. But well-written qualitative research reports can be captivating to the extent that some persons may mistakenly believe that reading about how to do qualitative research should be enough to enable them to conduct a qualitative research study. With that caveat in mind, the objective of this chapter is to build on the information presented in Chapter 6 on appraising qualitative research. This time, however, it is assumed that readers might be thinking about practice-based research questions that they would like to pursue in collaboration with an experienced qualitative researcher. This chapter is designed for individuals interested in such collaborative experiences.

Not All Descriptive Research Is Qualitative

Descriptive studies are typically used in a preliminary way by quantitative researchers to establish the knowledge base and generate hypotheses for conducting correlational, quasi-experimental, and experimental studies (Powers & Knapp, 2011). Quantitative studies may use some of the same techniques used by qualitative researchers (e.g., observation, interviews, and descriptive statistics); however, the philosophical underpinnings, purposes, and methods of the research designs are not the same. Qualitative descriptive research reflects certain features that are common among other types of traditional qualitative research designs and differs from quantitative descriptive research in many ways.

Multiple Purposes Focus on Understanding and Meaning
Qualitative descriptive studies also are more interpretive than quantitative descriptive studies. Interpretation of quantitative descriptive studies often is limited by the expectations of the researchers. Examples of these preset limits include operational definitions of concepts and subsequent measures. These constrictive interpretations "limit what can be learned about the meanings participants give to events (Sandelowski, 2000, p.336)."

In contrast, the different purposes of qualitative studies include discovering meaning, explaining meaning in context, promoting understanding, raising awareness, and challenging misconceptions about the nature of human experiences. These purposes are different from those of research designs needed to test theory/hypotheses and answer questions related to treatment or risk.

Openness and Flexibility Accommodate the Unexpected
Qualitative researchers cast a wider net. They consider all that happens in "the field" (i.e., all that is observed or brought to their awareness in any way) as data. In addition, they expect, welcome, and accommodate the unexpected in the process of data collection. "[I]n quantitative research, there is a sharper line drawn between exploration (finding out what is there) and description (describing what has been found)" (Sandelowski, 2000, p. 336). Qualitative procedures are more flexible to allow for decision making about new directions in data gathering influenced by simultaneous collection and analysis of incoming data.

Distinctive Procedures Assure Depth, Accuracy, and Completeness
Sampling in qualitative studies is purposeful to ensure data quality and completeness (i.e., the concept of **saturation**) and to enhance theoretical generalizability (Morse, 1999). Sample size varies, and samples are often comparatively small; however, data sets are very large and dense. Use of multiple data sources (e.g., participant observation, interview, and material artifacts) is common and ongoing. Qualitative researchers also rely on the discovery of multiple means of validation in the data collection and analysis process to ensure that findings are complete and accurate.

Presentation of Findings Involves Multiple Reporting Styles
Presentation of findings in qualitative research does not follow a uniform format. It involves multiple reporting styles. It is not structured around preselected variables and is more fully elaborated from

participants' points of view and in their own words. Varied writing techniques may be used to sensitize readers to the real-life complexities and feeling tones of participants' experiences. Full narrative descriptions seek to establish descriptive validity through accurate portrayals of events and interpretive validity by accounting for the meanings that participants attribute to those events (Sandelowski, 2000, citing Maxwell, 1992).

Conclusions Are Not Based on Prior Assumptions

Qualitative researchers do not limit conclusions to those based on prior assumptions about a phenomenon (e.g., in the form of predetermined measures and items on surveys and other data collection instruments) or drawn from "the results of statistical tests, which are themselves based on sets of assumptions" (Sandelowski, 2000, p. 336). The prior assumptions of qualitative researchers are reflected upon, temporarily set aside, and ultimately treated as data to be analyzed along with study participants' accounts.

Qualitative Research Is Complete and Nonhierarchical

Qualitative descriptive research may generate basic knowledge, hypotheses, and theories to be used in the design of other types of qualitative or quantitative studies. However, qualitative descriptive research, like all types of qualitative studies, is not necessarily a preliminary step to some other type of research (Morse, 1996). It is "a complete and valued end-product in itself" (Sandelowski, 2000, p. 335). This reflects the nonhierarchical nature of all qualitative research. It has no fixed counterpart to quantitative researchers' linear continuum that conceptualizes knowledge development as a progression upward from preliminary descriptive research designs to experiments and clinical trials. Therefore, more often it is assumed that "[n]o method is absolutely weak nor strong, but rather more or less useful or appropriate in relation to certain purposes" (Sandelowski, p. 335).

....

Don't let the fear of the time it will take to accomplish something stand in the way of your doing it. The time will pass anyway, we might just as well put that passing time to the best possible use.
—Earl Nightingale

....

Not All Qualitative Research Is Descriptive

Some qualitative research studies are interpretive, involving a higher degree of analytic complexity. Kearney (2001) along with Sandelowski and Barroso (2003) provide useful discussions about different features and degrees of complexity in qualitative research reports. All research involves interpretation in the natural course of describing what the findings signify and their perceived relevance. But not all research is interpretive in intent. "The defining feature of findings [characteristic of interpretive explanation] is the transformation of data to produce … science- or narrative-informed clarification or elucidation of conceptual or thematic linkages that re-present the target phenomenon in a new way" (Sandelowski & Barroso, p. 914).

Interpretive Nature of Qualitative Designs

Qualitative research designs, in varying degrees, involve the use of deliberate interpretive strategies seeking to describe a phenomenon more completely. As a result, qualitative descriptive studies are more interpretive than quantitative descriptive studies because of their purposes and the ways in which they are conceptualized, designed, and carried out. However, they are less interpretive than other qualitative approaches (Sandelowski, 2000). Although all qualitative research studies involve description, there are certain types of studies that are not solely descriptive, such as the traditional designs of

♦ *Ethnography*—when the purpose is to explain human experience in cultural context, as an interpretation or in theoretical terms
♦ *Grounded theory*—when the purpose is to generate a theory that explains the ways in which persons move through an experience (e.g., in stages or phases)
♦ *Phenomenology* or *hermeneutics*—when the purpose is to produce an interpretation of what an experience is like (i.e., how it feels and its meaning for individuals in the context of their everyday lives)

Qualitative descriptive studies differ from other qualitative studies that represent one of the interpretive traditions in several ways. First, qualitative descriptive studies do not move as far *into* the data in terms of producing "thick" descriptions. Geertz (1973) used the term **thick description** as a metaphor for the use of interpretative devices to deepen ethnographic descriptions and, specifically, to make them more eloquently revealing of taken-for-granted, hidden meanings, and symbols within everyday events. Second, qualitative descriptive studies do not move as far *away from* the data in their interpretations of findings. That is, they involve "a kind of interpretation that is low-inference, or likely to result in easier consensus among … most observers" (Sandelowski, 2000, pp. 335–336) about how closely description captures the actual reality of a situation or human experience.

Description Versus Interpretation as an End Product

Finally, in qualitative descriptive studies, description is the end product. The purely descriptive study employs "a straight descriptive summary of the informational contents of data [that are] organized in a way that best fits the data" (Sandelowski, 2000, pp. 338–339). In qualitative interpretive studies, description is the means to an end. In these types of studies, researchers are expected to "put much more of their own interpretive spin on what they see and hear," re-presenting and transforming the data by "deliberately choos[ing] to describe an event in terms of a conceptual, philosophical, or other highly abstract framework or system" (Sandelowski, p. 336).

No Single Set of Procedural Steps for Designing Qualitative Research Studies

Different types of qualitative research have unique methodological approaches that determine how researchers think about a phenomenon of interest, as well as what they do to understand it better. Creswell (2007) discusses how study designs differ across qualitative traditions, focusing on a small subset, specifically *phenomenology*, *narrative*, *grounded theory*, *ethnography*, and *case study*.

In addition to having external diversity, qualitative traditions also exhibit significant internal diversity. For example, Creswell (2007) observed "a lack of orthodoxy in ethnography [due to] a number of subtypes . . . with different theoretical orientations and aims, [which] has resulted in pluralistic approaches" (p. 69). In like manner, grounded theory has been described as "a family of methods" in which "scholars invoke differences of approach and substance" (Bryant & Charmaz, 2007, pp. 11, 12). Differences across schools of phenomenological inquiry have also been noted, such as, the descriptive Husserlian-focused Duquesne School of phenomenological psychology, the interpretive emphasis of Heideggerian hermeneutics, van Manen's (1990/1997) humanistic pedagogical approach, and the transcendental phenomenology of Moustakas (1994). Significant differences in approaches within the same school of phenomenology have also been documented, as in Beck's (1994) comparison of methodologies of Duquesne School phenomenologists Colaizzi, Giorgi, and VanKaam.

Consequently, the diversity, complexity, and dynamic nature of the field of qualitative inquiry require that individuals be specific about the research tradition and style that they will be following. In addition, the description of procedural steps to be used needs to be consistent with standards for that particular design. Providing practical assistance in matching research question to method and within-method procedures is an important part of the mentor or qualitative coresearcher role.

Qualitative Studies Designed and Conducted by Researchers Mentored in a Specified Approach Will Have the Best Outcomes

Rising interest in conducting qualitative studies has been fueled by increased awareness of their usefulness as well as the greater availability of textbooks and articles about the various qualitative methods. Textbooks in particular, however, largely fail to communicate:

◆ The extent of diversity within traditions
◆ The limitations of written descriptions that attempt to reconstruct the more creative, reflective, and cognitive processing aspects of interpretive qualitative methodologies
◆ Distinctions between quantitative and qualitative descriptive research
◆ Distinctions between descriptive and interpretive qualitative work

Sandelowski's (2000) presentation of qualitative description is especially helpful in addressing confusion and misperceptions related to choice of direction in qualitative research design. One of the confusions discussed is when a study has overtones of a particular qualitative approach (e.g., phenomenology, grounded theory, ethnography) but is not a pure example of that kind of study. Discussed misperceptions include mislabeling of research and "erroneous references to or misuses of methods or techniques" (p. 337).

Articles like Sandelowski's can do what textbooks do not do, as well—focus on select issues in closer detail. However, there is an abundance of resources on a wide range of topics. Therefore, the best approach to designing and conducting qualitative studies of any type is in partnership with a qualified researcher who can differentiate between what information will be more or less useful, who understands the clinical question and can propose possible research directions, and who has been mentored in the specific method to be used.

GENERAL PRINCIPLES OF QUALITATIVE RESEARCH DESIGN

All researchers, qualitative or quantitative, must address certain areas when designing a research study. The general principles that guide the development of qualitative research projects can be found in Box 20.2.

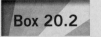 **Box 20.2**   General Principles of Qualitative Research Design

1. Identify a study question.
2. Review the literature.
3. Define the theoretical perspective.
4. Select an appropriate research design.
5. Formulate a purpose statement.
6. Establish study significance.
7. Describe the research procedures.
8. Discuss study limitations.

Identifying a Study Question

In qualitative research, the primary study question is the one that summarizes, in its most general form, what the study is about. Accompanying subquestions lend further focus, as in the following example from the literature. The primary study question is italicized for emphasis.

> *How do older adults with numerous chronic health issues perceive their bodies in terms of aesthetics and in terms of physical functioning?* (Clarke et al., 2008, p. 1086). How do gender norms, ageism, and illness experiences shape and constrain their body evaluations?

Often, identification of research questions such as these evolves from curiosity about some phenomenon in the clinical arena (e.g., what the "struggle between physical abilities and disabilities and personal goals, values, and priorities" is like for persons as they age, Clarke et al., 2008, p. 1084), hunches based on observation and experience (e.g., issues related to loss of independence and social pressures to maintain young-looking bodies), and knowledge of some literature (e.g., studies of the embodied experience of singular chronic conditions viewed from the perspective [or through the lens] of literature on body image and ageism).

Reviewing the Literature

A systematic literature review provides information about existing evidence related to study questions. It is used as a framework to explain why the study is important, to indicate what it may contribute to knowledge about the topic, and to set the stage for presentation of results in published reports. For example, Wainwright, Donovan, Kavadas, Cramer, and Blazeby (2007) described the literature framing their work as:

> The extent to which loss of appetite and body weight result from the progress of disease (cancer cachexia), the physiological changes that result from surgery (iatrogenesis), or psychosocial factors is poorly understood, and the three factors might be linked (Van Knippenberg et al., 1992) . . . In an important study, Kelly (1992) explored the experiences of ulcerative colitis patients who underwent radical surgery (total colectomy and ileostomy) . . . Esophagectomy patients have much in common with ileostomists. They, too, must adapt to profound physical change that affects a major bodily function . . . Clinical studies describing outcomes after esophagectomy focus on survival, mortality, morbidity, and dysphagia (difficulty swallowing). Some quantitative researchers have attempted to measure changes in quality of life after esophagectomy . . . but other aspects of recovery have been less well explored . . . Qualitative accounts of patients' experiences are particularly lacking yet provide valuable insights that might inform changes in service provision. (pp. 759–760)

This example illustrates that citing an absence of literature on a topic is not enough. Exploring what about the phenomenon is poorly understood, the wider literature about recovery from illness and treatment, and the state of the science regarding studies of outcomes after espohagectomy provided evidence to support the need for further study.

Defining the Theoretical Perspective

Theoretical perspectives that guide qualitative research range from the basic philosophical assumptions that are implicit in methodological practices of all qualitative studies (Creswell, 2007) and social science theories associated with particular traditions (e.g., theories of culture in ethnographic research, symbolic interaction in grounded theory research) to particular ideological perspectives and theoretical frameworks. Implicit assumptions and embedded theories of a research tradition that guides methods may be demonstrated rather than explicitly discussed in the design of a study (i.e., through explanation of study procedures). Other theoretical or ideological perspectives that pertain to the research questions may be presented early in the design of some studies as orienting/sensitizing frameworks or at the end of others, as outcomes of the research.

In the following example, social support theories used to guide understanding in a narrative study of community social support for Cuban refugees in Texas are introduced at the beginning of the study.

> Social support has been defined . . . as a set of actions that assists a focal person in meeting personal goals or dealing with the demands of a particular situation . . . Unfortunately, this approach . . . places the attention and expectations on the individual . . . and can even lead to blame . . . for his or her inability to cope adequately. Historically, theorists also assumed that the immediate family was always a source of support, but that has not been supported by research with refugees . . . As an alternative to the focus on the individual and family, the interactional approach to social support defines support as a complex transactional process between the person and his or her social environment in which both the person and the situation must be considered. (Barnes & Aguilar, 2007, p. 226)

In contrast, discussion of theory occurs at the end of theory-generating studies, as in the following example:

> Mothers and fathers in this study demonstrated extraordinary parenting through a multifaceted process of safeguarding precarious survival as they pursued technologically advanced surgical treatment for their baby's lethal heart defect. Extraordinary parenting was characterized by unusual parenting activities that occurred in a taken-for-granted context of technology and family involvement. (Rempel & Harrison, 2007, p. 833)

Consequently, defining the theoretical perspective of a qualitative study involves choices about how theory will be used. The result is less uniformity than in the case of theory-testing and theory-verification research designs that consistently begin with a theoretical framework.

Selecting an Appropriate Research Design

Qualitative description is the design of choice for many basic clinical questions that involve the desire to facilitate an understanding of a human experience as a whole through in-depth engagement with study participants, most usually in their natural environments (i.e., the field). Styles and techniques typically involve researchers in field activities that may include active participation, observation, and/or interviews.

Pursuing questions that lead to choosing another type of qualitative design should be contingent on the availability of a researcher who is a specialist in that particular methodology. Commonly used possible choices, described in broad strokes, include ethnography, grounded theory, and phenomenology. In selecting a design, it is important to be sensitive to two important considerations. One is that a descriptive qualitative design may involve "hues, tones, and textures . . . [i.e.] the look, sound, and feel of other [qualitative] approaches" (Sandelowski, 2000, p. 337). However, these studies should not be confused with or mislabeled as examples of one of these approaches. Nor should such a study be referred to as "mixed-methods" research, because these designs are explicitly constructed to maximize the use of combined qualitative and quantitative approaches (Creswell, 2008; Teddlie & Tashakkori, 2008). The second consideration is that in choosing a traditional design one needs to consider the diversity in these fields and accurately reflect the chosen method in the study design description.

Formulating a Study Purpose

Purpose statements draw attention to the central research focus, study participants, and the nature and selected elements of the research design. The following example of a purpose statement identifies a style of counseling research (i.e., consensual qualitative research [CQR]) involving a prescribed set of interviewing and analysis techniques.

> The purpose of this qualitative study was to gain understanding of the potential career issues and concerns of childhood leukemia survivors. Firsthand accounts of the life and career development process as experienced by childhood leukemia survivors provide opportunity for helping professionals to identify the career needs of this population, as well as the challenges they encounter in their career development

and life planning. Thus, our methodological framework incorporated CQR to answer two main research questions: (a) What effect does a childhood cancer diagnosis have on the survivors' education and career plans? and (b) What is the role of family in the survivors' educational and career planning? (Brown et al., 2008, p. 21)

Establishing the Significance of the Study

Although activities up to and including establishing a study's significance have been described as six separate steps, in reality these efforts at laying the groundwork for a study evolve simultaneously. Identification of researchable clinical issues and literature reviews, in particular, help establish why a study is needed and how it will contribute to improving professional practice. Often, statements of significance are combined with purpose statements, as in the following example:

> The aim of the present study is to investigate [the] question: What sort of sense of self, if any, takes shape when the strategies of memory importation, memory appropriation, and memory compensation are used in autobiographical narratives by people who have had severe anterograde memory impairments for 1 year? It is a memory deficit that reduces the ability to form memories of events occurring after neurological harm, while at the same time memories occurring before are retained . . . More specifically, we wanted to find out whether they experienced a sense of Nochi's (1998) "lost self," or whether they experienced themselves in a different fashion altogether. This question bears important ramifications, not least for the rehabilitation services offered to these individuals . . . We believe as clinical professionals we need a better understanding of how people make sense of themselves, especially under extreme circumstances, before "reaffirming" or "reconstructing" a putatively damaged "self" in people of whom the only thing we know is that they have a damaged brain. (Medved & Brockmeier, 2008, p. 471)

Describing Research Procedures

There is no single set of procedural steps in qualitative research. What to do and how to do it are dictated by the topic plus background understandings and purposes of the selected study design. Typically, multiple common techniques are combined in various ways to achieve study outcomes. Areas to address include sampling and sampling strategy, ethical considerations, data collection and management, data analysis and interpretation, and standards of quality and scientific rigor.

Sample and Sampling Strategy

The sampling plan must describe the location and characteristics of the population from which a sample will be selected, the estimated sample size, inclusion/exclusion criteria, and recruitment procedures. A variety of sampling strategies may support purposeful selection of the best sources of information about an experience. Research questions, type of study, and previous studies or similar studies in the literature suggest rationales for estimating the size of the sample. Researchers must also explain how they will know when the necessary sample size has been reached, because this cannot be easily determined a priori. Commonly, this process involves monitoring the quality of databases as the research progresses. Decisions about when optimum sample size is achieved are based on judgments about (a) usefulness of the data in various informational categories, (b) types of additional data sources needed to capture an adequate view of the phenomenon, and (c) number of interviews and/or observations needed before informational categories are full and continued data collection produces no new information (concept of redundancy or saturation).

Ethical Considerations

Researchers need to keep up to date with the most current ethical guidelines for the protection of human subjects required by the federal government, funding agencies, and local institutions. Of note for qualitative researchers is the importance of addressing how use of common techniques involving close researcher–participant interaction (e.g., participant observation and in-depth interviews) over periods of time will take into account the issues of confidentiality, privacy, and concerns about nonconsenting members of a group and undue burden. Researchers need to realize that close attachments may develop between themselves and study participants, which will need to be monitored and managed kindly and professionally. They also need to be sensitive to the emotions of study participants who may experience distress at the baring of painful memories and be prepared to describe the steps the researcher will take if such distress occurs.

Data Collection and Data Management

Qualitative researchers may use multiple data collection strategies in a single study. Most important is matching and explaining how particular strategies will meet stated study aims. Examples of what will be observed, sample interview questions, and descriptions of other kinds of data sources (e.g., documents, artifacts, audiovisual materials) serve as indicators of the kinds of data that will be collected. Who will be collecting the data and how information will be recorded need to be described in detail. If there are multiple data collectors, how they are trained and supervised, as well as checks for interrater reliability (assessment of the extent to which two or more raters/evaluators of the data agree) also require explanation.

Data management systems for record keeping, storage, organization, and retrieval of information are an important consideration in research that typically generates large volumes of data. It is wise to lay out a plan prior to data collection. The plan may be a combination of a physical filing system for raw field notes, audiotapes, documents, and hard copy transcriptions and a computer software program, of which there are many varieties. The researcher needs to keep in mind that although some software programs support data analysis through features beyond storage and retrieval that enable manipulation and various displays of data, they do not actually perform analyses. Analysis of qualitative data is an intellectual process.

Data Analysis and Interpretation

Data analysis is an ongoing activity that occurs simultaneously with data collection. Therefore, description of procedures involves outlining approaches that will be used throughout the course of the research. For instance, it might be useful to describe the process for deciding about the need to modify the direction of questions and observation in response to new insights and informational needs. This will include how decisions and analytic thoughts and questioning of the data will be recorded and used. Specific analytic steps vary with different types of qualitative designs. Some of the more generic steps of data analysis involve:

- Reading through all the data to get a general sense of what is there and reflecting on possible meanings
- Coding/labeling, categorizing, and writing reflective notes about the data to examine it from all angles
- Generating detailed written descriptions
- Searching for recurring themes and patterns

Interpretive strategies move beyond description of what is there to reflection on the possible meaning of data (e.g., what it may suggest or symbolize, what there is to be learned as a result of new insights). An explanation of procedures might project how the interpretation will appear in the final written report. For example, meaning may be expressed by representing participants' perspectives within a new explanatory or sensitizing framework that reflects what the researcher has come to understand of the participants' reality. A researcher may also use reflection, intuition, and imaginative play (i.e., mentally stretching/varying different aspects of the data via the imagination) to arrive at a creative synthesis that produces a richly textured picture of the experience. Continuous writing and rewriting are a natural part of developing strong, oriented portrayals of all the experiential aspects of a phenomenon.

Whether the end product tends more toward description or interpretation, it is important to explain how data integration and conclusions will be reached, particularly in designs where more than one data source will be used. The importance and potential usefulness of findings need to be part of this discussion.

Standards of Quality and Scientific Rigor

How quality will be monitored and scientific rigor will be maintained needs to be directly addressed. Because general criteria for evaluating qualitative studies are discussed extensively in Chapter 6, comments here are limited to identifying broad areas to consider in designing a qualitative study. Greatest emphasis is usually placed on validity relating to concerns about accuracy, credibility, and confirmability (i.e., evidence in the data to support findings and interpretations). Researchers may choose the most appropriate steps for ensuring quality and rigor from among a variety of strategies.

Similarly, strategies for documenting how decisions were made throughout the course of the study (the concept of an audit trail) may be described. This is thought by some to be similar to quantitative researchers' notions of reliability. Most important is that selected criteria are consistent with study aims and chosen design because although there are common strategies, there are no hard and fast rules about what procedures must be followed in every research approach. And some quality measures that are effective for one approach may not serve well for another.

Discussing Study Limitations

All types of research are delimited/bounded and limited by their scope and degree of generalizability. Qualitative researchers engaged in theory generation most often refer to the need for further research to determine generalizability, for example:

> Although there is some agreement between the theory developed in this study [the dynamic nature of trust in the individual's nonphysical suffering experience] and existing literature (Kahn & Steeves, 1995; Morse, 2001), there are fundamental differences between what nonphysical suffering is and what the experience encompasses . . . but nursing has not developed any effective interventions to "move" the individual through the suffering experience across settings. Findings in this study suggest that establishing and supporting trust and developing relationships might be a future area of research or intervention when caring for a suffering individual. (Sacks & Nelson, 2007, p. 689)

In this instance, theory testing in intervention studies might lead to an estimate of statistical generalizability (i.e., the extent to which inferences based on this and/or other extant theoretical models may apply to a larger population). Verification, extension, or development of new theory, in turn, would need to be based on accumulated evidence of many studies.

Transferability, or **theoretical generalizability**, of qualitative research refers to the extent to which the evidence, knowledge, understandings, or insights gained may be thought to be meaningful and applicable to similar cases or other situations. For example, health professionals involved in caring for persons with AIDS dementia, on the basis of their own experience, will be able to judge the extent to which Kelly's (2007) interpretive ethnography of the lived experiences of hope and loss in the HAART era of treatments is theoretically generalizable. Clinicians can do this by asking such questions as:

- Does the description of ways in which treatments influence the experience of personal hope and "living loss" fit/make sense/ring true/resonate with my own observations?
- Does it provide insights or make me think differently or reflect more deeply on my own experiences?
- Would the understandings generated about what the experience is like be helpful to new practitioners or individuals/families undergoing this experience?
- Does it add new understandings to existing knowledge in this field?
- Can insights from this study also be valuable when applied to situations of persons with other types of life-threatening illnesses whose hopes are structured in accordance with evolutionary advances in treatments and new technologies?

In other words, "[t]he knowledge gained is not limited to demographic variables; it is the fit of the topic or the comparability of the problem that is of concern. Recall, it is the knowledge that is generalized" (Morse, 1999, p. 6).

Validation of study findings might come in the form of application of the knowledge in practice. Researchers often will describe their interpretation of findings based on sample selection as a natural limitation of the research. For example, Cristancho et al. (2008) stated, "Our use of purposive sampling is a limiting factor in our ability to generalize our findings beyond small rural Midwestern communities that have experienced a rapid increase in their Hispanic immigrant populations" (p. 644). Bogan, Powell, and Dudgeon (2007) indicated that purposive sampling of extreme cases provided information-rich experiences that shed light on what may have been expected and what may have been unexpected, in this case for individuals who had completed a lymphedema rehabilitation program in an inpatient setting for 2–3 weeks. However, the high rates of compliance described by participants may have been related to the participants' inpatient treatment occurring within the previous 5 years. Furthermore, Bogan and colleagues indicated that the patients' experiences with years of living with severe and debilitating lymphedema may have served as motivation for compliance with self-management whereas patients with less complicated and less advanced presentations may not have been so inspired.

Other research limitations include potential pitfalls in chosen methods and issues related to the nature of the study topic. For example, researchers investigating the so-called sensitive topics (e.g., drug cultures, deviance, crime, and abuse) or working with vulnerable populations (e.g., children or persons who are mentally ill, cognitively impaired, institutionalized, or incarcerated) must address limitations in terms of anticipated ethical, practical, and methodological issues associated with their research plans.

CONCLUSIONS

This chapter offers broad considerations for generating qualitative evidence within the context of a research world that comprises both qualitative and quantitative approaches to evidence-based practice. Because neither approach exists in a vacuum, some necessary distinctions have been drawn in the interests of promoting clearer communication. However, the primary focus has been on general principles that guide the development of qualitative research projects. This discussion does not take the place of more specific guidance that researchers planning an actual study would need to obtain through training and consultation, as appropriate.

....

Use what talent you possess: The woods would be very silent if no birds sang except those that sang best.
—Henry Van Dyke

....

EBP FAST FACTS

◆ Qualitative research studies can help clinicians understand how they can care for their patients to maximize their health.
◆ There are different qualitative approaches to discovery of knowledge, including:
   ● *Qualitative description*—to understand persons' experiences from new and information-enriched points of view
   ● *Ethnography*—to understand persons' experiences within their cultural context
   ● *Grounded theory*—to understand how persons move through an experience
   ● *Phenomenology*—to understand how a person assigns meaning to it an experience
◆ Conducting a qualitative study requires advanced training. Point of care clinicians need to partner with experienced nurse researchers if they wish to learn more about the research process through active participation.

Acknowledgment

The author wishes to thank Jeanne T. Grace, PhD, RN, WHNP, and anonymous reviewers for reading and commenting on earlier drafts of this chapter.

References

Barnes, D. M., & Aguilar, R. (2007). Community social support for Cuban refugees in Texas. *Qualitative Health Research, 17*, 225–237.

Beatson, J. (2013). Supporting Refugee Somali Bantu mothers with children with disabilities. *Pediatric Nursing, 39*(3), 142–145.

Beck, C. T. (1994). Reliability and validity issues in phenomenological research. *Western Journal of Nursing Research, 16*, 254–267.

Bogan, L. K., Powell, J. M., & Dudgeon, B. J. (2007). Experiences of living with non-cancer-related lymphedema: Implications for clinical practice. *Qualitative Health Research, 17*, 213–224.

Brown, C., Pikler, V. I., Lavish, L. A., Keune, K. M., & Hutto, C. J. (2008). Surviving childhood leukemia: Career, family, and future expectations. *Qualitative Health Research, 18*, 19–30.

Bryant, A., & Charmaz, K. (2007). *The SAGE handbook of grounded theory.* London: Sage.

Carroll, L., Rothe, J., & Ozegovic, D. (2013). What does coping mean to the worker with pain-related disability? A qualitative study. *Disability & Rehabilitation, 35*(14), 1182–1190.

Clarke, L. H., Griffin, M., & PACC Research Team. (2008). Failing bodies: Body image and multiple chronic conditions in later life. *Qualitative Health Research, 18*, 1084–1095.

Creswell, J. W. (2007). *Qualitative inquiry and research design: Choosing among five approaches* (3rd ed.). Thousand Oaks, CA: Sage.

Creswell, J. W. (2008). *Research design: Qualitative, quantitative, and mixed methods approaches* (3rd ed.). Thousand Oaks, CA: Sage.

Cristancho, S., Garces, D. M., Peters, K. E., & Mueller, B. C. (2008). Listening to rural Hispanic immigrants in the Midwest: A community-based participatory assessment of major barriers to health care access and use. *Qualitative Health Research, 18*, 633–646.

Geertz, C. (1973). Thick description: Toward an interpretive theory of culture. In C. Geertz (Ed.). *The interpretation of cultures* (pp. 3–30). New York: Basic Books.

Gjengedal, E., Ekra, E., Hol, H., Kjelsvik, M., Lykkeslet, E., Michaelsen, R., … Wogn-Henriksen, K. (2013). Vulnerability in health care—reflections on encounters in every day practice. *Nursing Philosophy, 14*(2), 127–138.

Grace, J. T., & Powers, B. A. (2009). Claiming our core: Appraising qualitative evidence for nursing questions about human response and meaning. *Nursing Outlook, 57*(1), 27–34.

Higginbotham, G., Safipour, J., Mumtaz, Z., Chiu, Y., Paton, P. & Pillay, J. (2013). 'I have to do what I believe': Sudanese women's beliefs and resistance to hegemonic practices at home and during experiences of maternity care in Canada. *BMC Pregnancy and Childbirth, 13*, 51. Retrieved from http://www.biomedcentral.com/1471-2393/13/51

Kahn, D. L., & Steeves, R. H. (1995). The significance of suffering in cancer care. *Seminars in Oncology Nursing, 11*, 9–16.

Kearney, M. H. (2001). Levels and applications of qualitative research evidence. *Research in Nursing & Health, 24*, 145–153.

Kelly, M. (1992). Self, identity, and radical surgery. *Sociology of Health & Illness, 14*, 390–415.

Kelly, A. (2007). Hope is forked: Hope, loss, treatments, and AIDS dementia. *Qualitative Health Research, 17*, 866–872.

Martin, D., Bulmer, S., & Pettker, C. (2013). Childbirth expectations and sources of information among low- and moderate-income nulliparous pregnant women. *The Journal of Perinatal Education, 22*(2), 103–112.

Maxwell, J. A. (1992). Understanding and validity in qualitative research. *Harvard Educational Review, 62*, 279–299.

Medved, M. I., & Brockmeier, J. (2008). Continuity amid chaos: Neurotrauma, loss of memory, and sense of self. *Qualitative Health Research, 18*, 469–479.

Morse, J. M. (1996). Is qualitative research complete? *Qualitative Health Research, 6*, 3–5.

Morse, J. M. (1997). Learning to drive from a manual? *Qualitative Health Research, 7*, 181–183.

Morse, J. M. (1999). Qualitative generalizability. *Qualitative Health Research, 9*, 5–6.

Morse, J. M. (2001). Toward a praxis theory of suffering. *Advances in Nursing Science, 24*, 47–59.

Moustakas, C. (1994). *Phenomenological research methods.* Thousand Oaks, CA: Sage.

Nochi, M. (1998). "Loss of self" in the narratives of people with traumatic brain injuries: A qualitative analysis. *Social Science and Medicine, 46*, 869–878.

Papadopoulou, C., Johnston, B., & Themessl-Huber, M. (2013). The experience of acute leukaemia in adult patients: A qualitative thematic synthesis. *European Journal of Oncology Nursing, 17*(5), 640–648.

Patton, M. Q. (2002). *Qualitative research and evaluation methods* (3rd ed.). Thousand Oaks, CA: Sage.

Powers, B. A., & Knapp, T. R. (2011). *Dictionary of nursing theory and research* (4th ed.). New York: Springer.

Probst, S., Arber, A., & Faithfull, S. (2013). Coping with an exulcerated breast carcinoma: An interpretative phenomenological study. *Journal of Wound Care, 22*(7), 352–360.

Rempel, G. R., & Harrison, M. J. (2007). Safeguarding precarious survival: Parenting children who have life-threatening heart disease. *Qualitative Health Research, 17*, 824–837.

Sacks, J. L., & Nelson, J. P. (2007). A theory of nonphysical suffering and trust in hospice patients. *Qualitative Health Research, 17*, 675–689.

Sandelowski, M. (2000). Whatever happened to qualitative description? *Research in Nursing & Health, 23*, 334–340.

Sandelowski, M., & Barroso, J. (2003). Classifying the findings in qualitative studies. *Qualitative Health Research, 13*, 905–923.

Sellevold, G., Egede-Nissen, V., Jakobsen, R., & Sørlie, V. (2013). Quality care for persons experiencing dementia: The significance of relational ethics. *Nursing Ethics, 20*(3), 263–272.

Teddlie, C., & Tashakkori, A. (2008). *Foundations of mixed methods research: Integrating quantitative and qualitative techniques in the social and behavioral sciences.* Thousand Oaks, CA: Sage.

Van Knippenberg, F. C. E., Out, J. J., Tilanus, H. W., Mud, H. J., Hop, W. C. J., & Verhage, F. (1992). Quality of life in patients with resected esophageal cancer. *Social Science & Medicine, 35*, 139–145.

van Manen, M. (1990/1997). *Researching lived experience: Human science for an action sensitive pedagogy.* London, Ontario: University of Western Ontario & State University of New York Press.

Wainwright, D., Donovan, J. L., Kavadas, V., Cramer, H., & Blazeby, J. M. (2007). Remapping the body: Learning to eat again after surgery for esophageal cancer. *Qualitative Health Research, 17*, 759–771.

Chapter 21

Writing a Successful Grant Proposal to Fund Research and Evidence-Based Practice Implementation Projects

Bernadette Mazurek Melnyk and Ellen Fineout-Overholt

There's always a way if you are willing to pay the price of time, energy, or effort.

—Robert Schuller

Although grant writing can be "character-building," it is a worthwhile means to an end dream of being able to conduct a study or project that is meaningful to you and one that can lead to substantial improvements in the quality of care and patient outcomes. Once a decision has been made to conduct a study to generate evidence that will guide clinical practice or to implement and evaluate a practice change as part of an evidence-based practice (EBP) implementation or outcomes management project, the feasibility of conducting such an initiative must be assessed. Although small pilot studies or outcome management projects can be conducted with relatively few resources, most studies (e.g., randomized controlled trials or RCTs) typically require funding to cover items such as research assistants, staff time, instruments to measure outcomes of interest, intervention materials, and data management and analyses. This chapter focuses on strategies for developing a successful grant proposal to fund research as well as EBP implementation or outcome management projects. Many of these grant-writing strategies are similar, whether applying for large-scale grants from federal agencies, such as the National Institutes of Health (NIH) or the Agency for Healthcare Research and Quality (AHRQ), or more small-scale funding from professional organizations or foundations. Potential funding sources and key components of a project budget will also be highlighted.

PRELIMINARY STRATEGIES FOR WRITING A GRANT PROPOSAL

A grant proposal is a written plan outlining the specific aims, background, significance, methods, and budget for a project that is requesting funding from sources such as professional organizations, federal agencies, or foundations. It is not uncommon for the process of planning, writing, and revising a rigorous detailed grant proposal for certain funding sources (e.g., NIH, AHRQ, the Centers for Disease Control and Prevention [CDC]) to take several months. In contrast, other sources (e.g., foundations and professional organizations) may require only the submission of a concise abstract or two- to three-page summary of the project for funding consideration. When embarking on the road to writing a successful grant proposal, whether for a large or small project, there are five critical qualities that the writer must possess—the five "Ps": (1) passion, (2) planning, (3) persuasion, (4) persistence, and (5) patience.

The Five Ps

The first quality is *passion* for the proposed initiative. Passion for the project is essential, especially because many character-building experiences (e.g., writing multiple drafts, resubmissions) will surface along the road to successful completion.

Second, detailed *planning* must begin. Every element of the project needs to be carefully considered, along with strategies for overcoming potential obstacles. Developing a strong team to carry out the project as well as plan and write the grant facilitates success.

The third element for successful grant writing is *persuasion*. The grant application needs to be written in a manner that excites the reviewers and creates a compelling case for why the project should be funded.

Finally, *persistence* and *patience* are indispensable qualities, especially because the grant application process is very competitive across federal agencies, professional organizations, and foundations. In many cases, repeated submissions are required to secure funding. Therefore, resubmitting applications and being patient and receptive to grant reviewers' feedback are crucial ingredients for success. One tip for success is to surround yourself with uplifting motivational quotes to inspire and encourage you through the writing process (Box 21.1).

First Impressions

Remember that you never get a second chance to make a great first impression. Paying attention to details and being as meticulous as possible for the first grant submission will be well worth the effort when your grant is reviewed.

Once the idea for a study project is generated, the literature searched and critically appraised, and a planning meeting conducted to determine the design and methods (see Chapters 19 and 20), it's time to begin a search for potential funding sources.

Credentials

To obtain grants from most national federal funding agencies (e.g., NIH and AHRQ), Doctor of Philosophy (PhD) degree is usually the minimum qualification necessary for the principal or lead investigator (PI) on the project. However, many clinicians with master's degrees make substantial contributions to federally funded studies as members of research teams that are spearheaded by clinicians with doctorates. For many professional organization and foundation funding sources, a master's degree is usually sufficient to obtain grant funding, although it typically fares well in the peer review of the grant proposal to have a researcher with a PhD as part of the team.

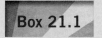 **Box 21.1**   Motivational Quotes for Success With Grant Writing

....

Failures are only temporary setbacks and "character-building" experiences.
—Les Brown

Most people give up just when they're about to achieve success. They quit on the one-yard line. They give up at the last minute of the game, one foot from a winning touchdown.
—H. Ross Perot

I do not think there is any other quality so essential to success of any kind as the quality of perseverance. It overcomes almost everything, even nature.
—John D. Rockefeller

....

Potential Funding Sources

Academic medical centers, schools within university settings, and healthcare organizations frequently have internal mechanisms available to fund small research projects (e.g., pilot and feasibility studies), often through a competitive grants program. External funding agencies, such as NIH and AHRQ; foundations, such as the W.T. Grant Foundation, the Robert Wood Johnson Foundation, or Josiah Macy Jr. Foundation; for-profit corporations, such as pharmaceutical companies; and professional organizations, such as the Society of Critical Care Medicine and the American Heart Association, often list priorities or areas that they are interested in supporting (e.g., palliative care, pain management for critically ill patients, symptom management, and HIV risk reduction).

Establishing a list of potential funding agencies whose priorities are matched with the type of study or project that you are interested in conducting will enhance chances for success. Grants.gov is an outstanding site that lists all current discretionary funding opportunities from 26 agencies of the U.S. government, including NIH and the National Science Foundation along with all of the most important funders of research in the U.S. Internet links to various potential funding agencies/organizations are listed in Table 21.1.

Table 21.1 Internet Links to Various Potential Funding Agencies

Type	Organization	Internet Link
V	U.S. Department of Health and Human Services	http://grants.gov
M	National Institute of Mental Health	http://gopher.nimh.nih.gov/
V	National Institutes of Health	http://www.nih.gov/
M	National Alliance on Mental Illness	http://www.nami.org/research/policy.html
V	National Institute of Nursing Research	http://www.ninr.nih.gov/
N	American Nurses Foundation (American Nurses Association)	http://www.anfonline.org/
V	Sigma Theta Tau International	http://www.nursingsociety.org/Research/Grants/Pages/small_grants.aspx
N	American Academy of Nursing	http://www.aannet.org/
V	Agency for Healthcare Research and Quality	http://www.ahrq.gov/fund/
V	Centers for Disease Control and Prevention	http://www.cdc.gov/
M	Substance Abuse and Mental Health Services Administration	http://www.samhsa.gov/
G	National Institute on Aging	http://www.nia.nih.gov/
M	National Institute on Drug Abuse	http://www.drugabuse.gov/funding
V	National Center for Complementary and Alternative Medicine	http://nccam.nih.gov/research/
M	Alzheimer's Association	http://www.alz.org/

M	American Academy of Child & Adolescent Psychiatry	http://www.aacap.org/
N	National League for Nursing	http://www.nln.org/researchgrants/index.htm
M	American Psychiatric Association	http://www.psych.org/
V	Foundation Center	http://www.foundationcenter.org
V	Robert Wood Johnson Foundation	http://www.rwjf.org/
P	The Annie E. Casey Foundation	http://www.aecf.org/
O	Oncology Nursing Society	http://www.ons.org/
O	American Cancer Society	http://www.cancer.org/

N, nursing issues (e.g., recruitment/retention, competencies); G, geriatric; M, mental health; O, oncology; P, pediatric; V, multi-type (nonspecific, general categories).

Additional helpful resources are databases that match a clinician's interests with federal and foundation research grant opportunities. Two databases that most universities have available to provide this type of matching include the Sponsored Programs Information Network (SPIN) and Genius Smarts. With information from thousands of different sponsoring agencies, SPIN facilitates the identification of potential grants in an individual's area of interest, once specified in the database. Genius Smarts sends e-mail messages to people who are registered in the SPIN database whenever there is a match between the identified areas of interest and potential funding opportunities.

Foundation Center is an Internet site that assists individuals in learning about and locating foundations that match with their individual interests. The Center's mission is to support and improve institutional philanthropic efforts by promoting public understanding of the field and assisting grant applicants to succeed. Helpful online education and tutorials on grant writing are also available at this website. Registration is free for Foundation Center.

The Foundation Center can be found at **http://foundationcenter.org**

Application Criteria

Before proceeding with an application to a specific funding agency or organization, the criteria required to apply for a grant need to be identified. For example, to be eligible for a research grant from some professional organizations, membership in the organization is required. In addition, some foundations require that the grant applicant live in a particular geographical area to apply for funding. Obtaining this type of information as well as conducting a background investigation on a particular organization or foundation will save precious time and energy in that grant applications will be submitted only to sources that match your interest area and qualifications.

Some grant writers find it helpful to contact an individual from the agency or to write a letter of inquiry that contains an abstract of the proposed project before actually writing and submitting the full proposal for funding. The names and contact information for program officers (i.e., the program development/administration contact personnel for grant applicants) are typically listed on an agency's home page. Although some individuals prefer to write the grant abstract after the entire proposal is completed, others find it worthwhile to develop the abstract first and seek up-front consultation about the project's compatibility with a potential funding agency's interests.

Importance of the Abstract

The proposal's abstract is key to the success of the proposal and should create a compelling case for why the project needs to be funded. Important components of the abstract should include:

◆ Clinical significance of the project, including the **"so what?" factor** (i.e., the potential impact of the project) (Melnyk & Morrison-Beedy, 2012)
◆ Study's aims or hypotheses/study questions
◆ Conceptual or **theoretical framework**
◆ Design and methods, including sample and outcome variables to be measured, as well as the intervention if the study is a clinical trial
◆ Approach to analyses

Finding a Match

If the preconsultation indicates that the proposed work is not a good match for the potential funding agency, fight off discouragement. Much time and energy will be saved in developing a grant proposal for an agency that is interested in the project as opposed to one that is not. Because grant funding is very competitive, consider targeting several potential funding sources to which your proposal can be submitted simultaneously. However, first determine whether multiple submissions of essentially the same proposal to different funding agencies are allowable by carefully reading the guidelines for submission or asking the program officer from the funding source. Also, keep in mind that various agencies may be willing to fund specific parts of the overall project budget.

Once potential funding agencies are identified, it is extremely beneficial to obtain copies of successfully funded proposals if available. Review of these proposals for substantive quality as well as layout and formatting often strengthens the proposal, especially for first-time grant applicants. Federal agencies (e.g., NIH, AHRQ) will provide copies of successfully funded proposals upon request.

 Copies of well-written NIH grant applications along with the summary statements from the review can be accessed at http://www.niaid.nih.gov/ncn/grants/app/default.htm. In addition, abstracts of past and currently funded federal proposals are available at NIH RePORTER at http://projectreporter.nih.gov/reporter.cfm

For copies of grants funded by professional organizations and foundations, requests should be made directly to the investigator(s). Abstracts of currently funded projects from professional organizations and foundations are often available on their websites or publicized in their newsletters.

Guidelines for Submission

Before writing the proposal, guidelines for grant submission should be obtained from each potential funding source (e.g., length of the proposal, desired font, specifications on margins), reviewed carefully, and followed meticulously. Some funding agencies will return grants if all directions are not followed, which may delay evaluation of the grant proposal until the next review cycle. Also, be sure that the grant proposal looks pleasing aesthetically and does not contain grammatical and typographical errors. A well-organized proposal that is clear and free of errors indicates to reviewers that the actual project will be carried out with the same meticulous detail (Cummings, Holly, & Hulley, 2006).

 Tips and answers to frequently asked questions for new applicants who are applying to the NIH for grant funding can be obtained at http://www.nigms.nih.gov/Research/Application/Tips.htm

Criteria for Rating and Reviewing

In addition to obtaining the guidelines for grant submission, ask whether the funding agency provides grant applicants with the criteria on which grants are rated and reviewed.

 The NIH publishes the review criteria on which grant applications are rated by reviewers at **http://grants.nih.gov/grants/peer_review_process.htm.** In addition to overall impact of the project, the following core criteria are fairly typical of other rating systems used by multiple funding agencies and include:

- ◆ **Significance of the study:** Does the project address an important problem or a critical barrier to progress in the field? How will successful completion of the aims change the concepts, methods, technologies, treatments, services, or preventive interventions that drive this field?
- ◆ **Investigator(s):** Are the project directors (PDs)/PIs, collaborators and other researchers well suited to the project?
- ◆ **Innovation:** Does the application challenge and seek to shift current research or clinical practice paradigms by using novel theoretical concepts, approaches or methodologies, instrumentation, or interventions?
- ◆ **Approach:** Are the overall strategy, methodology, and analyses well reasoned and appropriate to accomplish the specific aims of the project? Are potential problems, alternative strategies, and benchmarks for success presented?
- ◆ **Environment:** Will the scientific environment in which the work will be done contribute to the probability of success? Are the institutional support, equipment, and other physical resources available to the investigators adequate for the project proposed?
- ◆ Additional review criteria include (a) protection for human subjects and (b) inclusion of women, minorities, and children

From: National Institutes of Health. Peer review process. Retrieved July 1, 2013, from http://grants.nih .gov/grants/peer_review_process.htm

Develop the Outline

Before writing the proposal, it is helpful to develop an outline that includes each component of the grant application with a timeline and deadline for completion. If working within a team, the PI can then assign specific sections of the grant proposal to various team members. Team members should be informed that before the final product is ready for submission, the document may require several revisions.

As a rule of thumb, it is important to avoid the "old and predictable." Grant reviewers look favorably on projects that are innovative. In addition, never assume that the reviewers will know what you mean when you are writing the grant. Writing with clarity and providing rationales for the decisions that you have made about your design and methods are instrumental in receiving a positive grant review.

At the same time, avoid promising too much or too little within the context of the grant. Thinking that it is advantageous to accomplish a multitude of goals within one study is a commonly held belief, but projects that are so ambitious in scope that feasibility is in question tend to fare poorly in review.

Any time your team lacks a particular expertise related to your project, it is important to obtain expert consultants who can provide guidance in needed areas. These individuals can critique the proposal to strengthen the application before it is submitted. Of additional benefit is a mock review in which successful grant writers and others with expertise in the project area are convened to critique the grant's strengths and limitations. With this type of feedback, you can strengthen the grant application before it is ever submitted for funding consideration. Another strategy is to ask individuals with no expertise in the project area to read the grant proposal and provide feedback on its clarity.

> ### Box 21.2 — General Strategies for Writing and Funding Grant Proposals
>
> ◆ Possess the five Ps: (1) passion, (2) planning, (3) persuasion, (4) persistence, and (5) patience.
> ◆ Remember, you never get a second chance to make a first great impression. Submit a high-quality proposal the first time.
> ◆ Formulate a great team with the expertise needed to successfully conduct the project.
> ◆ Write a concise, compelling abstract of the project that addresses the "so what" factor.
> ◆ Identify potential funding sources that are a match with your project.
> ◆ Obtain presubmission consultation from staff at the potential funding agency to determine whether the project is a good match with the agency's priorities.
> ◆ Obtain and meticulously follow the guidelines for grant submission from the potential funding agency.
> ◆ Review successfully funded proposals from the same funding agency.
> ◆ Obtain the criteria on which grants are rated if available from the funding agency.
> ◆ Develop a topical outline of the proposal with a timeline for when specific components will be completed.
> ◆ Be innovative; avoid the "old and predictable."
> ◆ Write with clarity and provide rationales for your decisions; always justify!
> ◆ Do not promise too much or too little.
> ◆ Conduct a mock review of the proposal in which both experts and nonexperts in the area to provide critique.
> ◆ Make the document look aesthetically pleasing.
> ◆ Spell check and also personally review the document for grammatical and typographical errors.
> ◆ Obtain editorial review before the proposal is submitted.
> ◆ Celebrate successful completion of the grant!

Some individuals find it helpful to place a draft of the grant aside for a few days, then read it again. A fresh perspective a few days later is often invaluable in making final revisions. Additionally, obtaining an editorial review of the grant proposal before submitting it is important in achieving the strongest possible product. See Box 21.2 for a summary of general strategies for successful grant writing.

SPECIFIC STEPS IN WRITING A SUCCESSFUL GRANT PROPOSAL

The typical components of a grant proposal are listed in Box 21.3. Although not all of these components may be required for every grant, it is helpful to consider each one when planning the project.

The Abstract

A large amount of time should be invested in developing a clear, compelling, comprehensive, and concise abstract of the project. Because it is a preview of what is to come, the abstract needs to pique the interest and excitement of the reviewers so that they will be compelled to read the rest of the grant

Box 21.3 Typical Components of a Grant Application

- Abstract
- Table of contents
- Budget
- Biosketches of investigators (usually a condensed two-page to three-page curriculum vitae or resume)
- Specific aims
- Introduction to the problem
- Goals or objectives of the study
- Research hypotheses or research questions
- Background for the study, including background and innovation of the project
- Critical review and synthesis of the literature (consider the inclusion of a table that summarizes findings from prior studies)
- Discussion on how the proposed work will fill a gap in prior work or extend what is known
- Theoretical/conceptual framework
- Prior research experience of the investigators
- Inclusion of prior studies by the PI and research team as well as professional experience
- Research methods
- Design (e.g., experimental, nonexperimental)
- Methods
- Sample and setting (selection criteria, sampling design, plans for recruitment of subjects)
- Intervention if applicable (detailed descriptions of experimental and control or comparison interventions)
- Variables with measures (validity and reliability information for each measure)
- Procedure for data collection
- Approach to data analysis
- Potential limitations with alternative strategies
- Timetable for the proposed work
- Human subjects and ethical considerations
- Consultants
- References
- Appendix
- Letters of support
- Instruments
- Resources available and environment
- Prior publications

application. A poorly written abstract will immediately set the tone for the review and may bias the reviewers to judge the full proposal negatively or dissuade them from reading the rest of the proposal, given that reviewers typically review multiple grant applications simultaneously. See Box 21.4 for two examples of grant abstracts from funded grants that are clear and comprehensive but concise and compelling.

Box 21.4   Examples of Grant Abstracts From Two
Funded Studies

Example #1: FUNCTIONAL OUTCOMES AFTER INTENSIVE CARE AMONG ELDERS

Funded by the American Nurses Foundation (Principal investigator: Diane Mick, PhD, RN, CCNS, GNP; Total costs = $2,700).

Objective: Both age and probability of benefit have been suggested as criteria for allocation of healthcare resources. This study will evaluate elders' functional outcomes after intensive care in an effort to discern benefit or futility of interventions.

Methods: A descriptive correlational design will be used. Subjects who are 65 years of age will be identified as "elderly" or "frail elderly" on admission to the Intensive Care Unit (ICU), using Katz's Index of Activities of Daily Living scale. Illness severity will be quantified using the Acute Physiology and Chronic Health Evaluation II Scale. Functional status at admission and at discharge from the ICU, and at 1-month and 3-month post-ICU discharge intervals will be quantified with the Medical Outcomes Study 36-Item Short-Form Health Survey (SF-36). Significance of relationships among age, frailty, gender, illness severity, and functional outcomes will be determined, as well as which patient characteristics and clinical factors are predictive of high levels of physical functioning after ICU discharge.

Significance: Findings may be useful as an adjunct to clinical decision making. As the clinicians who are closest to critically ill elderly patients, nurses are positioned to facilitate dialogue about elderly patients' wishes and expectations.

Example #2: COPE/HEALTHY LIFESTYLES FOR TEENS: A SCHOOL-BASED RCT

Funded by the NIH/National Institute of Nursing Research (Principal Investigator: Bernadette Mazurek Melnyk, PhD, RN, CPNP/PMHNP, FAANP, FNAP, FAAN; Co-investigators: Diana Jacobson, PhD, RN, CPNP, Stephanie Kelly, PhD, RN, FNP, Michael Belyea, PhD, Gabriel Shaibi, PhD, Leigh Small, PhD, RN, FAANP, FAAN, Judith O'Haver, PhD, RN, CPNP and Flavio F. Marsiglia, PhD. [R01NR012171]; Total costs = $2.3 million).

The prevention and treatment of obesity and mental health disorders in adolescence are two major public health problems in the United States today. The incidence of adolescents who are overweight or obese has increased dramatically over the past 20 years, with approximately 17.1 percent of teens now being overweight or obese. Furthermore, approximately 15 million children and adolescents (25 percent) in the U.S. have a mental health problem that is interfering with their functioning at home or at school, but less than 25 percent of those affected receive any treatment for these disorders. The prevalence rates of obesity and mental health problems are even higher in Hispanic teens, with studies suggesting that the two conditions often coexist in many youth. However, despite the rapidly increasing incidence of these two public health problems with their related health disparities and adverse health outcomes, there has been a paucity of theory-based intervention studies conducted with adolescents in high schools to improve their healthy lifestyle behaviors as well as their physical and mental health outcomes. Unfortunately, physical and mental

(continued)

health services continue to be largely separated instead of integrated in the nation's healthcare system, which often leads to inadequate identification and treatment of these significant adolescent health problems.

Therefore, the goal of the proposed randomized controlled trial is to test the efficacy of the COPE (Creating Opportunities for Personal Empowerment)/Healthy Lifestyles TEEN (Thinking, Feeling, Emotions & Exercise) Program, an educational and cognitive-behavioral skills building intervention guided by cognitive behavior theory, on the healthy lifestyle behaviors and depressive symptoms of 800 culturally diverse adolescents enrolled in Phoenix, Arizona high schools. The specific aims of the study are to: (1) Use a randomized controlled trial to test the short- and more long-term efficacy of the COPE TEEN Program on key outcomes, including healthy lifestyles behaviors, depressive symptoms and body mass index percentage, (2) Examine the role of cognitive beliefs and perceived difficulty in leading a healthy lifestyle in mediating the effects of COPE on healthy lifestyle behaviors and depressive symptoms; and (3) Explore variables that may moderate the effects of the intervention on healthy lifestyle behaviors and depressive symptoms, including race/ethnicity, gender, SES, acculturation, and parental healthy lifestyle beliefs and behaviors. Six prior pilot studies support the need for this full scale clinical trial and the use of cognitive-behavioral skills building in promoting healthy lifestyles beliefs, behaviors and optimal mental health in teens.

This study is consistent with the NIH roadmap and goals of improving people's health and preventing the onset of disease and disability as well as promoting the highest level of health in a vulnerable population.

Table of Contents

The table of contents containing the components of the grant and corresponding page numbers must be completed accurately so that a reviewer who wants to refer back to a section of the grant can easily identify and access it.

Budget

Many hospitals and universities have research centers or offices with an administrator specifically skilled in developing budgets for grant proposals. It is helpful to seek the assistance of this person, if available, when developing the budget for your project to avoid overestimating or underestimating costs. Knowing which expenses the funding organization will and will not cover is important before developing the budget. This information is often included in the potential funder's guidelines for grant submission.

Most budgets are delineated into two categories: personnel and nonpersonnel (e.g., travel, costs associated with purchasing instruments, honoraria for the subjects). Many professional organizations pay only for **direct costs** (i.e., those costs directly required to conduct the study, such as personnel, travel, photocopying, instruments, and subject fees) and not for **indirect costs** (i.e., those costs that are not directly related to the actual conduct of the study but are associated with the "overhead" in an organization, such as lights, telephones, office space). Reviewers will critically analyze whether there are appropriate and adequate personnel to carry out the study and whether the costs requested are allowable and reasonable. In applying for small grants from professional organizations and foundations, which may not provide enough funds to cover a portion of the salaries for the investigators/clinicians who will implement the project, it is important to negotiate release time with administrators during the preparation of the grant so that there will be ample time to successfully complete the project if funded. Typically, subscriptions to journals, professional organization memberships, and entertainment are examples of nonallowable costs. See Table 21.2 for an example of a grant application's proposed budget.

Biosketches of the Principal Investigator and Research Team Members

For the review panel to assess the qualifications of the research team so that it can make a judgment about the team's ability to conduct the proposed project, **biosketches** are typically required as part of the grant application. A biosketch is a condensed two- to three-page document, similar to a resumé or brief curriculum vita, which captures the individual's educational and professional work experience, honors, prior research grants, and publications.

Introduction and Specific Aims

The significance of the problem should be immediately introduced in the grant proposal so that the reviewers can make the judgment that the project is worth funding right from the beginning of the proposal. The **"so what?" factor**, which is a term used to describe the development and conduct of a study or project with high-impact potential, should be discussed in the introduction (Melnyk & Morrison-Beedy, 2012) (see Chapter 19). Key questions that every individual needs to reflect upon as they begin to develop a study or project include:

- ◆ "So what" is the prevalence of the problem?
- ◆ "So what" will be the end outcome of the study or project once completed?
- ◆ "So what" difference will the study or project make in improving health, education or healthcare quality, costs, and, most importantly, patient, family or community outcomes? (Melnyk & Morrison-Beedy, 2012)

For example, the following introduction is quickly convincing of the "so what?" outcome factor and the need for more intervention studies with teenagers who use tobacco:

> *Approximately 3,000 adolescents become regular tobacco users every day. Evidence from prior studies indicates that teens who smoke are more likely to abuse other substances, such as alcohol and drugs, than teens who do not smoke. There is also accumulating evidence that morbidities associated with cigarette smoking include hypertension, hypercholesteremia, and lung and heart disease.*

In the introduction to the grant, it is also important to be clear about what it is that the study will accomplish (i.e., the goals or objectives). For example, "This proposal will evaluate the effects of a conceptually driven, reproducible intervention program on smoking cessation in 15- to 18-year-old adolescents."

Background and Significance

In this section of the grant proposal, it is important to convince the reviewers that the problem being presented is worthy of study because the findings are likely to improve the clinical practice and/or health outcomes of a specific population. How the proposal will extend the science in the area or have a positive impact on clinical practice should be explicitly stated. In addition, a comprehensive but concise review of prior studies in the area should be presented, along with a critical analysis of their major strengths and limitations, including the gaps of prior work. It is beneficial to use a table to summarize the sample, design, measures, outcomes, and major limitations of prior studies. The literature review must clearly provide justification for the proposed study's aims, hypotheses, and/or research questions.

The inclusion of a well-defined conceptual or theoretical framework is important in guiding the study and explaining findings of the study. If a separate section devoted to the conceptual or theoretical framework is not specified in the guidelines for grant submission, it is typically included in the background section of

Table 21.2 Example of a Grant Application's Proposed Budget

Principal Investigator

Funding Agency

Submission Date

Earliest Start Date

Personnel	Role of project	First Year Type of Appointment	% of Effort	Base Salary ($)	Salary ($)	Benefit Rate (%)	Benefits ($)	Total Salary & Benefits ($)
Mary Smith	Principal investigator	12	5	68,000	3,400	28.50	969	4,369
Roberta Picarazzi	Co-investigator	12	5	68,000	3,400	28.50	969	4,369
TBA (24 hours @ $38/hr)	Research associate	12			912	28.50	260	1,172
TBA (49 hours @ $18/hr)	Research assistant	12			882	31.00	273	1,155
					0		0	0
					8,594		2,471	11,065
Consultant costs								0
NA								
Equipment								0
NA								
Supplies								50
General office supplies		50						
Travel								0
Local								
Domestic								

(continued)

Table 21.2 Example of a Grant Application's Proposed Budget *(Continued)*

Other expenses					4,350
Lab supplies					
Pharmacy setup fee	500				
Drug/material costs and labor	$15/day × 3 days	3,600	Sample size = 80		
Photocopying		50			
Instrument for data collection					
Patient satisfaction tool					
Human subjects consent form					
Presentation materials (poster & slides)		200			
Subtotal direct costs for initial budget period					15,465
Consortium/contractual costs					
Direct costs					
Indirect costs					
Total direct costs for initial budget period					15,465
Less equipment costs					15,465
Indirect costs					—

NA, not applicable; TBA, to be announced.

the proposal. When crafted appropriately, it is clear how the theoretical/conceptual framework is driving the study hypotheses, the intervention if applicable, and/or the relationship between the proposed study variables. This section of the grant should also include definitions of the constructs being measured, along with a description of how the constructs to be studied relate to one another.

For example, if an individual is using a coping framework to study the effects of a stress-reduction intervention program with working women, it would be important in the theoretical framework to state that coping comprises two functions: emotional coping, which regulates emotional responses (e.g., anxiety and depression), and functional coping, which is the solving of problems (e.g., the ability to demonstrate high-quality work performance). Therefore, a study of working women that uses this coping framework should evaluate the effects of the stress-reduction program on the outcome measures of anxiety, depression, and work performance.

The background section should conclude with the study's **hypotheses**, which are statements about the predicted relationships between the **independent** and **dependent** or **outcome variables**. Hypotheses should be clear, testable, and plausible. The following is an example of a well-written hypothesis:

> *Family caregivers who receive the CARE program (i.e., the independent variable or treatment) will report less depressive symptoms (i.e., the dependent variable) than family caregivers who receive the comparison program at 2 months following their relative's discharge from the hospital.*

When there is not enough prior literature on which to formulate a hypothesis, the investigator may instead present a research question to be answered by the project. For example, if no prior intervention studies have been conducted with family caregivers of hospitalized older adults, instead of proposing a hypothesis, it may be more appropriate to ask the following research question: "What is the effect of an educational intervention on anxiety and depressive symptoms in family caregivers of hospitalized older adults?"

Prior Research Experience

A summary of professional experience and/or prior work conducted by the PI or project coordinator as well as the research team members should be included in the grant application. Inclusion of this type of information demonstrates that a solid foundation has been laid on which to conduct the proposed study and leaves the reviewers feeling confident that the research team will be able to complete the work that it is proposing.

Study Design and Methods

The design of the study should be clearly described. For example, "This is a **randomized controlled trial** with repeated measures at 3 and 6 months following discharge from the neonatal intensive care unit." Another example might be, "The purpose of this 6-month project is to determine the effect of implementing transdisciplinary rounds on care delivery and patient outcomes in the burn/trauma unit of a large tertiary hospital."

In discussing the study's methods, it is important to provide rationales for the selected methods so that the reviewers will know that you have critically thought about potential options and made the best decision, based on your critical analysis. Nothing should be left to the reviewers' imagination, and all decisions should be justified.

If the proposed study is an intervention trial, it is very important to discuss the strategies that will be undertaken to strengthen the **internal validity** of the study (i.e., the ability to say that it was the independent variable or the treatment that caused a change in the dependent variable, not other extraneous factors). See Chapter 19 for a discussion of strategies to minimize threats to internal validity in **quantitative studies**.

The sample should be described in this section of the proposal, including its inclusion criteria (i.e., who will be included in the study) and exclusion criteria (i.e., who will be excluded from participation), as well as exactly how the subjects will be recruited into the study. The feasibility of recruiting the targeted number of subjects should also be discussed, and support letters confirming access to the sample should be included in the grant application's appendix. In addition, it is essential to have a description of how subjects from both genders as well as diverse cultural groups will be included. If people younger than 21 years will not be a part of the research sample, it is imperative to provide a strong rationale for their exclusion because Public Law 103–43 requires that women and children be included in studies funded by the federal government. In quantitative studies, a **power analysis** (i.e., a procedure for estimating sample size) should always be included (Cohen, 1992). This calculation is critical so that the reviewers will know that there is an adequate sample size for the statistical analysis. Remember, **power** (i.e., the ability of a study to detect existing relationships among variables and thereby reject the null hypothesis that there is no relationship [Polit & Beck, 2011]) in a study increases when sample size increases. Many clinical research studies do not obtain significant findings solely because the sample size is not large enough and the study does not have adequate power to detect significant relationships between variables.

Next, the sampling design (e.g., **random** or **convenience sampling**) should be described. When it is not possible to randomly sample subjects when conducting a study, strategies to increase representativeness of the sample and enhance **external validity** (i.e., **generalizability**) should be discussed. For example, the investigators might choose to recruit subjects from a second study site.

For intervention studies/clinical trials, all components of the intervention must be clearly described (Melnyk & Morrison-Beedy, 2012). Discussion about how the theoretical/conceptual framework guided the development of the intervention is beneficial in assisting the reviewers to see a clear connection between them. Issues of reproducibility and feasibility of the proposed intervention should also be discussed. In addition, it is important to include information about what the comparison or **attention control group** will receive throughout the study.

For intervention studies, it is important to provide details regarding how the integrity of the intervention will be maintained (i.e., the intervention will be delivered in the same manner to all subjects), as well as assurance that the intervention will be culturally sensitive. Additionally, it is important to include a discussion about what type of **manipulation checks** (i.e., assessments to determine whether subjects actually processed the content of the intervention or followed through with the activities prescribed in the intervention program) will be used in the study. **"Booster" interventions** (i.e., additional interventions at timed intervals after the initial intervention) are a good idea to include in the study's design if long-term benefits of an intervention are desired.

It is important to include how outcomes of the study will be measured. If using formal instruments, description of each measure must be included in the grant proposal, including **face, content,** and **construct validity** (i.e., does the instrument measure what it is intended to measure?) and **reliability** (i.e., does the instrument measure the construct consistently?). In addition, a description of the scoring of each of the instruments should be included, along with their cultural sensitivity. Justification for why a certain measure was selected is important, especially if there are multiple valid and reliable instruments available that tap the same construct. If collecting patient outcomes, descriptions of how, when, and by whom the data will be collected should be included in the proposal. Incorporating outcomes in studies and projects that the current healthcare system is most concerned about (e.g., patient complications, rehospitalizations, length of stay, costs) is especially important to speed the translation at which findings are incorporated into real-world practice settings.

Internal consistency reliability (i.e., the degree to which all the subparts of an instrument are measuring the same attribute of an instrument [Polit & Beck, 2011]) should be at least 80%, whereas **interrater reliability** (i.e., the degree to which two different observers assign the same ratings to an attribute being measured or observed [Polit & Beck, 2011]) should be at least 90% and assessed routinely to correct for any **observer drift** (i.e., a decrease in interrater reliability) (Melnyk & Morrison-Beedy, 2012). For intervention studies, it is important to include measures that are sensitive to change over time (i.e., those with low test–retest reliabilities) so that the intervention can demonstrate its ability to affect the study's outcome variables.

When conducting research, both self-report and nonbiased observation measures should be included whenever possible because convergence on both of these types of measures will increase the credibility of the study's findings. In addition, the use of valid and reliable instruments is preferred whenever possible over the use of instruments that are newly developed and lacking established validity and reliability.

The procedure or protocol for the study should be clearly described. Specific information about the timing of data collection for all measures should be discussed. Using a table helps to summarize the study protocol in a concise snapshot so that reviewers can quickly grasp when the study's measures will be collected (Table 21.3).

The description of data analysis must include specific and clear explanations about how the data to answer each of the study hypotheses or research questions will be analyzed. Adding a statistical consultant to your study team who can assist with the writing of the statistical section and the analysis of the study's data will fare favorably in the review process.

Even if the guidelines for the proposal do not call for it, it is very advantageous to include a section in the grant that discusses potential limitations of the proposal with alternative approaches. By doing so, it demonstrates to the reviewers that potential limitations of the study have been recognized, along with plans for alternative strategies that will be employed to overcome them. For example, inclusion of strategies to guard against study attrition (i.e., loss of subjects from your study) would be important to discuss in this section.

A timetable that indicates when specific components of the study will be started and completed should be included in the grant application (Figure 21.1). This projected timeline should be realistic and feasible.

Human Subjects

When writing a research proposal, it is essential to discuss the risks and benefits of study participation, protection against risks, and the importance of the knowledge to be gained from the study. The demographics of the sample that you intend to recruit into your study are also very important to describe in the proposal. In addition, the process through which informed consent will be obtained needs to be discussed, along with how confidentiality of the data will be maintained. Some funding agencies require the proposal to be reviewed and approved by an appropriate research subjects review board, and others require proof of approval if funding is awarded before commencement of the project.

In addition, if a study is a clinical trial, federal agencies (e.g., NIH) require a **data and safety monitoring plan,** which outlines how adverse effects will be assessed and managed.

If applying to the NIH for funding, Public Law 103–43 requires that women and minorities be included in all studies unless there is acceptable scientific justification provided as to why their inclusion is not feasible or appropriate with regard to the health of the subjects or the purpose of the research. NIH also requires that children younger than 21 years be included in research unless there are ethical or scientific reasons for their exclusion.

 More specific information on the protection and inclusion of human subjects can be found in Chapter 22 and at http://grants.nih.gov/grants/frequent_questions.htm

Consultants, References, and Appendices

A section for consultants is often included in grant applications. The expertise and role of each consultant on the project should be described.

Each citation referenced in the grant proposal should be included in the reference list. All references should be accurate, complete, and formatted according to the guidelines for submission (e.g., American Psychological Association [APA] or American Medical Association [AMA] formatting).

Grant applications typically require or allow the investigator to include letters of support from consultants or study sites, copies of instruments that will be used in the study, lists of resources available, and publications of the research team that support the application. Support letters from consultants

Table 21.3 Summary of a Study's Protocol

Variables	Measures	Cronbach's Alphas	1	2	3	4	5	6	7	8	9
Maternal Emotional Outcomes											
State anxiety	State anxiety inventory (A-State)	0.94–0.96	●		●	●		●	●	●	●
Negative mood state	Profile of mood states (POMS, short form)	0.92–0.96	●	●	●	●		●	●	●	●
Depression	Depression subscale, POMS	0.92–0.96	●	●	●	●	●	●	●	●	
Stress related to PICU	Parental stressor scale: PICU (PSS:PICU)	0.90–0.91	●	●							
Posthospitalization stress	Posthospitalization stress index for parents	0.83–0.85	●	●	●	●					
Maternal Functional Outcomes											
Parent participation in care	Index of parent participation	0.85	●	●							
Other Key Maternal Variables											
Parental beliefs	Parental beliefs scale	0.91	●								
Manipulation checks evaluation	Manipulation checks Self-report questionnaire	NA	●	●	●	●					
		NA	●	●	●	●					
Child Adjustment Outcomes											
Posthospitalization stress	Posthospitalization stress index for children	0.78–0.85	●	●	●	●					
Child behavior	Behavioral assessment scale for children	0.92–0.95	●	●			●				

Notes: Example of a study protocol for a randomized controlled trial to determine the effects of an intervention program on the coping outcomes of young critically ill children and their mothers. Time 1, phase I intervention (6–16 hours after Pediatric Intensive Care Unit (PICU) admission); Time 2, phase II intervention (16–30 hours after PICU admission); Time 3, phase III intervention (2–6 hours after transfer to pediatric unit); Time 4, observation contact (24–36 hours after transfer to pediatric unit); Time 5, phase III intervention (2–3 days following hospital discharge); Time 6, 1 month postdischarge follow-up (1 month following hospital discharge); Time 7, 3 months postdischarge follow-up (3 months following hospital discharge); Time 8, 6 months postdischarge follow-up (6 months following hospital discharge); Time 9, 12 months postdischarge follow-up (12 months following hospital discharge).

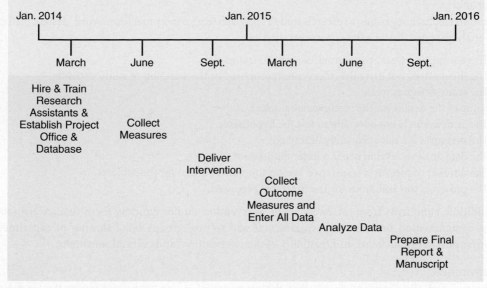

Figure 21.1: Sample timetable for a project's proposed work.

indicate to the reviewers that they are enthusiastic about the proposed study or project and that they are committed to their role on the project. Letters of support from study sites are helpful to indicate enthusiasm for the study and permission for subjects to be recruited from those sites.

Common Feedback From Grant Reviews

This section of the chapter describes feedback that is commonly provided by reviewers of federal grants and some professional organizations. It is organized according to typical categories used for rating grant applications. Feedback from a grant review should help to strengthen the proposed study and facilitate the professional growth of the investigator.

Significance
Reviewers typically judge the significance of a project by whether the study addresses an important problem or extends what is known in the area. Common feedback in this category may include statements such as:

◆ The literature does not capture the entire body of information on the selected concepts.
◆ The argument for why an intervention in this particular population is needed is not strong.
◆ It is not clear how this study or project builds on prior work in the area.

Investigators
Comments about the investigator and research team frequently discuss whether the investigators are appropriately skilled and suited to conduct the work being proposed.

Innovation
In rating a project's innovation (i.e., whether the project employs novel approaches or methods), common feedback from reviewers may include statements such as:

◆ This is a traditional, individual-focused intervention.
◆ The investigator is not convincing in the presentation of evidence that this study needs to be done.
◆ The use of a CD-ROM to deliver the intervention is not necessarily innovative, given the wide array of media currently available.

Approach

Common feedback regarding a research study's approach (e.g., conceptual framework, design, methods, and analyses) typically includes statements such as:

◆ There is no, or a weak, conceptual/theoretical framework.
◆ The theory does not drive the intervention proposed or the selection of study variables.
◆ The study design is weak.
◆ Some of the details for the methods are unclear.
◆ The sample size is not adequate to test the hypotheses.
◆ The measures are not adequately described.
◆ The data analysis section needs a fuller discussion.
◆ The number of measures being used creates too much burden for the subjects.
◆ The project is too ambitious for the timetable proposed.

In addition, comments from reviewers about intervention studies typically focus on concerns about cross-contamination between the experimental and control groups (e.g., sharing of experimental information), reproducibility and feasibility of the intervention, and cultural sensitivity.

Environment

Reviewers typically comment on whether the environment is conducive to support the work being proposed (e.g., whether there is evidence of enough resources and institutional support for the project).

Major Pitfalls of Grant Proposals

There are numerous weaknesses in grant proposals that limit their ability to fare well during the review process. Box 21.5 outlines these common pitfalls.

Major Characteristics of Funded Grant Proposals

Unlike proposals that are weak, strong proposals have characteristics that enhance their fundability. These characteristics include:

◆ Creativity and innovation
◆ High scientific quality
◆ Clarity

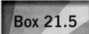 **Box 21.5**   Major Pitfalls of Grant Proposals

◆ Lack of new or original ideas
◆ Failure to acknowledge published relevant work
◆ Fatal flaws in the study design or methods
◆ Applications that are incomplete or do not contain enough detail about the methods
◆ Unrealistic amount of work
◆ Uncritical approach
◆ Human subjects concerns
◆ Absence of a theory or conceptual framework
◆ Absence of links to current literature
◆ Lack of significance
◆ Inappropriate or weak data analysis plan
◆ Promising too much or too little

◆ Excellent technical quality (e.g., organized, easy to read, and free of grammatical and spelling errors)
◆ Potential to make an impact in the clinical field
◆ Greater depth in thinking about conceptual issues

Successful grant proposals also include a thoughtful discussion about the limitations of the proposed work as well as strategies for dealing with potential problems without overemphasizing these issues (Cummings et al., 2006). Copies of successful grant applications funded by NIH are posted on the NIH website and various professional organization funded applications may be able to be obtained on request.

A Nonfunded Grant: Strategies for Resubmission

Many individuals feel dejected when their proposals are not successful in securing funding. However, openness to constructive feedback, continued belief in one's ability to be successful, and persistence are often necessary to turn a nonfunded proposal into a funded one.

. . . .

The only limit to our realization of tomorrow will be our doubts of today.
—Franklin Delano Roosevelt

If you believe you can, you probably can. If you believe you won't, you most assuredly won't. Belief is the ignition switch that gets you off the launching pad.
—Dr. Dennis Waitley

. . . .

Even the most successful grant writers face rejection at times during their careers. When confronted with a rejected proposal, being able to seek the advice of a seasoned mentor who has faced and overcome grant rejections is invaluable in addressing how you will handle the revisions and further pursuit of funding.

Once a grant proposal is rejected, it is important to determine whether a resubmission will be allowed by the funding agency. If permitted, it is important to ask whether there are specific guidelines for resubmission and, if so, to obtain them. For example, the NIH allows one resubmission of a grant proposal. Individuals who are resubmitting are allowed a certain number of pages as an introduction to the revised proposal in which they specifically respond to how they have addressed the reviewers' concerns and suggestions.

If a resubmission is allowed, it is helpful to discuss the plans for addressing the reviewers' comments with the appropriate program officer or contact person at the funding agency. Individuals from the funding agency can often provide insights into the critique and make suggestions for revision.

After reading the reviewers' feedback, recognize that it is normal to feel sad, frustrated, and/or angry about the critique. It is also common to believe that the reviewers did not read your grant thoroughly or to feel that they did not understand your work and were overly critical of it. After reading the review comments, it is helpful to file them away for a week or two until you can come back to them with an open mind to begin the process of revising the proposal.

In the introduction to the revised application, first inform the review committee that its critique has assisted you in clarifying and strengthening your proposed work. It is critical to respond point by point to the major issues raised by the review panel, without a defensive posture. If you disagree with a recommendation from the review panel, do so gently and astutely. Be sure to include a good rationale, as in the following example:

> We agree that cross-contamination is always a concern in clinical intervention studies and have given it thoughtful consideration. However, we believe that this potential problem can be minimized by taking several precautions. For example, we will administer the interventions to the subjects in a private room adjacent to the intensive care unit so that the staff nurses will not overhear the content of the interventions and begin to share it with the families.

Finally, revise the text enough so that reviewers will note that you took their suggestions seriously, but do not completely rewrite the application as though it were new. Guidelines for resubmission will often inform applicants to use a boldface or italic font to identify the content that has been changed within the context of the grant proposal.

Unhelpful responses in the resubmission process include not taking the reviewers' critique seriously by ignoring their suggestions, as well as denigrating the review panel's criticisms. In addition, changing the research design in an attempt to please the review panel without critical thought and analysis will not fare well in the re-review of the grant proposal.

SPECIFIC CONSIDERATIONS IN SEEKING FUNDS FOR OUTCOMES MANAGEMENT OR QUALITY IMPROVEMENT PROJECTS

EBP implementation and outcomes management projects as well as quality improvement initiatives that focus on improving practice performance, including changes in care delivery modalities (e.g., primary nursing versus team nursing), system supports for the healthcare team (e.g., electronic health record with clinical decision support system), and evaluation of the effect of a practice change on patient outcomes within a particular environment (e.g., how substance abusers respond to education about drug rehabilitation and the subsequent effect on the recurrence of abuse in a small county rehabilitation program), are usually not funded by federal agencies. Internal funding sources and foundations are typically the most viable places to obtain funding for these types of endeavors. The application process for a foundation can range in rigor from a one-page to two-page abstract to a full-scale NIH-style grant proposal.

For internal sources of funding within one's institution (e.g., colleges/schools of nursing, academic health centers, hospitals), guidelines are usually available upon request from the research office, if one exists, or from the department that handles professional, educational, or research affairs. As with other types of grant applications, obtaining and explicitly following the guidelines for submission are essential for success. In both cases, one of the primary tenets of securing funding is that the project reflects the mission and stated goals of the organization or foundation. Specifically, the grant application needs to be an excellent match, often between what the funding source desires and what can be provided. Generally, foundations are very clear about the specific areas in which they are willing to provide fiscal support. For example, a major funding area for the Kellogg Foundation is ensuring that children obtain the education they need to be successful in life.

 More specific information about the foundation and a list of recent grant awards can be found on the foundation's website at **http://www.wkkf.org/**

Many universities and medical centers have a foundation relations office that can assist individuals in locating a good foundation match and pursuing funding for their proposals. In fact, some universities and medical centers require that all requests for foundation funds be streamlined through their foundation relations office so that multiple applications from various departments are not submitted simultaneously to the same foundation.

One way to determine whether the foundation that you wish to query about funding is a good match with your project is to peruse projects that were recently funded, which can typically be found on the foundation's website. Scanning the list of these funded projects can provide a sense of the types of projects that are currently being funded. If few to no healthcare projects are funded, realize that this may not be a good match and that more inquiry is necessary before soliciting funding from that organization. If you determine that a foundation is a good match for your project, carefully study the requirements for proposal submission. Some foundations require that the first step in the application process include only an abstract of the proposed project. If the abstract matches the organization's goals and is reviewed favorably, the applicant may be asked to provide a more detailed proposal. However, some foundations or organizations may provide funding based on the abstract alone, especially if the budget request is small (e.g., less than $10,000). Other foundations require a full-scale proposal, including detailed budgets and biographical sketches for the project director and team members. By carefully following the guidelines provided by the organization, the chance of funding will increase.

Keep in mind that most foundations require that the sponsoring organization meet the regulations of the U.S. Internal Revenue Service as a 501c3 organization (i.e., tax exempt). When preparing to seek foundation funding, be aware that many foundations seldom provide large funding relative in size to federal grants. In perusing foundation websites, you may note that, on average, most foundation grants range between $500 and $50,000.

An example of an organization that funds initiatives such as outcomes management or quality improvement projects is the American Association of Critical-Care Nurses (AACN).

 Information about AACN's small grant opportunities along with specific requirements for submission can be found at http://www.aacn.org

FUNDING FOR EVIDENCE-BASED PRACTICE IMPLEMENTATION PROJECTS

EBP implementation projects are typically clinical projects that use research findings to improve clinical practice. They are usually conceived in response to an identified clinical problem. Unlike research studies that have a goal to generate new knowledge, EBP implementation projects are usually meant to solve clinical problems through the application of existing research-based knowledge (e.g., evidence-based clinical practice guidelines).

The application of the pain management guidelines developed by AHRQ to healthcare settings nationwide is a good example of an EBP implementation project in action. These guidelines were based on sound scientific evidence and developed by nationally known clinical experts. Managers, clinical specialists, and educators then implemented the published guidelines in their clinical settings, measuring clinical outcomes preimplementation and postimplementation.

Sources that fund EBP implementation projects, such as AACN's Small Project Grants, do not generally require the scientific rigor of a typical research proposal. Because the nature of this type of funding is small (i.e., usually $500 to $1,500), the timeline from funding to project implementation is short (usually less than 12 months), and the project usually involves the application of well-established research evidence (e.g., guidelines, procedures, and protocols). Thus, the application process is modified accordingly and typically includes:

- Cover letter
- Grant application form
- Timetable for the project
- **Budget:** Funding requested and justification for funding requested
- **Evidence of ethical review**: If an institutional review board is not available in the institution, a letter of approval from facility administration should be requested, indicating that they are aware of the project and its implications for their patients.
- **Participant consent**: All subjects in the project must give written consent, especially if the eventual publication of project results is anticipated (exception: data abstraction from medical records with elimination of all patient-specific identifying data).
- **Program questions**: Specific to each grant, these questions should be answered in detail. When describing the project, use the information outlined in the methods section of this chapter as a general guide.

Remember that many organizations require membership or registration on their websites to be eligible to apply for funding or to gain access to funding guidelines.

Foundations typically restrict their focus to certain populations or service areas (e.g., rural nursing homes). For example, the Washington Square Health Foundation focuses on funding grants to promote and maintain access to adequate health care for all people in the Chicagoland area regardless of race, sex, creed, or financial need. This foundation awards funding to medical and nursing educational programs, medical research institutions, and direct healthcare services (e.g., outcomes management initiatives). General guidelines for submitting a grant proposal to the Washington Square Health Foundation include:

- Collected assessment data about the healthcare needs of high-risk, underserved, and/or disadvantaged populations in the service area
- Implemented targeted activities to increase the accessibility of healthcare services to one or more high-risk, underserved, and/or disadvantaged populations
- Designed and implemented with community involvement, new or expanded services to address the healthcare needs of one or more high-risk, underserved, and/or disadvantaged populations
- Identified opportunities to increase assets of high-risk, underserved, and/or disadvantaged communities, such as by employing community members as staff in health programs, locating health service delivery sites in the community, and negotiating purchasing contracts with local businesses for health service–related products

    The Washington Square Health Foundation can be found at **http://www.wshf.org**

Some foundations fund demonstration and quality improvement projects as well as community initiatives versus research because of the desire to influence practice or healthcare improvements quickly. For example, the Fan Fox & Leslie R. Samuels Foundation has shifted the focus of its healthcare program from applied research to patient-based and social service activities that assist older adults in New York City. The refocused program is designed to improve the mechanism for health and social services to be delivered through support to organizations that reflect inventive, useful, competent, and thoughtful care to their patients. Requirements for a grant application to the Fan Fox & Leslie R. Samuels Foundation include the following:

- The program will improve the overall quality of life or healthcare service delivery to New York City's older adult population.
- The program has a realistic, achievable work plan and a rational, well-justified budget.
- The program staff members who will perform the work are experienced and highly qualified.
- The sponsoring organization is stable, competent, and committed.

To submit an abstract for funding to the Fan Fox & Leslie R. Samuels Foundation, applicants must compile a cover sheet with the following information: legal name, address, phone, fax, and e-mail and website addresses (if available) of the institution or organization; the program director's name, address, phone, fax, and e-mail (if available); the name and exact title of the organization's CEO; the program title and its duration; the total dollar amount requested; and a one paragraph summary of the proposed program. In addition, a three-page letter (1-inch margins, 12-point font) that clearly states the following must be submitted:

- The general problems and issues being addressed and their importance
- A brief description of the nature of the program and its significance, with clear goals and objectives
- The recommended approach to care or services that represents an improvement over how services are delivered now; how the proposed program makes care or service provision better
- A description of the anticipated benefit of the program to older adults, including the number of individuals who will be impacted
- The program's overall significance
- A summary of the critical activities to be performed, the timeframe for the proposed program, and a brief breakdown of the projected budget

◆ If successful, the likelihood that the program will be continued by the institution
◆ The commitment of the sponsoring institution (e.g., contribution of salaries, space, overhead) during and after the grant term

The Fan Fox & Leslie R. Samuels Foundation can be found at http://www.samuels.org/

The pursuit of foundation funding is a good option to follow for EBP implementation or quality improvement projects and outcomes management initiatives. Most requirements for foundation applications are readily available on the Internet, which enhances the timeliness of application submission. As with any other funding endeavor, assuring that the foundation or organization's goals are a good match for your project, carefully following the supplied guidelines, and providing the clearest and most informative presentation of the project, whether that be only an abstract or a full proposal, will increase chances for successful funding.

CONCLUSION

The process of writing a grant proposal is a challenging but rewarding experience. Formulating a great team, judicious planning, careful attention to the detailed requirements of the grant application, and background homework on potential funding sources as well as prior work in the area will facilitate the writing of an innovative, compelling, clear proposal that is matched appropriately for the potential funding agency.

It is helpful to remember that the process of writing a grant proposal resembles the eating of a 2-ton chocolate elephant. If you sit on a stool in front of the elephant and look up, the whole elephant appears too large to consume. However, if you sit on the stool looking straight ahead and consume the part of the elephant that is directly in front of you, then move the stool to the next parts in sequential order and consume them one at a time, soon the whole chocolate elephant will be eaten! In addition, when writing a grant proposal, it is helpful to remember the following individuals who succeeded in their endeavors as the result of not being afraid to take risks in combination with strong belief in themselves and sheer persistence:

◆ *Babe Ruth struck out 1,330 times. In between his strikeouts, he hit 714 home runs.*
◆ *R. H. Macy failed in retailing seven times before his store in New York became a success.*
◆ *Abraham Lincoln failed twice in business and was defeated in six state and national elections before being elected president of the United States.*
◆ *Theodor S. Geisel wrote a children's book that was rejected by 23 publishers. The 24th publisher sold six million copies of it—the first "Dr. Seuss" book—and that book and its successors are still staples of every children's library (Kouzes & Posner, 2012, p. 214).*

Remember, successful people often fail their way to success with enthusiasm. This also applies to the process of grant writing. Therefore, keep your dream of the impact that you want to make alive and focus on it every day, prepare well, believe in yourself and your team's ability to write a great grant proposal, seek mentorship and critique, and stay persistent through the "character-builders" to resubmit until your project is funded!

EBP FAST FACTS

◆ You never get a second chance to make a great impression, so make sure that your grant application follows directions precisely and is of high quality when submitted for the first time.
◆ Comprise a great team for the project that builds upon each other's strengths.

◆ Review grants that were funded by the organization or agency to which you intend to submit your grant application.

◆ Write a clear compelling abstract that gets reviewers excited about the project.

◆ Obtain reviews of your grant from experts before it is officially submitted.

◆ Do Not Give Up! Persist through the character-builders until your project is funded.

References

Cohen, J. (1992). A power primer. *Psychological Bulletin, 112*(1), 155–159.

Cummings, S. R., Holly, E. A., & Hulley, S. (2006). Writing and funding a research proposal. In S. B. Hulley, S. R. Cummings, & W. S. Browner, (Eds.), *Designing clinical research: An epidemiologic approach* (2nd ed., pp. 285–299). Philadelphia, PA: Lippincott Williams & Wilkins.

Kouzes, J. M., & Posner, B. Z. (2012). *The leadership challenge* (5th ed.). San Francisco, CA: Jossey-Bass.

Melnyk, B. M., & Morrison-Beedy, D. (2012). *Intervention research: Designing, conducting, analyzing and funding.* New York: Springer Publishing Company.

Polit, D. F., & Beck, C. T. (2011). *Nursing research: Generating and assessing evidence for nursing practice* (9th ed.). Philadelphia, PA: Lippincott, Williams & Wilkins.

Chapter 22

Ethical Considerations for Evidence Implementation and Evidence Generation

Dónal P. O'Mathúna

In great affairs men show themselves as they wish to be seen; in small things they show themselves as they are.

—Nicholas Chamfort

CONNECTING EVIDENCE-BASED PRACTICE AND ETHICS

Evidence-based practice (EBP) involves applying evidence to practice, which should lead to improved outcomes. The outcomes resulting from evidence implementation should be carefully evaluated, otherwise our confidence in applying the evidence can be weak. The impetus for evaluating the implementation of evidence may arise from a commitment to EBP itself or from a commitment to ethical practice and improving outcomes. "How evidence and ethics interrelate is an often neglected and overlooked dimension of evidence-based approaches to health care" (Upshur, 2013, p. 86). Ethical principles influence both the importance of evaluating the impact of evidence on patients and the way those evaluations are conducted.

Ethics examines issues of right and wrong, good and bad, in any area of human interaction. Various sets of ethical principles have been articulated to guide healthcare practice. Beauchamp and Childress (2012) developed one widely used approach that focuses on four core ethical principles. Beneficence captures the importance of doing good for patients. Nonmaleficence addresses the importance of not harming patients. Autonomy acknowledges that patients have the right to make decisions about their health, lives, and bodies. Justice declares that resources should be distributed fairly among people and without prejudice. The principle of fidelity is often added to capture the importance of trust and honesty. Other ethical principles have been proposed to capture the diverse range of situations in which disagreements arise over the right thing to do, or the right way to be (Box 22.1). Ethical decision making can be seen as a method of balancing such principles when they conflict in the complex situations encountered in life and, particularly, in health care.

As with any area of health care, EBP raises ethical issues. Some of the motivations underlying the advancement of EBP are, at their core, ethical. Organizations in the United States, such as the Institute of Medicine (IOM) and the Agency for Healthcare Research and Quality (AHRQ), have found evidence of problems with the quality of American health care (IOM, 2006). Important progress has been made in various areas in recent years (NCQA, 2012). However, problems remain, raising concerns about whether practice is beneficent or just. For example, overuse of medical services is believed to be common and costly, with some estimates attributing 30% of U.S. health spending to overuse (Korenstein, Falk, Howell, Bishop, & Keyhani, 2012). This is both a matter of using evidence appropriately and also an ethical issue of using resources wisely and justly.

Other countries also report serious problems with their healthcare systems. A survey of primary care doctors in 10 developed countries (i.e., Australia, Canada, France, Germany, the Netherlands, New Zealand, Norway, Switzerland, the United Kingdom, and the United States) identified strengths and weaknesses in each system (Schoen et al., 2012). In another survey of eight developed countries, patients with chronic illnesses reported system-wide problems with their healthcare systems in the areas of access, safety, and care (Schoen, Osborn, How, Doty, & Peugh, 2009). These involve the ethical principles of justice, nonmaleficence, and beneficence. In addition, problems in developing countries raise a host of other ethical issues that will not be addressed in this chapter (O'Mathúna, 2007).

515

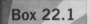

Box 22.1   Fifteen Ethical Principles of the *Universal Declaration on Bioethics and Human Rights*

1. Human dignity and human rights
2. Benefit and harm
3. Autonomy and individual responsibility
4. Consent
5. Persons without the capacity to consent
6. Respect for human vulnerability and personal integrity
7. Privacy and confidentiality
8. Equality, justice, and equity
9. Nondiscrimination and nonstigmatization
10. Respect for cultural diversity and pluralism
11. Solidarity and cooperation
12. Social responsibility and health
13. Sharing of benefits
14. Protecting future generations
15. Protection of the environment, the biosphere, and biodiversity

Source: United Nations Educational, Scientific and Cultural Organization (2008).

The IOM has developed a conceptual framework to help understand healthcare quality and how it can be improved practically. It defines quality as "the degree to which health services for individuals and populations increase the likelihood of desired health outcomes and are consistent with current professional knowledge" (IOM, 2009). The core dimensions of quality, as articulated in several IOM reports, are safety, effectiveness, patient-centeredness, timeliness, equity, and efficiency (Baily, Bottrell, Lynn, & Jennings, 2006).

Each of these dimensions is underpinned by ethical principles (Box 22.1). For example, the ethical principle of increasing benefit and reducing harm promotes safety. The ethical principle of equality, justice, and equity promotes the use of resources according to effectiveness in a timely, equitable fashion. The ethical principle of human dignity (i.e., respect for persons) promotes patient-centeredness and equity. Thus, promotion of healthcare quality can be seen as an ethical enterprise. EBP, as the backbone of all quality initiatives, is also underpinned by the same ethical principles. However, that does not mean that every approach to improving quality is necessarily ethical (or evidence-based).

Situations where evidence-based quality improvement (EBQI) initiatives (for more information on EBQI see Chapter 10) could conflict with ethical principles include (a) attempts to improve quality for some patients that may inadvertently cause harm for others, for example, if people or resources are diverted away from them; (b) strategies intended to improve quality that may turn out to be ineffective or even lower the quality of care; and (c) activities declared to be quality improvement (QI) that may be more accurately described as clinical research or vice versa. The term *clinical research* will be used here, although *human subjects research* is also used, especially in regulatory contexts.

Clinical research is defined as research where investigators directly interact with human subjects or material of human origin (National Institutes of Health, 2005). If research activities are carried out without patient informed consent, they may be seen as an unethical use of patients as research subjects (Baily et al., 2006). Research participation is viewed as an optional activity, and therefore informed consent is required to respect the ethical principle of autonomy. In contrast, it may be seen as unethical to require patients to provide their consent for care that is known to provide them with better outcomes compared to their acceptance of mediocre care that does not have that guarantee. Despite these issues, if efforts are not made to improve quality, healthcare professionals may violate their ethical responsibility to promote beneficence and nonmaleficence by providing patients with the most safe and effective clinical care possible. When this violation happens, patients will continue to be put at risk from lower quality health care.

One approach to improving the quality of health care is referred to as performance improvement (PI) or QI. Such projects can be defined as "systematic, data-guided activities designed to bring about immediate improvements in healthcare delivery in particular settings" (Lynn et al., 2007, p. 667). These activities include an array of methods designed to solve practical clinical problems and to bring about and evaluate change, sometimes based on evidence. Some similarity between QI and EBP can be seen in the description of QI as an approach that "means encouraging people in the clinical care setting to use their daily experience to identify promising ways to improve care, implement changes on a small scale, collect data on the effects of those changes, and assess the results" (Baily et al., 2006, p. S5). This is much like the EBP paradigm that requires clinicians to bring their expertise as well as empiric knowledge into innovative clinical decision making. However, the QI approach does not explicitly require the participation of the patient as does EBP.

The EBP implementation approach can be centered on an issue arising in a unit, an institution, or a system. Evidence can be applied to bring about change for one patient, or it may be intended to effect change across a system or profession. Documenting the change is imperative. Here is where the EBP implementation approach is often confused with clinical research. These two enterprises involve human participants and sometimes use similar methods to evaluate outcomes. For some, EBP implementation activities are seen as a form of clinical research that should come under the same ethical and regulatory requirements, particularly the ethical requirement for informed consent. Others claim that some EBP implementation activities are sufficiently different that they should not be considered clinical research. They would thus fall under general clinical care and not require explicit informed consent; however, specific ethical principles still apply. One issue that often distinguishes these two approaches is the generalizability of their findings. Clinical research should be conducted with samples that are representative of the population of interest so that the findings can be applied to that population. This is the more just approach since the group that takes on the additional risks of research participation also benefits from the results. Implementation of evidence in practice is the application of interventions, practices, or approaches that are known to produce outcomes with some degree of confidence; however, the people to whom the care is provided are not usually representative of a population. Rather they are the patients under that provider's care, no matter what the setting (e.g., hospital, community, primary care practice, or long-term care facility). This type of process often occurs when trying to improve the quality of care; however, to generalize the process or the findings (i.e., outcomes) from EBP implementation is not the goal. Rather the goal is to initiate and sustain meaningful change within the clinicians' practice and for particular patients or clients.

Confusion still exists around the ethical issues surrounding EBP implementation and how it compares and contrasts with clinical research. The formal processes often seem to be a confusing factor for institutional review boards (IRBs; otherwise known as research ethics committees). Some IRBs and regulators view the EBP implementation process as research based on descriptions of the deliberate application of an evidence-based protocol across all patients and the evaluation of outcomes. However, if clinicians withheld known beneficial treatment from patients, this could be considered unethical. In addition, collection of data, in and of itself, should not be viewed as clinical research. To follow that logic would require that daily intake and output values that are totaled and described would be considered research that produced generalizable knowledge. Research produces knowledge in such a way that it can be applied to a broader population than those from whence it came. EBP implementation is applying research, with internal evidence, to improve care. To guard against this issue hindering best practice for patients and violating beneficence, clinicians and IRBs must use caution to ensure that unique ethical requirements for research are applied to research and that the ethical requirements fitting to EBP implementation are appropriately applied.

This ethical debate has raged in the literature for a number of years. Given that the answers accepted will significantly impact efforts to improve the quality of health care, it is important to understand these ethical issues. While much of the debate has been triggered by how these issues have been dealt with in the United States, the ethical issues have relevance for other jurisdictions. Two cases are presented in the following section to highlight the issues involved.

....

It is not fair to ask of others what you are unwilling to do yourself.
—Eleanor Roosevelt

....

TWO ETHICAL EXEMPLARS

Michigan ICU Study

In the United States, 80,000 bloodstream infections related to catheters occur each year in intensive care units (ICUs) leading to increased lengths of stay and costs (Miller & O'Grady, 2012). Researchers continue to investigate interventions to reduce morbidity and costs (Kim, Holtom, & Vigen, 2011). In 2004, clinicians from Johns Hopkins University coordinated a prospective cohort study to examine the impact of introducing evidence-based strategies to reduce infection rates in all ICUs in Michigan (to be referred to in this chapter as the Michigan ICU study). Just over 100 ICUs participated in the 18-month study (Pronovost et al., 2006). A large and sustained reduction in rates of catheter-related infections occurred (up to 66% reduction). The median number of infections per 1,000 catheter-days decreased from 2.7 at baseline to 0 during the final study period ($P <0.002$).

The study involved a number of educational interventions targeted at ICU personnel to improve patient safety. This included designating one physician and one nurse as team leaders in each ICU. The researchers developed a checklist to promote clinicians' use of five evidence-based procedures recommended by the Centers for Disease Control and Prevention. These were (a) hand washing; (b) using full-barrier precautions during insertion of central venous catheters; (c) cleansing the skin with chlorhexidine prior to catheter insertion; (d) avoiding, where possible, the femoral site for catheter insertion; and (e) removing unnecessary catheters. Neither expensive technology nor additional ICU staff was required, though each hospital provided adequate staff to implement the educational intervention.

The study had limitations and, as with any study, required critical appraisal (Daley, 2007; Jenny-Avital, 2007). Nonetheless, the results were praised in *The New York Times* as "stunning" because of how the study saved more than 1,500 lives during its 18 months (Gawande, 2007). However, a few weeks after the study results were published, the Office for Human Research Protections (OHRP), the federal agency charged with protecting people involved in research in the United States, ordered an investigation into possible ethical violations in the study (Miller & Emanuel, 2008). In November 2007, the OHRP ruled that the project had violated ethics regulations and should be shut down, including planned expansions in other states (Gawande, 2007).

The OHRP held that the Michigan ICU study had violated two ethics regulations. The study was submitted to the Johns Hopkins University IRB, which deemed it exempt from review. The IRB viewed the project as an EBP implementation and QI initiative, not clinical research. The OHRP disagreed and held that it was research. Informed consent was not obtained in the project because it was considered exempt from IRB review (Pronovost et al., 2006). OHRP held that informed consent should not have been waived for this reason because it viewed the project as clinical research.

Wide application of OHRP's approach could mean that "whole swaths of critical work to ensure safe and effective care would either halt or shrink" (Gawande, 2007). In the resolution to the situation, both the parties agreed that the study was clinical research because an educational intervention of unknown efficacy was being tested on clinicians (OHRP, 2008). At the same time, it is most likely that the study would have satisfied the regulations for expedited IRB review since it involved no more than minimal risks (Miller & Emanuel, 2008). The IRB review could also have determined that informed consent was not ethically required since the five infection-control guidelines were evidence-based (i.e., their expected outcomes previously had been demonstrated through research) and patients were not being put at additional risks (OHRP). The protocol could have been introduced as part of standard clinical practice and covered by patients' general consent to treatment. Thus, their autonomy would still be respected even though explicit informed consent was not obtained. The OHRP also concluded that since the Michigan ICU study demonstrated the effectiveness of its interventions, future implementation and monitoring of the checklists would not be research but improving clinical care.

Spanish ICU Study

The importance of establishing whether a project is research or evidence implementation is revealed by another exemplar, this time in Spain. An educational program on compliance with evidence-based guidelines in patients with severe sepsis was prospectively evaluated for its impact on mortality (Ferrer, Artigas, Levy, et al., 2008). About 20% of Spain's ICUs participated. Based on the results, the authors concluded that if the educational program was implemented in all Spanish hospitals, 490 lives might be saved each year. As with any project or study, this one had limitations and should be critically appraised, especially as its design falls at a lower level of evidence in the study hierarchy for interventions (Kahn & Bates, 2008). This makes causation difficult to establish, but the project remains a good example of an educational program introduced to promote evidence-based guidelines on a national level while also including an objective evaluation of its impact. It would appear to be ethically sound based on its promotion of beneficence and nonmaleficence.

The project was subsequently criticized for ethical reasons similar to those of the Michigan ICU study. Based on viewing the Spanish project as clinical research, the project coordinators were criticized for not obtaining informed consent from the patients involved and thus not respecting their autonomy (Lemaire, 2008). The authors defended their decision on the basis that the project was EBQI and thus part of good clinical care (Ferrer, Artigas, & Levy, 2008). They gave several reasons for not viewing their project as clinical research. Foremost among these was that the educational program taught previously established evidence-based guidelines and did not expose patients to test interventions. In particular, they noted that the project was reviewed by the research ethics committee at every participating hospital and in that way ensured that appropriate ethical standards were maintained.

> If the people who make the decisions are the people who will also bear the consequences of those decisions, perhaps better decisions will result.
> —John Abrams

PRACTICAL CONSEQUENCES

Much of the controversy has revolved around establishing whether evidence implementation activities fall within the definition of clinical research. The focus of this chapter is on the ethical aspects of this distinction, which have important practical and regulatory implications. The OHRP can impose severe penalties on organizations found to be in violation of U.S. regulations. The OHRP has regularly defined research very broadly and thereby often included QI activities within its oversight (Lynn et al., 2007). Similar regulatory uncertainty and confusion can exist in the United Kingdom (Hill & Small, 2006) and elsewhere in Europe (Lemaire, Ravoire, & Golinelli, 2008).

Another practical consequence of "getting it wrong" can arise if clinicians decide to pursue publication of their findings. Many journals will not publish articles they deem to be clinical research if they have not already had IRB review (Lynn et al., 2007). Sometimes clinicians conducting evidence implementation activities decide to pursue publication only after the project is completed and the findings are viewed as having broader interest (Hill & Small, 2006). Some journals evaluate the ethics of a study or project themselves regardless of whether or not an ethics committee reviewed the original proposal, but not all take the time and effort this requires (Abbasi & Heath, 2005).

The more significant consequences relate to patients. Since responsibility for classifying a project or study as research currently rests with the investigators, inappropriate classification could avoid ethical review or lead to less intensive review and miss the opportunity to identify ethical or methodological concerns (Abbasi & Heath, 2005). If, however, EBP project coordinators view an ethics application as an onerous, lengthy, and perhaps nonrelevant process, they may decide to forgo conducting important practice evaluations. Given that current practice can always be improved, this may leave practitioners unwilling to make evidence-based changes, putting patients at risk for continued lower quality care, or to promote the introduction of practice changes without monitoring their effects (Lynn et al., 2007). It is important that the ethical considerations that apply to EBP initiatives, such as protection of privacy, be addressed by project coordinators; however, other ethical safeguards designed for clinical research, such as individual informed consent, may not be feasible or appropriate for EBP implementation projects.

PIERS (Pre-eclampsia Integrated Estimate of RiSk) Project

Research ethics review itself is beginning to be empirically evaluated, leading to some evidence that applying research standards to QI projects can have detrimental effects. The PIERS project was a multicenter international study of a standardized assessment tool for women admitted to hospital with preeclampsia (Firoz, Magee, Payne, Menzies, & von Dadelszen, 2012). The tool was designed to monitor maternal and fetal predictors of adverse outcomes based on established evidence-based criteria. A project was designed to introduce the tool and evaluate its impact by examining the outcomes in patients' medical records. The project was submitted for ethical approval at all seven participating sites. Three ethics committees viewed it as continuous quality improvement (CQI) that did not require individual informed consent, while four viewed it as research requiring informed consent from the women to have their medical records examined by the researchers. The investigators found that when informed consent was required, those with more severe preeclampsia were less likely to enroll. This biased their sample and risked compromising the scientific validity at the research sites compared to the CQI sites where all women's data were analyzed. In addition, obtaining informed consent required additional time and resources, which sometimes were not available, leading to lower enrollment.

Informed consent should not be abandoned just because it restricts research or takes time. However, the type of informed consent required in clinical research may not always be necessary or appropriate for evidence-based QI. Different approaches to consent may be more appropriate with different types of studies or projects and forms of data collection and analysis (Hansson, 2010). Before examining this more closely, the ethically relevant differences between research and QI will be reviewed.

DISTINGUISHING RESEARCH, EVIDENCE IMPLEMENTATION, AND QUALITY IMPROVEMENT

Research can be viewed as generating the evidence upon which practice should be based, that is, the *why* of practice. Rigorous methodology is key to the conduct of a research study. Evidence-based implementation projects use the EBP process to bring about change in practice to improve patient outcomes. Attending rigorously to the EBP process is imperative for an evidence implementation project to be successful and ethical. Poorly designed research and EBP projects will waste valuable resources (violating the principle of justice) and may lead to practice that is neither effective nor beneficent. Through the EBP process, clinicians find, evaluate, apply, and re-evaluate the impact of the evidence-based intervention on an outcome, that is, the *what* of practice. For clinicians to know if the processes they are employing are reliable for obtaining consistent outcomes, they use QI methods. Two terms must be mentioned when discussing EBQI: **quality assurance** and **audit**. Both the terms are designed to assess how well current practice compares with best practice (Casarett, Karlawish, & Sugarman, 2000). Quality assurance involves planned, systematic processes, which should have been established using evidence, that is, the *how* of practice. These processes are the core of QI and are designed to assure patients and providers that quality of care is addressed in a systematic and reliable manner. An audit evaluates whether or not current (or past) practice is based on the best available evidence. Different methods are also used within QI projects. EBQI includes a set of processes designed to align with the best available evidence; therefore in this chapter, audit and quality assurance will be subsumed under the term EBQI (Casarett et al., 2000).

Evidence implementation and EBQI involve methodologies that are also used in clinical research, which is why distinctions can be difficult. A spectrum of methods is involved in these approaches to problem solving. Randomized controlled trials are on the clinical research end of the spectrum. These require specific protection of study participants from harm due to unknown outcomes. Across the spectrum, practitioners may use similar data collection methods to evaluate outcomes before and after they introduce something new to their practice; this generates internal evidence. In this instance, there are no comparison or control groups or sample sizes. For example, consider a group of practitioners caring for some middle-aged male patients who are not taking their blood pressure medication consistently. When the practitioners review the patients' current (baseline) blood pressures (i.e., internal evidence), they realize that some intervention is necessary to improve this parameter. To make a practice change and improve the quality of care, they discuss what they would recommend and conduct a preliminary search for evidence regarding other interventions that may impact blood pressure in middle-aged males. In our example, let's say the clinicians find a well-done systematic review of the benefits of exercise on multiple outcomes, including blood pressure. They consider how to introduce the intervention so that everyone in the clinic is aware of the outcomes of their plan as well as how to achieve them. They offer the exercise intervention to all middle-aged male patients with elevated blood pressure, collect data on how the intervention was used by the men, and record their blood pressures to evaluate whether the intervention achieved the expected outcome. As the clinicians review the data, they note some positive changes. As a result, they talk about how well the evidence-based exercise intervention worked, what adjustments they need to make so that it might work better and how they can incorporate the intervention into their routine clinical discussions with patients. An EBQI activity like this would lead to higher quality of care for patients and produce evidence that this change led to better outcomes in practice.

Along this spectrum of EBQI and research are a range of activities. A practitioner might tell colleagues about an evidence-based change that improved care. They decide to introduce this change across the unit. Others hear about it and decide to evaluate the outcomes from units that applied the evidence and compare them to outcomes from other units that did not implement the change. Someone then suggests that the activities should be written up and submitted for publication. When considered from an ethical viewpoint, the question arises whether at some point the project has become one that should be submitted for ethical approval because patient information is being used in a way for which it was not originally collected. However, for EBQI and evidence implementation projects, ethical review could be useful to ensure patient information is managed appropriately, for example, that all appropriate steps were being taken to protect patient privacy. The question then arises about who should provide such ethical review, which is a matter we will consider later in the chapter.

EBQI and evidence implementation (the EBP process) meet only a portion of the U.S. regulatory definition of research as "a systematic investigation, including research development, testing and evaluation, designed to develop or contribute to generalizable knowledge" (Baily et al., 2006, p. S28). While EBQI and the EBP process are systematic and involve evaluation and testing, only research methods contribute to generalizable knowledge. Nevertheless, the methods of research, QI, and EBP can be similar, which triggers much of the ethical debate about these different approaches to problem solving. Bailey goes on to comment:

> QI uses the kind of reasoning that is inherent in the scientific method, it involves systematic investigations of working hypotheses about how a process might be improved, and it frequently employs qualitative and quantitative methods and analytic tools that are also used in research projects. (Baily et al., 2006, p. S11)

Since there are no established criteria for distinguishing these approaches unambiguously, people can review the same QI project and come to different conclusions as to whether or not it should be classified as research and fall under the ethical requirements of research studies. Two articles by research ethicists came to the opposite conclusions regarding whether the Michigan ICU study should have been regulated as clinical research and required to obtain informed consent. Miller and Emanuel (2008) held that the project was research because it prospectively implemented a protocol, tested hypotheses, and had a goal of contributing to generalizable knowledge (inferred only from its publication). However, Baily (2008) concluded that it was not clinical research because it was designed to promote clinicians' use of evidence-based procedures and placed patients at no additional risk than the original ethically reviewed studies.

Clear distinctions between research, EBQI, and the EBP process are sometimes difficult to determine. However, there are differences, and some of them are ethically significant, particularly regarding informed consent. When examining a study or project, these factors must be taken into account in determining what ethical issues may arise and how they should be addressed. From an ethical perspective, classifying a study or project as research, QI, or EBP is not the most important factor, as this can lead to an overly simplistic approach to ethics. The OHPR criticized Johns Hopkins University for its general conclusion that all EBQI or EBP projects were not clinical research and were therefore exempt from review (OHRP, 2007). Instead, OHRP held that each project needed to be evaluated individually as to whether or not it warranted exemption. Several ethical issues must be addressed no matter how a project or study is classified. Overall, protecting and promoting the well-being of everyone involved (beneficence and nonmaleficence) in a project or a study, including how their patient data are protected (privacy and confidentiality), should be paramount. This suggests that some ethical evaluation of EBQI and EBP projects is important.

Research is focused on questions for which answers are not known. When we don't know whether intervention A is better than intervention B, research in the form of a randomized controlled trial may be conducted. When we don't know how diet influences the risk of cancer, epidemiological research is conducted. When we don't know how patients experience and cope with a disability, qualitative research is carried out. Research is focused on *generating* evidence *for* practice, EBP is focused on *implementing* evidence *in* practice, and EBQI is focused on *evaluating* how well practice is working. Activities should be regarded as EBP when clinicians take a body of established evidence and use this to improve outcomes. In this way, the EBP process falls within good clinical management (Figure 22.1). Both EBP and EBQI seek to promote use of the best available evidence with the best processes so that practice outcomes are improved.

Research is not an integral part of routine clinical practice. In evidence-based care, clinical practice relies on knowledge generated by research to provide best care; however, patients do not need to be involved in research projects to receive quality clinical care. Research may occur in clinical settings, but if so, patients should only be enrolled if they volunteer for research. "In contrast, QI is *an integral part of the ongoing management of the system for delivering clinical care*, not an independent, knowledge-seeking enterprise" (Baily et al., 2006, p. S12). EBP is integral to the ongoing improvement (versus management) of quality care. This distinction among research, EBP, and EBQI is crucial and will be discussed in more detail later in the chapter.

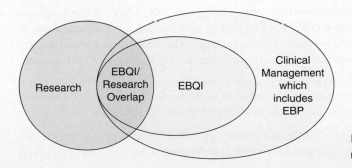

Figure 22.1: Distinguishing between research and EBQI projects.

Research often carries risks for patient safety, which is one of the reasons for informed consent. Research on interventions involving risk is justified when researchers do not know which alternative is best. The risks may be side effects, known or unknown. The risks may be that a patient receives an intervention that turns out to be less effective. Because research is pursuing knowledge that is not known, risks are inherent. The risks with EBP, since it is based on previously reviewed research, are primarily in the area of patient information. EBQI activities are also usually associated with very low risks, such as revealing personal information in questionnaires or interviews. As patient information is collected for evaluation, privacy and confidentiality must be protected. Some EBQI activities may carry some risk of harm because there is insufficient external evidence to guide the project and internal evidence becomes paramount, which must be evaluated when designing the project. However, sometimes the risks may be greater if the EBQI activities are *not* implemented and the old way of doing things remains in place or important outcomes are never reviewed (Hansson, 2010).

Researchers conducting studies are often not part of the clinical team caring for patients, whereas EBP and EBQI are almost always carried out by clinicians involved in caring for patients in the project. This supports the notion that EBP and EBQI are part of routine clinical practice and can foster a culture of continual improvement toward the highest quality care and outcomes. Another distinction between EBP, EBQI, and research is that the former two often use data that practitioners have regular access to in their clinical roles, whereas research data are usually distinct from clinical care and generated primarily for the study.

Funding for research is often generated externally, while EBP and EBQI projects are usually conducted using the resources available to the clinical team. External funding can generate conflicts of interest for researchers. The research study itself may put researchers' interests at odds with those of the participants (the patients), which is one reason for IRB review. In contrast, EBP and EBQI projects, by their nature, are intended to improve the quality of care the patients receive.

Research, EBP, and EBQI have been distinguished on the basis of generalizability, but this may not be as clear-cut as desired. One perspective is that the goal of publication is an indicator of generalizability, but that is not necessarily the case. EBP and EBQI projects, just as case reports, are helpful to clinicians. As discussed in Chapter 5, case reports should not be considered generalizable information, but they remain valuable to practitioners. Case reports, and case series, describe clinical practice in a systematic way, yet they are reports of clinical practice, not research. They reflect on what has happened in clinical practice and help others to learn from those experiences.

In the same way, publication of EBP and EBQI projects provide opportunities for others to learn from those experiences. A desire to share the findings of these projects should be seen as part of the ethical commitment to help others improve patient outcomes, either by introducing the same evidence-based changes or by avoiding them if they turn out to be unhelpful. Publication of the results of these projects should not change the nature of the original EBP or EBQI activities. However, the context-dependent nature of these projects must be taken into account if others choose to consider implementing these processes elsewhere.

In research, publication is usually envisioned as one of the outcomes expected, if not required, for the project to be successful. For EBP and EBQI, this is not always the case, and publication is unlikely to be a strong motivation for the project. In some cases publication may be preplanned, but in others, "it is more likely that a successful project will prompt its instigators to tell others what they have done, [and] that there will be a retrospective decision to seek publication" (Hill & Small, 2006, p. 103). Though not a major motivator for an EBP or EBQI project, the final step in the EBP process is the dissemination of results, which can be viewed as an ethical obligation no matter what the results are.

Overall, clinicians must carefully consider whether a project is best classified as clinical research, EBP, or EBQI. Figure 22.1 is an adaptation of a diagram used to represent the distinctions (Baily et al., 2006). This also offers the opportunity for some studies to be classified as overlapping research and EBQI. For example, a systematic QI investigation designed to bring about local clinical improvements may also develop generalizable knowledge as part of the evolution of the work (Baily et al., 2006). The Michigan ICU study and the Spanish sepsis project could be placed in this overlapping region, while the preeclampsia study was originally intended to be generalizable given its multicenter, international design.

This serves to highlight that the important factor for ethical review is not how a project or study is classified, but whether the activity is ethically appropriate. EBP does not fall into this overlapping region as the basis for all EBP projects is an already ethically reviewed body of evidence that has been deemed safe for patients; however, the ethical responsibility to protect patient information still remains.

ETHICAL PRINCIPLES AS APPLIED TO RESEARCH, EBP, AND EBQI

Much has been written on research ethics (Emanuel et al., 2008). A set of seven ethical requirements have been proposed as the ethical foundations upon which clinical research should be based (Emanuel, Wendler, & Grady, 2000):

1. Social or scientific value
2. Scientific validity
3. Fair subject selection
4. Favorable risk–benefit ratio
5. Independent review
6. Respect for potential and enrolled subjects
7. Informed consent

They are summarized in the following sections as originally proposed for clinical research, and their relevance for EBQI activities is also described, where appropriate (Baily et al., 2006). All the seven principles are ethically important and are not listed in any order of priority.

Social or Scientific Value

For research to be ethical, it should be worth doing. Appropriate use of resources is an ethical issue because of the principle of justice. Further research on questions that have been adequately answered by prior studies is ethically questionable. Exposing human subjects to any level of risk is unethical if the research does not have value to society or health care. This also places an ethical obligation on researchers to share their results and findings with others so that they can benefit from the new knowledge.

Similarly, EBP and EBQI activities are only ethical if they are worth doing. The value of the activity may initially be very local. Practitioners should identify significant clinical outcomes that could benefit from improvements. The value of different proposed activities may need to be compared to determine which have the potential to improve care the most, which is the essence of EBP. After conducting a local project or study, its wider value may be noted. For example, the results of the Michigan ICU study were extremely valuable worldwide, and it would have been unethical not to disseminate them broadly.

Scientific Validity

To be ethical, a research project must be methodologically rigorous to ensure a well-done study that can produce generalizable, valid findings. In addition, nonadherence to the EBP process or various processes of QI can result in poorly designed or implemented projects that waste resources and the time of those involved. The goal of EBQI is usually local improvement, not generalizable knowledge, so different methods may be used, but they should still be rigorously applied. Context and local factors are embedded in EBP and EBQI, while they are usually minimized in research by its methodological rigor. Nevertheless, exposing people to any risk in a flawed study or project is unethical.

Fair Subject Selection

The selection of subjects for research studies should be fair so that risks and benefits are shared equally. Inclusion and exclusion criteria for recruiting study participants should be based on good scientific reasons, not convenience or vulnerability. People should not be selected *because* they are marginalized, powerless, or poor. Such groups may become human subjects or participants, but only if the research is relevant to people in those groups. Those groups that bear the risks and burdens of research should have the potential to benefit from the results.

The same criteria should apply in EBP and EBQI activities. Those involved in an EBP or EBQI project should be determined more by where the project is conducted and a population of patients than recruitment techniques aimed at representative sampling. If resources prevent improving care in all areas, decisions about where to focus should be made fairly and not based on people's status or other irrelevant factors. EBP and EBQI should be present across health care, including clinics or services that serve the underprivileged. Funding for services for the underprivileged should include resources for EBP and EBQI, just as they should for fee-paying or profitable services.

Favorable Risk–Benefit Ratio

Both research and EBQI should be committed to minimizing the risks and maximizing the gains of all studies and projects. Risks in research can range from very high to none, while risks in EBQI are usually low. Risks may be physical but can also include risks to privacy and respect. Wherever possible, the risk–benefit ratio should be improved as much as possible. This way both beneficence and nonmaleficence are promoted. With EBP, risks are known because of the body of evidence that guides practice and defines expected outcomes. No new risks should be associated with EBP when the fidelity (how the evidence is implemented) is high.

Independent Review

Independent review of research is ethically required because of the potential conflicts of interest. Research subjects are inherently used as means to a goal of securing new knowledge. They may be placed at risk of harm for the good of others. In clinical contexts, the potential exists to exploit patients as research subjects because what is best for the research project may not be what is best for patients.

Different views exist on the nature of the review that EBP and EBQI activities ethically require. The author's view is that different types of ethical review are best for different types of EBP and EBQI activities. The reasons for this will be developed in the following sections and will be brought together in the chapter's conclusion.

Respect for Potential and Enrolled Subjects

Research has scientific goals, with respect for the participants involved in the research remaining paramount. As the Declaration of Helsinki states, "In medical research involving human subjects [participants], the well-being of the individual research subject must take precedence over all other interests" (World Medical Association, 2008). This respect applies to those who are asked to participate in the research and decide not to do so. It includes protecting privacy and confidentiality, maintaining participants' welfare during the project, keeping them informed of significant changes during the research, and allowing them to withdraw from research.

In EBP and EBQI activities, respect for patients must also take precedence. Improving their outcomes is the goal of EBQI and inherent to the nature of the activities. As with research, it includes protecting privacy and confidentiality, maintaining welfare, and keeping patients informed. However, the issue of withdrawing from EBQI (i.e., initiatives designed to produce known improvement in outcomes) is tied up with informed consent and its appropriateness to EBQI is discussed later in this chapter. The focus of EBP is best care for patients to achieve best outcomes. It does not seem logical or ethical to exclude patients from these projects or to allow them to remove themselves. However, refusal of treatment is always a right of patients and should be respected in these EBP projects as well.

Informed Consent

Informed consent is one of the bedrocks of clinical ethics and research ethics. Participating in research is viewed as voluntary, and this places an ethical obligation on researchers to provide information so that people can make informed decisions to enroll or not. This requirement is based on the importance of respecting an individual's autonomy over his or her body and health. Researchers must provide information regarding the risks and benefits of participation and help people understand this information. Informed consent is a process that often must be revisited as subjects engage in the research and understand its expectations and implications more fully.

The issue of informed consent for EBP and EBQI is one of the more widely debated ethical issues. Informed consent is not necessary for involvement in EBP as such projects fall within good clinical practice, are supported by a body of external evidence (i.e., research), and are covered by a patient's consent to clinical care. However, EBQI is driven usually by internal evidence and a small amount of external evidence, and therefore informed consent for EBQI will be examined in depth in the following section.

....

The bravest thing you can do when you are not brave is to profess courage and act accordingly.
—Corra Harris

....

INFORMED CONSENT AND EVIDENCE-BASED QUALITY IMPROVEMENT

One of the important issues debated within EBQI is whether informed consent is necessary. This was a central ethical issue in the two projects discussed in detail in this chapter. Part of the reason for informed consent is to protect patients, both from harm and from ways they might not be respected as persons. People who come to health services do not usually expect to become participants of research. Therefore, to respect them as individuals, they are offered the opportunity to participate or not in the research. If they agree, a *process* of informed consent will be initiated. From an ethical perspective, this process is not simply one of getting an informed consent form signed but an ongoing dialogue between researcher and participant about the research study.

Many activities happen when patients are within the health services. These activities are designed to restore or maintain optimal health for those patients. Patients enter the healthcare system trusting that clinicians are there to assist them toward health and minimize their risks while in their care. Therefore, obtaining informed consent for each individual action or intervention would not be practical. Collecting multiple informed consents likely would be unethical if this took away from the care patients received because so much time would be spent garnering informed consents. Consequently, separate informed consent is usually not expected when patients engage in what they might normally anticipate to be part of usual care. Furthermore, patients, whether in primary care or in acute care, sign a consent for treatment with the understanding that their best interest will be most important when decisions are made regarding what interventions are provided to them.

Debate over informed consent can be seen as a question of whether patients should expect EBQI and EBP to be seen as part of standard healthcare practice. Some argue that "much of QI is simply good clinical care combined with systematic, experiential learning. Individual practitioners are constantly learning by doing and taking steps to improve their own practice" (Baily et al., 2006, p. S8). The ethical commitment to care for and do good for patients (beneficence), coupled with an avoidance of harm (nonmaleficence), implies a commitment to improve clinical practice whenever possible. Taking steps to improve one's own practice includes evaluating whether or not improvement has occurred. This can be done through formal examinations, peer feedback, and other methods. A commitment to improve care more generally should similarly include steps to evaluate the quality of care (i.e., outcomes) in formal and informal ways. EBQI and EBP play a role in this, and as such, professionals and organizations have an ethical responsibility to conduct these types of projects to demonstrate whether or not change in process or implementation of evidence demonstrates sustainable improvement in outcomes.

This understanding of EBQI also places a responsibility on patients to participate in such activities. In that case, informed consent would not be necessary. This can be seen as similar to the responsibilities of teachers and students. If teachers have a responsibility to evaluate and improve their teaching, feedback from students is vital. This could be viewed as a mutual ethical responsibility, so students should provide feedback in response to the teaching. Certainly, protections need to be put in place, such as ensuring that the feedback is anonymous so that students who point out problems need not fear reprisal. Since students benefit from improved teaching, students have a responsibility to provide accurate information that will contribute to improved learning, and therefore signed informed consent is not necessary. In fact, it may be counterproductive, as such forms may be the only items that identify which students provided feedback and which did not.

This understanding of health care (and education) may not sit well with the current emphasis on autonomy and individualism. Individual rights should be valued in health care, but sometimes individual autonomy is prioritized over all other ethical principles. A culture can exist in which patients see themselves primarily as customers, purchasing the services they desire. This can foster an environment in which patients feel little or no obligation to the service or system that provides their care. They may feel they are paying for a service and can go elsewhere if they are not satisfied.

An individualistic paradigm brings a significant loss of the sense of a social commitment to improve the healthcare services that will be available to everyone. Viewing health care as primarily a business can have this same effect. Customers rightly feel little sense of responsibility to improve the quality of a local hardware store or the goods they buy from the store. The market is supposed to take care of that. But health care is not the same type of commodity as hardware.

In addition, such individualism is not realistic in health care and does not produce quality care. Patients are part of a social network and benefit from the experiences of others who have participated in prior clinical research, EBP, and EBQI. What is needed is an appropriate balance between individual autonomy and group responsibility (Greaney, O'Mathúna, & Scott, 2012). Patients should be able to see with gratitude how others have contributed to the care and service they receive and be willing to become involved in helping improve healthcare outcomes. We can all do this by accepting responsibility to participate in EBP and EBQI activities and managing our own health to maximize limited resources. Such a sense of moral obligation to the quality of our healthcare services is vital if the outcomes are to improve. Paradoxically, a commitment by everyone to improve the health care available for everyone should mean that we will each individually receive higher quality health care when we need to avail of those services and resources.

Such a view of health care places ethical responsibilities on healthcare organizations, professionals, and patients to participate in improving the quality of healthcare processes as well as outcomes. Patients may be unaware of this responsibility. For a long time, patients were afforded little opportunity to give feedback to healthcare professionals. In some cases, such feedback was overlooked, and in some, the feedback was actively rejected. The necessity of improving health care means that the voices of patients must be heard. This also places an ethical responsibility on patients to engage with improvement processes. And it will require strategies to inform the general public that healthcare organizations are committed to improving outcomes through implementing evidence and that their help is needed to do so.

This means that someone seeking care from a healthcare organization cannot insist on the freedom to opt out completely from efforts to improve the quality of care in that organization without jeopardizing the very benefits he or she seeks. In fact, it is in the best interest of patients to cooperate with EBP and EBQI activities and even to seek out the healthcare organizations that are the most committed to improving processes and outcomes. As an ethical matter, the responsibility of patients to cooperate in healthcare improvement activities is justified by the benefits that each patient receives because of the cooperation of others in the collective enterprise (Baily et al., 2006).

REVIEWING RESEARCH, EBP, AND EBQI PROJECTS

Review of research studies by an IRB is imperative and safeguards people who are participating in research. Some ethical review activities involve an overlap between research and EBQI. These situations could continue to be sent to IRBs for review, but the IRB has an obligation to examine them with the distinctions between EBQI and research in mind. The majority of EBQI is low risk and could be reviewed within clinical management and supervision structures. This is based on the view that EBQI is part of normal healthcare activities and is thus "a systematic, data-guided form of the clinical and managerial innovation and adaptation that has always been an integral part of clinical and managerial practice" (Baily et al., 2006, p. S28). Also, EBP projects should be ethically reviewed to ensure that patient privacy is maintained.

Various practical structures could be put in place to facilitate an ethical review. In some cases, external review may be necessary, for example, when projects involve more risk or seem to become more like research. Clinicians and ethical review boards need flexibility and knowledge of the purpose of the project or study. One benefit of keeping the review in the clinical setting would be that it could contribute to fostering a culture of evidence implementation in practice. This may also prevent ethical review from being seen as unwelcome scrutiny, or a bureaucratic hurdle to be overcome. What is needed is

> *... a scrutiny process that can recognise when a light hand is needed. We have to be able to deconstruct projects, be they research audit or QI, such that appropriate scrutiny is imposed—to improve the proposed activities and to defend the interests of those subjected to them.* (Hill & Small, 2006, p. 105)

Bringing EBQI review into the normal routine of clinical management offers an opportunity to enhance quality, ethical care. It gives everyone the opportunity to become more familiar with the review of EBQI activities and how ethical standards can be upheld. This is also true for appropriate ethical review of EBP projects. These reviews require adequate knowledge and skills in critical appraisal and ethical reflection. Ethical reviews are also an opportunity to remind everyone of the importance of implementing evidence in practice, continual practice improvement, monitoring of change, and ethical practice. The idea of a one-size-fits-all ethical review does not apply to the current complex culture that incorporates EBP, EBQI, and generation of research.

EBP FAST FACTS

◆ Research is focused on *generating* evidence *for* practice, EBP is focused on *implementing* evidence *in* practice, and EBQI is focused on *evaluating* how well practice is working.

◆ EBP and EBQI can be ethically justified by the intent to benefit patients and use resources wisely.

◆ EBQI has some similarities with research and may have unknown risks and should therefore be ethically reviewed and implemented. It also differs from research, and this should be taken into account in ethical review.

◆ The key ethical principles of good research are applicable and important for EBQI.

◆ Ethical considerations that apply to EBP initiatives, such as protection of privacy, are important to address; however, other ethical safeguards designed for clinical research, such as individual informed consent, may not be feasible or appropriate for EBP implementation projects.

◆ What is most important is not how a study or project is classified, but whether the activity is ethically appropriate.

References

Abbasi, K., & Heath, I. (2005). Ethics review of research and audit. *BMJ, 330*, 431–432.

Baily, M. A. (2008). Harming through protection? *New England Journal of Medicine, 358*(8), 768–769.

Baily, M. A., Bottrell, M., Lynn, J., & Jennings, B. (2006). The ethics of using QI methods to improve health care quality and safety. *Hastings Center Report, 36*(4), S1–S408.

Beauchamp, T. L., & Childress, J. F. (2012). *Principles of biomedical ethics* (7th ed.). New York: Oxford University Press.

Casarett, D., Karlawish, J. H. T., & Sugarman, J. (2000). Determining when quality improvement initiatives should be considered research: Proposed criteria and potential implications. *Journal of the American Medical Association, 283*(17), 2275–2280.

Daley, M. R. (2007). Catheter-related bloodstream infections [letter]. *New England Journal of Medicine, 356*(12), 1267–1268.

Emanuel, E. J., Grady, C., Crouch, R. A., Lie, R., Miller, F., & Wendler, D. (Eds.). (2008). *The Oxford textbook of clinical research ethics.* New York: Oxford University Press.

Emanuel, E. J., Wendler, D., & Grady, C. (2000). What makes clinical research ethical? *Journal of the American Medical Association, 283*(20), 2701–2711.

Ferrer, R., Artigas, A., & Levy, M. (2008). Informed consent and studies of a quality improvement program [letter]. *Journal of the American Medical Association, 300*(15), 1762–1763.

Ferrer, R., Artigas, A., Levy, M. M., Blanco, J., González-Díaz, G., Garnacho-Montero, …de la Torre-Prados, M. V. (2008). Improvement in process of care and outcome after a multicenter severe sepsis educational program in Spain. *Journal of the American Medical Association, 299*(19), 2294–2303.

Firoz, T., Magee, L. A., Payne, B. A., Menzies, J. M., & von Dadelszen, P. (2012). The PIERS experience: Research or quality improvement? *Journal of Obstetrics and Gynaecology Canada, 34*(4), 379–381.

Gawande, A. (2007). A lifesaving checklist. *The New York Times.* Retrieved March 10, 2009, from http://www.nytimes.com/2007/12/30/opinion/30gawande.html

Greaney, A.-M., O'Mathúna, D. P., & Scott, P. A. (2012). Autonomy and choice in healthcare: Self-testing devices as a case in point. *Medicine, Health Care and Philosophy, 15*(4), 383–395.

Hansson, M. (2010). Do we need a wider view of autonomy in epidemiological research? *BMJ, 340,* 1172–1174.

Hill, S. L., & Small, N. (2006). Differentiating between research, audit and quality improvement: Governance implications. *Clinical Governance: An International Journal, 11*(2), 98–107.

Institute of Medicine. (2006). *Preventing medication errors.* Washington, DC: National Academy Press.

Institute of Medicine. (2009). *Crossing the quality chasm: The IOM health care quality initiative.* Retrieved March 10, 2009, from http://www.iom.edu/CMS/8089.aspx

Jenny-Avital, E. R. (2007). Catheter-related bloodstream infections [letter]. *New England Journal of Medicine, 356*(12), 1267.

Kahn, J. M., & Bates, D. W. (2008). Improving sepsis care: The road ahead. *Journal of the American Medical Association, 299*(19), 2322–2323.

Kim, J. S., Holtom, P., & Vigen, C. (2011). Reduction of catheter-related bloodstream infections through the use of a central venous line bundle: Epidemiologic and economic consequences. *American Journal of Infection Control, 39*(8), 640–646.

Korenstein, D., Falk, R., Howell, E. A., Bishop, T., & Keyhani, S. (2012). Overuse of health care services in the United States: An understudied problem. *Archives of Internal Medicine, 172*(2), 171–178.

Lemaire, F. (2008). Informed consent and studies of a quality improvement program [letter]. *Journal of the American Medical Association, 300*(15), 1762.

Lemaire, F., Ravoire, S., & Golinelli, D. (2008). Non-interventional research and usual care: Definition, regulatory aspects, difficulties and recommendations. *Thérapie, 63*(2), 103–106.

Lynn, J., Baily, M. A., Bottrell, M., Jennings, B., Levine, R. J., Davidoff, F., … James, B. (2007). The ethics of using quality improvement methods in health care. *Annals of Internal Medicine, 146*(9), 666–673.

Miller, D. L., & O'Grady, N. P. (2012). Guidelines for the prevention of intravascular catheter-related infections: Recommendations relevant to interventional radiology for venous catheter placement and maintenance. *Journal of Vascular and Interventional Radiology, 23*(8), 997–1007.

Miller, F. G., & Emanuel, E. J. (2008). Quality-improvement research and informed consent. *New England Journal of Medicine, 358*(8), 765–767.

National Committee for Quality Assurance (NCQA). (2012). *The state of health care quality report 2012.* Retrieved July 1, 2013, from http://www.ncqa.org/ReportCards/HealthPlans/StateofHealthCareQuality.aspx

National Institutes of Health. (2005). *Glossary: Clinical research.* Retrieved May 8, 2009, from http://grants.nih.gov/grants/policy/hs/glossary.htm

Office for Human Research Protections. (2007). *RE: Human subject research protections under federalwide assurances FWA-5752, FWA-287, and FWA-3834.* Retrieved March 9, 2009, from http://www.hhs.gov/ohrp/detrm_letrs/YR07/nov07c.pdf

Office for Human Research Protections. (2008). *RE: Human subject research protections under federalwide assurances FWA-5752, FWA-287, and FWA-3834.* Retrieved March 2, 2009, from http://www.hhs.gov/ohrp/detrm_letrs/YR08/feb08b.pdf

O'Mathúna, D. P. (2007). Decision-making and health research: Ethics and the 10/90 gap. *Research Practitioner, 8*(5), 164–172.

Pronovost, P., Needham, D., Berenholtz, S., Sinopoli, D., Chu, H., Cosgrove, S., … Goeschel, C. (2006). An intervention to decrease catheter-related bloodstream infections in the ICU. *New England Journal of Medicine, 355*(26), 2725–2732.

Schoen, C., Osborn, R., How, S. K. H., Doty, M. M., & Peugh, J. (2009). In chronic condition: Experiences of patients with complex health care needs, in eight countries, 2008. *Health Affairs, 28*(1), w1–w16.

Schoen, C., Osborn, R., Squires D., Doty, M., Rasmussen, P., Pierson, R., & Applebaum, S. (2012). A survey of primary care doctors in ten countries shows progress in use of health information technology, less in other areas. *Health Affairs, 31*(12), 2805–2816.

United Nations Educational, Scientific and Cultural Organization. (2008). *Bioethics core curriculum.* Paris: United Nations Educational, Scientific and Cultural Organization. Retrieved May 8, 2009, from http://unesdoc.unesco.org/images/0016/001636/163613E.pdf

Upshur, R. E. G. (2013). A call to integrate ethics and evidence-based medicine. *Virtual Mentor, 15*(1), 86–89.

World Medical Association. (2008). *Declaration of Helsinki.* Retrieved March 14, 2009, from http://www.wma.net/e/policy/b3.htm

Making EBP Real: Selected Excerpts from a Funded Grant Application

COPE/Healthy Lifestyles for Teens: A School-Based RCT

Bernadette Mazurek Melnyk, Principal Investigator

Co-Investigators: Diana Jacobson, Stephanie Kelly, Michael Belyea, Gabriel Shaibi, Leigh Small, and Flavio Marsiglia

Funded by the NIH/National Institute of Nursing Research (#1RO1NRO12171)

Specific Aims

The prevention and treatment of overweight/obesity and mental health disorders in adolescence are two major public health problems in the United States today [11, 12]. The incidence of adolescents who are overweight or obese has increased dramatically over the past 20 years, with approximately 17.1% of teens now being overweight (i.e., a gender- and age-specific body mass index [BMI] at or above the 85th percentile) or obese, which is defined as a gender- and age-specific body mass index at or above the 95th percentile [13, 14]. Furthermore, approximately 15 million children and adolescents in the United States have a mental health problem that is interfering with their functioning at home or at school, but less than 25% receive treatment for these disorders [21, 25]. Depression among adolescents is associated with disabling morbidity, significant mortality, and substantial healthcare costs [26, 27]. The prevalence rates of obesity and mental health problems are even higher in Hispanic teens, with the two conditions often coexisting [13, 32–35].

Despite the rapidly increasing incidence and adverse health outcomes associated with both overweight and mental health problems, very few theory-based intervention studies have been conducted with adolescents to improve both their healthy lifestyle behaviors and mental health outcomes [36]. Unfortunately, physical and mental health services continue to be largely separated instead of integrated in the nation's healthcare system, which often leads to inadequate identification and treatment of these significant adolescent health problems. Furthermore, most obesity treatment and prevention trials have focused on school-age children [37–45].

Findings from our recent pilot studies of the feasibility and efficacy of the COPE/Healthy Lifestyles TEEN Program, a theory-driven, cognitive behavioral skills building (CBSB) healthy lifestyles intervention program, with overweight and normal weight culturally diverse adolescents have indicated promising short-term positive physical and mental health outcomes (e.g., an increase in healthy lifestyle behaviors, decrease in weight, decrease in depressive symptoms) (see preliminary studies). Therefore, the primary goal of the proposed study is to test the short-term and more long-term efficacy of the COPE/Healthy Lifestyles TEEN Program on the healthy lifestyle behaviors and depressive symptoms of *800* culturally diverse teens enrolled in Phoenix, Arizona, high schools for the ultimate purpose of preventing overweight and mental health disorders.

Specific Aim 1

Use a randomized controlled trial (RCT) to test the short-term and more long-term efficacy of the COPE/Healthy Lifestyles TEEN Program to improve healthy lifestyle behaviors and depressive symptoms of 14- to 16-year-old culturally diverse adolescents enrolled in Phoenix, Arizona, high schools.

◆ **Hypotheses 1a** *(primary outcomes)*. Immediately following the COPE program and at 6 and 12 months postintervention, teens who receive the COPE program versus teens who receive an attention control program (i.e., Healthy Teens) will report:

◆ more healthy lifestyle behaviors
◆ less depressive symptoms

◆ **Hypothesis 1b** *(subgroup analysis: secondary outcome)*. Immediately following the COPE program and at 6 and 12 months postintervention, among teens with elevated depressive symptoms at baseline, those who receive the COPE program versus teens who receive the attention control program will have less depressive symptoms.

◆ **Hypotheses 1c** *(subgroup analysis: secondary outcome)*. Immediately following the intervention and at 6 and 12 months postintervention, overweight teens at baseline who receive the COPE program versus teens who receive an attention control program will have less weight gain.

◆ **Hypothesis 1d** *(subgroup analysis: secondary outcome)*. Fewer normal weight teens in COPE versus the attention control program will convert to *overweight* at 6 and 12 months postintervention.

Specific Aim 2

Examine the role of cognitive beliefs and perceived difficulty in leading a healthy lifestyle in mediating the effects of the COPE program on healthy lifestyle behaviors and depressive symptoms in 14- to 16-year-old adolescents.

◆ **Hypothesis 2** *(theory building exploratory)*. The effects of the COPE program on the teens' healthy lifestyle behaviors and depressive symptoms will be mediated by their beliefs about their ability to make healthy lifestyles choices and perceived difficulty in leading a healthy lifestyle.

Specific Aim 3

Explore variables that may moderate the effects of the intervention on healthy lifestyle behaviors and depressive/anxiety symptoms (e.g., race/ethnicity, gender, SES, family composition, acculturation, structural barriers to activity, and parental healthy lifestyle beliefs and behaviors).

Background and Significance

The prevalence of unhealthy lifestyle behaviors leading to overweight and obesity as well as mental health problems in adolescents continues to be significant public health concerns. Data from the National Health and Nutrition Examination Survey (NHANES) from 2003 to 2004 indicate that, in all youth aged 12 to 19 years, 34.3% had a BMI percentile greater than or equal to the gender- and age-adjusted 85th percentile (overweight). For all adolescents, the prevalence of obesity (>95th percentile) was 17.4. Mental health/psychosocial problems, risk-taking behaviors, and injuries, many of which are preventable, currently cause more morbidity and mortality in the pediatric and adolescent population than do physical diseases and disorders [30]. Children and adolescents who are affected by depression often have lower self-esteem, underdeveloped social skills, and poor academic functioning [30]. Depression in adolescents also has been associated with risk-taking behaviors, such as alcohol and drug use, cutting behaviors, and high-risk sexual behaviors. Unfortunately, childhood and adolescent mental health is often underestimated as the foundation for adult health. Less than 25% of teens with a significant mental health disorder are seen by an appropriate mental health service provider [30, 60]. As most of the major mental health disorders begin in adolescence, intensified efforts must be placed on preventing and treating these disorders during this critical time in development [12].

Theoretical Framework for the Proposed Study

Driven by cognitive behavior theory (CBT), the COPE/Healthy Lifestyles TEEN Program is a series of 15 educational and CBSB sessions that focuses on empowering teens to engage in healthy lifestyle behaviors (i.e., nutrition, physical activity, positive strategies to cope with stress, problem-solving, regulation of negative mood, and goal setting). It is designed to be easily integrated into high-school health education classes. Based on cognitive theory, we teach the teens how to cognitively restructure their thinking when negative events/interpersonal situations arise that tend to lead them into negative thought patterns and how to turn that thinking into a more positive interpretation of the situation/interpersonal interaction so that they will emotionally feel better and behave in more healthy ways. Emphasis is placed on how patterns of thinking have an impact on behavior and emotions (i.e., the thinking, feeling, and behaving triangle). The program also includes educational content to increase teens' knowledge of how to lead a healthy lifestyle and homework activities to reinforce skills that are being learned in the classroom, *which assists them with putting into daily practice what they are learning in the educational sessions*. Brief bouts of physical activity (i.e., 15 to 20 minutes) also are incorporated into each of the 16 sessions to assist the teens in raising their beliefs/confidence in their ability to develop regular activity patterns (see the COPE Conceptual Model.)

Conclusion, Significance, and Innovation of the Proposed Study

School is an ideal environment in which to test innovative interventions designed to increase healthy lifestyle behaviors and ultimately prevent or treat overweight/obesity as well as to enhance the highest level of mental health outcomes in adolescents. Preventive interventions that are

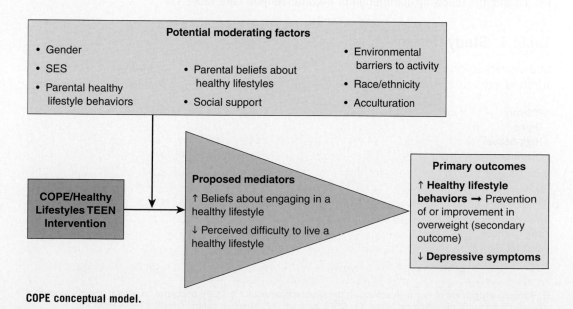

COPE conceptual model.

implemented in schools need to be reproducible, teacher-friendly, and inexpensive to implement. There is some evidence indicating that healthy lifestyle interventions that incorporate education, physical activity, and behavior modification may be the most promising strategies for preventing and treating overweight and obesity in teens; however, more long-term efficacy of these interventions is unknown [140]. Furthermore, the processes through which these interventions work are not known and moderating variables that could shed light upon under which circumstances or for whom the interventions work best have not been studied. Use of CBSB is a novel conceptual approach to targeting two of the most pressing public health problems in teens. Another innovative aspect of our proposed study is that we have powered it so that we have a large enough sample to study subgroups of the teens (i.e., those who are already overweight; those who are mildly to moderately depressed) where the effects of COPE may have the greatest impact.

Research Design and Methods

Overview of Design

This study is a prospective, blinded, randomized controlled test of the efficacy of the COPE/Healthy Lifestyles TEEN Program and the mediational roles of cognitive beliefs and perceived difficulty in leading a healthy lifestyle in improving the healthy lifestyle behaviors and depressive symptoms of culturally diverse adolescents in high school. Participants ($N = 800$) will be recruited from teens, aged 14 to 16 years, who are freshmen and sophomores enrolled in health education courses at eight high schools in Phoenix, Arizona (i.e., four high schools in the Phoenix Union School District and four high schools in the Paradise Valley School District). Two of the four schools within each of the two school districts will be randomly assigned by a random number generator to receive either the COPE/Healthy Lifestyles TEEN Program or the Healthy Teens Program. All teens in the health education courses in the *eight* high schools will be invited to participate in the study. The teens in the health education courses will receive either: (1) an 8-week, 15-session (i.e., an average of two sessions per week) multicomponent educational and CBSB program with physical activity (i.e., COPE/Healthy Lifestyles), or (2) an 8-week, 15-session attention control program (Healthy Teens). In addition to baseline assessments, outcomes will be measured at three time points: (1) immediately following completion of the 8-week intervention, (2) 6 months following completion of the intervention, and (3) 12 months following completion of the intervention (see Table 1).

Table 1 **Study Design**

		Baseline	Intervention	Postintervention	6-Month Follow-Up	12-Month Follow-Up
Phoenix Union High-School District	R	O1	X1	O2	O3	O4
	R	O1	X2	O2	O3	O4
Paradise Valley High-School District	R	O1	X1	O2	O3	O4
	R	O1	X2	O2	O3	O4

R, Random assignment of four high schools in the same school district to COPE or control for a *total of eight randomly assigned schools*; O, measurement times; X1, COPE program; X2, attention control (Healthy Teens Program).

Rationale for Three Follow-Up Assessments (Postintervention, 6 Months, 12 Months) Follow-up at three times is important to determine whether the effects of COPE can be sustained over time and to determine the appropriate timing of booster interventions if needed for future studies.

Intervention Conditions (Independent Variable)

COPE/Healthy Lifestyles TEEN Program COPE is a manualized 15-session educational and cognitive behavioral skills building program guided by CBT with physical activity as a component of each session (see Appendix B). It was first developed by the primary investigator (PI) in 2002 and has been pilot tested three times with White, Hispanic, and African-American adolescents as a group intervention in high-school settings and once with 18- and 19-year-old college freshmen.

Each session of COPE contains 15 to 20 minutes of physical activity (e.g., walking, dancing), not as an exercise training program, but rather to build beliefs/confidence in the teens that they can engage in and sustain some level of physical activity on a regular basis. Those healthy lifestyle intervention programs that have employed exercise interventions only have not led to sustained changes in healthy lifestyle behaviors. Our program is designed to enhance healthy lifestyle behaviors and sustain them because lifelong cognitive behavioral skills are taught in the program. Because the COPE/Healthy Lifestyles TEEN Program is completely manualized for the teens and instructors, it can be easily implemented by health teachers in high-school settings. COPE sessions are detailed in Table 2.

Rationale for the Healthy Teens Attention Control Program An attention control program that controls for the time spent with the adolescents in the COPE group is essential to determining the efficacy of the experimental program. The Healthy Teens Program will assist in ruling out alternative explanations of the mechanism by which the intervention works. It will be standardized like the COPE program to ensure that it can be evaluated. It will be administered in a format like that of the COPE intervention program and will include the same number and length of sessions, except for that it will not include the theoretical active components of CBT and will not include theoretical mechanisms to produce our hypothesized changes in outcomes. Teens in the attention control group also will receive the sessions in their required health class. The difference between the two programs will lie in the content of the sessions, with the Healthy Teens Program being focused on safety and common health topics/issues for teens (e.g., road safety, skin care, acne, sun safety). Workbook activities and homework assignments will focus on the topics being covered in class as well.

Assessment of Fidelity of the Intervention Monitoring fidelity of the intervention program is essential to having greater confidence in the findings, being able to explain the results obtained, and in helping to ensure internal validity of the study

Measures

Rationale for the Study Instruments Instruments fall into four categories, including those administered: (1) to identify potential covariates/moderators, (2) to define outcomes, (3) to quantify proposed mediators, and (4) to evaluate the experimental process. Teens who participate in the program will complete outcome instruments on four occasions (Weeks 0, 9, 34, and 58). Outcome and mediator instruments were chosen because they measure key components of the theoretical framework on which the intervention is based. Process instruments will be used to inform the design of future research and dissemination studies.

Overview of Analysis Plan

Statistical analysis of data from this first full-scale test must serve several purposes beyond simply demonstrating the efficacy of COPE; for example, estimating effect sizes, mapping

Table 2 COPE/Healthy Lifestyles TEEN Program Content[a]

Session #	Session Content	Key Constructs From the Conceptual Model and COPE Intervention
1	Introduction of the COPE Healthy Lifestyles TEEN Program and goals.	
2	Healthy Lifestyles and the Thinking, Feeling, Behaving triangle.	Cognitive behavioral skills building (CBSB)
3	Self-esteem. Positive thinking/self-talk.	CBSB
4	Goal setting. Problem solving.	CBSB
5	Stress and Coping.	CBSB
6	Emotional and behavioral regulation.	CBSB
7	Effective communication. Personality and communication styles.	CBSB
8	Barriers to goal progression and overcoming barriers. Energy balance. Ways to increase physical activity and associated benefits.	CBSB and physical activity information
9	Heart rate. Stretching.	Physical activity information
10	Food groups and a healthy body. Stoplight diet: Red, yellow & green.	Nutrition information
11	Nutrients to build a healthy body. Reading labels. Effects of media and advertising on food choices.	Nutrition information
12	Portion sizes. "super size." Influence of feelings on eating.	Nutrition information
13	Social eating. Strategies for eating during parties, holidays, and vacations.	Nutrition information
14	Snacks. Eating out.	Nutrition information
15	Integration of knowledge and skills to develop a healthy lifestyle plan; Putting it all together	CBSB

[a]Fifteen to 20 minutes of physical activity also is a component of each COPE session to build beliefs/confidence in the teens that they can engage in and sustain some level of physical activity on a regular basis.

the trajectory of group differences over time, and identifying subgroup differences. Analysis will begin with careful characterization of the sample with descriptive statistics that identify (a) potential problems due to skewed sampling, (b) differences between intervention and control groups that are evident at baseline despite randomization, and (c) differences between groups that appear at follow-up due to differential attrition.

The second phase of the analysis will use linear hierarchical models (also referred to as random coefficient and mixed models) to explore the effect of the intervention over time because these models incorporate random effects to reflect the correlation among observations from members of the same group [163, 164].

The entire grant application may be accessed at http://thepoint.lww.com/Melnyk3e.

Appendix A
Templates for Asking Clinical Questions

INTERVENTION In _____ (P), how does _____ (I) compared to _____ (C) affect _____ (O) within _____ (T)?
ETIOLOGY Are _____ (P), who have _____ (I) compared with those without _____ (C) at _____ risk for/of _____ (O) over _____ (T)?
DIAGNOSIS OR DIAGNOSTIC TEST In _____ (P) are/is _____ (I) compared with _____ (C) more accurate in diagnosing _____ (O)?
PROGNOSIS/PREDICTION In _____ (P), how does _____ (I) compared to _____ (C) influence _____ (O) over _____ (T)?
MEANING How do _____ (P) with _____ (I) perceive _____ (O) during _____ (T)?

SHORT DEFINITIONS OF DIFFERENT TYPES OF QUESTIONS

Intervention: Questions addressing the treatment of an illness or disability.
Etiology: Questions addressing the causes or origin of disease, the factors that produce or predispose toward a certain disease or disorder.
Diagnosis: Questions addressing the act or process of identifying or determining the nature and cause of a disease or injury through evaluation.
Prognosis/Prediction: Questions addressing the prediction of the course of a disease.
Meaning: Questions addressing how one experiences a phenomenon.

SAMPLE QUESTIONS

Intervention: In African American female adolescents with hepatitis B (P), how does acetaminophen (I) compared to ibuprofen (C) affect liver function (O)?
Etiology: Are 30- to 50-year-old women (P) who have high blood pressure (I) compared with those without high blood pressure (C) at increased risk for an acute myocardial infarction (O) during the first year after hysterectomy (T)?
Diagnosis: In middle-aged men with suspected myocardial infarction (P), are serial 12-lead ECGs (I) compared with one initial 12-lead ECG (C) more accurate in diagnosing an acute myocardial infarction (O)?

Prognosis/Prediction: (1) For patients 65 years and older (P), how does the use of an influenza vaccine (I) compared to not received the vaccine (C) influence the risk of developing pneumonia (O) during flu season (T)?

(2) In patients who have experienced an acute myocardial infarction (P), how does being a smoker (I) compared to a nonsmoker (C) influence death and infarction rates (O) during the first 5 years after the myocardial infarction (T)?

Meaning: How do 20-something men (P) with a diagnosis of below the waist paralysis (I) perceive their interactions with their romantic significant others (O) during the first year after their diagnosis (T)?

Appendix B
Rapid Critical Appraisal Checklists

General Appraisal Overview for All Studies

Date: Reviewer(s) Name(s):

Article Citation (APA):

PICOT Question:

General Description of Study

Overview of Study
◆ **Purpose of study:**

◆ **Study design:**

◆ **Research question(s) or hypotheses:**

◆ **Study aims:**

◆ **Sampling technique, sample size, and characteristics:**

◆ **Major variables studies:**
  ● **Independent variable:**
  ● **Dependent (outcome) variable(s):**

◆ **Statistical analysis (include whether appropriate to answer research questions/hypothesis):**

RAPID CRITICAL APPRAISAL CHECKLIST FOR DESCRIPTIVE STUDIES

VALIDITY

Are the results of the study valid?

◆ Were study/survey methods appropriate for the question?	Yes	No
◆ Was sampling methods appropriate for the research question?	Yes	No
◆ Was sample size implications on study results discussed?	Yes	No
◆ Were variables studied appropriate for the question?	Yes	No

- Dependent variables are:
- Independent (outcome) variables are:

◆ Were outcomes appropriate for the question?	Yes	No
◆ Were valid and reliable instruments used to measure outcomes?	Yes	No
◆ Were the chosen measures appropriate for study outcomes?	Yes	No
◆ Were outcomes clearly described?	Yes	No
◆ Did investigators and/or funding agencies declare freedom from conflict of interest?	Yes	No

RELIABILITY

What are the results?

- ◆ What were the main results of the study?
  - Was there statistical significance? Explain.
  - Was there clinical significance? Explain.

◆ Were safety concerns including adverse events and risk/benefit described?	Yes	No

APPLICABILITY

Will the results help me in caring for my patients?

◆ Are the results applicable to my patient population?	Yes	No
◆ Will my patients' and families' values and beliefs be supported by the knowledge gained from the study?	Yes	No

Reflection prompts: Would you use the study results in your practice to make a difference in patient outcomes?

- ◆ If yes, how?
- ◆ If yes, why?
- ◆ If no, why not?

Additional comments/reflections:

Recommendation for article use within a body of evidence:

RAPID CRITICAL APPRAISAL OF EVIDENCE-BASED PRACTICE (EBP) IMPLEMENTATION OR QUALITY IMPROVEMENT (QI) PROJECTS

Indicate the extent to which the item is met in the published report of the EBP or QI project.

Validity of Evidence Synthesis (i.e., good methodology)	1 No	2 A Little	3 Somewhat	4 Quite a Bit	5 Very Much
1. The title of the publication identifies the report/project as an EBP implementation or QI project					
2. The project report provides a structured summary that includes, as applicable: data to establish the existent and background of the clinical issue, inclusion and exclusion criteria, and source(s) of evidence, evidence synthesis, objective(s) and setting of the EBP or QI project, project limitations, results/outcomes, recommendations and implications for policy					
3. Report includes existing internal evidence to adequately describe the clinical issue					
4. Provides an explicit statement of the question being addressed with reference to participants or population/intervention/comparison/outcome (PICO)					
5. Explicitly describes the search method, inclusion and exclusion criteria, and rationale for search strategy limits					
6. Describes multiple information sources (e.g., databases, contact with study authors to identify additional studies, or any other additional search strategies) included in the search strategy and date					
7. States the process for title, abstract, and article screening for selecting studies					
8. Describes the method of data extraction (e.g., independently or process for validating data from multiple reviewers)					
9. Includes conceptual and operational definitions for all variables for which data were abstracted (e.g., define blood pressure as systolic blood pressure, diastolic blood pressure, ambulatory blood pressure, automatic cuff blood pressure, or arterial blood pressure)					

10. Describes methods used for assessing risk of bias of individual studies (including specification of whether this was done at the study or outcome level)

11. States the principal summary measures (e.g., risk ratio, difference in means)

12. Describes the method of combining results of studies including quality, quantity, and consistency of evidence

13. Specifies assessment of risk of bias that may affect the cumulative evidence (e.g., publication bias, selective reporting within studies)

14. Describes appraisal procedure and conflict resolution

15. Provides number of studies screened, assessed for eligibility, and included in the review, with reasons for exclusion at each stage, ideally with a flow diagram

16. For each study, presents characteristics for which data were extracted (e.g., study size, design, method, follow-up period) and provides citations

17. Presents data on risk of bias of each study and, if available, any outcome-level assessment

18. For all outcomes considered (benefit or harms), includes a table with summary data for each intervention group, effect estimates, and confidence intervals, ideally with a forest plot

19. Summarizes the main findings including the strength of evidence for each main outcome; considering their relevance to key groups (i.e., healthcare providers, users, and policy makers)

20. Discusses limitations at study and outcome levels (e.g., risk of bias) and at review level (e.g., incomplete retrieval of identified research, reporting bias)

21. Provides a general interpretation of the results in the context of other evidence and implications for further research, practice, or policy changes

Validity of Implementation (i.e., well-done project)

1. Purpose of project flows from evidence synthesis

2. Stakeholders (active and passive) are identified and communication with them is described

3. Implementation protocol is congruent with evidence synthesis (fidelity of the intervention)

4. Implementation protocol is sufficiently detailed to provide for replication among project participants

5. Education of project participants and other stakeholders is clearly described

6. Outcomes are measured with measures supported in the evidence synthesis

Reliability of Implementation Project (i.e., I can learn from or implement project results)

1. Data are collected with sufficient rigor to be reliable for like groups to those participants of the project

2. Results of evidence implementation are clinically meaningful (statistics are interpreted as such)

Application of Implementation (i.e., this project is useful for my patients)

1. How feasible is the project protocol?

2. Have the project managers considered/included all outcomes that are important to my work?

3. Is implementing the project safe (i.e., low risk of harm)?

Summary Score

Recommendations with consideration of this type of level IV intervention evidence:
32–64: consider evidence with extreme caution
65–128: consider evidence with caution
128–160: consider evidence with confidence

© 2011 Fineout-Overholt. This form may be used for educational purposes without permission from the author. Other uses, please informe the author of your intent to use the form.

RAPID CRITICAL APPRAISAL QUESTIONS FOR COHORT STUDIES

1. Are the results of the study valid?

a. Was there a representative and well-defined sample of patients at a similar point in the course of the disease?	Yes	No	Unknown
b. Was follow-up sufficiently long and complete?	Yes	No	Unknown
c. Were objective and unbiased outcome criteria used?	Yes	No	Unknown
d. Did the analysis adjust for important prognostic risk factors and confounding variables?	Yes	No	Unknown

2. What are the results?

a. What is the magnitude of the relationship between predictors (i.e., prognostic indicators) and targeted outcome?	_____
b. How likely is the outcome event(s) in a specified period of time?	_____
c. How precise are the study estimates?	_____

3. Will the results help me in caring for my patients?

a. Were the study patients similar to my own?	Yes	No	Unknown
b. Will the results lead directly to selecting or avoiding therapy?	Yes	No	Unknown
c. Are the results useful for reassuring or counseling patients?	Yes	No	Unknown

RAPID CRITICAL APPRAISAL CHECKLIST FOR A RANDOMIZED CLINICAL TRIAL (RCT)

1. Are the results of the study valid?

a. Were the subjects randomly assigned to the experimental and control groups?	Yes	No	Unknown
b. Was random assignment concealed from the individuals who were first enrolling subjects into the study?	Yes	No	Unknown
c. Were the subjects and providers blind to the study group?	Yes	No	Unknown
d. Were reasons given to explain why subjects did not complete the study?	Yes	No	Unknown
e. Were the follow-up assessments conducted long enough to fully study the effects of the intervention?	Yes	No	Unknown
f. Were the subjects analyzed in the group to which they were randomly assigned?	Yes	No	Unknown
g. Was the control group appropriate?	Yes	No	Unknown
h. Were the instruments used to measure the outcomes valid and reliable?	Yes	No	Unknown
i. Were the subjects in each of the groups similar on demographic and baseline clinical variables?	Yes	No	Unknown

2. What are the results?

a. How large is the intervention or treatment effect (NNT, NNH, effect size, level of significance)?	_____
b. How precise is the intervention or treatment (CI)?	_____

3. Will the results help me in caring for my patients?

a. Were all clinically important outcomes measured?	Yes	No	Unknown
b. What are the risks and benefits of the treatment?	_____		
c. Is the treatment feasible in my clinical setting?	Yes	No	Unknown
d. What are my patient's/family's values and expectations for the outcome that is trying to be prevented and the treatment itself?	_____		

RAPID CRITICAL APPRAISAL OF SYSTEMATIC REVIEWS OF CLINICAL INTERVENTIONS/TREATMENTS

1. Are the results of the review valid?

a. Are the studies contained in the review randomized controlled trials?	Yes	No
b. Does the review include a detailed description of the search strategy to find all relevant studies?	Yes	No
c. Does the review describe how validity of the individual studies was assessed (e.g., methodological quality, including the use of random assignment to study groups and complete follow-up of the subjects)?	Yes	No
d. Were the results consistent across studies?	Yes	No
e. Were individual patient data or aggregate data used in the analysis?	Individual	Aggregate

2. What were the results?

a. How large is the intervention or treatment effect (OR, RR, effect size, level of significance)?	_____
b. How precise is the intervention or treatment (CI)?	_____

3. Will the results assist me in caring for my patients?

a. Are my patients similar to the ones included in the review?	Yes	No
b. Is it feasible to implement the findings in my practice setting?	Yes	No
c. Were all clinically important outcomes considered, including risks and benefits of the treatment?	Yes	No
d. What is my clinical assessment of the patient and are there any contraindications or circumstances that would inhibit me from implementing the treatment?	Yes	No
e. What are my patient's and his or her family's preferences and values about the treatment that is under consideration?	Yes	No

RAPID CRITICAL APPRAISAL OF QUALITATIVE EVIDENCE

1. Are the results of the study valid (i.e., trustworthy and credible)?

a. How were study participants chosen?

b. How were accuracy and completeness of data assured?

c. How plausible/believable are the results?

i. Are implications of the research stated?	Yes	No	Unknown
1. May new insights increase sensitivity to others' needs?	Yes	No	Unknown
2. May understandings enhance situational competence?	Yes	No	Unknown

d. What is the effect on the reader?

1. Are results plausible and believable?	Yes	No	Unknown
2. Is the reader imaginatively drawn into the experience?	Yes	No	Unknown

2. What were the results?

a. Does the research approach fit the purpose of the study?	Yes	No	Unknown
i. How does the researcher identify the study approach?	Yes	No	Unknown
1. Are language and concepts consistent with the approach?	Yes	No	Unknown
2. Are data collection and analysis techniques appropriate?	Yes	No	Unknown
ii. Is the significance/importance of the study explicit?	Yes	No	Unknown
1. Does review of the literature support a need for the study?	Yes	No	Unknown
2. What is the study's potential contribution?			
iii. Is the sampling strategy clear and guided by study needs?	Yes	No	Unknown
1. Does the researcher control selection of the sample?	Yes	No	Unknown
2. Do sample composition and size reflect study needs?	Yes	No	Unknown

b. Is the phenomenon (human experience) clearly identified?

i. Are data collection procedures clear?	Yes	No	Unknown
1. Are sources and means of verifying data explicit?	Yes	No	Unknown
2. Are researcher roles and activities explained?	Yes	No	Unknown
ii. Are data analysis procedures described?	Yes	No	Unknown
1. Does analysis guide direction of sampling and when it ends?	Yes	No	Unknown

2. Are data management processes described?	Yes	No	Unknown

c. What are the reported results (description or interpretation)?

  i. How are specific findings presented?

1. Is presentation logical, consistent, and easy to follow?	Yes	No	Unknown
2. Do quotes fit the findings they are intended to illustrate?	Yes	No	Unknown

  ii. How are overall results presented?

1. Are meanings derived from data described in context?	Yes	No	Unknown
2. Does the writing effectively promote understanding?	Yes	No	Unknown

3. Will the results help me in caring for my patients?

a. Are the results relevant to persons in similar situations?	Yes	No	Unknown
b. Are the results relevant to patient values and/or circumstances?	Yes	No	Unknown

c. How may the results be applied in clinical practice?

RAPID CRITICAL APPRAISAL OF EVIDENCE-BASED GUIDELINES

Credibility

1. Who were the guideline developers?	_____		
2. Were the developers representative of key stakeholders in this specialty (interdisciplinary)?	Yes	No	Unknown
3. Who funded the guideline development?	_____		
4. Were any of the guidelines developers funded researchers of the reviewed studies?	Yes	No	Unknown
5. Did the team have a valid development strategy?	Yes	No	Unknown
6. Was an explicit (how decisions were made), sensible and impartial process used to identify, select, and combine evidence?	Yes	No	Unknown
7. Did its developers carry out a comprehensive, reproducible literature review within the past 12 months of its publication/revision?	Yes	No	Unknown
8. Were all important options and outcomes considered?	Yes	No	Unknown
9. Is each recommendation in the guideline tagged by the level/strength of evidence upon which it is based and linked with the scientific evidence?	Yes	No	Unknown
10. Do the guidelines make explicit recommendations (reflecting value judgments about outcomes)?	Yes	No	Unknown
11. Has the guideline been subjected to peer review and testing?	Yes	No	Unknown

Applicability/Generalizability

12. Is the intent of use provided (e.g., national, regional, local)?	Yes	No	Unknown
13. Are the recommendations clinically relevant?	Yes	No	Unknown
14. Will the recommendations help me in caring for my patients?	Yes	No	Unknown
15. Are the recommendations practical/feasible (e.g., resources—people and equipment) available?	Yes	No	Unknown
16. Are the recommendations a major variation from current practice?	Yes	No	Unknown
17. Can the outcomes be measured through standard care?	Yes	No	Unknown

Modified from Slutsky, J. (2005). *Using Evidence-Based Guidelines: Tools for Improving Practice*, In B.M. Melnyk & E. Fineout-Overholt (Eds). *Evidence-Based Practice in Nursing & Healthcare. A Guide to Best Practice*. (pp. 221–236). Philadelphia: Lippincott, Williams & Wilkins. This form may be used for educational, practice change & research purposes without permission.

Evaluation Table Template and Synthesis Table Template for Critical Appraisal

EVALUATION TABLE TEMPLATE

Caveats

1. The **only studies** you should put in these tables are the ones that **you know answer your question** after you have done rapid critical appraisal (i.e., the keeper studies).
2. Use abbreviations and create **a legend** for readers and yourself.
3. Keep your descriptions brief—there should be **NO complete sentences.**
4. This evaluation is for the purpose of knowing your studies to synthesize.

Citation: Author(s), Date of Publication & Title	Conceptual Framework	Design/ Method	Sample/Setting	Major Variables Studied and Their Definitions	Measurement of Major Variables	Data Analysis	Study Findings	Appraisal of Worth to Practice Strength of the Evidence (i.e., level of evidence + quality [study strengths and weaknesses])
***								
Author, year, title	Theoretical basis for study	Indicate design & briefly describe what was done in the study	Number, characteristics, attrition rate & why?	Independent variables (e.g., IV1 = IV2 =) Dependent variables (e.g., DV =)	What scales were used to measure the outcome variables (e.g., name of scale, author, reliability info [e.g., Cronbach alphas])	What stats were used to answer the clinical question (i.e., all stats do not need to be put into the table)	Statistical findings or qualitative findings (i.e., for every statistical test you have in the data analysis column, you should have a finding)	<ul><li>Strengths and limitations of the study</li><li>Risk or harm if study intervention or findings implemented</li><li>Feasibility of use in your practice</li><li>Remember: level of evidence + quality of evidence = strength of evidence & confidence to act</li><li>Use the USPSTF grading schema http://www.ahrq.gov/clinic/3rduspstf/ratings.htm</li></ul>

***These prompts are listed for each column to help you with what to list there—please do not repeat the headings, just provide the data.
Used with permission, © 2007 Fineout-Overholt.

EVIDENCE SYNTHESIS TABLES

(e.g., Comparisons of Variable of Interest: Outcome, Intervention, Measurement, Definition of Variable, Levels of Evidence [design] Across Studies)

The table below is **one template/example** for how you could construct a synthesis table for interventions across studies.

Studies	A	B	C	D	E	F
Interventions						
1	X	X			X	X
2			X	X		X
3			X	X		X

Legend: A = study author & year; B = study author & year; C = study author & year; etc. X indicates presence of the intervention.

The table below is **another template** for a synthesis table focused on design, sample, and outcome across studies. There could be many more. Choose your information carefully that you will include in your syntheses tables. Create your **OWN** synthesis table—remember the studies are telling the story about your issue! Your studies should indicate what is important to put in the synthesis table.

Studies	Design	Sample	Outcome
A	RCT	$N = 450$ Age: 60–90 Ethnicity: 80% Asian 20% Caucasian	Falls ⇩
B	Quasi-experimental, Correlational	$N = 35$ Age: 75–85 Ethnicity: 73% Caucasian 10% African American 17% Hispanic	Falls ⇩
C	EBP Implementation Project	$N = 50$ Age: 55–90 Ethnicity: 100% Caucasian	Falls ⇩

Appendix D
Walking the Walk and Talking the Talk: An Appraisal Guide for Qualitative Evidence

QUALITATIVE DESCRIPTION

1 Sword, W., Busser, D., Ganann, R., McMillan, T., & Swinton, M. (2008). Women's care-seeking experiences after referral for postpartum depression. *Qualitative Health Research, 18*, 1161–1173.

Question: What were women's experiences of seeking care after referral from public health nurse for probable postpartum depression, including responses to being referred, specific factors that hindered or facilitated care seeking, experiences seeking care, and responses to interventions offered?

Design: **Qualitative description** … is "the method of choice [for describing] … phenomena [that entail] … the presentation of the facts of the case in everyday language … [It] is less interpretive than phenomenological, theoretical, ethnographic, or narrative descriptions … [but] more interpretive than quantitative description, which typically entails surveys or other pre-structured means to obtain a common dataset on pre-selected variables … " (Sandelowski, 2000, pp. 336,339).

Sample: New mothers (*N* = 18) recruited from an early prevention and intervention initiative (Healthy Babies, Healthy Children) who accepted, as part of the program, the offer of a home visit by a public health nurse.

Procedures: In-depth, semistructured telephone interviews conducted approximately 4 weeks after screening for postpartum depression were thought to be less burdensome on new mothers than asking for face-to-face interviews in their homes or another location. Two trained research assistants used an interview guide containing broad, open-ended questions about women's feelings about being referred for probable postpartum depression and their subsequent care-seeking experiences. The conversational interview style included probes and reflective statements to obtain clarification and encourage more detailed description. The interviews, averaging 40 to 50 minutes in length, were audiotaped and transcribed verbatim. In addition, participants' demographic data were obtained from the women's completion of a structured questionnaire.

Data entry and management in NVivo qualitative data software supported conventional content analysis as described by Hsieh and Shannon (2005). Preliminary codes were assigned to meaningful units of data (sentences or phrases). Further data reduction occurred over the course of the analysis, as related codes were subsumed under broader emergent categories. Focusing on the research questions led to development of a rich description of women's care seeking after referral for postpartum depression.

Appraisal:
◆ *Are the results valid/trustworthy and credible?* Yes. [**Sample Selection**]: English-speaking women in the public health program, Healthy Babies, Healthy Children, with an Edinburgh Postnatal Depression Scale (EPDS) score of 12 or higher, indicative of probable depression (Cox & Holden, 2003), were eligible to participate in the study. "The EPDS is a well-validated and widely used instrument to assess the presence of depressive symptoms" (p. 1163). [**Accuracy and Completeness**]: Accuracy (credibility) was assured through analysis of each interview by multiple independent coders followed by research team review and the arrival at initial and final

coding schemes through a process of discussion and consensus. Transcripts were reviewed to ensure that the final coding scheme had been consistently applied to all the data. Completeness of data (credibility) was assured by a search for negative cases (outliers/exceptions to identified informational categories and concepts). Goodness of fit between analysis and data from which it was generated (confirmability) was demonstrated by the use of quotes and examples. Reliability (dependability) was assured by careful documentation of the research process (the audit trail), including a record of evolving and finalized coding decisions and data analysis procedures. **[Plausibility/Believability]:** Quotes that give voice to study participants and illustrate different aspects of the phenomenon are well chosen and appropriately introduced. These representations of the women's thoughts and feelings illuminate and draw the reader into their experience.

◆ *What were the results of the study?* **[Approach/Purpose/Phenomenon]:** Qualitative description accomplishes the intended purpose to produce a detailed and straightforward report of women's experiences related to seeking care following referral for probable postpartum depression. "A socioecological framework of health services utilization was used as an orienting framework for data collection" (p. 1163). **[Reported Results]:** Specific barriers and facilitators of care seeking were identified at individual, social network, and health system levels of influence. At the *individual level*, women's normalizing of symptoms, limited understanding, waiting for symptoms to improve, discomfort discussing mental health concerns, and fears deterred care seeking. Symptom awareness and not feeling like oneself prompted women to seek care. At the *social network level*, normalizing of symptoms and limited understanding of postpartum depression on the part of family and friends posed barriers; while expressions of worry or concern and encouragement to seek care facilitated women's care seeking. *Health system–level* barriers included normalizing of symptoms, offering unacceptable interventions, and disconnected care pathways (communication and timing disruptions). Care seeking was facilitated by having established and supportive relationships, legitimization of postpartum depression, outreach and follow-up, and timeliness of care.

◆ *Will the results help me in caring for my patients?* **[Relevance]:** Promotion of knowledge and awareness of postpartum depression is needed among both the general public and healthcare professionals, since normalizing symptoms and limited understanding were found to be barriers to care seeking at all three levels of influence. The research reflects patient values (preferences, concerns, and expectations) and circumstances (clinical state). **[Application]:** All care providers coming in contact with new mothers should be alert for symptoms; and consistent use of screening instruments should be considered. Findings also highlight the importance of interpersonal skills in establishing trust and supportive relationships that include acknowledgement of women's fears about discussing mental health concerns, assistance to making informed decisions, and efforts to learn about various treatment modalities that may be used to more effectively match interventions with women's individual needs and preferences. Analysis further suggests that improved coordination of care would broaden opportunities for appropriate assessment and treatment of women with postpartum depression.

ETHNOGRAPHY

2 Scott, S. D., Estabrooks, C. A., Allen, M., & Pollock, C. (2008). A context of uncertainty: How context shapes nurses' research utilization behaviors. *Qualitative Health Research, 18,* 347–357.

Question: How do characteristics of the work environment context and culture influence nurses' research utilization behaviors?

Design: **An ethnographic study**…Cultural understanding obtained through ethnographic fieldwork requires researcher presence in study participants' environments. Participant observation is the central fieldwork technique combined with in-depth interviewing and also collection of artifacts as appropriate to the purposes of the research.

Sample: A maximum variation sampling strategy (i.e., selection of persons, events, and/or settings that offer or represent a wide variety of perspectives related to the phenomenon of interest) was used to purposefully sample events where research use occurred (e.g., patient care rounds and reports) and providers ($N = 29$ nurses, nurse leaders, physicians, and allied health care professionals) on a pediatric critical care unit. The majority of patients, aged from 1 month to 16 years, had recently undergone cardiac surgery, were sedated and ventilated, and required one-on-one care.

Procedures: Systematic observations of approximately 2 hours in length were recorded in fieldnotes and completed over a 7-month period. Observation on all nursing shifts and on all days of the week focused on everyday communication patterns associated with unit routines, patient care rounds, nursing report times, and breaks. Interviews of purposefully selected unit members were 1 to 4 hours in length (average length = 75 minutes). Interviews were tape-recorded and transcribed verbatim. Analysis, guided by Fetterman's (1998) description of ordering (coding and grouping) and interpreting (identifying patterns in) the data, led to identification of uncertainty ("a cognitive state of being unable to anticipate the meaning and/or outcome of an experience," p. 350) as the unit's primary characteristic that shaped nurses' work and the nature of valued knowledge (i.e., a higher value and reliance placed on immediately available knowledge gained through clinical experience and advanced practice than the value placed on research knowledge).

Appraisal:
- ◆ *Are the results valid/trustworthy and credible?* Yes. [**Sample Selection**]: Events and intensive care unit (ICU) personnel were selected purposefully to ensure comprehensive observations of organizational patterns and a broad representation of views, as described above. [**Accuracy and Completeness**]: Credibility was assured by prolonged engagement in the field, documentation of researcher biases and preconceptions, broad sampling for diverse variations and common patterns, and triangulation of data sources. Dependability and confirmability were addressed by documentation of research materials, research processes, and decisions (an audit trail). And rich descriptions of the nursing unit were provided in sufficient detail to allow readers to make judgments about transferability. [**Plausibility/Believability**]: A table of data excerpts supporting each source of uncertainty and well-staged examples provides a realistic/authentic cultural portrait of study participants' work world (see authenticity criteria—Guba & Lincoln, 1989).
- ◆ *What were the results of the study?* [**Approach/Purpose/Phenomenon**]: An ethnographic research design is well suited to research purposes such as this one that sought to understand how context and organizational culture shape the phenomenon of interest—nurses' research utilization behaviors. [**Reported Results**]: In this high-intensity technology-driven work environment, uncertainty was reported to shape nurse study participants' behaviors to an extent that research use was seen as irrelevant. Four major sources of uncertainty were described and illustrated by excerpts from the data. Sources of uncertainty included (a) the precarious status of seriously ill patients, (b) the inherent unpredictability of nurses' work, (c) the complexity of teamwork in a highly sophisticated environment, and (d) a changing management. "In response to the context of uncertainty on this unit, these nurses chose to retreat to a zone of safety, doing what they were told, focusing on routine, and deferring to the authority of others ... [They] did not perceive that managers expected them to use research ... [and although] they believed research was important... they did not believe that accessing and assessing research was part of their role" (p. 355).
- ◆ *Will the results help me in caring for my patients?* [**Relevance**]: The influence of context and organizational culture on research utilization in complex organizational structures is an important and understudied phenomenon. "Clearly, the concepts of culture and context overlap. In this article [the authors] use the term context to signify those aspects of the work setting that extend beyond the unit examined. [They] use the term culture to refer to aspects that are particular, but not unique, to the unit examined" (p. 348). [**Application**]: In this research, the perceived arbitrariness and unpredictability of physicians' and/or administrators' responses to nurses' actions produced a lack of confidence in their own decision making, thus affecting their willingness to use research in their

practice. The authors suggest that "particular organizational qualities or features (i.e., certainty) must be present to create and sustain clinical environments that are ideal for research utilization. [Consequently,] uncertainty must be controlled or reduced [before attempting to introduce] research utilization interventions … ." Efforts to do so may be facilitated by an appreciation for how organizational context influences research utilization behaviors and an understanding of possible sources of uncertainty that could be " … prevent[ing] nurses from going outside of the 'safe zone' " (p. 356).

VIDEO-ASSISTED ETHNOGRAPHY

3   Carroll, K., Iedema, R., & Kerridge, R. (2008). Reshaping ICU ward round practices using video-reflexive ethnography. *Qualitative Health Research, 18,* 380–390.

Question: What are the ways in which clinicians can enhance their communication processes through the use of video-ethnographic and reflexive research methodology?

Design: **Video-reflexive ethnography** … a combination of an ethnographic focus on observation and interviewing with video filming and analysis of video-reflexive sessions (involving study participants' responses to viewings of the video recordings).

Sample: Medical ICU ward rounds and planning meetings in a metropolitan 800-bed tertiary referral and teaching hospital (*N* = 1) was the field site for this study.

Procedures: The medical communication reflexive session held with staff was preceded by 12 days (approximately 193 hours) of participant observation and interviewing to establish trust relationships and orient to the culture of the unit. Observations captured medical ward rounds, planning meetings, nursing handovers, and organizational aspects such as staffing allocation and assignments, allied health practice, and work-related informal hallway conversations. Observations and opportunistic interviews with medical, nursing, allied health, and clerical staff were recorded in handwritten fieldnotes and stored in computerized files. Eight hours of video data capturing formal medical communication were coded by the primary researcher, and analysis was guided by two key questions: Who is or is not speaking? What information is being communicated? Selected footage, representative of three themes emerging from the analysis, was used to produce a 10-minute DVD for the feedback component of the study. In the video-reflective session, which lasted 90 minutes and was attended by 10 intensivists, clinicians engaged in problem solving their own communication difficulties.

Appraisal:
◆   *Are the results valid/trustworthy and credible?* Yes. [**Sample Selection**]: The selection of ICU ward rounds and daily planning meetings was based on the agreed upon importance of these communication mechanisms to patient care and clinician-identified tensions surrounding their purposes, length, and complexities. [**Accuracy and Completeness**]: Credibility was assured by prolonged engagement and persistent observation in the field, triangulation of data sources and methods, and validation of study outcomes in partnership with study participants. [**Plausibility/ Believability**]: Detailing of significant participant responses before and after the video-reflexive session demonstrates how the method may both empower individuals to act (tactical authenticity) and stimulate action (catalytic authenticity) (Guba & Lincoln, 1989).
◆   *What were the results of the study?* [**Approach/Purpose/Phenomenon**]: Use of video data for reflexive feedback narrows and strengthens the ethnographic focus on details of the research phenomenon (communication processes in cultural context) while offering "interventionist possibilities … [b]y creating a space for inquiry that goes beyond epidemiological and descriptive approaches to health service provision … (Shojania & Grimshaw, 2005)" (p. 381). [**Reported Results**]: The first theme ("the big picture"), including talk of patient trajectory and medical

diagnosis, was generally communicated by senior intensivists with little input from junior and other staff. The second theme ("small detail"), involving current physiologic knowledge of each patient, was communicated by junior doctors. The third theme was the lack of multidisciplinary voice, evidenced by the absence of talk time for other health professionals in the recorded video data. The article focuses on one feedback meeting that catalyzed changes in morning rounds and planning meetings. Changes included greater time efficiency, a greater presence of intensivists in the ICU, increased nursing staff satisfaction, and a handover sheet to improve the structure of clinical information exchanges.

◆ *Will the results help me in caring for my patients?* [**Relevance**]: This type of video-assisted research, by emphasizing the role of participants as partners, is directly responsive to their immediate interests and concerns. [**Application**]: The authors suggest that taking an interventionist rather than a descriptive approach, by using video-ethnographic and reflexive research methodology, enhances clinicians' and researchers' understanding of the complexity of contemporary hospital-based work, thus enabling clinicians to appraise and reshape existing practices as in this example of enhancing communication processes.

GROUNDED THEORY

4   **Marcellus, L. (2008). (Ad)ministering love: Providing family foster care to infants with prenatal substance exposure. *Qualitative Health Research, 18*, 1220–1230.**

Question: What is the process of becoming and providing family foster care giving in the context of caring for infants with prenatal drug and alcohol exposure?

Design: **A constructivist approach to grounded theory (Charmaz, 2006).** "A number of the disputes among grounded theorists and critiques by other colleagues result from where various authors stand between interpretive and positivist traditions … Constructivist grounded theory is part of the interpretive tradition … Constructivists study *how*—and sometimes *why*—participants construct meanings and actions in specific situations … to show the complexities of particular worlds, views, and actions" (pp. 129, 130, 132).

Sample: Foster families ($N = 11$) in five different communities; all but one with at least one foster child in the home; and 10 of whom had their own children participating in the study, with ages ranging from 5 to 31 years.

Procedures: The primary data collection strategy was open-ended, semistructured family interviews lasting between 1 and 2 hours. Interviews were recorded, transcribed, and mailed back to family participants for editing and elaboration on further thoughts they may have had while reading the transcript. Researcher observations and reactions were recorded after each interview. Additional data collection strategies included follow-up telephone calls and e-mails, attendance at foster parent events and child welfare conferences, examination of relevant government documents related to child-in-care policies and guidelines, and review of professional and lay literature and media. Three social workers, all with at least 10 years of experience supporting foster families, were also interviewed. Data analysis involved grounded theory techniques of constant comparison, increasingly abstract consideration of the data, and identification of a basic social process.

Appraisal:

◆ *Are the results valid/trustworthy and credible?* Yes. [**Sample Selection**]: Families were recruited through the Guardianship Branch of the British Columbia Ministry for Child and Family Development, a Canadian government agency responsible for administering foster care services. The initial goal of locating families at different time points (to represent families waiting for their first placement, novice and experienced families) was limited by the gatekeeper role of resource workers, reluctance of all family members to participate, and the effect of overall low morale of families in the child welfare system. Within these constraints, "following identification of the initial group of participants, recruitment decisions were then based on the emerging theory and the principles of theoretical sampling" (p. 1221). [**Accuracy and Completeness**]: Validation strategies included periodic review of and discussion about the emerging analysis with an interdisciplinary grounded theory seminar group (peer debriefing), study participants (member checking), and other foster parents and social workers (triangulation of sources of information). [**Plausibility/Believability**]: Depiction of a model/diagram of the theory and selective use of quotes enhance plausibility and direct reader attention to the phases of this experiential process (starting out, living as a foster family, and moving on).

♦ *What were the results of the study?* [**Approach/Purpose/Phenomenon**]: Use of a grounded theory approach suits the theory-generating purpose of this research on the phenomenon of family foster care of infants with prenatal substance exposure. [**Reported Results**]: The basic social process—*(Ad)ministering Love*—is described as having several phases that represent the tension families experience between providing love and guidance for a special needs infant within the restrictions and scrutiny of a child protective system. *Phase 1* (starting out) involves determining family readiness to foster, meeting the requirements of the system, immersing (plunging into the experience) for the first time, and finding their niche (discovering age and gender preferences for foster children that were good fits with the strengths and demands of the family). *Phase 2* (living as a foster family), the middle phase of this process, is depicted as circular and ongoing. Key elements of this phase include rebalancing family life with each placement (being expected to suddenly care for and integrate the infant into family life in addition to being ready to let go with little notice), honoring limits (such as family need for respite), experiencing an emotional double bind (developing attachments and experiencing grief and loss when having to let go), working (i.e., navigating rules of) the child welfare system, feeling a powerless responsibility (responsibility over day-to-day decisions with no control over the long-term decisions affecting the child's future), and public parenting (living with pressure to meet a high level of parenting expertise and effectiveness under supervision by the state). *Phase 3* (moving on) involves relinquishing the role of foster family (no longer actively accepting new placements for various reasons, e.g., to commit to long-term foster placements or adoption of the foster children), losing fit (because of changes in family focus, needs, or composition), and transferring child focus (moving away from full-time active fostering while continuing to be connected to caring for children in some way, e.g., volunteering with child-related activities).

♦ *Will the results help me in caring for my patients?* [**Relevance**]: The varied aspects of the described process of fostering an infant with special needs bring families into contact with many persons, including, nurses, physicians, and infant development specialists. However, in spite of ongoing oversight by the system, families' work within their homes along with its demands and rewards "remain generally unseen, unknown, and unacknowledged by others" (p. 1230). [**Application**]: Understanding the nature and consequences of this type of care giving is an important factor in being able to effectively support foster families and the infants and children in their care.

GROUNDED THEORY

5 **Denz-Penhey, H., & Murdoch, J. C. (2008). Personal resiliency: Serious diagnosis and prognosis with unexpected quality outcomes.** *Qualitative Health Research, 18,* 391–404.

Question: What is common in stories of persons with serious disease who have less than a 10% chance of survival and have a good quality of life at the time of first interview?

Design: **A Glaserian grounded theory approach (Glaser, 1978, 1992)** in which attention is focused on emergence of theory from data without the use of a preestablished formula. Theoretical sensitivity (Glaser, 1978) is emphasized in Glaserian grounded theory. This acquired or enhanced natural personal quality of the researcher is exemplified by the ability to grasp subtleties of meaning in empirical data, to interact or dialog with the data, to reflect on interactions between data with the help of theoretical terms and concepts, and to consider boundaries of emerging interpretations (i.e., the possibilities for alternative interpretations) in developing theoretical understanding of a phenomenon. Glaser argues that the acquisition and use of theoretical sensitivity is what makes the development of a grounded, well-integrated, and conceptually dense theory possible. The authors of this article comment on an initial attempt to use Strauss and Corbin's (1990) paradigm model approach to grounded theory without success before deciding on a Glaserian approach.

Sample: Participants ($N = 11$) varied in age from 20 to 77 at first diagnosis and from 23 to 89 at first interview, which was conducted between 2 and 40 years after the first illness. Each had a life-threatening disease: seven had metastatic cancer, one had acute myeloid leukemia, one had Eisenmenger syndrome (congenital heart disease), one had multiorgan failure, and one had congestive heart failure with multiple chronic conditions.

Procedures: A total of 26 open-ended, semistructured interviews were conducted, with each participant interviewed between two and four times. First interviews averaged 2.5 hours in length and 1 hour for follow-up interviews (with one lasting 5 hours at the first interview and 3.5 hours at the second). Participants determined the length of time they wished to speak. A constant comparative method of data analysis was used, with participants' reported information compared for similarities, variations, and differences; creation of categories; and reflection on the bigger picture and the core category that links categories together.

Appraisal:

◆ *Are the results valid/trustworthy and credible?* Yes. [**Sample Selection**]: Selection criteria included (a) participants who, in their own and their doctors' opinions, were exhibiting a good quality of life at first contact with the interviewer; (b) participants who had recovered, were in remission, or whose medical condition had stabilized when this was not expected given the diagnosis, prognosis, and treatment; (c) participants with less than 10% chance of survival with their conditions, according to their attending physicians, at the time of the first interview; and (d) participants whose less than 10% chance of survival, in each case, was confirmed, on the basis of documented evidence, by a medical practitioner with specialty expertise in their condition but no prior knowledge of them. "The first six participants accepted were the first to be referred to the study by their doctors. The final five participants were [purposefully] chosen in an attempt to find disconfirming data [negative case analysis] to modify the developing theory" (p. 392). [**Accuracy and Completeness**]: Sampling was purposeful with theoretical sampling proceeding after analysis of data from the first six participants to seek excellent examples for the evolving theory and to check for disconfirming data. Member checks were performed to assure accuracy of information and plausibility of information categories and interpretations. Participants were provided with verbatim transcripts for confirmation and correction. Confirmation of fit among data, categories, and conceptual development of the theoretical framework was achieved by the primary analyst working with a second analyst, frequent and extensive memoing, creation of an audit trail, and peer debriefing (consensus building with two project supervisors). [**Plausibility/Believability**]: A table illustrating the various dimensions and dimensional aspects of the theory draws together the variables of interest whose relationships are logically laid down in the reporting and discussion of study results. There are some well-selected quotes that illustrate points that the authors wish to make. But these are limited because "there is no mandate in grounded theory write-ups [as in some other studies] to foreground the perspectives and voices of individual participants…Data are used only to show how a theory was constructed, and that it was indeed constructed from these data" (Sandelowski, 1998, p. 377).

◆ *What were the results of the study?* [**Approach/Purpose/Phenomenon**]: The selection of a grounded theory approach was used to sort out the variables, relationships, and content relevant to the phenomenon of personal resiliency. The authors explain that " … in the field of patient care in serious illness we do not yet know the full range of variables that need to be explored … the basic exploratory study of allowing the data to define the variables common to the stories of people who have had unexpectedly good outcomes in terminal disease has not yet been done, and this study attempts to do so" (p. 392). [**Reported Results**]: The core category in stories of persons who had survived unexpectedly was *Personal resiliency: The illness as secondary to a quality-connected life.* The five dimensions of this "way of being and acting in the world" (p. 394) were *social connectedness* (friendships, community, and group participation), *connectedness to family* (giving, receiving, participating, belonging), *connectedness to the physical environment* (enjoying/appreciating multiple aspects of place, i.e., home, landscape, nature, animals, and/or plants), *connectedness to experiential inner wisdom* (wisdom of bodily needs and tolerances, life-changing insights, intuitive inner wisdom), and *connectedness to a strong psychological self—"This is Me"* (values providing a sense of meaning and purpose in their lives and positive mindsets that supported a way of being that included a strong sense of acceptance, mental flexibility, ability to change activities and lifestyles in response to new information, mental stamina, and active participation in decisions related to their disease treatment and management).

◆ *Will the results help me in caring for my patients?* [**Relevance**]: Healthcare professionals need to be as attentive to advising patients on life activities and relationships as they are to prescribing biomedical interventions. Knowledge of how resiliency has helped other persons faced with similar circumstances may be useful to patients and their families. [**Application**]: The authors say: "Patient-directed quality of life is an ethical way to practice and medical carers can use this information to support patient autonomy. Improved quality of life is a beneficial outcome in itself, and if increased longevity should occur as well, that can be regarded as an additional bonus" (pp. 402–403).

DESCRIPTIVE PHENOMENOLOGY

6 Wongvatunyu, S., & Porter, E. (2008). Helping young adult children with traumatic brain injury: The life-world of mothers. *Qualitative Health Research, 18,* 1062–1074.

Question: What is the personal–social context of the experience of mothers who are helping young adult survivors of moderate or severe traumatic brain injury (TBI)?

Design: Porter's (1995) descriptive phenomenological method based on Husserlian phenomenology and the phenomenological sociology of Schutz and Luckman (1973). This involved bracketing (avoiding ideas and use of language that suggest preconceptions of the experience) and asking mothers, in an open neutrally worded way, simply to talk about their experiences as caregivers and to describe what their lives were like before and after the TBI. Probes were employed to encourage clarification and elaboration. Example: "When the mothers related an intention basic to the helping experience, the first author asked them to explain their reason(s) for having that intention" (p. 1064). Thus, the authors explain (p. 1064), in differentiating data pertaining to lifeworld from data pertaining to intentions (Porter, 1995), reasons (rationales) for intentions (particular things mothers did to help their children) were identified as reflections of the mothers' lifeworld to be described in "objectivated categories" (Schutz & Luckman, 1973, p. 180).

Sample: Participants ($N = 7$) were recruited by posting notices in local clinics for TBI survivors and in meeting rooms of family support groups at the local rehabilitation center. Mothers' ages ranged from 46 to 64 years ($M = 53$) and their young adult TBI survivors (five men and two women) ranged in age from

20 to 36 years. The young adults had been injured at least 6 months earlier and lived with their mothers, with the exception of one man who recently had left his mother's home to live with his wife and children.

Procedures: Three in-depth, tape-recorded interviews were conducted with each mother over a 2-month period. Most of the 1-hour interviews took place at the mothers' homes, with some done in private meeting rooms at the university for the mothers' convenience. Each interview was transcribed immediately so that discussion of ideas generated by them could be used to guide exploratory questions in subsequent interviews. In the analysis, a three-level classification scheme was used to document consistencies among the mothers' lifeworlds. "From specific to general, the levels of the lifeworld were (a) 'element' (Porter, 1995, p. 35), (b) 'descriptor' (Porter, 1995, p. 35), and (c) feature (Spiegelberg, 1994) (Wongvatunyu & Porter, 2008, p. 1064)." An element was common to some or all the women. Descriptors were coined to capture the similarities that pertained to particular lifeworld features. Feedback from each mother was obtained in the third interview to determine if labels for phenomena and lifeworld features were descriptive of her experience.

Appraisal:

◆ **Are the results valid/trustworthy and credible?** Yes. [**Sample Selection**]: The focus on mothers of young adults allows for examination of what happens when young adults return to the parental home as TBI survivors. "Mothers ... engage in supportive and emotional activities (Francis-Connolly, 2000) rather than basic caregiving such as youngsters need ... [but] factors relevant to developmental tasks can resurface, such as functional status, history of the mother–child relationship (Verhaeghe, Defloor, & Grypdonck, 2005), and reintegration into the community (Winstanley, Simpson, Tate, & Myles, 2006)" (p. 1063). [**Accuracy and Completeness**]: Accuracy of data and plausibility of interpretations were assured by member checking (repeating several key questions at second and third interviews to check reliability and soliciting feedback on labels and features used in the interpretation of findings) and prompt discussion of each interview. [**Plausibility/Believability**]: A table of lifeworld features and their component descriptors is accompanied by quotes that faithfully capture study participants' values (preferences, concerns, and expectations) and unique circumstances. These lend authenticity (Guba & Lincoln, 1989) to and provide validation of the reported research findings.

◆ **What were the results of the study?** [**Approach/Purpose/Phenomenon**]: A descriptive (Husserlian) phenomenologic study is the method of choice when exploration is directed toward uncovering and illuminating the empirical essence of the lifeworld ... in this case, the lifeworld of mothers helping young adult children with TBI. [**Reported Results**]: Five lifeworld features basic to the maternal experience of helping young adult TBI survivors and their accompanying descriptors were identified. *Having a child who survived a TBI as a young adult* was characterized as "particularly complex" (p. 1065), involving nine descriptors of mothers' common experience which included *feeling unprepared to take it all in, looking for answers that no one has, thinking positively about my child's situation, holding on to the child who has been mine all this time, getting to know my child now, knowing all about my child, starting over with my baby, continuing to mother my child, and hoping for the best for my child.* Six months or more after the injury, mothers were aware of *perceiving that life has really changed,* involving *living with changes in my relationship with my child, living with changes in my own life, putting my life on hold, and perceiving the changes as part of my life and as lifelong. Having sufficient support/feeling bereft of any help* pertained to situations of either *receiving that kind of support or lacking that kind of support from health professionals* where the support was that which was consistent with what was needed at various times during the postinjury period. Descriptors of the lifeworld feature—*believing that my child is still able*—reflected mothers' common experience of *perceiving that my child can work on that issue, perceiving that my child is trying hard to progress, and perceiving that my child is able to do more in life.* Mothers' faith in their own helping abilities—*believing that I can help my child*—were "basic facets of the lifeworld" (p. 1070). Mothers mentioned *having personality traits* and *having previous experience that are relevant to helping my child now.* Most mothers talked about the importance of having patience or trying to become more patient.

◆ *Will the results help me in caring for my patients?* [**Relevance**]: TBI is noted to be a leading cause of death and disability among young persons in the United States. Thus, caregivers need to understand the personal–social factors affecting involved family members. The authors claim to report what they believe is "the first study to illuminate the lifeworld of … mothers" of young adult TBI survivors (p. 1063), the rationale for which is described earlier under "sample selection." [**Application**]: The authors suggest that during conversations with mothers of TBI survivors, healthcare professionals could adopt some of the phrases used to characterize these findings to offer support (e.g., "mothers of TBI survivors can feel as though they are looking for nonexistent answers") and recognize mothers' unique expertise (e.g., "What are special things about your child that you feel I should know?" … "To broach discussion of changed relationships, practitioners can ask mothers about ways in which their children seem like different people" (p. 1071). Sensitivity to the different types of support needed at different times postinjury should involve making sure that mothers are aware of opportunities for help that they might not be aware of needing in the aftermath of the injury as they focus their concentration on the injured child. Finally, findings about the importance of patience and the never-ending nature of the experience should encourage healthcare professionals to provide opportunities at each encounter for mothers to talk about the impact of the injury on their lives rather than asking only about the progress of the young adult.

HERMENEUTIC PHENOMENOLOGY

7 Woodgate, R. L., Ateah, C., & Secco, L. (2008). Living in a world of our own: The experience of parents who have a child with autism. *Qualitative Health Research, 18,* 1075–1083.

Question: What is the lived experience of parents who have a child with autism?

Design: **Hermeneutic phenomenology as described by van Manen.** According to van Manen (1990): "Hermeneutic phenomenology tries to be attentive to both terms of its methodology: it is a *descriptive* (phenomenological) methodology because it wants to be attentive to how things appear, it wants to let things speak for themselves; it is an *interpretive* (hermeneutic) methodology because it claims that there are no such things as uninterpreted phenomena" (p. 180). Phenomenologists using this approach are especially interested in how the phenomenon of interest is related to the everyday world of human experience. That is, they adhere to a theory of interpretation that assumes the need to explain meaning in relation to context. An understanding of the meaning of the phenomenon is revealed through analysis and interpretation of the texts created from conversations with persons who know what it is like to be living the experience as well as other informational sources that support reflection on essential themes that characterize it.

Sample: Participants ($N = 21$) were parents from 16 families of children with autism (16 mothers and 5 fathers) all but 2 of whom had at least one other child. The children with autism (all boys except for two girls) ranged in age from 3 to 9 years, with age at initial diagnosis ranging from 2.5 to 3.5 years.

Procedures: Data collection involved tape-recorded open-ended interviews during which participants were asked to tell what life was like for them before, during, and after their child was diagnosed with autism. Probes were used as needed to facilitate the telling of stories in a conversational manner. Interviews were between 1.5 and 3 hours in length. Observations of the contexts of interviews were recorded in fieldnotes. Tapes were transcribed and the interview and fieldnote texts were analyzed, using van Manen's selective highlighting approach. This involved selecting and highlighting sentences or sentence clusters suggestive of thematic content, writing notes (analytic memos) about themes related to the experience, and reducing all textual data (through processes of writing and rewriting) until "essential themes" emerged which were defined as "unique to the phenomenon of parents who have a child with autism and … fundamental to the overall shared description of living the experience" (pp. 1077–1078).

Appraisal:

◆ *Are the results valid/trustworthy and credible?* Yes. [**Sample Selection**]: "The only legitimate informants in phenomenological research are those who have lived the reality … " (p. 1077). Participants were recruited through a support group. Children's conditions, as described by their parents, varied in terms of difficulties with communication, social relations, and repetitive, stereotypical behavior. "The extent of treatment the children received was dependent both on what services were available to them and what parents could afford" (p. 1077). [**Accuracy and Completeness**]: Accuracy was addressed by rigorous writing and rewriting to include all meaningful themes and ensure that they were presented as disclosed. In van Manen's (1990) approach to phenomenology, writing and rewriting are a vital part of the analytic process that helps produce a heightened awareness of the phenomenon and deepen the interpretation. "Writing is a reflexive activity that involves the totality of our physical and mental being … To be able to do justice to the fullness and ambiguity of the experience of the lifeworld, writing may turn into a complex process of rewriting (rethinking, reflecting, recognizing) … Writing and rewriting are the thing (van Manen, 1990, pp. 131, 132)." Other measures to ensure rigor were prolonged engagement with participants and the data, careful line-by-line analysis of transcripts, and detailed memo writing. Accuracy and credibility were also enhanced by discussion of preliminary interpretations with participants during and following each interview. [**Plausibility/Believability**]: Themes were fully explained and supported by examples and well-selected quotes. Quotes were used strategically to validate findings and establish a mood (Sandelowski, 1994) reflective of parents' values/concerns and actions/reactions.

◆ *What were the results of the study?* [**Approach/Purpose/Phenomenon**]: The human science approach of this phenomenologic method is a good fit with the study interest in stimulating reflection on lived experiences in the everyday lives of parents of children with autism, with the intent to increase thoughtfulness (pedagogic understanding) about how best to respond and offer support to such families. [**Reported Results**]: *The essence (essential nature) of the parents' experiences (i.e., what the experiences were like) was "living in a world of our own"* that left them feeling isolated. Their sense of isolation was attributed to four main sources: society's lack of understanding, missing a "normal" way of life, being disconnected from their families, and dealing with an unsupportive "system" (bureaucracies of child-related agencies, healthcare facilities, and educational settings). "Parents expressed feeling completely defeated and on their own when they felt that family members, friends, professionals within the system, and others in their lives were not there to support their sense of hope that things would get better for their child" (p. 1079). *Three themes support the essence* in terms of demonstrating how parents struggled to remove the isolation that they felt enveloped themselves and their children. *Theme 1: vigilant parenting*, incorporated strategies of (a) *acting sooner rather than later*/keeping abreast of care needs, (b) *doing all you can*, and (c) *staying close to your gut feelings. Theme 2: sustaining the self and family*, involved sustaining family integrity while enhancing protective measures for the child with autism through (a) *working toward a healthy balance* of self-needs and the child's needs, (b) *cherishing different milestones* in the child's development, and (c) *learning to let go*/accepting and allowing situations that cannot be changed play out. *Theme 3: fighting all the way*, referred to making "the system" work for parents and their children by (a) *learning all you can* and (b) *educating others.*

◆ *Will the results help me in caring for my patients?* [**Relevance**]: What was found to be unique about these research findings was that, from parents' perspectives, their sense of isolation mainly resulted from lack of understanding and support from external sources (society, family, and the conglomerate structure of child health/assistance systems). [**Application**]: Thus, the study reinforces the need to educate persons who lack understanding of the impact of autism on children and parents and to address gaps in helping services in order to create "a seamless system that will help foster more enduring relationships between parents and all professionals involved in the care of children with autism" (p. 1082). Additionally, "given [their] expertise, … parents [themselves] could become invaluable assets in helping professionals understand human relationships and responses" (p. 1083).

NARRATIVE/LIFE STORY METHODS

8 Thomas, S. P., & Hall, J. M. (2008) **Life trajectories of female child abuse survivors thriving in adulthood.** *Qualitative Health Research, 18*, 149–166.

Question: How have thriving female adult survivors of child abuse been able to achieve success in their lives?

Design: **Narrative/life story methods.** Life story/life history approaches represent a form of biographical research that involves the recording of a person's life story as told to the researcher by the person himself/herself. The researcher then may use different investigative strategies to explore this recorded record of the individual's life. Narrative methods (the study of stories or narratives of human experiences) involve "an analysis of meaning in context through interpretation of persons' life experiences … for the purpose of evoking a response from readers and promoting dialog" (Powers & Knapp, 2006, p. 110).

Sample: Participants were women ($N = 27$) ranging in age from 29 to 79 years who had experienced childhood abuse, beginning as early as infancy and continuing, in most cases, until they left home. A majority (74%) experienced sexual abuse, combined with other forms (physical/emotional abuse and neglect), with adult men commonly the sexual/physical aggressors and mothers tending to be nonprotective and/or verbally abusive. Nearly all had experienced depression, anxiety-related symptoms, and other signs of post-traumatic stress disorder. However, the study's exclusion criteria prohibited women who were currently in crisis—those experiencing severe depression, psychotic symptoms, suicidality, interpersonal violence, drug or alcohol abuse, or acute physical illness—from participation in the study. "Provision for psychiatric care was made and a referral list was given to each participant, in the event that an interview caused distress" (p. 151).

Procedures: Three open-ended interviews were conducted by the same interviewer (a graduate-level psychiatric nurse) across a time span of 6 to 12 months in settings of the women's choice (home, workplace, university office). Free-flowing storytelling was encouraged, with little use of interviewer probes, in order to allow women to share details of their lives in their own words and in their own ways. Analysis of interview transcripts occurred in three phases. *Phase I* involved content mapping, through development and use of a concept list, to reduce and summarize the texts in accordance with the aims of the study. Summary Narrative Assessment (SNA) forms were also developed to enable the research team to shift analytic focus between the SNAs and the original transcripts in a dialectical (conversational style of reasoning) process. "Women were classified into four groups: 'thrivers' who made upward progress since their 20s ($n = 8$), 30s ($n = 8$), or 40s ($n = 6$) and 'strugglers' ($n = 5$) who had made some progress but were hindered by frequent thinking about abusive dynamics and were less successful in work and relationships" (p. 152). Graphs of healing trajectories showed no predominant pattern. Identified turning points were also diverse with aftermaths that were often negative (brought about by crises such as divorce, death in the family, and others related to women's personal thoughts or epiphanies). *Phase II* involved a systematic examination of the direction and nature of the aftermath of turning points, using a coding scheme to identify the redemption (a painful event made better) and contamination (a good experience ruined/undermined) sequences that followed. The full transcripts (rather than the SNAs) were read and analyzed line-by-line to enhance understanding. *Phase III* involved creation of "detailed trajectories of exemplar cases, to highlight turning points and the most significant redemptive sequences in [the women's] lives; they often explicitly identified those as lifesaving. A new concept, *setbacks*, was incorporated in Phase III, to differentiate adverse events that had lesser impact and duration than turning points, not necessarily changing the direction of a life trajectory" (p. 152).

Appraisal:

◆ *Are the results valid/trustworthy and credible?* Yes. [**Sample Selection**]: The majority of participants responded to a feature article in a local newspaper about the study and its focus on success stories rather than problems associated with the abuse. Flyers and network sampling were other means of recruitment. Telephone screening was used to determine that potential participants were not currently in crisis. [**Accuracy and Completeness**]: "Throughout the analysis, the larger multidisciplinary team was used as a sounding board for … emergent discoveries. In addition to weekly or biweekly evening meetings over a 4-year period, the team held half-day retreats; notes taken at these meetings constitute an audit trail for the project. Critique and consensual validation by team members from varied disciplines (psychology, psychiatry, nursing) and by several experiential consultants (CM survivor not in the study) enhanced the rigor and credibility of the analysis" (p. 153). [**Plausibility/Believability**]: Verisimilitude (a criterion of good literary style—evocative, creative writing) was established through multiple figures illustrating the report's storied turning points, redemption and contamination sequences, setbacks, and life trajectories (steady upward progression, roller-coaster, and struggler patterns).

◆ *What were the results of the study?* [**Approach/Purpose/Phenomenon**]: Narrative/life story methods are a good fit with research aims to examine surviving and thriving after childhood maltreatment (CM). The authors explain that this methodology was chosen "because it permits us to learn how people interpret their own traumatic experiences. 'Telling narratives is a major way that individuals make sense of disruptive events in their lives' (Riessman, 1990, p. 1199)" (p. 149). [**Reported Results**]: *Diverse patterns of healing* included a roller-coaster pattern, patterns of steady upward progress, and patterns of continued struggle. *Four types of redemption narratives* were found: redemption by counseling or psychotherapy, redemption by a loving relationship, redemption by God, and self-redemption. *Three common threads* interwoven throughout all of the women's narratives were issues related to telling/not telling, remembering/not remembering, and forgiving/not forgiving.

◆ *Will the results help me in caring for my patients?* [**Relevance**]: The article foregrounds participants' voices that "command attention of clinicians and policy makers because earlier and more efficacious interventions could have fostered earlier thriving and mitigated years of suffering" (p. 164). [**Application**]: The authors advise "patience, gentleness, and sensitivity … in working with CM survivors, not pressuring women to remember abuse, not urging them to confront (or forgive) abusers if they do not wish to do so" (p. 163). To foster thriving, earlier and longer, rather than short-term, therapies are needed as well as tolerance for some distortion of the early experience that may be a healthy self-protective mechanism commonly observed among trauma survivors.

FOCUS GROUP ANALYSIS

9   Morgan, D. G. et al. (2008). Taking the hit: Focusing on caregiver "error" masks organizational-level risk factors for nursing aide assault. *Qualitative Health Research, 18,* 334–346.

Question: What are nursing aide (NA) perceptions of the characteristics of incidents of physical aggression against themselves by nursing home residents?

Design: **Focus group analysis.** Focus groups generate data on a particular topic through discussion and interaction. Sessions are moderated by a group leader and are conducted as informal, semistructured interviews. In this research, as in many studies, the group interview technique was used in conjunction with other forms of data collecting. The study plan involved use of structured prospective event-reporting logs (diaries) in which NAs were to document consecutive incidents of resident aggression (time, place, type of activity taking place, views on what caused it, and their emotions and behavior) followed by focus groups to further explore the NAs' perceptions of these events. This article is limited solely to reporting outcomes of the focus group analysis.

Sample: Participating nursing homes included eight with special care units (SCUs) for persons with dementia and three non-SCU facilities, since comparison of perceptions of employees in nursing homes with and without SCUs was of interest. All NAs were eligible to participate. A total of 19 focus groups were conducted with 138 NAs. The focus groups were of two types. Those necessitated by a need to understand barriers to participation in the study (*N* = 9) were conducted in five facilities with a total of 74 NAs. Those aimed at exploring physical aggression, as originally planned (*N* = 10), were conducted in the remaining six facilities with a total of 63 NAs. An individual interview was also conducted in one facility where staffing levels limited formation of a second group.

Procedures: A semistructured interview guide was designed as a follow-up to questions in the diary. Due to NAs' discomfort with sessions being tape-recorded, a flip chart was used to document discussion points. Researchers also wrote detailed notes, including verbatim quotes, which were entered into a word processing program. Concurrent data collection and analysis enabled subsequent interviews to be guided by the analysis of those that had gone before. The narrative text data were analyzed using grounded theory techniques to identify themes.

Appraisal:
♦ *Are the results valid/trustworthy and credible?* Yes. [**Sample Selection**]: The research design called for follow-up in-depth interviews (focus groups) in approximately half of the participating facilities to deepen understanding of the larger study findings. This plan was modified to include focus group follow-up in all nursing homes in order to address low response rates to the structured event-reporting log/diary approach. Posters, brochures, and unit communication books were used to publicize the focus groups, groups were scheduled for ease of attendance by workers on different shifts, and funding was offered for staff relief during meeting times. [**Accuracy and Completeness**]: Explanation of sampling strategies and facilitation of the group process are thorough, and the purpose of focus groups in the overall study, to enhance accuracy and credibility through triangulation of data sources, is established. [**Plausibility/Believability**]: Sets of quotes are sequenced and contextualized around NA responses to reports of physical aggression (feeling blamed, lack of acknowledgment and action, desire for respect and involvement, and factors influencing risk of exposure). The effect intensifies the feeling and mood of study participants' contributions at the same time that the quotes support plausible arguments about organizational conditions that underlie NAs' reactions.

♦ *What were the results of the study?* [**Approach/Purpose/Phenomenon**]: This study was part of a larger study on rural dementia care in the midwestern Canadian province of Saskatchewan. A focus group format fit the researchers' need to further explore and follow up on NA perceptions of barriers to study participation and views on the phenomenon of physical aggression they experienced at the hands of nursing home residents. [**Reported Results**]: Although each of the two sets of focus groups was conducted for a different purpose, the analysis converged around consistent themes. Specifically, NAs' reluctance to participate in the diary component of the study was directly linked to perceptions of their experiences in caring for residents demonstrating physically aggressive behavior. *Consistent themes that were the cause of frustration* were (a) NAs' perceptions of being blamed when they reported resident aggression, (b) lack of acknowledgment and action in response to reports of aggression, and (c) NAs' desire for respect and involvement in decision and policy making within the organization. The third theme derived from a perception of themselves "at the bottom of the organizational hierarchy" even though they were the caregivers who had "extensive knowledge of individual residents and their needs" (p. 340). *Factors influencing risk of exposure to physical aggression* included workload, inflexible routines, limited access to specialized programs and personnel for behavior management assessment, and inadequate education for NAs, RNs, and physicians. "Rushing care" for residents, particularly those with dementia who need a slower pace, was the most frequently cited problem. Rigid institutional routines (care according to predetermined schedules) contributed to rushing of care that led to resident agitation and aggression. NAs also reported that poorly controlled pain led to resident aggression as well as difficulty to get aggressive residents assessed for a behavioral medication management solution "because the nurses were concerned about medication cost and side effects" (p. 342). There was little difference between reports of NAs who worked on SCUs and those who did not.

◆ **Will the results help me in caring for my patients?** [**Relevance**]: Resident aggression in nursing homes is a serious problem. NAs, because they provide the majority of care, are most at risk for both verbal aggression and physical assault. Small rural nursing homes, in particular, may have fewer resources, including specialized dementia care programs, which places even higher job-related strain on personnel, especially NAs. [**Application**]: The authors suggest that "to fully address the issue of NA assault there must be a shift in focus away from the behavior of individual NAs to the broader system level ... The analysis points to the need for multiple changes at the organizational level ... the difficulties of finding effective strategies should not prevent organizations from acknowledging and responding more actively to the plight of NAs who are 'taking the hit,' both literally and figuratively, for the current situation in long-term care" (pp. 342–344).

METASYNTHESIS/META-ETHNOGRAPHY

10 Yick, A. G. (2008). **A metasynthesis of qualitative findings on the role of spirituality and religiosity among culturally diverse domestic violence survivors.** *Qualitative health Research,* *18,* 1289–1306.

Question: What can a synthesis of existing qualitative findings tell us about the role of culture, spirituality, and religion on domestic violence? Specifically (a) How do domestic violence victims and survivors use religious and spiritual resources to cope and find meaning? (b) How do religion and spirituality overtly and covertly promote abuse? (c) How does culture affect the intersection of religion or spirituality and domestic violence?

Design: **Metasynthesis as outlined by Noblit and Hare.** Noblit and Hare (1988) provide a step-by-step approach to performing meta-ethnography, a metasynthesis approach in the anthropologic/ethnographic tradition. It involves a systematic comparison of qualitative research reports on a designated topic to obtain a full understanding of the phenomenon and a determination of how the key metaphors of each study relate to one another (i.e., translating the studies into one another). Synthesis of these multiple translations refers to the researcher's formulation of overarching metaphors that remains faithful to the interpretations found in the original research sources and accurately portrays their shared and unique findings.

Sample: The sample consisted of *six qualitative research studies* (i.e., eight articles, taking into account three studies that were published from the same dataset). Table 1 summarizes the characteristics of each study. All studies met the following criteria: (a) use of a qualitative design, (b) use of direct quotes from participants from the original study, (c) use of English language, and (d) examination of women who were (or were at the time of the original study) affected by domestic violence. "This study focused solely on male perpetrators and female spouses or intimate partners. A decision was made to focus on heterosexual relationships because the dynamics are different in gay and lesbian domestic violence and domestic violence perpetrated by females" (p. 1293). *Women who were participants in the original studies (N = 62)* were from diverse racial/ethnic and religious backgrounds: more than half (*n* = 34) African American, nine Asian women, nine White women, and several from other ethnic groups with Catholic, Protestant, Muslim, and Buddhist backgrounds. (The demographics of this population are displayed in Table 4.)

Procedures: Each study was read in its entirety to obtain a sense of it as a whole. In subsequent readings, words and terms were highlighted to capture concepts. Table 2 shows how meanings from units of text were condensed and then summarized into an interpretation with an underlying meaning and subthemes. Table 3 shows how nine identified overarching themes were linked back to the concepts in the original studies.

Appraisal:

◆ *Are the results valid/trustworthy and credible?* Yes. [**Sample Selection**]: Diverse databases were used in the library search, including Ebscohost, PsyArticles, CINAHL, ProQuest, Medline, SocIndex, and Sage Sociology and Psychology Collections. [**Accuracy and Completeness**]: The researcher identified and used a recognized approach (Noblit & Hare, 1988). Search strategies and sample selection are described. Strengths and limitations of the study are discussed. Tables reflect the approach that was used. They also support the rigor and credibility of the analysis by reducing explanation of procedures and outcomes to easy-to-understand visual displays. This helps readers to focus on the key ideas contained in the report. [**Plausibility/Believability**]: Tables tracking and organizing the characteristics of the studies and the stages of the analytic process illustrate and increase confidence in the plausibility of the reported results.

◆ *What were the results of the study?* [**Approach/Purpose/Phenomenon**]: In this research, metasynthesis addresses what the researchers describe as "the problem with findings from individual studies … that end up as 'little islands of knowledge' (Glaser & Strauss, 1971, p. 181) or what Paterson, Thorne, Canam, and Jillings (2001) coined 'many individual pieces of the jigsaw puzzle' (p. 4). Because of minimal efforts to examine, synthesize, and draw inferences from a line of similar studies, advancement of the knowledge base is often precluded (Finfgeld, 2003; Walsh & Downe, 2005)" (p. 1290). [**Reported Results**]: The main themes and concepts from the six studies were reduced to nine themes. (a) *Strength and resilience stemming from a spiritual or religious base* was expressed as an intangible form (invoking God or a higher being) and also as tangible forms of support from organizational and nonorganizational spiritual or religious resources. (b) *Tension stemming from the definitions or standards of an ideal family* by their church/religion/culture "might [have been] deeply woven into these women's makeup, making it difficult for them to leave abusive relationships" (p. 1299). (c) *Tension stemming from religious or cultural definitions of gender role expectations* may also "trigger confusion and guilt" (p. 1300). (d) *The experience of a spiritual vacuum* described in four of the six studies "[did] not seem to revolve around religion but rather that transcendent dimension that guides an individual's life … [a loss of] personhood" (p. 1300). (e) *Reconstruction as part of the spiritual journey* involved spiritual growth and changing views on life's meaning with religious connotations. (f) *Recouping (or recovering) the spirit and self* "included learning interpersonal skills and self-awareness capacities and establishing personal boundaries … an integration process [for the women's previously fragmented identities]" (p. 1301). (g) *New interpretations of definitions of "submission"* involved decision making about what practices and beliefs were disempowering to women and noting features within religious guidelines (e.g., the context of scriptures) that might make deviation from particular tenets appropriate. (h) *Forgiveness as healing* was a theme in four studies that included not only forgiving abusive husbands or partners but also satisfying a need to feel forgiven. "Because of gender role expectations and the church community's disapproval of divorce, self-blame was prevalent, which made the need to feel forgiven that much stronger … [The need for God's forgiveness helped women] move on and heal" (p. 1302). (i) *Giving back—social activism* "was a product of these women's spiritual awakening and their recouping their sense of self and spirit … Sharing their stories [to reach out to other women and girls and instill values in their children was] at the heart of their social activism" (p. 1302).

◆ *Will the results help me in caring for my patients?* [**Relevance**]: The premise underlying the importance of developing knowledge in this area is that the effect of culture, spirituality, and religion on domestic violence may be one that enables victims to cope and find meaning or one that overtly and covertly promotes the abuse. Thus, it is important to develop a better understanding of how differences among these orientations may be harnessed or reframed by pulling together women's reported views on the topic.

[**Application**]: The author observes a need for collaboration on the part of practitioners, churches, and faith communities "to develop culturally competent best practices in working with domestic violence victims and survivors" (p. 1303). Healthcare providers could work with survivors and victims on rebuilding a "sense of self"; explore how race, culture, and ethnicity influence definitions of forgiveness; and find ways to connect individuals with their communities "so they can give back and recoup their sense of self" (pp. 1303–1304).

References

Carroll, K., Iedema, R., & Kerridge, R. (2008). Reshaping ICU ward round practices using video-reflexive ethnography. *Qualitative Health Research, 18*, 380–390.

Charmaz, K. (2006). *Constructing grounded theory: A practical guide through qualitative analysis.* Thousand Oaks, CA: Sage.

Cox, J., & Holden, J. (2003). *Perinatal mental health: A guide to the Edinburgh Postnatal Depression Scale (EPDS).* London: Gaskell.

Denz-Penhey, H., & Murdoch, J. C. (2008). Personal resiliency: Serious diagnosis and prognosis with unexpected quality outcomes. *Qualitative Health Research, 18*, 391–404.

Fetterman, D. (1998). *Ethnography: Step-by-step* (2nd ed.). Thousand Oaks, CA: Sage.

Finfgeld, D. L. (2003). Metasynthesis: The state of the art—So far. *Qualitative Health Research, 13*, 893–904.

Francis-Connolly, E. (2000). Toward an understanding of mothering: A comparison of two motherhood stages. *American Journal of Occupational Therapy, 54*, 281–289.

Glaser, B. (1978). *Theoretical sensitivity: Advances in the methodology of grounded theory.* Mill Valley, CA: Sociology Press.

Glaser, B. (1992). *Basics of grounded theory analysis: Emergence vs. forcing.* Mill Valley, CA: Sociology Press.

Glaser, B., & Strauss, A. (1971). *Status passage: A formal theory.* Chicago: Aldine.

Guba, E. G., & Lincoln, Y. S. (1989). *Fourth generation evaluation.* Newbury Park, CA: Sage.

Hsieh, H. F., & Shannon, S. E. (2005). Three approaches to qualitative content analysis. *Qualitative Health Research, 15*, 1277–1288.

Marcellus, L. (2008). (Ad)ministering love: Providing family foster care to infants with prenatal substance exposure. *Qualitative Health Research, 18*, 1220–1230.

Morgan, D. G., Crossley, M. F., Stewart, N. J., D'Arcy, C., Forbes, D. A., Normand, S. A., & Cammer, A. L. (2008). Taking the hit: Focusing on caregiver "error" masks organizational-level risk factors for nursing aide assault. *Qualitative Health Research, 18*, 334–346.

Noblit, G. W., & Hare, R. D. (1988). *Meta-ethnography: Synthesizing qualitative studies.* Newbury Park, CA: Sage.

Paterson, B. L., Thorne, S. E., Canam, C., & Jillings, C. (2001). *Meta-study of qualitative health research: A practical guide to meta-analysis and meta-synthesis.* Thousand Oaks, CA: Sage.

Porter, E. J. (1995). The life-world of older widows: The context of lived experience. *Journal of Women & Aging, 7*(4), 31–46.

Powers, B. A., & Knapp, T. R. (2006). *Dictionary of nursing theory and research* (3rd ed.). New York: Springer.

Riessman, C. K. (1990). Strategic uses of narrative in the presentation of self and illness. *Social Science and Medicine, 30*, 1195–1200.

Sandelowski, M. (1994). The use of quotes in qualitative research. *Research in Nursing & Health, 17*, 479–482.

Sandelowski, M. (1998). Writing a good read: Strategies for re-presenting qualitative data. *Research in Nursing & Health, 21*, 375–382.

Sandelowski, M. (2000). Whatever happened to qualitative description? *Research in Nursing & Health, 23*, 334–340.

Schutz, A., & Luckman, T. (1973). *The structures of the life-world* (R. M. Zaner & H. T. Engelhardt, Jr., Trans.). Evanston, IL: Northwestern University Press.

Scott, S. D., Estabrooks, C. A., Allen, M., & Pollock, C. (2008). A context of uncertainty: How context shapes nurses' research utilization behaviors. *Qualitative Health Research, 18*, 347–357.

Shojania, K. G., & Grimshaw, J. M. (2005). Evidence-based quality improvement: The state of the science. *Health Affairs, 24*, 138–151.

Spiegelberg, H. (1994). *The phenomenological movement: A historical introduction* (3rd revised and enlarged ed.). Dordrecht, the Netherlands: Kluwer Academic Press.

Strauss, A., & Corbin, J. (1990). *Basics of qualitative research: Grounded theory procedures and techniques.* Newbury Park, CA: Sage.

Sword, W., Busser, D., Ganann, R., McMillan, T., & Swinton, M. (2008). Women's care-seeking experiences after referral for postpartum depression. *Qualitative Health Research, 18*, 1161–1173.

Thomas, S. P., & Hall, J. M. (2008). Life trajectories of female child abuse survivors thriving in adulthood. *Qualitative Health Research, 18*, 149–166.

van Manen, M. (1990). *Researching lived experience: Human science for an action sensitive pedagogy.* London, Canada: Althouse.

Verhaeghe, S., Defloor, T., & Grypdonck, M. (2005). Stress and coping among families of patients with traumatic brain injury: A review of the literature. *Journal of Clinical Nursing, 14*, 1004–1012.

Walsh, D., & Downe, S. (2005). Meta-synthesis method for qualitative research: A literature review. *Journal of Advanced Nursing, 50*(2), 204–211.

Winstanley, J., Simpson, G., Tate, R., & Myles, B. (2006). Early indicators and contributors to psychological distress in relatives during rehabilitation following severe traumatic brain injury: Findings from the brain injury outcomes study. *Journal of Head Trauma Rehabilitation, 21*, 453–466.

Wongvatunyu, S., & Porter, E. J. (2008). Helping young adult children with traumatic brain injury: The life-world of mothers. *Qualitative Health Research, 18*, 1062–1074.

Woodgate, R. L., Ateah, C., & Secco, L. (2008). Living in a world of our own: The experience of parents who have a child with autism. *Qualitative Health Research, 18*, 1075–1083.

Yick, A. G. (2008). A metasynthesis of qualitative findings on the role of spirituality and religiosity among culturally diverse domestic violence survivors. *Qualitative Health Research, 18*, 1289–1306.

Appendix E
Example of a Health Policy Brief

ENSURING ACCESS TO SAFE, QUALITY, AND AFFORDABLE HEALTH CARE THROUGH A ROBUST NURSING WORKFORCE

Making the Case for Healthcare Reform

America's healthcare delivery system is in desperate need of reform. Since the early 1990s, health care appeared to shift from a system based on providing quality care to one driven by market-based economic models. Demands by the customers (business and government) to lower costs and adhere to a structured business plan overrode the public's ideal of health care as a humanitarian service.[1] The shift received significant attention. In 1995 the American Hospital Association referred to the changes as the "worst disaster to hit US hospitals," explaining that patient errors, malpractice suits, and union activities all increased under this flawed model.[1] Within the next six years, institutions such as the Health Research and Services Administration (HRSA) and the Institute of Medicine (IOM) looked critically at the failing system. Landmark IOM studies such as *"To Err Is Human"* and *"Crossing the Quality Chasm"* showed that the healthcare system was in crisis (Institute of Medicine).[2,3] Adverse outcomes were on the rise with as many as 98,000 Americans dying each year from avoidable medical errors (Institute of Medicine).[2] These numbers sent shockwaves throughout the healthcare community and on Capitol Hill. The basic premises of health care—quality and safety—were being compromised.

The national healthcare system is at a crossroads. It can no longer continue to function under the current circumstances, but there are positive aspects that must be retained. It is the role of the new Administration, Congress, and vested stakeholders to differentiate what must be kept, from what must be reformed. The nursing workforce fits squarely in both of these categories. Registered Nurses (RNs) are the backbone of the healthcare system representing the largest group of healthcare professionals with 2.4 million practicing nurses in the United States. Yet, the ongoing shortage of nurses is contributing to the breakdown of the nation's ability to ensure access to safe, quality, and affordable health care. Unfortunately, the demand for RNs continues to outpace the supply of new nurses entering the healthcare system each year.

As a stakeholder in healthcare reform, the American Association of Colleges of Nursing (AACN) offers its expertise by recommending that a significant investment be made to increase the capacity of nursing schools to educate more nurses. Without a robust nursing workforce, the healthcare system will not be able to offer safe, affordable, and quality health care. Outlined below is an overview of the nursing shortage crisis and AACN's specific recommendations of healthcare reform from the nursing education perspective.

Nursing Shortage

◆ According to the latest projections from the U.S. Bureau of Labor Statistics, more than one million new and replacement nurses will be needed by 2016.[4] This estimate takes into consideration the overburdened healthcare system, the growing complexity of nursing care, and the basic demand for nurses as the baby boomer population ages. However, the perception that "just more nurses" are needed is flawed. The greatest need is for nurses prepared at the baccalaureate and graduate levels.

Demand for a Highly Educated Nursing Workforce

◆ RNs provide services along the entire spectrum, including lifesaving interventions and preventative care. Patients who enter the nation's hospitals and healthcare facilities typically suffer from multiple comorbidities such as obesity, diabetes, and hypertension. More acute patients have fundamentally changed the intensity of nursing care. The changes in how health care is delivered have created demand for nursing personnel who can function with more independence in clinical decision making and case management, perform the traditional role of clinical caregiver, and teach patients how to comply with treatment regimens and maintain good health. Knowing that patients today are more complex and require an advanced level of specialized care, the need for nurses who are highly educated is critical. Therefore, the nursing shortage and its impact on patient care cannot be solved by simply increasing the pipeline. The workforce must be fortified with more highly educated and well-qualified nurses, specifically nurses with a baccalaureate degree or higher.

◆ Unlike graduates of diploma or associate-degree nursing programs, the nurse with a baccalaureate degree is prepared to practice in all healthcare settings—critical care, outpatient care, public health, and mental health. In addition to the liberal learning and global perspective gained from a four-year baccalaureate education, the curriculum includes clinical, scientific, decision-making, and humanistic skills, including preparation in community health, patient education, as well as nursing management and leadership. Such skills are essential for today's professional nurse who must make quick, sometimes life-and-death decisions; design and manage a comprehensive plan of nursing care; understand a patient's treatment, symptoms, and danger signs; supervise other nursing personnel and support staff; master advanced technology; guide patients through the maze of healthcare resources in a community; and educate patients on healthcare options and how to adopt healthy lifestyles.

◆ The National Advisory Council on Nurse Education and Practice, policy advisors to Congress and the U.S. Secretary for Health and Human Services on nursing issues, has urged that at least two-thirds of the nurse workforce hold baccalaureate or higher degrees in nursing by 2010. Currently, only 47.2% of nurses hold degrees at the baccalaureate level and above.[5] Organizations such as AACN, the American Nurses Association, and the American Organization of Nurse Executives are calling for all professional registered nurses to be educated at the baccalaureate level in an effort to adequately prepare nurses for their challenging and complex roles. However, this task is not easily achieved.

The Nurse Faculty Shortage

◆ The nursing educational system in the United States is significantly strained. Despite marked increases in nursing school enrollment and graduations, capacity barriers have prohibited schools from accepting more students. Last year AACN reported that 40,285 qualified applicants were turned away from baccalaureate and graduate nursing programs. The top reason cited by schools of nursing for not increasing enrollment was a lack of faculty. According to a *Special Survey on Vacant Faculty Positions* released by AACN in July 2008, data show a national nurse faculty vacancy rate of 7.6% (American Association of Colleges of Nursing, 2008).[6] Most of the vacancies (88.1%) were faculty positions requiring or preferring a doctoral degree (American Association of Colleges of Nursing, 2008).[6] Yet, enrollment in research-focused doctoral nursing programs was up by only 0.9% from the 2006-2007 academic year (American Association of Colleges of Nursing, 2008).[6] More concerning, only one in ten of our nation's registered nurse hold master's or doctoral degrees, which are required to teach. If action is not taken to educate the next generation of nurses and nurse faculty, health care in America will continue to suffer.

The Solution

As Congress looks towards healthcare reform, AACN strongly suggests that the nursing workforce be increased. A robust nursing workforce is needed before quality, access, and affordability of health care can be addressed. AACN is committed to working with Congress to address the nursing and nurse faculty shortage through legislative efforts that not only increase the number of nurses but ensure that they are qualified to practice in a demanding healthcare environment. Provided below are AACN's top recommendations to Congress as they address the nursing shortage as a component of healthcare reform:

◆ **Reauthorize the Title VIII Nursing Workforce Development Programs, which are authorized under the Public Health Service Act (42 U.S.C. 296 et seq.).**

  ● Over the last 44 years, Nursing Workforce Development programs have addressed all aspects of nursing shortages—education, practice, retention, and recruitment. As the largest source of federal funding for nursing education, these programs bolster RN education from entry-level preparation through graduate study. The Title VIII programs award grants to schools of nursing, as well as direct support to nurses and nursing students through loans, scholarships, traineeships, and programmatic grants. By supporting the supply and distribution of qualified nurses, these programs help to ensure that nurses are available to provide care to individuals in all healthcare settings. Additionally, the Title VIII programs also favor institutions that educate nurses for practice in rural and medically underserved communities. However, authorization of all Title VIII programs has expired.

◆ **Increase funding for the Title VIII Nursing Workforce Development Programs.**

  ● During the nursing shortage of the 1970s, Congress addressed the problem by providing increased levels of funding for Title VIII programs. Specifically, in 1973 Congress appropriated $160.61 million to the authorities; the largest appropriation of funds Title VIII has ever received. In today's dollars this would be a commitment of over $763 million. Currently, Title VIII receives $156.05 million to focus on a similar, critical national nursing shortage. Compounding the impact of this low appropriation level is the stagnant nature of Title VIII funding in the face of escalating education costs. In FY 2006 and 2007, $149.68 million was appropriated to Title VIII. This allocation supported 75,946 nursing students and nurses in 2006 while only 71,729 in 2007, due in part to increased tuition costs and inflation.

References

1. Curtin, L. L. (2007). The perfect storm: Managed care, aging adults, and a nursing shortage. *Nursing Administration Quarterly, 31*(2), 105–110.
2. Institute of Medicine. (2002). *To err is human: Building a safer health system.* Washington, DC: The National Academies Press.
3. Institute of Medicine. (2001). *Crossing the quality chasm: A new health system for the 21st century.* Washington, DC: The National Academies Press.
4. Bureau of Labor and Statistics. (2007). *Occupational projections to 2016.* Accessed July 29, 2008, from www.bls.gov/opub/mlr/2007/11/art5full.pdf
5. Health Resources and Services Administration. (2004). *National sample survey of registered nurses.* Accesssed February 19, 2008, from http://bhpr.hrsa.gov/healthworkforce/reports/rnpopulation/preliminaryfindings.htm
6. American Association of Colleges of Nursing. (2008). *Special survey on vacant faculty positions.* Washington, DC.

Appendix F
Example of a Press Release

NIH ⟩ **National Institutes of Health**
Turning Discovery Into Health

For Immediate Release: Tuesday, September 10, 2013
Lifestyle intervention improves high schoolers' health, social skills, grades

NIH-supported research shows promise for teens at risk of becoming overweight, obese

A teacher-delivered intervention program promoting healthy lifestyles improved health behaviors, social skills, severe depression, and academic performance in high school adolescents, a study has found. Routine integration of such programs into health education curricula in high school settings may be an effective way to prevent high-risk teen populations from becoming overweight or obese, and could lead to improved physical health, psychosocial skills, and academic outcomes, according to the study.

The study, supported by the National Institute of Nursing Research (NINR), part of the National Institutes of Health, appears in the online September issue of the American Journal of Preventive Medicine. It is one of the first studies to report multiple immediate improvements that were sustained over time using a teacher-delivered, cognitive-behavioral skills-building intervention program incorporated into a high school health education class. Cognitive-behavioral skills training teaches coping techniques, social functioning skills, and problem solving skills.

The randomized controlled trial examined the short- and long-term effects of the COPE (Creating Opportunities for Personal Empowerment) Healthy Lifestyles (TEEN) Thinking, Emotions, Exercise, Nutrition Program. The COPE TEEN program is an intervention targeting obesity, social skills, and mental health. The study was led by Bernadette Melnyk, Ph.D., R.N., The Ohio State University's chief wellness officer and dean of the College of Nursing.

"Nutrition and physical activity-based interventions are often tested when it comes to preventing obesity, but mental and psychosocial health can also be contributing factors," said NINR Director Dr. Patricia Grady. "This NINR-supported study highlights the importance of an evidence-based lifestyle intervention that addresses the complex interplay of these factors."

The researchers measured healthy lifestyle behaviors, body mass index (BMI), depressive symptoms, social skills, and the academic performance of 779 culturally diverse 14- to 16-year-old high school students, randomized to receive the COPE TEEN program or an attention control program. At the end of the program, COPE TEEN participants had significantly higher levels of physical activity, as measured by daily pedometer steps (an average of 13,861 steps per day compared to an average of 9,619 steps per day), and had a significantly lower mean BMI than the control group.

COPE TEEN adolescents scored higher averages on a social skills scale measuring cooperation, assertion, and academic competence, and earned higher grades in the health course in which the intervention was given. They also reported significantly lower levels of alcohol use than teens not receiving the intervention (13 percent vs. 20 percent, respectively). Students with high depression scores prior to the intervention showed significantly lower depression scores that dropped from severe depressive symptoms into the normal range following COPE compared to similar students in the control group.
S. Department of Health & Human Services

575

The COPE TEEN intervention program consisted of a 15-session education and cognitive-behavioral skills-building program taught by teachers once-a-week in a required health class. Each session consisted of 15 to 20 minutes of physical activity (e.g., walking, dancing, and kick boxing movements). The pedometers reinforced the physical activity component of the COPE program; students were asked to increase their step counts each week and to track their daily steps.

Six months after completing the intervention program, COPE teens retained a significantly lower BMI, and were less likely to have moved from the healthy weight category to an overweight or obese category relative to control group participants. For the COPE teens, 143 teens remained in the healthy weight category at six months, only four moved into the overweight category and none of the students progressed to the obese category. In the control group, 187 remained in the healthy weight category while 15 progressed to the overweight category; and three moved into the obese category.

Overall, the study results suggest that combining health education with cognitive-behavioral skills-building may be an effective way to prevent and treat overweight and obesity in teens.

"Further research is needed to continue to evaluate the effectiveness of the COPE program on a wider scale, including other groups of high-risk teens and an adapted version for middle-school children" said Dr. Melnyk. "But this study shows that the intervention can be a promising approach for promoting healthy lifestyles, improving psychosocial health and enhancing academic outcomes in a setting where teens spend a significant amount of time — in the classroom — and by teachers, who have been shown to be able to sustain longer-term, positive outcomes."

Dr. Melnyk noted that the practical nature of the intervention, financially and in its ease of implementation, is a particular strength.

"In light of school budget reductions and challenges, it is critical that the intervention be feasible, cost-effective and sustainable," said Dr. Melnyk. "By delivering the program through high school teachers, hiring additional health professionals to deliver the program is not necessary. Long after the study ends, trained teachers can continue to deliver the COPE program and improve a variety of important outcomes in their students."

NINR supports basic and clinical research that develops the knowledge to build the scientific foundation for clinical practice, prevent disease and disability, manage and eliminate symptoms caused by illness, and enhance end-of-life and palliative care. For more information about NINR, visit the website at http://www.ninr.nih.gov.

About the National Institutes of Health (NIH): NIH, the nation's medical research agency, includes 27 Institutes and Centers and is a component of the U.S. Department of Health and Human Services. NIH is the primary federal agency conducting and supporting basic, clinical, and translational medical research, and is investigating the causes, treatments, and cures for both common and rare diseases. For more information about NIH and its programs, visit www.nih.gov.

NIH...Turning Discovery Into Health

Appendix G

An Example of a Successful Media Dissemination Effort: Patient-Directed Music Intervention to Reduce Anxiety and Sedative Exposure in Critically Ill Patients Receiving Mechanical Ventilatory Support

Linda L. Chlan and Kathryn Kelley

If an intriguing story with strong evidence appears in a top medical journal, will anyone still pay attention to it? What follows is an example of a media dissemination effort and the media attention that emanated from a research paper published in a major medical journal that highlights a coordinated, team-based approach between the paper's author and communications professionals at The Ohio State University (OSU).

PUBLICATION NOTIFICATION AND INITIATION OF MEDIA DISSEMINATION EFFORTS

Linda Chlan, PhD, RN, FAAN, who arrived at The Ohio State University College of Nursing in January 2013 as a distinguished professor of Symptom Management Research, contacted Kathryn Kelley, chief advancement officer at the Ohio State College of Nursing, in early May 2013 to confidentially inform her of a research manuscript that would be posted 2 weeks later in *JAMA: The Journal of the American Medical Association* but would be embargoed until that time. In an introductory conversation, Kathryn had informed Linda of the approach she had recommended during faculty meetings; offering advance notice of a published article meant that she could employ the central University Communications media relations staff with robust resources available at their fingertips. Their staff boast a strong reputation for their research writing and hold the primary university license for EurekAlert! an online scientific news service operated by the American Association for the Advancement of Science and enjoy established relationships with large networks of national media who cover scientific, medical, and other academic research.

For a story of this magnitude, Kathryn reached out to provide a general overview of the research study and findings to Emily Caldwell, assistant director of Research and Innovation Communications within University Communications at Ohio State, who immediately contacted Linda to set up a face-to-face appointment. She reviewed the research being published and took notes to capture the personality of the story through Linda's passion, dedication, and focus toward music therapy as a means to lower anxiety and reduce the need for sedative medications while patients are on mechanical ventilators.

Dear Dr. Chlan,

Congratulations on your JAMA paper. Kathryn has filled me in on some of the info. I would like to write a news release about the paper. Ideally, we would send that release out under embargo, password protected so only reporters who honor embargoes can access it, on or about May 15 to give reporters a chance to work on it in advance of the publication on the following Monday…I am happy to contact JAMA directly to ask for it. We work with embargoed material in high-profile journals routinely—Nature, Cell, etc. But even if for some reason I can't get the paper, may I interview you—possibly Monday? I am wide open that day and could be at your doorstep whenever you prefer. Tuesday is also a possibility, after about 10:30.

I believe I saw in the email thread that you'll be at a meeting on the day of publication—this is another good reason to have the release available earlier, so reporters can reach you to prepare their stories in advance. I will also be on vacation that day, but colleagues of mine will be able to assist with reporter requests for the paper or efforts to contact you remotely.

Many thanks,
Emily

Linda wanted to make sure that the embargo was upheld, so Kathryn took extra care to validate the research communications group, whom she had collaborated with for over a decade, and their expertise in working with The *JAMA* Network. In short, all publication rules and regulations were followed.

By May 15, Emily had finished her draft for review by Linda and Kathryn. The method that research communications staff take with stories is that they use an "inverted pyramid" to prioritize the content with a summary of the main findings in the first few paragraphs in as layperson-friendly language as possible. Emily included a quote from Linda and provided information about the journal in which the research is cited. Then more details were provided about the research that media might cut from the news story due to space limitations. That approach allowed the essential information at the top to remain in the story. In this case, Emily included mention of *JAMA* closer to the top of the story because of the journal's prestige.

As stated above, any media story about the article was not to be published until after the May 20, 2013, 2 PM embargo. The embargo date coincided with an invited paper presentation at the American Thoracic Society (ATS) international conference by Linda on the main findings contained in the *JAMA* article. *JAMA*'s policy is that any pre-embargo dissemination of the paper should come from their office. That would provide a valid media outlet with a copy prior to the embargo, in addition to the abstract that was available on a website link. A reporter could receive a copy 5 days prior to publication. The password-protected posting of the release would allow enough time for reporters to contact Linda for comments before the story broke.

Emily posted the story under password protection on EurekAlert! and Newswise online media distribution services on May 16, 2013. Kathryn has a media distribution account, as well, although the decision was made to go with the university-wide primary accounts. *JAMA*'s press office was informed that the news release would be offered on the password-protected sites with prominent language about the embargo. Reporters were directed to the *JAMA* site to request copies of the original research study until the embargo lifted.

The press release written by Emily Caldwell of OSU was posted on the Ohio State Research News and the College of Nursing websites on May 20, 2013, as follows:

Listening to Favorite Music Lowers Anxiety, Sedation in ICU Patients on Ventilators

Clinical Trial Shows Benefits of Non-Medication Strategy to Address Potential Side Effects

COLUMBUS, Ohio (May 20, 2013)—New research suggests that for some hospitalized ICU patients on mechanical ventilators, using headphones to listen to their favorite types of music could lower anxiety and reduce their need for sedative medications.

In a clinical trial, the option to listen to music lowered anxiety, on average, by 36.5 percent, and reduced the number of sedative doses by 38 percent and the intensity of sedation by 36 percent compared to ventilated intensive care unit patients who did not receive the music intervention. These effects were seen, on average, five days into the study.

The research is published online in the *Journal of the American Medical Association*.

Researchers first assessed the patients' musical preferences and kept a continuous loop of music running on bedside CD players. When patients wished to listen to music, they were able to put on headphones that were equipped with a system that time- and date-stamped and recorded each use.

Professional guidelines recommend that pain, agitation and delirium be carefully managed in the ICU, with the goal of keeping mechanically ventilated patients comfortable and awake. However, the researchers acknowledged that over-sedation is common in these patients, which can lead to both physiological problems linked to prolonged immobility and psychological issues that include fear and frustration over not being able to communicate, and even post-traumatic stress disorder.

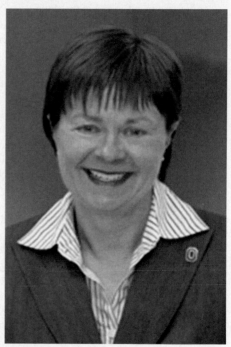

"We're trying to address the problem of over-sedation from a very different perspective, by empowering patients. Some patients do not want control, but many patients want to know what is going on with their care," said Linda Chlan, distinguished professor of symptom management research in The Ohio State University's College of Nursing and lead author of the study.

"But I'm not talking about using music in place of the medical plan of care. These findings do not suggest that clinicians should place headphones on just any ICU patient. For the intervention to have the most impact and to have the desired effect of reducing anxiety, the music has to be familiar and comforting to the patient—which is why tailoring the music collection for the patient to listen to was key to the success of this study."

Chlan also presented the research Monday (5/20) at the American Thoracic Society International Conference in Philadelphia.

Chlan and colleagues conducted the study with 373 patients in 12 ICUs at five hospitals in the Minneapolis–St. Paul area. Of those, 126 patients were randomized to receive the patient-directed music intervention, 125 received usual care and 122 were in an active control group and could self-initiate the use of noise-canceling headphones. All patients had to be alert enough to give their own consent to participate.

A music therapist assessed each patient in the music group to develop a collection that met the patient's preferences. This was no easy task, as the patients are not able to speak when they are on a ventilator. The research team developed a screening method specifically for this part of the study. Researchers purchased downloadable files and placed up to 1,000 selections on each patient's mp3-compatible CD player.

Researchers instructed patients to use the intervention if they were feeling anxious, wanted to relax, or needed quiet time. Nurses were asked to prompt patients twice during each shift about their interest in listening to music. In weaker patients, nurses helped with placement of the headphones.

In all patients, researchers performed daily assessments of anxiety and two measures of sedative exposure to any of eight commonly used medications: intensity of the medication and frequency of doses. Anxiety was measured with a visual analog scale that asked patients to describe their anxiety by pointing to a chart anchored by the statements "not anxious at all" and "most anxious ever." Patients remained in the study as long as they were on ventilators, up to a maximum of 30 days.

Study patients were hospitalized for a variety of conditions that primarily included lung problems or infections. The main reasons for ventilation were respiratory failure or respiratory distress. The study showed that patients in the music group listened to music, on average, for almost 80 minutes per day, and patients with noise-canceling headphones used them for an average of 34 minutes per day. No relationship was found between time spent using the device and anxiety, but researchers did note that more patients listening to music were liberated from the mechanical ventilator than were patients from either other group at the end of the study.

A complex statistical analysis of the data showed that significant reductions in anxiety and sedation could be seen in patients in the music intervention within five days when they were compared to patients who received usual care. Patients using noise-canceling headphones showed some improvements in anxiety and lower sedation intensity, but the effects were not as strong as those seen in the music group.

"There is something there with noise-canceling headphones, but the music is so much more powerful. With the music, we were able to show a simultaneous reduction in anxiety and in sedation," Chlan said. "When we listen to music, our entire brain lights up. We want to capitalize on the pleasant, comforting memories associated with music because it occupies brain channels that otherwise would be occupied by an anxiety-producing stimulus. That's why music is so much more than just something nice to listen to."

A former medical intensive care unit nurse, Chlan now leads a research program that emphasizes testing treatment strategies that complement traditional medical approaches to ICU care.

"I think about tackling the modifiable risk factors. And sedation is directly modifiable because it is controlled by the clinician. Nonpharmacological, integrative interventions like music bring in a piece that does not induce adverse side effects and does not contribute to ICU-acquired problems," she said.

She and colleagues now are working on making the highly controlled research protocol more friendly to standard hospital practices. "If this is going to have wide clinical impact, that really has to be done," she said.

The most important outcome, Chlan said, would be measurable reduction in ventilated patients' anxiety.

"I think anxiety gets lost in the mix when we are assessing patients. We have federal guidelines about assessing pain. I would like us to have some guidelines about assessing anxiety because that is one of the most frequently occurring symptoms that patients report about being in an intensive care unit," she said.

This research was funded by a grant from the National Institute of Nursing Research. Chlan, who joined Ohio State in January, led this study while a member of the faculty at the University of Minnesota. Co-authors include Craig Weinert, Annie Heiderscheit, Mary Fran Tracy, Debra Skaar and Kay Savik, all of the University of Minnesota, and Jill Guttormson of Marquette University.

COORDINATION OF MEDIA REQUESTS FOR INTERVIEWS

Media requests came fast and furious in the days and weekend leading up to Linda's paper presentation at the ATS international conference and the *JAMA* article posting. Kathryn was responsible for fielding requests and prioritizing them for Linda, which required determining the reporter's deadline and the demographic scope of the media outlet. As is standard these days, most questions were emailed, which allowed for more time and convenience in responding to reporter queries.

The *JAMA* network staff was also informed of the primary media contacts for reporters to contact, in addition to Linda. Since both Emily and Kathryn were going on vacation the weekend before the ATS presentation and *JAMA* online journal posting, a schedule was arranged that allowed for no downtime in responding quickly to journalists.

Kathryn responded to the reporters as quickly as possible to let them know Linda's schedule and that she would try to get to the answers or provide her availability as soon as she was able, given her travel to the ATS conference. When Kathryn was not available, she forwarded the requests to Emily to handle. Coincidentally, on the way to her flight to Richmond, VA, Kathryn noticed Linda waiting in line to board her flight to Philadelphia, PA, for the ATS international conference, offering a few minutes to hash out more details on prioritization and to determine available times in between flight and conference schedules. The national news reporters who had requested interviews within the last 24 hours were highlighted and prioritized for follow-up at the earliest available moment. The first media representative to enquire about Linda's research was from a freelance writer in New Mexico. CBS Radio conducted an interview during a 5-minute break in Linda's conference schedule, and then *US News & World Report* made contact. *Huffington Post* also ran the story. Given the large national reach of these particular media outlets and the possible snowball effect of them running the story on other news organizations, Kathryn considered these as top priorities for immediate response.

Another important element is the need to promote a research story internally—the dean, associate deans, administrators, faculty, and staff within the college and throughout the university are primary audiences, as they have the greatest potential for to spark further collaboration and promotion of fellow researchers based in their home court. OSU is the only campus in the nation to combine seven health sciences colleges and a comprehensive academic medical center, The Ohio State University Wexner Medical Center, so opportunities for interprofessional collaboration is par for the course. An e-mail with the press release and link was sent out to the College of Nursing, the health sciences colleges, and the university's faculty and staff newsletters.

In June, several other journalists from *Psychiatric News* and the American College of Physicians *Hospitalist* magazine also contacted Linda, as well as a reporter from *Reader's Digest*. A local public radio program director read the research story in the faculty and staff newspaper and requested an interview.

Some reporters, such as the host of the public radio music program, asked if Linda envisioned the music therapy approach sometimes taking the place of drugs. Others asked questions about the standard practice that this therapy might enhance. Many requested that the answers be provided in layperson's terms; Linda did an excellent job of explaining the impact of her study and the effects observed in patients. They also asked the "so what" questions: why is this work important, what is the impact on patients, and what can be learned in this study? And they wanted to know next steps—would this propel Linda toward a follow-up study on music therapy for ICU patients?

The media placements were tracked by Google news alerts and an online media monitoring service. This list is still not exhaustive, since the media tracking service may not have registered multiple stories that resulted from the UPI wire service or reprints from some of the major news outlets in journals and local papers with more limited readership.

Media placements that have been recorded as of July 5, 2013:

- CBS Radio
- Toronto's The Globe and Mail
- MedPage Today
- State of Health blog
- AACN Critical Care
- American Thoracic Society News
- UPI wire services
- MDLinx
- US News & World Report
- Philadelphia Inquirer

◆ Huffington Post
◆ Nurse Practitioner News
◆ Critical Care SmartBrief
◆ WOSU—Music in Mid-Ohio
◆ MENAFN News (Middle East North Africa Financial Network)

Pending placements from reporter inquiries:

◆ American College of Physicians Hospitalist magazine (Success Story)
◆ Psychiatric News
◆ Reader's Digest

Internal Ohio State media outlets:

◆ OSU Today (faculty and staff e-newsletter)
◆ onCampus (faculty and staff biweekly newspaper)
◆ OneSource (Ohio State Wexner Medical Center intranet)

NEXT STEPS

Any media relations person loves a story that has "legs," and this story continues to generate media interest. Since the initial release in May 17, separate media outlets have requested information and/or published the story in their respective newspaper, radio shows, and magazines. The "evergreen" quality of this story bears continued promotion; the next step will be to set up an appointment with the director of national broadcast news at Ohio State's University Communications to interview Linda. These video clips will be distributed to TV and radio journalists in the field, especially when the topic is trending, which means that a topic has become popular or is the cause of much discussion on a news or social media website.

BE PREPARED: LESSONS LEARNED TO DISSEMINATE AND APPLY TO YOUR RESEARCH FINDINGS

How can you achieve this level of success to promote your research? Lessons for those writing research papers can consider the following tips:

◆ Before the paper is submitted to the journal, find out what media relations resources and staff are available at your university, if you don't already know.
◆ Trust the professionals—we had to take a leap of faith with all parties involved in the proper dissemination of the story and fielding of media relations queries.
◆ Make sure you have established an internal mechanism for reporter queries—both the college and the university media relations staff persons were going on vacation, yet they worked out a schedule that still allowed for quick responses to journalists.
◆ Work to build a relationship between the journal editors and your media relations staff for clear communication about media embargoes and quick turnaround for releasing journal articles once that embargo clears.
◆ Build availability into your schedule—there are fewer reporters with the closing of major newspapers nationally, and they are definitely struggling under the "make do with less" environment. In short, they may have as little time as you do. The rule of thumb is to acknowledge their initial inquiry in 15 to 30 minutes; if you delay the response, they may move on to another story. Also, make sure you allow time for interviews as Linda did, even if the time available is only 5 to 10 minutes in the midst of a busy conference.

- Relationships with media can grow over time—you never know if a local reporter may work for a national news outlet in the future.
- You may ask to review any written material before it is published to check for accuracy. If a reporter has a generous deadline, such as for a magazine, this may be possible; sometimes, they do not have this luxury or are not willing to share their materials.
- Provide your cell phone number and e-mail to make it easier for reporters to contact you, while making sure the appointed media relations staffer is also included as back up to provide background information and statistics.
- Media coaching—every researcher and faculty member could use even a little—allows you to learn about organizing your responses in layperson-friendly language and how to correspond with media. Invite a media relations staff person to explain the process and offer tips/techniques at a faculty meeting.

CONCLUSION

Garnering media attention from the publication of research findings can be thrilling for the researcher. However, responding to multiple media requests in lay language can be a daunting experience for a majority of faculty members lacking media savvy without any media training. We hope that our experiences and lessons learned can provide the researcher with some useful information to promote one's research and the significance of those research findings while effectively dealing with multiple media outlets using a team-based approach.

Appendix H
Approved Consent Form for a Study

CONSENT

Behavioral/Social Science

IRB Protocol Number: 2012B0367

IRB Approval Date: August 21, 2012

Version: 2

The Ohio State University Consent to Participate in Research

Study Title: Coping in College Students: A Pilot Study

Researchers: Bernadette Melnyk, PhD, RN, CPNP/PMHNP, FAAN; Megan Amaya, PhD

This is a consent form for research participation. It contains important information about this study and what to expect if you decide to participate.

Your participation is voluntary.

Please consider the information carefully. Feel free to email questions to Dr. Megan Amaya at Amaya.13@ osu.edu before making your decision whether or not to participate. If you decide to participate, you will be asked to indicate your consent to participate in this study. You may print a copy of this electronic form for your records.

Purpose:

The purpose of this study is to describe stress and coping in college students before and after they take their freshman survey course. You will be completing questionnaires in week 1 of your survey course, week 14, and approximately 4 and 12 months after you take your survey course. You will answer a demographic questionnaire along with three surveys about stress and coping and an evaluation questionnaire about your freshman survey course.

Procedures/Tasks:

If you participate in this study, you will consent to participate in the study via Carmen, answer a demographic questionnaire and three online survey questionnaires about your stress and coping at four time points, and receive a $5 gift certificate each time that you complete the questionnaires.

Duration:

You will be in the study for a total of 15 months. You will complete the survey at the beginning of the semester, toward the end of the semester, at the end of spring semester (April), and 1 year later (April 2015). Each survey you complete should take approximately 15 to 20 minutes in duration, for approximate total of 2 hours for 15 months.

You may leave the study at any time. If you decide to stop participating in the study, there will be no penalty to you, and you will not lose any benefits to which you are otherwise entitled. Your decision will not affect your future relationship with The Ohio State University.

Risks and Benefits:

The benefits of participating in the study include increasing participant awareness of their own thoughts, feelings, stress, emotional health state, and coping skills.

The potential risk to the participant may include sharing personal and sensitive information in the online questionnaire.

Confidentiality:

Efforts will be made to keep your study-related information confidential. However, there may be circumstances where this information must be released. For example, personal information regarding your participation in this study may be disclosed if required by state law. Also, your records may be reviewed by the following groups (as applicable to the research):

◆ Office for Human Research Protections or other federal, state, or international regulatory agencies

◆ The Ohio State University Institutional Review Board or Office of Responsible Research Practices

◆ The sponsor, if any, or agency (including the Food and Drug Administration for FDA-regulated research) supporting the study

In addition, an investigator on the research team will score your survey within 24 to 48 hours after you complete them to make sure students who have high anxiety or depression are referred to their necessary medical personnel if they need it. In the event that you indicate any potential for self-harm, it will be necessary to break confidentiality for your safety and student counseling services will be notified.

We will work to make sure that no one sees your survey responses without approval. But, because we are using the Internet, there is a chance that someone could access your online responses without permission. In some cases, this information could be used to identify you.

Your data will be protected with a code to reduce the risk that other people can view the responses.

Incentives:
To compensate you for participating in this study, each participant in the College of Social Work and College of Nursing will receive a $5 gift card to Bruegger's Bagels every time they complete the survey. Each participant at the Newark and Mansfield campus will receive a $5 gift card to Starbucks every time they complete the survey. This totals to $20 per participant over the course of the study. Your gift cards will be mailed to your preferred place of residence. You will need to state your preferred address in the demographic questions located in the initial survey, conducted through a secure, online, Checkbox survey. The gift card will be placed in an envelope and sent through US postal service to your preferred address.

Participant Rights:
You may refuse to participate in this study without penalty or loss of benefits to which you are otherwise entitled. If you are a student or employee at Ohio State, your decision will not affect your grades or employment status.

If you choose to participate in the study, you may discontinue participation at any time without penalty or loss of benefits. By signing this form, you do not give up any personal legal rights you may have as a participant in this study.

An Institutional Review Board responsible for human subjects research at The Ohio State University reviewed this research project and found it to be acceptable, according to applicable state and federal regulations and University policies designed to protect the rights and welfare of participants in research.

Contacts and Questions:
For questions, concerns, or complaints about the study you may contact **Dr. Megan Amaya, co-investigator**.

For questions about your rights as a participant in this study or to discuss other study-related concerns or complaints with someone who is not part of the research team, you may contact Ms. Sandra Meadows in the Office of Responsible Research Practices at 1-800-678-6251.

If you are injured as a result of participating in this study or for questions about a study-related injury, you may contact Dr. Megan Amaya.

Signing the Consent Form:
I have read (or someone has read to me) this form and I am aware that I am being asked to participate in a research study. I have had the opportunity to ask questions and have had them answered to my satisfaction. I voluntarily agree to participate in this study.

Subject's Signature_____

Printed first and last name_____

Date_____

I am not giving up any legal rights by signing this form. I will be given a copy of this form.

Appendix I

System-Wide ARCC Evidence-Based Practice Mentor Role Description

ORGANIZATIONAL CULTURE	1. Role Responsibilities: Assesses organization for readiness & sustainability of an EBP culture with valid & reliable instruments
	Activities include, but are not limited to:
	  ▪ **Evaluates decision making pattern across disciplines**
	  ▪ **Reviews and leads revision of philosophy to reflect EBP**
	  ▪ **Establishes a critical mass of healthcare providers with knowledge & skills in EBP**
	  ▪ **Conducts other ARCC interventions (e.g., journal club, EBP rounds) to foster an EBP culture**

	Feedback:

PROFESSIONAL PRACTICE	2. Role Responsibilities: Stimulates, facilitates, and educates nursing staff toward a culture of evidence-based practice.
	Activities include, but are not limited to:
	  • **Leads regularly scheduled classes with varying levels of complexity to educate point-of-care staff about using evidence in practice**
	  • **Provides in-house projects to foster point-of-care staff's use of external & internal evidence in making clinical decisions**

	Feedback:

INTERNAL & EXTERNAL EVIDENCE	3. Role Responsibilities: Mentors point-of-care staff in generating evidence through participating in studies and outcome management, evidence-based QI, and EBP implementation projects.
	Activities include, but are not limited to:
	  • **Assists with study or project design and proposal development**
	  • **Facilitates data analysis for research and evidence-based implementation & QI projects**
	  • **Develops and sustains processes that facilitate corroboration of internal & external evidence**

	Feedback:

TEAMWORK	4. Role Responsibilities: Acts as Chair or Co-chair for House-Wide Evidence-Based Practice z Committee
	Activities include, but are not limited to:
	  • **Collaborates with co-chair in planning agenda that is focused on house-wide clinical issues**
	  • **Reviews ongoing research and QI projects at each meeting**
	  • **Facilitates teamwork on house-wide evidence-implementation projects**
	  • **Discusses implications of project outcome data for future practice & policy change**

	Feedback:

INTER-DISCIPLINARY TEAM COLLABORATION	5. Role Responsibilities: Collaborates & fosters collaboration among healthcare providers in the use of evidence in clinical decision-making.
	Activities include, but are not limited to:
	  • **Discusses practice concerns with various clinician groups to foster best practices**
	  • **Participates in interdisciplinary groups in relation to use of research in decision-making activities**

	Feedback:

ACADEMIC & SERVICE PARTNERSHIP	6. Role Responsibilities: Serves as a liaison between hospital and university professors.
	Activities include, but are not limited to:
	  • **Solicits and facilitates collaborative research opportunities with university professors**
	  • **Partners with university professors in development of nursing research proposals**

	Feedback:

KNOWLEDGE TRANSLATION	7. Role Responsibilities: Uses external & internal evidence to foster best practice.
	Activities include, but are not limited to:
	  • **Translates external & internal evidence for point-of-care staff in clinical decision-making**
	  • **Uses external & internal evidence to stimulate change in standards of practice**

	Feedback:

RETURN ON INVESTMENT (ROI) FOR EBP	8. Role Responsibilities: Fosters & assists with measurement of outcomes based on evidence.
	Activities include, but are not limited to:
	  • **Administers budget for EBP implementation (QI) & research generation**
	  ▪ **Generates income through contributions/grants/ participation in research generation with various academic and other partners**

	Feedback:

Appendix J

ARCC Timeline for an EBP Implementation Project

ARCC Timeline for an EBP Implementation Project

PICOT Question:		
Team Members:		
EBP Mentor & Contact Info:		
Preliminary Checkpoint A	• Describe the chosen EBP model(s) and how it/they will guide the implementation project	Notes:
Preliminary Checkpoint B	• Who are the stakeholders for your project • Active (on the implementation team) & supportive (not on the team, but essential to success) • Identify project team roles & leadership • Begin acquisition of any necessary approvals for project implementation and dissemination (e.g., system leadership, unit leadership, ethics board [IRB]) • *Consult with EBP mentor*	Notes & Progress:
Checkpoint One	• Hone PICOT question & assure team is prepared • Build EBP knowledge & skills • *Consult with EBP mentor*	Notes & Progress:
Checkpoint Two	• Conduct literature search & retain studies that meet criteria for inclusion • Connect with librarian • Meet with implementation group— TEAM BUILD • *Consult with EBP mentor*	Notes & Progress:
Checkpoint Three	• Critically appraise literature • Meet with group to discuss how completely evidence answers question; pose follow-up questions and re-review the literature as necessary • *Consult with EBP mentor*	Notes & Progress:
Checkpoint Four	• Meet with group • Summarize evidence with focus on implications for practice & conduct interviews with content experts as necessary to benchmark • Begin formulating detailed plan for implementation of evidence • Include who must know about the project, when they will know, how they will know • *Consult with EBP mentor*	Notes & Progress:

Checkpoint Five	• Define project purpose—connect the evidence & the project • Define baseline data collection source(s) (e.g., existing dataset, electronic health record), methods, & measures • Define post project outcome indicators of a successful project • Gather outcome measures • Write data collection protocol • Write the project protocol (data collection fits in this document) • Finalize any necessary approvals for project implementation & dissemination (e.g., system leadership, unit leadership, IRB) • *Consult with EBP mentor*	Notes & Progress:
Checkpoint Six (about mid-way)	• Meet with implementation group • Discuss known barriers & facilitators of project • Discuss strategies for minimizing barriers & maximizing facilitators • Finalize protocol for implementation of evidence • Identify resources (human, fiscal, & other) necessary to complete project • Supply EBP mentor with written IRB approval & managerial support • Begin work on poster for dissemination of initiation of project & progress to date to educate stakeholders about project—get help from support staff • Include specific plan for how evaluation will take place: who, what, when, where, & how and communication mechanisms to stakeholders • *Consult with EBP mentor*	Notes & Progress:
Checkpoint Seven	• Meet with implementation group to review proposed poster • Make final adjustment to poster with support staff • Inform stakeholders of start date of implementation & poster presentation • Address any concerns or questions of stakeholders (active & supportive) • *Consult with EBP mentor*	Notes & Progress:
Checkpoint Eight	• Poster presentation (preferred event is a system-wide recognition of quality, research, or innovation) • LAUNCH EBP implementation project • *Consult with EBP mentor*	Notes & Progress:

continued

Checkpoint Nine	• Mid-project meet with all key stake-holders to review progress & provide outcomes to date. • Review issues, successes, aha's, & triumphs of project to date. • *Consult with EBP mentor*	Notes & Progress:
Checkpoint Ten	• Complete final data collection for project evaluation • Present project results via poster presentation—locally & nationally • *Celebrate with EBP mentor & agency leadership*	Notes & Progress:
Checkpoint Eleven	• Review project progress, lessons learned, new questions generated from process • *Consult with EBP mentor about new questions*	Notes, Progress, & Next Steps:

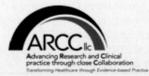

Appendix K

Sample Instruments to Evaluate Organizational Culture and Readiness for Integration of EBP, EBP Beliefs, and EBP Implementation in Clinical and Academic Settings

Organizational Culture & Readiness for System-Wide Integration of Evidence-based Practice Survey

Below are 19 questions about evidence-based practice (EBP). Please consider the culture of your organization and its readiness for system wide implementation of EBP and indicate which answer best describes your response to each question. There are no right or wrong answers.

Item	None at All	A Little	Somewhat	Moderately	Very Much
1. To what extent is EBP clearly described as central to the mission and philosophy of your institution?	1	2	3	4	5
2. To what extent do you believe that EBP is practiced in your organization?	1	2	3	4	5
3. To what extent is the nursing staff with whom you work committed to EBP?	1	2	3	4	5
4. To what extent is the physician team with whom you work committed to EBP?	1	2	3	4	5
5. To what extent are there administrators within your organization committed to EBP (i.e., have planned for resources and support [e.g., time] to initiate EBP)?	1	2	3	4	5
6. In your organization, to what extent is there a critical mass of nurses who have strong EBP knowledge and skills?	1	2	3	4	5
7. To what extent are there nurse scientists (doctorally prepared researchers) in your organization to assist in generation of evidence when it does not exist?	1	2	3	4	5
8. In your organization, to what extent are there Advanced Practiced Nurses who are EBP mentors for staff nurses as well as other APNs?	1	2	3	4	5
9. To what extent do practitioners model EBP in their clinical settings?	1	2	3	4	5
10. To what extent do staff nurses have access to quality computers and access to electronic databases for searching for best evidence?	1	2	3	4	5
11. To what extent do staff nurses have proficient computer skills?	1	2	3	4	5
12. To what extent do librarians within your organization have EBP knowledge and skills?	1	2	3	4	5
13. To what extent are librarians used to search for evidence?	1	2	3	4	5
14. To what extent are fiscal resources used to support EBP (e.g., education-attending EBP conferences/workshops, computers, paid time for the EBP process, mentors)?	1	2	3	4	5
15. To what extent are there EBP champions (i.e., those who will go the extra mile to advance EBP) in the environment among:					
a. Administrators?	1	2	3	4	5
b. Physicians?	1	2	3	4	5
c. Nurse Educators?	1	2	3	4	5
d. Advanced Practice Nurses?	1	2	3	4	5
e. Staff Nurses?	1	2	3	4	5
16. To what extent is the measurement and sharing of outcomes part of the culture of the organization in which you work?	1	2	3	4	5

Item	None	25%	50%	75%	100%
17. To what extent are decisions generated from:					
a. Direct care providers?	1	2	3	4	5
b. Upper administration?	1	2	3	4	5
c. Physician or other healthcare provider groups?	1	2	3	4	5

Item	Not Ready	Getting Ready	Been Ready but Not Acting	Ready to Go	Past Ready & onto Action
18. Overall, how would you rate your institution in readiness for EBP	1	2	3	4	5

19. Compared to 6 months ago, how much movement in your organization has there been toward an EBP culture?	None at All	A Little	Somewhat	Moderately	Very Much
	1	2	3	4	5

Organizational Culture & Readiness for School-wide Integration of Evidence-based Practice Survey for Students (OCRSIEP-ES)

Below are 19 questions about evidence-based practice (EBP). Please consider the state of your educational organization for the readiness of EBP and indicate which answer best describes your response to each question. There are no right or wrong answers.

Item	None at All	A Little	Somewhat	Moderately	Very Much
1. To what extent is EBP clearly described as central to the mission and philosophy of your educational agency?	1	2	3	4	5
2. To what extent do you believe that evidence-based education is practiced in your organization?	1	2	3	4	5
3. To what extent are the faculty who teach you committed to EBP?	1	2	3	4	5
4. To what extent are the community partners in which you have clinical practicum committed to EBP?	1	2	3	4	5
5. To what extent are there administrators within your educational organization committed to EBP (i.e., have planned for resources and support [e.g., time] to teach EBP across your courses)?	1	2	3	4	5
6. In your educational organization, to what extent is there a critical mass of faculty who have strong EBP knowledge and skills?	1	2	3	4	5
7. To what extent is there ongoing research by nurse scientists (doctorally prepared researchers) in your educational organization to assist in generation of evidence when it does not exist?	1	2	3	4	5
8. In your educational organization, to what extent are there faculty who are EBP mentors?	1	2	3	4	5
9. To what extent do faculty model EBP in your didactic and clinical settings?	1	2	3	4	5
10. To what extent do students have access to quality computers and access to electronic databases for searching for best evidence?	1	2	3	4	5
11. To what extent do students have proficient computer skills?	1	2	3	4	5
12. To what extent do librarians within your educational organization have EBP knowledge and skills?	1	2	3	4	5
13. To what extent are librarians used to search for evidence?	1	2	3	4	5
14. To what extent are fiscal resources used to support EBP (e.g., education-attending EBP conferences/workshops, computers, paid time for the EBP process, mentors)?	1	2	3	4	5
15. To what extent are there EBP champions (i.e., those who will go the extra mile to advance EBP) in the environment among:					
a. Dean?	1	2	3	4	5
b. Associate Deans?	1	2	3	4	5
c. Didactic Course Faculty?	1	2	3	4	5
d. Clinical Course Faculty?	1	2	3	4	5
e. Students?	1	2	3	4	5
16. To what extent is the measurement and sharing of outcomes part of the culture of your educational organization?	1	2	3	4	5

Item	None	25%	50%	75%	100%
17. To what extent are decisions generated from:					
a. Faculty?	1	2	3	4	5
b. Dean?	1	2	3	4	5
c. Students?	1	2	3	4	5

Item	Not Ready	Getting Ready	Been Ready but Not Acting	Ready to Go	Past Ready & onto Action
18. Overall, how would you rate your educational organization in readiness for EBP (how ready is it)?	1	2	3	4	5

Item	None at All	A Little	Somewhat	Moderately	Very Much
19. Compared to 6 months ago, how much movement in your educational organization has there been toward an EBP culture?	1	2	3	4	5

Organizational Culture & Readiness for School-wide Integration of Evidence-based Practice Survey (OCRSIEP-E)
Below are 19 questions about evidence-based practice (EBP). Please consider the state of your educational organization for the readiness of EBP and indicate which answer best describes your response to each question. There are no right or wrong answers.

Item	None at All	A Little	Somewhat	Moderately	Very Much
1. To what extent is EBP clearly described as central to the mission and philosophy of your educational agency?	1	2	3	4	5
2. To what extent do you believe that evidence-based education is practiced in your organization?	1	2	3	4	5
3. To what extent is the faculty with whom you work committed to EBP?	1	2	3	4	5
4. To what extent is the community partners with whom you work committed to EBP?	1	2	3	4	5
5. To what extent are there administrators within your organization committed to EBP (i.e., have planned for resources and support [e.g., time] to initiate EBP)?	1	2	3	4	5
6. In your organization, to what extent is there a critical mass of faculty who have strong EBP knowledge and skills?	1	2	3	4	5
7. To what extent is there ongoing research by nurse scientists (doctorally prepared researchers) in your organization to assist in generation of evidence when it does not exist?	1	2	3	4	5
8. In your organization, to what extent are there faculty who are EBP mentors?	1	2	3	4	5
9. To what extent do faculty model EBP in their educational and clinical settings?	1	2	3	4	5
10. To what extent do faculty have access to quality computers and access to electronic databases for searching for best evidence?	1	2	3	4	5
11. To what extent do faculty have proficient computer skills?	1	2	3	4	5
12. To what extent do librarians within your organization have EBP knowledge and skills?	1	2	3	4	5
13. To what extent are librarians used to search for evidence?	1	2	3	4	5
14. To what extent are fiscal resources used to support EBP (e.g., education-attending EBP conferences/workshops, computers, paid time for the EBP process, mentors)?	1	2	3	4	5
15. To what extent are there EBP champions (i.e., those who will go the extra mile to advance EBP) in the environment among:					
a. Administrators?	1	2	3	4	5
b. Community Partners?	1	2	3	4	5
c. Clinical Faculty?	1	2	3	4	5
d. Junior Faculty?	1	2	3	4	5
e. Senior Faculty?	1	2	3	4	5
16. To what extent is the measurement and sharing of outcomes part of the culture of the organization in which you work?	1	2	3	4	5
Item	None	25%	50%	75%	100%
17. To what extent are decisions generated from:					
a. Faculty?	1	2	3	4	5
b. College administration?	1	2	3	4	5
c. University administration?	1	2	3	4	5
Item	Not Ready	Getting Ready	Been Ready but Not Acting	Ready to Go	Past Ready & onto Action
18. Overall, how would you rate your institution in readiness for EBP?	1	2	3	4	5
Item	None at All	A Little	Somewhat	Moderately	Very Much
19. Compared to 6 months ago, how much movement in your educational organization has there been toward an EBP culture?	1	2	3	4	5

EBP Beliefs Scale

Below are 16 statements about evidence-based practice (EBP). Please circle the number that best describes your agreement or disagreement with each statement. There are no right or wrong answers.

	Strongly Disagree	Disagree	Neither Agree nor Disagree	Agree	Strongly Agree
1. I believe that EBP results in the best clinical care for patients.	1	2	3	4	5
2. I am clear about the steps of EBP.	1	2	3	4	5
3. I am sure that I can implement EBP.	1	2	3	4	5
4. I believe that critically appraising evidence is an important step in the EBP process.	1	2	3	4	5
5. I am sure that evidence-based guidelines can improve clinical care.	1	2	3	4	5
6. I believe that I can search for the best evidence to answer clinical questions in a time efficient way.	1	2	3	4	5
7. I believe that I can overcome barriers in implementing EBP.	1	2	3	4	5
8. I am sure that I can implement EBP in a time efficient way.	1	2	3	4	5
9. I am sure that implementing EBP will improve the care that I deliver to my patients.	1	2	3	4	5
10. I am sure about how to measure the outcomes of clinical care.	1	2	3	4	5
11. I believe that EBP takes too much time.	1	2	3	4	5
12. I am sure that I can access the best resources in order to implement EBP.	1	2	3	4	5
13. I believe EBP is difficult.	1	2	3	4	5
14. I know how to implement EBP sufficiently enough to make practice changes.	1	2	3	4	5
15. I am confident about my ability to implement EBP where I work.	1	2	3	4	5
16. I believe the care that I deliver is evidence-based.	1	2	3	4	5

EBP Beliefs Scale for Educators (EBPB-E)

Below are 21 statements about evidence-based practice (EBP). Please circle the number that best describes your agreement or disagreement with each statement. There are no right or wrong answers.

	Strongly Disagree	Disagree	Neither Agree nor Disagree	Agree	Strongly Agree
1. I believe that EBP results in the best clinical care for patients.	1	2	3	4	5
2. I am clear about the steps of EBP.	1	2	3	4	5
3. I am sure that I can implement EBP.	1	2	3	4	5
4. I believe that critically appraising evidence is an important step in the EBP process.	1	2	3	4	5
5. I am sure that evidence-based guidelines can improve clinical care.	1	2	3	4	5
6. I believe that I can search for the best evidence to answer clinical questions in a time efficient way.	1	2	3	4	5
7. I am sure that I can teach how to search for the best evidence.					
8. I believe that I can overcome barriers in implementing EBP.	1	2	3	4	5
9. I am sure that I can implement EBP in a time efficient way.	1	2	3	4	5
10. I am sure that implementing EBP will improve the care that my students deliver to patients.	1	2	3	4	5
11. I am sure about how to measure the outcomes of clinical care.	1	2	3	4	5
12. I believe that EBP takes too much time.	1	2	3	4	5
13. I am sure that I can access the best resources in order to integrate EBP in the curriculum.	1	2	3	4	5
14. I believe EBP is difficult.	1	2	3	4	5
15. I know how to implement EBP sufficiently enough to make curricular changes.	1	2	3	4	5
16. I am confident about my ability to implement EBP where I work.	1	2	3	4	5
17. I believe the care that I deliver is evidence-based.	1	2	3	4	5
18. I am sure that I can teach EBP in a time efficient way.	1	2	3	4	5
18. I am sure that integrating EBP into the curriculum will improve the care that students deliver to their patients.	1	2	3	4	5
19. I am sure that I can teach EBP.	1	2	3	4	5
20. I am sure that I can teach how to develop a PICOT question.	1	2	3	4	5
21. I know how to teach EBP sufficiently enough to impact students' practice.	1	2	3	4	5

EBP Implementation Scale

Below are 18 questions about evidence-based practice (EBP). Some healthcare providers do some of these things more often than other healthcare providers. There is no certain frequency in which you should be performing these tasks. Please answer each question by circling the number that best describes **how often each item has applied to you in the past 8 weeks**.

In the **past 8 weeks**, I have:

	0 times	1-3 times	4-5 times	6-7 times	8 or more times
1. Used evidence to change my clinical practice…	0	1	2	3	4
2. Critically appraised evidence from a research study…	0	1	2	3	4
3. Generated a PICO question about my clinical practice…	0	1	2	3	4
4. Informally discussed evidence from a research study with a colleague...	0	1	2	3	4
5. Collected data on a patient problem...	0	1	2	3	4
6. Shared evidence from a study or studies in the form of a report or presentation to more than 2 colleagues…	0	1	2	3	4
7. Evaluated the outcomes of a practice change…	0	1	2	3	4
8. Shared an EBP guideline with a colleague…	0	1	2	3	4
9. Shared evidence from a research study with a patient/family member…	0	1	2	3	4
10. Shared evidence from a research study with a multi-disciplinary team member…	0	1	2	3	4
11. Read and critically appraised a clinical research study…	0	1	2	3	4
12. Accessed the Cochrane database of systematic reviews…	0	1	2	3	4
13. Accessed the National Guidelines Clearinghouse…	0	1	2	3	4
14. Used an EBP guideline or systematic review to change clinical practice where I work…	0	1	2	3	4
15. Evaluated a care initiative by collecting patient outcome data…	0	1	2	3	4
16 Shared the outcome data collected with colleagues…	0	1	2	3	4
17. Changed practice based on patient outcome data…	0	1	2	3	4
18. Promoted the use of EBP to my colleagues…	0	1	2	3	4

EBP Implementation Scale for Educators (EBPI-E)

Below are 18 questions about evidence-based practice (EBP). Some healthcare professions educators do some of these things more often than other healthcare professions educators. There is no certain frequency in which you should be performing these tasks. Please answer each question by circling the number that best describes <u>how often each item has applied to you in the past 8 weeks</u>.

In the **past 8 weeks**, I have:

	0 times	1–3 times	4–5 times	6–8 times	>8 times
1. Used evidence to change my teaching...	0	1	2	3	4
2. Critically appraised evidence from a research study…	0	1	2	3	4
3. Generated a PICO question about my teaching/practice specialty …	0	1	2	3	4
4. Informally discussed evidence from a research study with a colleague...	0	1	2	3	4
5. Collected data on a clinical/educational issue...	0	1	2	3	4
6. Shared evidence from a study or studies in the form of a report or presentation to more than 2 colleagues…	0	1	2	3	4
7. Evaluated the outcomes of an educational change...	0	1	2	3	4
8. Shared an EBP guideline with a colleague…	0	1	2	3	4
9. Shared evidence from a research study with a student …	0	1	2	3	4
10. Shared evidence from a research study with a multi-disciplinary team member…	0	1	2	3	4
11. Read and critically appraised a clinical research study…	0	1	2	3	4
12. Accessed the Cochrane database of systematic reviews…	0	1	2	3	4
13. Accessed the National Guidelines Clearinghouse…	0	1	2	3	4
14. Used an EBP guideline or systematic review to change educational strategies where I work…	0	1	2	3	4
15. Evaluated an educational initiative by collecting outcomes...	0	1	2	3	4
16 Shared the outcome data collected with colleagues…	0	1	2	3	4
17. Changed curricular policies /materials based on outcome data...	0	1	2	3	4
18. Promoted the use of EBP to my colleagues…	0	1	2	3	4

A

Absolute risk increase (ARI): The absolute risk increase for an undesirable outcome is when the risk is more for the experimental/condition group than the control/comparison group.

Absolute risk reduction (ARR): The absolute risk reduction for an undesirable outcome is when the risk is less for the experimental/condition group than the control/comparison group.

Accountability (HIPAA) Act: The Health Insurance Portability and Accountability Act (HIPAA) was approved by the United States Congress in 1996 to protect the privacy of individuals. It enforces protections for works that improve portability and continuity of health insurance coverage.

Action research: A general term for a variety of approaches that aim to resolve social problems by improving existing conditions for oppressed groups or communities.

Adoption of research evidence: A process that occurs across five stages of innovation (i.e., knowledge, persuasion, decision, implementation, and confirmation).

Analysis: The process used to determine the findings in a study or project.

Analytic notes: Notes researchers write to themselves to record their thoughts, questions, and ideas as a process of simultaneous data collection and data analysis unfolds.

Applicability [of study findings]: Whether or not the results of the study are appropriate for a particular patient situation.

Article synopsis: A summary of the content of a single article.

Attrition: When subjects are lost from or drop their participation in a study (see loss of subjects to follow-up).

Audit: To examine carefully and verify the findings from a study or project.

Author name: The name of the person who wrote a paper.

Axial coding: A process used in grounded theory to relate categories of information by using a coding paradigm with predetermined subcategories (Strauss & Corbin, 1990).

B

Background questions: Questions that need to be answered as a foundation for asking the searchable, answerable foreground question. They are questions that ask for general information about a clinical issue.

Basic social process (BSP): The basis for theory generation—recurs frequently, links all the data together, and describes the pattern followed regardless of the variety of conditions under which the experience takes place and different ways in which persons go through it. There are two types of BSP, a basic social psychological process (BSPP) and a basic social structural process (BSSP).

Benchmarking: The process of looking outward to identify, understand, and adapt outstanding (best) practices and (high performance) to help improve performance.

Bias: Divergence of results from the true values or the process that leads to such divergence.

Biography: An approach that produces an in-depth report of a person's life. Life histories and oral histories also involve gathering of biographical information and recording of personal recollections of one or more individuals.

Biosketch: A two- to three-page document, similar to a resume or brief curriculum vitae, that captures an individual's educational and professional work experience, honors, prior research grants, and publications.

Blind review: A review process in which identification of the author/creator/researcher is removed and, likewise, the identity of the reviewers so that anonymity of both parties is assured.

Blocking: A strategy introduced into a study that entails deliberately including a potential extraneous intrinsic or confounding variable in a study's design in order to control its effects on the dependent or outcome variable.

Body of evidence: A group of keeper studies and lower level evidence retrieved by systematically searching all relevant databases using keywords, subject headings, and titles, as necessary.

Boolean operator AND: Defines the relationships between words, phrases, or subject headings. The Boolean operator AND is used for narrowing a search by retrieving records containing all of the words it separates.

Boolean operator OR: Defines the relationships between words, phrases, or subject headings. The Boolean operator OR is used to broaden a search by retrieving records containing any of the words, phrases, or subject headings that are specified.

Booster interventions: Interventions that are delivered after the initial intervention or treatment in a study for the purpose of enhancing the effects of the intervention.

Bracketing: Identifying and suspending previously acquired knowledge, beliefs, and opinions about a phenomenon.

C

Case–control study: A type of research that retrospectively compares characteristics of an individual who has a certain condition (e.g., hypertension) with one who does not (i.e., a matched control or similar person without hypertension); often conducted for the purpose of identifying variables that might predict the condition (e.g., stressful lifestyle, sodium intake).

Case reports: Reports that describe the history of a single patient, or a small group of patients, usually in the form of a story.

Case study: An intensive investigation of a case involving a person or small group of persons, an issue, or an event.

Categorical data/variables: Data that are classified into categories (e.g., gender, hair color) instead of being numerically ordered.

Ceiling effects: Participant scores that cluster toward the high end of a measure.

Clinical Expertise: Clinical expertise is more than the skills, knowledge, and experience of clinicians; rather it is expertise that develops from multiple observations of patients and how they react to certain interventions, with the central aspects of experiential learning and clinical judgment as main contributors and products.

Clinical decision support system: Computer programs with updated latest external evidence that interface with patient data from the electronic health record and through analysis assist healthcare providers in making clinical decisions.

Clinical inquiry: A process in which clinicians gather data together using narrowly defined clinical parameters; it allows for an appraisal of the available choices of treatment for the purpose of finding the most appropriate choice of action. Clinical inquiry in action includes problem identification and clinical judgment across time about the particular transitions of particular patient/family clinical situations. Four aspects of clinical inquiry in action include making qualitative distinctions, engaging in detective work, recognizing changing relevance, and developing clinical knowledge about specific patient populations.

Clinical practice guidelines: Systematically developed statements to assist clinicians and patients in making decisions about care; ideally, the guidelines consist of a systematic review of the literature, in conjunction with consensus of a group of expert decision makers, including administrators, policy makers, clinicians, and consumers who consider the evidence and make recommendations.

Clinical significance: Study findings that will directly influence clinical practice, whether they are statistically significant or not.

Cochrane Central Register of Controlled Trials: A database of controlled trials identified by contributors to the Cochrane Collaboration and others.

Cochrane Database of Systematic Reviews: A database containing reviews that are highly structured and systematic with explicit inclusion and exclusion criteria to minimize bias.

Cochrane Methodology Register: Studies prepared by the Cochrane Empirical Methodological Studies Methods Group that examine the methods used in reviews and more general methodological studies that could be used by anyone conducting systematic reviews.

Cohort study: A longitudinal study that begins with the gathering of two groups of patients (the cohorts), one that received the exposure (e.g., to a disease) and one that does not, and then following these groups over time (prospective) to measure the development of different outcomes (diseases).

Computer-assisted qualitative data analysis: An area of technological innovation that, in qualitative research, has resulted in uses of word processing and software packages to support data management.

Conceptual framework: A group of interrelated statements that provide a guide or direction for a study or project; sometimes referred to as a theoretical framework.

Confidence interval (CI): A measure of the precision of the estimate. The 95% confidence interval (CI) is the range of values within which we can be 95% sure that the true value lies for the whole population of patients from whom the study patients were selected.

Confirmability: Demonstrated by providing substantiation that findings and interpretations are grounded in the data (i.e., links between researcher assertions and the data are clear and credible).

Confounding: Occurs when two factors are closely associated and the effects of one confuses or distorts the effects of the other factor on an outcome. The distorting factor is a confounding variable.

Confounding variables: Those factors that interfere with the relationship between the independent and dependent variables.

Constant comparison: A systematic approach to analysis that is a search for patterns in data as they are coded, sorted into categories, and examined in different contexts.

Construct validity: The degree to which an instrument measures the construct it is supposed to be measuring.

Contamination: The inadvertent and undesirable influence of an experimental intervention on another intervention.

Content analysis: In qualitative analysis, a term that refers to processes of breaking down narrative data (coding, comparing, contrasting, and categorizing bits of information) and reconstituting them in some new form (e.g., description, interpretation, theory).

Content validity: The degree to which the items in an instrument are tapping the content they are supposed to measure.

Context: The conditions in which something exists.

Control group: A group of subjects who do not receive the experimental intervention or treatment.

Controlled vocabulary or thesaurus: A hierarchical arrangement of descriptive terms that serve as mapping agents for searches; often unique to each database.

Convenience sampling: Drawing readily available subjects to participate in a study.

Correlational descriptive study: A study that is conducted for the purpose of describing the relationship between two or more variables.

Correlational predictive study: A study that is conducted for the purpose of describing what variables predict a certain outcome.

Covariate: A variable that is controlled for in statistical analyses (e.g., analysis of covariance); the variable controlled is typically a confounding or extraneous variable that may influence the outcome.

Critical appraisal: The process of evaluating a study for its worth (i.e., validity, reliability, and applicability to clinical practice).

Critical inquiry: Theoretical perspectives that are ideologically oriented toward critique of and emancipation from oppressive social arrangements or false ideas.

Critical theory: A blend of ideology (based on a critical theory of society) and a form of social analysis and critique that aims to liberate people from unrecognized myths and oppression, in order to bring about enlightenment and radical social change.

Critique: An in-depth analysis and critical evaluation of a study that identifies its strengths and limitations.

Cronbach alpha: An estimate of internal consistency or homogeneity of an instrument that is comprised of several subparts or scales.

Cross-contamination: Diffusion of the treatment or intervention across study groups.

Cross-sectional study: A study designed to observe an outcome or variable at a single point in time, usually for the purpose of inferring trends over time.

Culture: Shared knowledge and behavior of people who interact within distinct social settings and subsystems.

D

Data and safety monitoring plan: A detailed plan for how adverse effects will be assessed and managed.

Database of Abstracts of Reviews of Effects (DARE): Database that includes abstracts of systematic reviews that have been critically appraised by reviewers at the NHS Centre for Reviews and Dissemination at the University of York, England.

Deep web: The part of the Internet that cannot be accessed by standard search engines. Search engines such as Google retrieve information from the surface web.

Dependent or **outcome variable:** The variable or outcome that is influenced or caused by the independent variable.

Descriptive studies: Those studies that are conducted for the purpose of describing the characteristics of certain phenomena or selected variables.

Design: The overall plan for a study that includes strategies for controlling confounding variables, strategies for when the intervention will be delivered (in experimental studies), and how often and when the data will be collected.

Dialogical engagement: Thinking that is like a thoughtful dialog or conversation.

Direct costs: Actual costs required to conduct a study (e.g., personnel, subject honoraria, instruments).

Discourse analysis: A general term for approaches to analyzing recorded talk and patterns of communication.

Dissemination: The process of distributing or circulating information widely.

E

EBP mentor: Typically, an advanced practice clinician with in-depth knowledge and skills in evidence-based practice (EBP) as well as in individual behavior and organizational change.

Educational prescription (EP): A written plan (usually self-initiated) for identifying and addressing EBP learning needs. The EP contains each step of the EBP process but may have a primary focus on one or two steps, such as searching or critical appraisal.

Effect size: The strength of the effect of an intervention.

Electronic health record (EHR): An electronic record of client information designed to provide comprehensive information that can be shared among all clinicians involved in a patient's care. The purpose is to have information travel with the patient across settings and locations; note an electronic medical record is the digital version of the paper charts in the clinician's office.

Emergence: Glaser's (1992) term for conceptually driven ("discovery") versus procedurally driven ("forcing") theory development in his critique of Strauss and Corbin (1990).

Emic and etic: Contrasting "insider" views of informants (emic) and the researcher's "outsider" (etic) views.

Environment: Surroundings.

Epistemologies: Ways of knowing and reasoning.

Essences: Internal meaning structures of a phenomenon grasped through the study of human lived experience.

Ethnographic studies: Studies of a social group's culture through time spent combining participant observation and in-depth interviews in the informants' natural setting.

Evaluation: An evaluation of worth.

Event rate: The rate at which a specific event occurs.

Evidence-based clinical practice guidelines: Specific practice recommendations that are based on a methodologically rigorous review of the best evidence on a specific topic.

Evidence-based decision making: The integration of best research evidence in making decisions about patient care, which should also include the clinician's expertise as well as patient preferences and values.

Evidence-based practice (EBP): A paradigm and lifelong problem-solving approach to clinical decision making that involves the conscientious use of the best available evidence (including a systematic search for and critical appraisal of the most relevant evidence to answer a clinical question) with one's own clinical expertise and patient values and preferences to improve outcomes for individuals, groups, communities, and systems.

Evidence-based quality improvement (EBQI): Quality improvement initiatives based on evidence.

Evidence-based theories: A theory that has been tested and supported through the accumulation of evidence from several studies.

Evidence summaries: Short summary of available evidence that generally provides recommendations for practice and research. Careful evaluation of how summaries are produced is warranted, ranging from comprehensive synthesis [e.g., systematic review] to simple listing of studies' findings.

Evidence user: Anyone who uses valid evidence to support or change practice; demonstrating skills in interpreting evidence, not generating evidence.

Excerpta Medica Online: A major biomedical and pharmaceutical database.

Exclusion criteria: Investigator-identified characteristics that are (a) possessed by individuals that would exclude them from participating in a study and (b) specified to exclude studies from a body of evidence.

Experiential learning: Experience requiring a turning around of preconceptions, expectations, sets, and routines or adding some new insights to a particular practical situation; a way of knowing that contributes to knowledge production; should influence the development of science.

Experimental design/experiment: A study whose purpose is to test the effects of an intervention or treatment on selected outcomes. This is the strongest design for testing cause-and-effect relationships.

External evidence: Evidence that is generated from rigorous research.

External validity: Generalizability; the ability to generalize the findings from a study to the larger population from which the sample was drawn.

Extraneous variables: Those factors that interfere with the relationship between the independent and dependent variables.

F

Face validity: The degree to which an instrument appears to be measuring (i.e., tapping) the construct it is intended to measure.

Factorial design: An experimental design that has two or more interventions or treatments.

False positive: A condition where the test indicates that the person has the outcome of interest when, in fact, the person does not.

False negative: A condition where the test indicates that the person does not have the outcome of interest when, in fact, the person does.

Feminist epistemologies: A variety of views and practices inviting critical dialogue about women's experiences in historical, cultural, and socioeconomic perspectives.

Fieldnotes: Self-designed observational protocols for recording notes about field observations.

Field studies: Studies involving direct, firsthand observation and interviews in informants' natural settings.

Fieldwork: All research activities carried out in and in relation to the field (informants' natural settings).

Fixed effect model: Traditional assumption that the event rates are fixed in each of the control and treatment groups.

Floor effects: Participant scores that cluster toward the low end of a measure.

Focus groups: This type of group interview generates data on designated topics through discussion and interaction. Focus group research is a distinct type of study when used as the sole research strategy.

Foreground questions: Those questions that can be answered from scientific evidence about diagnosing, treating, or assisting patients with understanding their prognosis, focusing on specific knowledge.

Forest plot: Diagrammatic representation of the results (i.e., the effects or point estimates) of trials (i.e., squares) along with their CIs (i.e., straight lines through the squares).

Frequency: The number of occurrences in a given time period.

Full-text: Any print resource that is available electronically.

Funnel plot: The plotting of sample size against the effect size of studies included in a systematic review. The funnel should be inverted and symmetrical if a representative sample has been obtained.

G

Generalizability: The extent to which the findings from a study can be generalized or applied to the larger population (i.e., external validity).

Gold standard: An accepted and established reference standard or diagnostic test for a particular illness.

Grey literature: Refers to publications such as brochures and conference proceedings.

(Grounded) formal theory: A systematic explanation of an area of human/social experience derived through meta-analysis of substantive theory.

(Grounded) substantive theory: A systematic explanation of a situation-specific human experience/social phenomenon.

Grounded theory: Studies to generate theory about how people deal with life situations that is "grounded" in empirical data and describes the processes by which they move through experiences over time.

H

Harm: When risks outweigh benefits.

Health Technology Assessment Database: Database containing information on evaluation of medical procedures and technologies in health care.

Health topic summaries: Concise overviews of a health topic.

Hermeneutics: Philosophy, theories, and practices of interpretation.

Hierarchy of evidence: A mechanism for determining which study designs have the most power to predict cause and effect. The highest level of evidence is systematic reviews of randomized controlled trials (RCTs), and the lowest level of evidence is expert opinion and consensus statements.

History: The occurrence of some event or program unrelated to the intervention that might account for the change observed in the dependent variable.

Hits: Studies obtained from a search that contain the searched word.

Homogeneous study population/Homogeneity: When subjects in a study are similar on the characteristics that may affect the outcome variable(s).

HSR Queries: Health and safety regulation questions.

Hyperlink: A connection to organized information that is housed in cyberspace and usually relevant to the site on which it was found.

Hypotheses: Predictions about the relationships between variables (e.g., adults who receive cognitive behavioral therapy will report less depression than those who receive relaxation therapy).

I

Incidence: New occurrences of the outcome or disorder within the at-risk population in a specified time frame.

Inclusion criteria: Essential characteristics specified by investigator that (a) potential participants must possess in order to be considered for a study and (b) studies must meet to be included in a body of evidence.

Independent variable: The variable that is influencing the dependent variable or outcome; in experimental studies, it is the intervention or treatment.

Indirect costs: Costs that are not directly related to the actual conduct of a study but are associated with the "overhead" in an organization, such as lights, telephones, and office space.

Informatics: How data, information, knowledge, and wisdom are collected, stored, processed, communicated, and used to support the process of healthcare delivery to clients, providers, administrators, and organizations involved in healthcare delivery.

Institutional Review Board (IRB): A committee that approves, monitors, and reviews research involving human subjects for the purpose of protecting the rights and welfare of research subjects.

Integrative reviews: Systematic summaries of the accumulated state of knowledge about a concept, including highlights of important issues left unresolved.

Integrity of the intervention: The extent to which an intervention is delivered as intended.

Internal consistency reliability: The extent to which an instrument's subparts are measuring the same construct.

Internal evidence: Evidence generated within a clinical practice setting from initiatives such as quality improvement, outcomes management, or EBP implementation projects.

Internal validity: The extent to which it can be said that the independent variable (i.e., the intervention) causes a change in the dependent variable (i.e., outcome), and the results are not due to other factors or alternative explanations.

Interpretive ethnography: Loosely characterized, a movement within anthropology that generates many hybrid forms of ethnographic work as a result of crossing a variety of theoretical boundaries within social science.

Interrater reliability: The degree to which two individuals agree on what they observe.

Interval data: Data that have quantified intervals and equal distances between points but without a meaningful zero point (e.g., temperature in degrees Fahrenheit); often referred to as continuous data.

Introspection: A process of recognizing and examining one's own inner state or feelings.

J

Journal title: The title of a journal.

K

Key informant: A select informant/assistant with extensive or specialized knowledge of his or her own culture.

Key stakeholder: An individual or institution that has an investment in a project.

Keyword: A word that is not a part of the database's controlled vocabulary/thesaurus. Keywords are sometimes searched only in titles and abstracts so caution should be used when searching only with keywords. Sometimes called textwords.

L

Level of evidence: A ranking of evidence by the type of design or research methodology that would answer the question with the least amount of error and provide the most reliable findings. Leveling of evidence, also called hierarchies, vary by type of question asked. An example is provided for intervention questions.

Level I evidence: Evidence that is generated from systematic reviews or meta-analyses of all relevant RCTs or evidence-based clinical practice guidelines based on systematic reviews of RCTs; the strongest level of evidence to guide clinical practice.

Level II evidence: Evidence generated from at least one well-designed randomized clinical trial (i.e., a true experiment).

Level III evidence: Evidence obtained from well-designed controlled trials without randomization.

Level IV evidence: Evidence from well-designed case–control and cohort studies.

Level V evidence: Evidence from systematic reviews of descriptive and qualitative studies.

Level VI evidence: Evidence from a single descriptive or qualitative study.

Level VII evidence: Evidence from the opinion of authorities and/or reports of expert committees.

Likelihood ratio: The likelihood that a given test result would be expected in patients with a disease compared to the likelihood that the same result would be expected in patients without that disease.

Lived experience: Everyday experience, not as it is conceptualized, but as it is lived (i.e., how it feels).

Loss of subjects to follow-up: The proportion of people who started the study but do not complete the study, for whatever reason.

M

Macro level change versus macrolevel: Change at a large-scale level (e.g., nationwide systems or large institutions).

Magnitude of effect: Expressing the size of the relationship between two variables or difference between two groups on a given variable/outcome (i.e., the effect size).

Manipulation checks: Assessments verifying that subjects have actually processed the experimental information that they have received or followed through with prescribed intervention activities.

Maturation: Developmental change that occurs, even in the absence of the intervention.

Mean: A measure of central tendency, derived by summing all scores and dividing by the number of participants.

Mediating variables and processes: The mechanisms through which an intervention produces the desired outcome(s).

Mediating variable: The variable or mechanism through which an intervention works to impact the outcome in a study.

Meta-analysis: A process of using quantitative methods to summarize the results from the multiple studies, obtained and critically reviewed using a rigorous process (to minimize bias) for identifying, appraising, and synthesizing studies to answer a specific question and draw conclusions about the data gathered. The purpose of this process is to gain a summary statistic (i.e., a measure of a single effect) that represents the effect of the intervention across multiple studies.

Meta-synthesis: A rigorous process of analyzing findings across qualitative studies. The results address a specific research question and are obtained through the synthesis of qualitative studies. The process allows researchers to find greater meaning through interpreting the qualitative data.

Method: The theory of how a certain type of research should be carried out (i.e., strategy, approach, process/overall design, and logic of design). Researchers often subsume description of techniques under a discussion of method.

MeSH®: Medline's controlled vocabulary: Medical Subject Headings.

Microlevel change: Change at a small-scale level (e.g., units within a local healthcare organization or small groups of individuals).

N

Narrative analysis: A term that refers to distinct styles of generating, interpreting, and representing data as stories that provide insights into life experiences.

Narrative review: A summary of primary studies from which conclusions are drawn by the reviewer based on his or her own interpretations.

National Guidelines Clearinghouse: A comprehensive database of up-to-date English language evidence-based clinical practice guidelines developed in partnership with the American Medical Association, the American Association of Health Plans, and the Association for Healthcare Research and Quality.

Naturalistic research: Commitment to the study of phenomena in their naturally occurring settings (contexts).

News embargo: A restriction on the release of any media information about the findings from a study before they are published in a journal article.

NHS Economic Evaluation Database: A register of published economic evaluation of health interventions.

Nominated/snowball sample: A sample obtained with the help of informants already enrolled in the study.

Nonexperimental study design: A study design in which data are collected but whose purpose is not to test the effects of an intervention or treatment on selected outcomes.

Null hypothesis: There is no relationship between or among study variables.

Number needed to harm (NNH): The number of clients, who, if they received an intervention, would result in one additional person being harmed (i.e., having a bad outcome) compared to the clients in the control arm of a study.

Number needed to treat (NNT): The number of people who would need to receive the experimental therapy to prevent one bad outcome or cause one additional good outcome.

O

Observation: Facts learned from observing.

Observation continuum: A range of social roles encompassed by participant observation and ranging from complete observer to complete participant at the extremes.

Observer drift: A decrease in interrater reliability.

Odds ratio (OR): The odds of a case patient (i.e., someone in the intervention group) being exposed (a/b) divided by the odds of a control patient being exposed (c/d).

Opinion leaders: Individuals who are typically highly knowledgeable and well respected in a system; as such, they are often able to influence change.

Ordinal data: Variables that have ordered categories with intervals that cannot be quantified (e.g., mild, moderate, or severe anxiety).

Outcomes management: The use of process and outcomes data to coordinate and influence actions and processes of care that contribute to patient achievement of targeted behaviors or desired effects.

Outcomes of healthcare delivery: The outcomes that are influenced by the delivery of clinical care.

Outcomes measurement: A generic term used to describe the collection and reporting of information about an observed effect in relation to some care delivery process or health promotion action.

Outcomes research: The use of rigorous scientific methods to measure the effect of some intervention on some outcome(s).

P

Paradigm: A worldview or set of beliefs, assumptions, and values that guide clinicians' and researchers' thinking. For example, where the researcher stands on issues related to the nature of reality (ontology), relationship of the researcher to the researched (epistemology), role of values (axiology), use of language (rhetoric), and process (methodology) (Creswell, 2007).

Participant observation: Observation and participation in everyday activities in study of informants' natural settings.

Participatory action research (PAR): A form of action research that is participatory in nature (i.e., researchers and participants collaborate in problem definition, choice of methods, data analysis, and use of findings); democratic in principle; and reformatory in impulse (i.e., has as its objective the empowerment of persons through the process of constructing and using their own knowledge as a form of consciousness raising with the potential for promoting social action).

Patient preferences: Values the patient holds, concerns the patient has regarding the clinical decision/treatment/situation, and choices the patient has/prefers regarding the clinical decision/treatment/situation.

Peer-reviewed: A project or paper or study is reviewed by a person(s) who is a peer to the author and has expertise in the subject.

Phenomenologic: Pertaining to the study of essences (i.e., meaning structures) intuited or grasped through descriptions of lived experience.

Phenomenological reduction: An intellectual process involving reflection, imagination, and intuition.

PICOT format: A process in which clinical questions are phrased in a manner that yields the most relevant information from a search; P = Patient population; I = Intervention or issue of interest; C = Comparison intervention or status; O = Outcome; T = Time frame for (I) to achieve the (O).

Placebo: A sham medical intervention or inert pill; typically given to subjects in experimental research studies to control for time and attention spent with subjects getting the experimental intervention.

Plan-Do-Study-Act cycle: Rapid cycle improvement in healthcare settings in which changes are quickly made and studied.

Power: The ability of a study design to detect existing relationships between or among variables.

Power analysis: Procedure used for determining the sample size needed for a study.

Practice-based data/evidence: Data that are generated from clinical practice or a healthcare system.

Pragmatism: A practical approach to solutions.

Prevalence: Refers to the persons in the at-risk population who have the outcome or disorder in a given "snapshot in time."

Principal investigator (PI): The lead person who is responsible and accountable for the scientific integrity of a study as well as the oversight of all elements in the conduct of that study.

Prognosis: The likelihood of a certain outcome.

Psychometric properties: The validity and reliability information on a scale or instrument.

Purposeful/theoretical sample: A sample intentionally selected in accordance with the needs of the study.

p value: The statistical test of the assumption that there is no difference between an experimental intervention and a control. p value indicates the probability of an event, given the assumption that there is no true difference. By convention, a p value of 0.05 is considered a statistically significant result.

Q

Qualitative data analysis: A variety of techniques that are used to move back and forth between data and ideas throughout the course of the research.

Qualitative data management: The act of designing systems to organize, catalogue, code, store, and retrieve data. System design influences, in turn, how the researcher approaches the task of analysis.

Qualitative description: Description that "entails a kind of interpretation that is low-inference (close to the 'facts'), or likely to result in easier consensus (about the 'facts') among researchers" (Sandelowski, 2000b, p. 335).

Qualitative evaluation: A general term covering a variety of approaches to evaluating programs, projects, policies, and so on using qualitative research techniques.

Qualitative studies: Research that involves the collection of data in nonnumeric form, such as personal interviews, usually with the intention of describing a phenomenon.

Quality assurance: The process of ensuring that initiatives or the care being delivered in an institution is of high quality.

Quality improvement data: Data that are collected for the purpose of improving the quality of healthcare or patient outcomes.

Quality improvement projects: Initiatives with a goal to improve the processes or outcomes of the care being delivered.

Quantitative research: The investigation of phenomena using manipulation of numeric data with statistical analysis. Can be descriptive, predictive, or causal.

Quantitative studies: Research that collects data in numeric form and emphasizes precise measurement of variables; often conducted in the form of rigorously controlled studies.

Quasi-experiments: A type of experimental design that tests the effects of an intervention or treatment but lacks one or more characteristics of a true experiment (e.g., random assignment; a control or comparison group).

R

Random assignment (also called randomization): The use of a strategy to randomly assign subjects to the experimental or control groups (e.g., tossing a coin).

Random error: Measurement error that occurs without a pattern, purpose, or intent.

Random sampling: Selecting subjects to participate in a study by using a random strategy (e.g., tossing a coin); in this method of selecting subjects, every subject has an equal chance of being selected.

Randomized block design: A type of control strategy used in an experimental design that places subjects in equally distributed study groups based on certain characteristics (e.g., age) so that each study group will be similar prior to introduction of the intervention or treatment.

Randomized controlled trial (RCT): A true experiment (i.e., one that delivers an intervention or treatment in which subjects are randomly assigned to control and experimental groups); the strongest design to support cause-and-effect relationships.

Rate of Occurrence: The rate at which an event occurs.

Ratio-level data: The highest level of data; data that have quantified intervals on an infinite scale in which there are equal distances between points and a meaningful zero point (e.g., ounces of water, height); often referred to as continuous data.

Reference population: Those individuals in the past, present, and future to whom the study results can be generalized.

Reflection: The act of contemplating.

Relative risk (RR): Measures the strength of association and is the risk of the outcome in the exposed group (Re) divided by the risk of the outcome in the unexposed group (Ru). RR is used in prospective studies such as RCTs and cohort studies.

Relative risk reduction (RRR): Proportion of risk for bad outcomes in the intervention group compared to the unexposed control group.

Reliability: The consistency of an instrument in measuring the underlying construct.

Reliability coefficients: A measure of an instrument's reliability (e.g., often computed with a Cronbach alpha).

Reliability of study findings: Whether or not the effects of a study have sufficient influence on practice, clinically and statistically; that is, the results can be counted on to make a difference when clinicians apply them to their practice.

Reliable measures: Those that consistently and accurately measure the construct of interest.

Representation: Part of the analytic process that raises the issue of providing a truthful portrayal of what the data represent (e.g., essence of an experience, cultural portrait) that will be meaningful to its intended audience.

Research design meeting: A planning meeting held for the purpose of designing a study and strategizing about potential funding as well as the roles of all investigators.

Research subjects review board (RSRB): Often referred to as an IRB; a group of individuals who review a study before it can be conducted to determine the benefits and risks of conducting the research to study participants.

Research utilization: The use of research knowledge, often based on a single study, in clinical practice.

return on investment: A measure of performance that demonstrates the efficiency of an investment/intervention; includes but is not limited to financial benefits of an evidence-based intervention.

Risk: The probability that a person (currently free from a disease) will develop a disease at some point.

Risk ratio: See relative risk.

Rules of evidence: Standard criteria for the evaluation of domains of evidence; these are applied to research evidence to assess its validity, the study findings, and its applicability to a patient/system situation.

S

Saturation: The point at which categories of data are full and data collection ceases to provide new information.

Saturation level: The level at which a searcher no longer finds any new references but, instead, is familiar and knowledgeable with the literature.

Search strategy: A process used to guide how a clinician will search a database. Involves identifying databases to search; keywords, subject headings to use; inclusion/exclusion criteria.

Semiotics: The theory and study of signs and symbols applied to the analysis of systems of patterned communication.

Semistructured interviews: Formal interviews that provide more interviewer control and question format structure but retain a conversational tone and allow informants to answer in their own ways.

Sensitivity: The probability of a diagnostic test finding disease among those who have the disease or the proportion of people with disease who have a positive test result (true positive).

SnNout: When a test has a high Sensitivity, a Negative result rules out the diagnosis.

Sociolinguistics: The study of the use of speech in social life.

Solomon four-group design: A type of experimental study design that uses a before–after design for the first two experimental groups and an after-only design for the second experimental and control groups so that it can separate the effects of pretesting the subjects on the outcome measure(s).

Specificity: The probability of a diagnostic test finding NO disease among those who do NOT have the disease or the proportion of people free of a disease who have a negative test (true negatives).

Spirit of inquiry: A persistent questioning about how to improve current practices; a sense of curiosity.

SpPin: When a test has a high Specificity, a Positive result rules in the diagnosis.

Standard error: An estimate due to sampling error of the deviation of the sample mean from the true population mean.

Statistical significance: The results of statistical analysis of data are unlikely to have been caused by chance, at a predetermined level of probability.

Stratification: A strategy that divides the study population into two or more subpopulations and then samples separately from each.

Structured, open-ended interviews: Formal interviews with little flexibility in the way that questions are asked but with question formats that allow informants to respond on their own terms (e.g., "What does…mean to you?" "How do you feel/think about…?").

Subject heading: A set of terms or phrases (known as controlled vocabulary) that classify materials.

Symbolic interaction: Theoretical perspective on how social reality is created by human interaction through ongoing, taken-for-granted processes of symbolic communication.

Synthesis: The process of putting together parts to make a whole (e.g., integrating the results of several studies to tell a story about an entire body of evidence).

Systematic review: A summary of evidence, typically conducted by an expert or expert panel on a particular topic, that uses a rigorous process (to minimize bias) for identifying, appraising, and synthesizing studies to answer a specific clinical question and draw conclusions about the data gathered.

T

Techniques: Tools or procedures used to generate or analyze data (e.g., interviewing, observation, standardized tests and measures, constant comparison, document analysis, content analysis, statistical analysis). Techniques are method-neutral and may be used, as appropriate, in any research design—either qualitative or quantitative.

Test–retest reliability: A test of an instrument's stability over time assessed by repeated measurements over time.

Thematic analysis: Systematic description of recurring ideas or topics (themes) that represent different, yet related, aspects of a phenomenon.

Theoretic interest: A desire to know or understand better.

Theoretical framework: The basis upon which a study is guided; its purpose is to provide a context for selecting the study's variables, including how they relate to one another as well as to guide the development of an intervention in experimental studies.

Theoretical generalizability: See transferability.

Theoretical sampling: Decision making, while concurrently collecting and analyzing data, about what further data and data sources are needed to develop the emerging theory.

Theoretical sensitivity: A conceptual process to accompany techniques for generating grounded theory (Glaser, 1978).

Thick description: Description that does more than describe human experiences by beginning to interpret what they mean, involving detailed reports of what people say and do, incorporating the textures and feelings of the physical and social worlds in which people move, with reference to that context (i.e., an interpretation of what their words and actions mean).

Transferability: Demonstrated by information that is sufficient for a research consumer to determine whether the findings are meaningful to other people in similar situations (analytic or theoretical vs. statistical generalizability).

True experiment: The strongest type of experimental design for testing cause-and-effect relationships: true experiments possess three characteristics: (a) a treatment or intervention, (b) a control or comparison group, and (c) a random assignment.

Truncation: The use of a symbol (e.g., * or ?) to shorten a word to its root. This results in additional words with the same root being found. For example, truncating child* will pick up the words child, childless, and children.

Type I error: Mistakenly rejecting the null hypothesis when it is actually true.

Type II error: Mistakenly accepting (not rejecting) the null hypothesis when it is false.

U

Unstructured, open-ended interviews: Informal conversations that allow informants the fullest range of possibilities to describe their experiences, thoughts, and feelings.

V

Valid measures: Those that measure the construct that they are intended to measure (e.g., an anxiety measure truly measures anxiety, not depression).

Validity [of study findings]: Whether or not the results of the study were obtained via sound scientific methods.

Volunteer/convenience sample: A sample obtained by solicitation or advertising for participants who meet study criteria.

Y

Yield: The number of hits obtained by a literature search. This can be per database and/or total yield; there can be several levels of yield (e.g., first yield and final yield, that is, only those studies that were kept for review).

All Cochrane definitions came from
http://www.update-software.com/cochrane/content.htm
All other sources of definitions cited in the glossary can be found in Chapter 6.

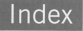

Index

Note: Page numbers followed by "b" denote boxes; those followed by "f " denote figures; those followed by "t" denote tables.

CCS1116